Advances in
Chromatographic Techniques for Therapeutic Drug Monitoring

Advances in

Chromatographic Techniques for Therapeutic Drug Monitoring

Edited by Amitava Dasgupta, PhD, DABCC

Professor of Pathology and Laboratory Medicine
University of Texas Health Sciences Center at Houston

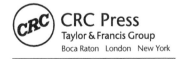

CRC Press
Taylor & Francis Group
Boca Raton London New York

CRC Press is an imprint of the
Taylor & Francis Group, an **Informa** business

CRC Press
Taylor & Francis Group
6000 Broken Sound Parkway NW, Suite 300
Boca Raton, FL 33487-2742

First issued in paperback 2017

ISBN 13: 978-1-138-11171-4 (pbk)
ISBN 13: 978-1-4200-6758-3 (hbk)

Library of Congress Cataloging-in-Publication Data

Advances in chromatographic techniques for therapeutic drug monitoring / editor, Amitava Dasgupta.
    p. ; cm.
  Includes bibliographical references and index.
  ISBN 978-1-4200-6758-3 (hardcover : alk. paper)
  1. Chromatographic analysis. 2. Drug monitoring. I. Dasgupta, Amitava, 1958- II. Title.
  [DNLM: 1. Drug Monitoring--methods. 2. Chromatography--methods. 3. Immunoassay--methods.
4. Pharmaceutical Preparations--analysis. WB 330 A2435 2010]

RS189.5.C48A38 2010
615'.7--dc22
                                                 2009026765

Visit the Taylor & Francis Web site at
http://www.taylorandfrancis.com

and the CRC Press Web site at
http://www.crcpress.com

Dedicated to my wife, Alice

Contents

Foreword

Analytical accuracy and precision are essential in order for therapeutic drug monitoring to achieve maximum efficacy and potential. Although immunoassays can be relatively easily automated, are more widely available in the diagnostic laboratory, and require less technical sophistication on the part of staff, they have historically been plagued with poor specificity and precision. Chromatographic techniques are not only more specific but can offer simultaneous measurements of clinically important metabolites as well as other drugs that may need to be monitored for therapeutic purposes.

This excellent book reviews not only those drugs for which chromatographic techniques have long been used but also drugs for which therapeutic monitoring is newer (e.g., antiretroviral agents, immunosuppressive drugs, antineoplastic compounds, antidepressant drugs, analgesics, cardioactive drugs, and antibiotics). An additional chapter focuses on the analysis of herbal supplements and the interaction of such supplements with the drugs being monitored. The authors are experts in their respective fields.

Edited by a distinguished authority on therapeutic drug monitoring, Amitava Dasgupta, this book should serve as both an invaluable reference text for analytical toxicologists and also as a practical guide for laboratory physicians and scientists involved in the monitoring of therapeutic agents.

David N. Bailey, MD
University of California at Irvine

Preface

As more new drugs are approved by the Federal Drug Administration, the need for therapeutic drug monitoring is also growing. Although many of the newer generations of drugs may not require therapeutic drug monitoring (for example, selective serotonin reuptake inhibitors (SSRIs) antidepressants) classical tricyclic antidepressants require routine monitoring, and many new drugs such as some new generations of anticonvulsants, protease inhibitors, and immunosuppressants such as sirolimus and everolimus require routine therapeutic drug monitoring. In addition, new research indicates that even for older antiretroviral drugs, when used along with protease inhibitors in highly active antiretroviral therapy (HARRT) to treat patients with AIDS, therapeutic drug monitoring may improve the clinical outcome. For newer drugs, chromatographic techniques (gas chromatography or high performance liquid chromatography) are the only available methods to determine the concentrations of these drugs in human serum or plasma for the purpose of therapeutic drug monitoring. Although immunoassays have been commercially available for over 25 drugs and most clinical laboratories use these assays for routine therapeutic drug monitoring, immunoassays suffer from many limitations, including interferences from drug metabolites, structurally similar drugs and, even under some circumstances, structurally unrelated drugs (such as hydroxyzine interference in some carbamazepine immunoassay) as well as endogenous compounds. Gas chromatography or high performance liquid chromatographic techniques are more specific than immunoassays especially when mass spectrometry is used as the detector. Such techniques are still considered as reference methods even for drugs where immunoassays are readily available.

This book is written to provide guidelines to toxicologists, pathologists, and laboratory scientists regarding the application of chromatographic techniques for therapeutic drug monitoring of both classical and newer drugs. For classical drugs for which immunoassays are readily available, clinical situations are presented where immunoassay results may be compromised and more sophisticated techniques such as chromatographic techniques are needed for therapeutic drug monitoring. Chromatographic methods for analyzing various drugs are discussed in each chapter and at the end of each chapter an extensive list of references has been provided so that anyone interested in implementing a new drug assay in his or her laboratory can find an appropriate method for the intended drug. In addition, detailed discussions on rationale for therapeutic drug monitoring of each class of drugs, and their basic pharmacology and toxicology have been discussed so that this book can be used as a complete guide for therapeutic drug monitoring.

I am grateful to all the contributors who took time from their busy schedules to write authoritative chapters for this book. Without their generous support and enthusiasm this book would have never materialized. I would like to thank Alice Wells, MT(ASCP) for her help in proofreading the entire manuscript. Many of our pathology residents read various chapters and made helpful comments and I thank them. Robert L. Hunter, MD, PhD, the chairman of our department, has been very supportive during the last one and a half years I spent on this book project and I would like to thank him. Professor David Bailey was very generous in writing a very kind foreword for this book, I would like to thank him from the bottom of my heart. Last but not least I would like to thank my wife Alice for putting up with me when I worked many late nights and weekends to get this project completed on time. I hope pathologists, clinicians, toxicologists, clinical chemists, and laboratory scientists will find this book helpful for their practice.

Amitava Dasgupta, PhD
University of Texas Health Sciences Center at Houston

Acknowledgments

I would like to thank all the contributors for their dedicated efforts and contributions to this ambitious project. Chemical structures were drawn using the ChemDraw® program. Dr. Hiroaki Taguchi has generously drawn many of the chemicals structures used in this book. Dr. Buddha D. Paul of the forensic toxicology division of the Armed Forces Institute of Pathology granted me permission to use several figures from his laboratory and I thank him for his kindness. I also thank the American Association for Clinical Chemistry, the copyright holder of *Clinical Chemistry Journal*, for generously granting us the permission to reprint free of charge many figures used in this book. Wolters Kluwer (Lippincott Williams and Wilkins), the copyright holder of the *Therapeutic Drug Monitoring Journal* and Preston Publications, the publisher of the *Journal of Analytical Toxicology*, also generously granted us permission to reprint free of charge figures published in the respective journals. I thank these publishers for their generous support in this educational project. All of the contributors made sincere efforts to acknowledge all sources of information used in this book in their respective reference sections. Any omission of credit is unintentional and if brought to our attention, we will quickly credit the proper sources in the reprint of the book.

Editor

Dr. Amitava Dasgupta is a professor of pathology and laboratory medicine at the University of Texas Health Sciences Center at Houston and also the director of clinical chemistry, toxicology, and point of care services at the Memorial-Hermann Hospital Laboratories, the major teaching hospital of the University of Texas Medical School at Houston. He received his PhD in chemistry from Stanford University and completed his fellowship in clinical chemistry from the University of Washington at Seattle. He is certified in both clinical chemistry and toxicology by the American Board of Clinical Chemistry. Dr. Dasgupta's major research interest is in the field of therapeutic drug monitoring and he has published 175 papers, many reviews and edited four books (including this one). He is on the editorial board of the *American Journal of Clinical Pathology, Archives of Pathology and Laboratory Medicine, Therapeutic Drug Monitoring, Clinica Chimica Acta,* and the *Journal of Clinical Laboratory Analysis.*

Contributors

John N. van den Anker, MD, PhD
Departments of Pediatrics, Pharmacology and
Physiology
The George Washington University School of
Medicine and Health Sciences
Washington, District of Columbia

Valerie Bush, PhD
Department of Clinical Laboratories
Bassett Healthcare
Cooperstown, New York

Anthony W. Butch, PhD
Department of Pathology and Laboratory
Medicine
Geffen School of Medicine
University of California at Los Angeles
Los Angeles, California

Amitava Dasgupta, PhD
Department of Pathology and Laboratory
Medicine
University of Texas Health Sciences Center at
Houston
Houston, Texas

Pradip Datta, PhD
Diagnostics Division
Siemens Healthcare Diagnostics
Tarrytown, New York

Roger Dean, PharmD
Clinical Pharmacist
University of Washington Medical Center
Seattle, Washington

Kimberly Napoli Eaton, PhD (Retired)
Department of Surgery
University of Texas Medical School at
Houston
Houston, Texas

Sean Ekins, PhD, DSc
Collaborations in Chemistry
Jenkintown, Pennsylvania

Uttam Garg, PhD
Department of Pathology and Laboratory
Medicine
Children's Mercy Hospitals and Clinics
Kansas City, Missouri

Glen L. Hortin, MD, PhD
Department of Pathology, Immunology, and
Laboratory Medicine
University of Florida College of Medicine
Gainsville, Florida

Saeed A. Jortani, PhD
Department of Pathology and Laboratory
Medicine
University of Louisville School of
Medicine
Louisville, Kentucky

JoEtta Juenke
Associated Regional and University
Pathologists (ARUP)
Laboratories Institute of Clinical and
Experimental Pathology
Salt Lake City, Utah

Kathleen A. Kelly, PhD
Department of Pathology and Laboratory
Medicine
Geffen School of Medicine
University of California at Los Angeles
Los Angeles, California

Matthew D. Krasowski, MD, PhD
Department of Pathology
University of Iowa Hospitals and Clinics
Iowa City, Iowa

Loralie J. Langman, PhD
Department of Laboratory Medicine and
    Pathology
Mayo Clinic College of Medicine
Rochester, Minnesota

Ronald W. McLawhon, MD, PhD
Division of Laboratory Medicine
Department of Pathology
School of Medicine
University of California, San Diego
San Diego, California

Gwendolyn A. McMillin, PhD
Department of Pathology
University of Utah
Salt Lake City, Utah

Natella Y. Rakhmanina, MD
Department of Pediatrics
The George Washington University School of
    Medicine and Health Sciences
Washington, District of Columbia

Mohamed G. Siam, MD, PhD
Toxicology and Therapeutic Drug Monitoring
    Laboratory
University of Pittsburgh Medical Center
    Presbyterian-Shadyside
Pittsburgh, Pennsylvania

and

Department of Forensic Medicine and
    Toxicology
Zagazig University
Zagazig, Egypt

Christine L.H. Snozek, PhD
Department of Laboratory Medicine and
    Pathology
Mayo Clinic College of Medicine
Rochester, Minnesota

Roland Valdes, PhD
Department of Pathology and Laboratory
    Medicine
University of Louisville School of
    Medicine
Louisville, Kentucky

Edward Peters Womack, MT(ASCP)
Department of Pathology and Laboratory
    Medicine
University of Louisville School of
    Medicine
Louisville, Kentucky

1 Introduction to Therapeutic Drug Monitoring and Chromatography

Amitava Dasgupta
University of Texas Medical School

CONTENTS

1.1 INTRODUCTION

The medications available in the market can be classified under two categories, over the counter (OTC) drugs and prescription medications. OTC drugs are relatively safe and none of these drugs are subjected to therapeutic drug monitoring except in patients with suspected overdose. However, an estimated 36 million Americans use OTC analgesic daily and there are numerous reports of drug interactions involving these OTC drugs [1]. In addition, suicide attempts using aspirin or acetamino-phen are common and in most hospitals both drugs are measured as a part of the toxicology panel. Many prescription medications have wide therapeutic windows and therapeutic drug monitoring is usually not recommended for these drugs. In contrast, a number of drugs demonstrate narrow therapeutic index and require routine monitoring in order to achieve maximum therapeutic benefit as well as to avoid unwanted drug toxicity.

Seven drugs; cyclosporine, digoxin, lithium, methotrexate, phenytoin, theophylline, and warfa-rin are among the most frequently encountered drugs in clinically significant adverse drug–drug interactions cases. All of these drugs have low therapeutic index (difference between a therapeutic dose and potentially lethal dose is relatively small) and a small increase in blood level due to inter-action with another drug may cause severe toxicity. This is the reason why all these drugs require therapeutic drug monitoring (for warfarin, a surrogate, international normalized ratio or INR is measured) [1].

Therapeutic drug monitoring has been used in clinical practice to individualize drug therapy in the 1970s. The objective of therapeutic drug monitoring is to optimize pharmacological responses of a drug therapy. In addition, therapeutic drug monitoring is also utilized to monitor a patient's compliance with a drug regimen and to identify potential drug–drug, drug–herb, or food–drug interactions.

Therapeutic drug monitoring is not limited to measuring the concentration of a drug in a bio-logical matrix but it also involves the proper interpretation of the drug concentration in serum or plasma using pharmacokinetic parameters so that appropriate conclusion can be reached regarding the progress of therapy and dose adjustment. The International Association for Therapeutic Drug Monitoring and Clinical Toxicology adopted the following definition, "Therapeutic drug monitor-ing is defined as the measurement made in the laboratory of a parameter that, with appropriate interpretation, will directly influence prescribing procedures. Commonly, the measurement is in a biological matrix of a prescribed xenobiotic, but it may also be of an endogenous compound pre-scribed as a replacement therapy in an individual who is physiologically or pathologically deficient in that compound" [2].

1.2   CHARACTERISTICS OF THE DRUGS THAT REQUIRE MONITORING

A drug may be administered to a patient via various routes including oral, rectal, intravenous, intramuscular, transdermal or through sublingual application. Each route of administration has its advantages and disadvantages. For example, oral route of administration is easiest for a patient, but the drug may suffer low bioavailability due to first pass metabolism or intake of food or the bioavailability may be higher if the patient consumes alcohol. Moreover, a peak drug level may be achieved after a long delay. In contrast, peak concentration can be achieved rapidly if the drug is administered intravenously or intramuscularly but that route of administration may result in patient discomfort. Rapid absorption of a drug can be achieved by sublingual application, but the drug may undergo first pass metabolism thus reducing efficacy of the drug. Usually a drug is poorly absorbed after transdermal application and absorption may also be low after rectal applica-tion of a drug.

Oral administration is a common route of administration of many drugs. Pharmacological response of a drug given in a selected dosing regimen depends on several factors, including com-pliance of the patient, bioavailability of the drug, rate of drug metabolism (depending on the genetic make up of the patient) as well as the protein binding ability of the drug. It has been well documented that only unbound (free) drug can bind with the receptor and produce the desired phar-macological effects. Although for a drug with relatively low protein binding, monitoring total drug concentration (free drug + bound drug) is sufficient for good patient management, for a strongly protein bound drug (protein binding > 80%), often a better correlation is observed between free drug concentration and efficacy of the drug as well as unwanted side effects. For example, adjusting phenytoin (protein binding approximately 90%) dosing in patients based on their serum phenytoin concentrations rather than seizure frequencies not only decrease the morbidity but also prevent unnecessary toxicity of phenytoin in these patients. Peterson et al. reported that in their study with 114 patients, total phenytoin concentrations provided as good an indication of clinical response as the free phenytoin concentrations in most patients, but in 14.2% patients, free phenytoin concentrations were better correlated with clinical picture than total phenytoin concentrations [3]. Another report indicated that quality of life improved in a group of patients with congestive heart failure where digoxin dosing was based on target therapeutic concentrations [4]. Pawinski et al. concluded that in order to achieve optimal drug concentrations for viral suppression of HIV-1 virus as well as to avoid drug toxicity, therapeutic drug monitoring of protease inhibitors is essential in treating patients with AIDS [5]. Criteria for drugs to be a candidate for therapeutic drug monitoring are listed below.

A. Narrow therapeutic range where the dose of a drug which produces the desired therapeutic concentrations is also closer to the dose that may also produce toxic serum concentration. For example, therapeutic range of digoxin is considered as 0.8–1.8 ng/ml, but toxicity can be encountered at a digoxin concentration of 2.0 ng/ml. Chugh et al. reported 22 cases over a four year time period where death occurred in these subjects from therapeutic levels of methadone (range of blood methadone levels: 0.1–0.9 mg/L) [6].
B. There is no clearly defined clinical parameter that allows dose adjustments. Serious toxicity may be encountered due to poorly defined clinical endpoint if the drug is not monitored.
C. There is an unpredictable relationship between dose and clinical outcome. For example, a certain dose may produce a desirable pharmacological response in one patient but the same dose may cause toxicity in another patient. Significant changes in metabolism due to genetic makeup, age, sex or disease for these drugs make them candidates for therapeutic drug monitoring.
D. Drugs that demonstrate nonlinear pharmacokinetic parameters are often candidates for therapeutic drug monitoring. For these drugs, a small change in dosage may cause disproportionate increases in serum concentration leading to toxicity. Moreover, accumulation of drugs may occur causing toxicity of significant interaction with another drug.
E. Toxicity of a drug may lead to hospitalization, irreversible organ damage and even death.
F. There is a correlation between serum concentration of the drug and its efficacy as well as toxicity.

1.3 DRUGS THAT REQUIRE THERAPEUTIC DRUG MONITORING

Usually the drugs with narrow therapeutic range are monitored and most of these drugs are used in treating chronic conditions. Patient compliance is a major issue for successful drug therapy and often patients do not take drugs as recommended especially when they are taking medications for treating chronic conditions. Gillisen reported that in patients with asthma, the adherence rates to medications are often below 50% [7]. In another study, authors concluded that therapeutic drug monitoring of anticonvulsant drugs is beneficial to assess compliance especially in patients with uncontrolled seizures and breakthrough seizures [8]. In addition to ensure patient compliance with a drug, therapeutic drug monitoring also has added benefits:

A. When a person reached a steady state, routine therapeutic drug monitoring is helpful to assess reasons for an altered drug response.
B. Dosage adjustments especially for children, elderly, pregnant women, critically ill patients where altered pharmacokinetic parameters of a drug may be observed.
C. Avoid drug toxicity.

D. Identify clinically significant drug-drug or drug-herb interaction and readjust dosage. For example, if quinidine is added to the drug regime of a patient taking digoxin, reduction in digoxin dosage is necessary in order to avoid digoxin toxicity because an increase in serum digoxin concentration occurs in 90% patients with initiation of quinidine therapy due to reduction in renal clearance of digoxin [9].

Usually anticonvulsants, cardioactive drugs, immunosuppressants, antiasthmatic drugs, antidepressants, antiretroviral drugs, antineoplastic drugs, ceratin analgesics, and antibiotics with narrow therapeutic windows are monitored. Commonly monitored therapeutic drugs along with their recommended therapeutic range are given in Table 1.1 except for antibiotics. Commonly monitored

TABLE 1.1
Commonly Monitored Therapeutic Drugs

Drug Class	Drug	Recommended Therapeutic Range (Trough Concentration)
Anticonvulsants	Phenytoin	10–20 μg/ml
	Carbamazepine	4–12 μg/ml
	Phenobarbital	15–40 μg/ml
	Primidone	5–12 μg/ml
	Valproic acid	50–100 μg/ml
	Methsuximide	10–40 μg/ml
Cardioactive drugs	Digoxin	0.8–1.8 ng/ml
	Procainamide and	4–10 μg/ml
	N-acetyl procainamide	4–8 μg/ml
	Quinidine	2–5 μg/ml
	Lidocaine	1.5–5.0 μg/ml
	Tocainide	5–12 μg/ml
Antiasthmatic	Theophylline	10–20 μg/ml
Antidepressants	Amitriptyline + nortriptyline	120–250 ng/ml
	Doxepin + nordoxepin	150–250 ng/ml
	Imipramine + desipramine	150–250 ng/ml
	Clomipramine	150–450 ng/ml
	Lithium	0.8–1.2 mEq/L
	Paroxetine	20–200 ng/ml
Immunosuppressants	Cyclosporine*	100–400 ng/ml
	Tacrolimus*	5–15 ng/ml
	Mycophenolic acid	1–3.5 μg/ml
Antineoplastic	Methotrexate	Varies with patient population
Analgesic	Acetaminophen	10–30 μg/ml
	Salicylate	150–300 μg/ml
Antiretroviral drugs	Amprenavir	150–400 ng/ml
	Indinavir	80–120 ng/ml
	Nevirapine	150–400 ng/ml
	Saquinavir	100–250 ng/ml

Note: Therapeutic ranges based on published literature and books. However, therapeutic ranges vary widely among different patient population and each institute should establish their own guidelines. These values are for purpose of example only.

* Whole blood trough concentrations are monitored. For all other drugs listed, serum or plasma trough concentrations are measured for therapeutic drug monitoring.

TABLE 1.2
Commonly Monitored Antibiotics

Drug	Recommended Therapeutic Range	
	Peak Concentration	Trough Concentration
Amikacin	15–25 µg/ml	< 5 µg/ml
Gentamicin	4–8 µg/ml	1–2 µg/ml
Tobramycin	4–8 µg/ml	1–2 µg/ml
Vancomycin	30–40 µg/ml	5–15 µg/ml
Ciprofloxacin	3–5 µg/ml	0.5–2 µg/ml

Note: Therapeutic ranges based on published literature and books. However, therapeutic ranges vary widely among different patient population and each institute should establish their own guidelines. These values are for purpose of example only.

TABLE 1.3
Less Frequently Monitored Drugs

Drug Class	Drug	Recommended Therapeutic Range (Trough Concentration)
Anticonvulsants	Clonazepam	10–50 ng/ml
	Gabapentin	2–12 µg/ml
	Zonisamide	10–40 µg/ml
	Lamotrigine	1–4 µg/ml
Cardioactive drugs	Amiodarone	1.0–2.5 ng/ml
	Flecainide	0.2–1.0 µg/ml
	Mexiletine	0.5–2.0 µg/ml
	Propanolol	50–100 ng/ml
	Verapamil	50–200 ng/ml
Antidepressants	Fluoxetine + norfluoxetine	300–1000 ng/ml
	Sertraline	30–200 ng/ml
	Haloperidol	2–15 ng/ml
Immunosuppressants	Sirolimus*	4–20 ng/ml
	Everolimus*	5–15 ng/ml
Antiretroviral drugs	Nelfinavir	700–1000 ng/ml
	Atazanavir	100 ng/ml
	Lopinavir	700 ng/ml
	Efavirenz	100 ng/ml

Note: Therapeutic ranges based on published literature and books. However, therapeutic ranges vary widely among different patient population and each institute should establish their own guidelines. These values are for purpose of example only.

* Whole blood concentration is monitored.

antibiotics are listed in Table 1.2 while less frequently monitored drugs are summarized in Table 1.3. In most instances, trough blood level (15 min prior to next dosage) is the preferred specimen for therapeutic drug monitoring. However, for certain antibiotics (vancomycin and aminoglycosides) both peak and trough drug levels are monitored due to very toxic nature of these drugs. Vancomycin and aminoglycoside can produce serious nephrotoxicity and ototoxicity. Peak serum concentrations for amikacin and kanamycin above 32–34 µg/ml are associated with a higher risk of nephrotoxicity and ototoxicity [10]. Vancomycin also has a low therapeutic index and both nephrotoxicity and ototoxicity can be encountered in patients undergoing vancomycin therapy [11]. It is also necessary to monitor both peak and trough concentration of vancomycin. Ranges for peak concentrations of 20–40 µg/ml have been widely quoted [12]. The given trough range of 5–10 µg/ml has reasonable literature support. Trough concentration above 10 µg/ml has been associated with an increased risk of nephrotoxicity [13,14].

1.4   PHARMACOKINETIC PARAMETERS AND THERAPEUTIC DRUG MONITORING

When a drug is administered orally it undergoes several steps in the body which eventually determine concentration of that drug in serum or whole blood.

1. Liberation: the release of a drug from the dosage form (tablet, capsule, extended release formulation).
2. Absorption: movement of drug from site of administration (for drugs taken orally) to blood circulation. Many factors affect this stage including gastric pH, presence of food particles, etc. Moreover, efflux mechanism if present in the gut may also dictate absorption of a drug for examples; aminoglycosides are poorly absorbed from the gut and can not be administered orally.
3. Distribution: movement of a drug from the blood circulation to tissues. This distribution in most cases is reversible. Certain drugs also cross the blood brain barrier.
4. Protein binding: drugs are bound to serum proteins in various degrees ranging from no protein binding to 99% protein binding. For example, lithium is not bound to serum protein at all while ceratin protease inhibitor such as ritonavir is 98% bound to serum proteins.
5. Metabolism: chemical transformation of a drug to the active and inactive metabolites. Cytochrome P450 enzyme system is the major drug metabolizing agent. Metabolism may follow linear or nonlinear kinetics and may be zero order, first order or may follow more complicated kinetics. Drug metabolites may be active further complicating the pharmacokinetic parameters.
6. Excretion: elimination of the drug from the body via renal, biliary or pulmonary mechanism.

Liberation of a drug after oral administration depends on the formulation of the dosage. Immediate release formulation releases the drugs at once from the dosage form when administered, while the same drug may also be available in sustained release formulation. The rationales for specialized oral formulations of drugs include prolongation of the effect for increased patient convenience and reduction of adverse effects through lower peak plasma concentrations. Local and systematic adverse effects of a drug can also be reduced by use of controlled release delivery systems. Controlled release dosage formulations include osmotic pumps and zero order kinetics system to control the release rate of a drug, bio-adhesive systems and gastric retention devices to control gastrointestinal transit of a drug, bio-erodible hydrogels; molecular carrier system such as cyclodextrin-encapsuled drugs, externally activated system and colloidal systems such as liposomes and microspheres [15]. Enteric coded formulations resist gastric acid degradation and deliver drugs into the distal small intestine and proximal colon. An enteric coded formulation of mycophenolic acid mofetil, a prodrug of immunosuppressant mycophenolic acid is commercially available [16].

Absorption of a drug depends on the route of administration. Generally, an oral administration is the route of choice but under certain circumstances (nausea, vomiting, and convulsion) rectal route may present a practical alternative for delivering anticonvulsants, nonnarcotic and narcotic analgesics, theophylline, antibacterial and antiemetic agents. This route can also be used for inducing anesthesia in children. Although rate of drug absorption is usually lower after rectal administration compared to oral administration, for certain drugs, rectal absorption is higher compared to oral absorption due to avoidance of the hepatic first pass metabolism after rectal delivery. These drugs include lidocaine, morphine, metoclopramide, ergotamine, and propranolol. Local irritation is a possible complication of rectal drug delivery [17]. When a drug is administered by direct injection, it enters the blood circulation immediately. Sometimes a drug may be administered by the intravenous or intramuscular route as a prodrug if the parent drug has potential for adverse drug reactions at the injection site, for example phenytoin. Fosphenytoin, a phosphate ester prodrug of phenytoin which is soluble in aqueous medium was developed as an alternative to intravenous phenytoin for acute treatment of seizure. The bioavailability of derived phenytoin from fosphenytoin relative to intravenous phenytoin administration is almost 100% [18].

When a drug enters the blood circulation, it is distributed throughout the body into various tissues and the pharmacokinetic parameter is called volume of distribution (V_d). This is the hypothetical volume to account for all drugs in the body and is also termed as the apparent volume of distribution

$$V_d = \text{dose/plasma concentration of drug}$$

The amount of a drug at a specific site (target receptor site), where it exerts its pharmacological activity is usually a very small fraction of the total amount of the drug in the body because most of the drug is distributed in tissue and blood. Protein binding of a drug also limits its movement into tissues. Muscle and fat tissues may serve as a reservoir for lipophilic drugs. For neurotherapeutics, penetration of the blood brain barrier is essential. Usually moderately lipophilic drugs can cross the blood brain barrier by passive diffusion and hydrogen bonding capacity of a drug can significantly influence the central nervous system uptake. However, drugs may also cross the blood brain barrier by active transport [19]. Many drugs do not effectively penetrate the blood brain barrier. Ningaraj et al. commented on challenges in delivering new anticancer drugs to brain tumors because most new anticancer drugs that are effective outside the brain have failed in clinical trials in treating brain tumors, in part due to poor penetration across the blood brain barrier and the blood brain tumor barrier [20]. However, there are also advantages when a drug does not effectively penetrate the blood brain barrier. Second generation antihistamines such as cetirizine have a low tendency to cross the blood brain barrier compared to its first generation counterpart, hydroxyzine, thus reducing sedation and impairment in patients taking cetirizine [21].

Drugs usually undergo chemical transformation (metabolism) before elimination. Drug metabolism may occur in any tissue including the blood. For example, plasma butylcholinesterase metabolizes drugs such as succinylcholine. The role of metabolism is to convert lipophilic nonpolar molecules to water soluble polar compounds for excretion in urine. Many drugs are metabolized in the liver in two phases by various enzymes but cytochrome P450 mixed function oxidase is the major liver enzyme responsible for the metabolism of a majority of drugs. Enzymes responsible for most Phase I and Phase II reactions are listed in Table 1.4.

Phase I reactions: this step involves manipulation of a functional group of a drug molecule in order to make the molecule more polar (increases water solubility) by enzyme induced chemical reactions such as oxidation, reduction, hydrolysis, etc.

Phase II reactions: this step may involve acetylation (adding acetate to polar site), sulfation (adding inorganic sulfate to polar site), methylation (adding methyl group to polar site), amino acid conjugation or glucuronidation (adding sugars to polar site).

The rate of enzymatic process that metabolizes most drugs is usually characterized by the Michaelis-Menten equation and follows first order kinetics (rate of elimination is proportional to drug concentration). However, for certain drugs for example, phenytoin, the metabolism is capacity limited.

The half-life of a drug is the time required for the serum concentration to be reduced by 50%. The fraction of a drug that remains in the body after five half-lives is approximately 0.03, while for repeated dosing of a drug, a steady state is reached after five to seven half-lives. Therapeutic drug

TABLE 1.4
Major Enzymes Responsible for Phase I and Phase II Metabolism of Drugs

Reaction	Phase	Name of Enzyme
Oxidation	Phase I	Cytochrome P450
		Alcohol dehydrogenase
		Aldehyde dehydrogenase
		Monoamine oxidase
Reduction	Phase I	Various reductase
Hydrolysis	Phase I	Esterases
		Epoxide Hydrolase
		Amidases
Glucuronidation	Phase II	Glucuronosyltransferase
Acetylation	Phase II	Acetyltransferase
Methylation	Phase II	Methyltransferase
Amino acid conjugation	Phase II	Glutathione transferase
Sulfation	Phase II	Sulfotransferase

monitoring is recommended when a drug reaches a steady state. Half-life of a drug can be calculated from the elimination rate constant (K) of a drug.

$$\text{Half-life} = \frac{0.693}{K}$$

Elimination rate constant can be easily calculated from the serum concentrations of a drug at two different time points using the formula where Ct_1 is the concentration of drug at a time point t_1 and Ct_2 is the concentration of the same drug at a later time point t_2:

$$K = \frac{\ln Ct_1 - \ln Ct_2}{t_2 - t_1}$$

A drug may also undergo extensive metabolism before fully entering the blood circulation. This process is called first pass metabolism. If a drug undergoes significant first pass metabolism, then the drug may not be delivered orally, for example, lidocaine.

Renal excretion is a major pathway for the elimination of drugs and their metabolites. Therefore, impaired renal function may cause accumulation of drugs and metabolites in serum thus, increasing the risk of adverse drug effect. This may be particularly important for drugs which have active metabolites, such as procainamide and carbamazepine. In renal failure N-acetylprocainamide (NAPA), the active metabolite of procainamide may accumulate causing drug toxicity. Moreover, other pathological conditions such as liver disease, congestive heart failure, and hypothyroidism may also decrease clearance of drugs. Drugs may also be excreted via other routes, such as biliary excretion. The factors which determine elimination of a drug through the biliary track include chemical structure, polarity, and molecular weight as well as active transport sites within the liver cell membranes for that particular drug. A drug excreted in bile may also be reabsorbed from the gastrointestinal track or a drug conjugate may be hydrolyzed by the bacteria of the gut, liberating the original drug, which can return into the blood circulation. Enterohepatic circulation may prolong the effects of a drug. Cholestatic disease states, in which flow of normal bile flow is reduced, will reduce bile clearance of a drug and may cause drug toxicity [22].

1.5 GENETIC VARIATIONS IN DRUG METABOLISM AND THERAPEUTIC DRUG MONITORING

Genetic differences between patients may significantly alter drug metabolism and therapeutic drug monitoring. Drugs are metabolized by various enzymes in the body including serum butylcholinesterase, thiopurine methyltransferase, N-acetyltransferase and most notably liver cytochrome P450 mixed function oxidase. The cytochrome P450 proteins (CYP) comprise a large group of heme-containing monooxygenase proteins that localize to the endoplasmic reticulum and mitochondrial membrane. Nicotinamide adenine dinucleotide phosphate (NADPH) is a required cofactor for CYP-mediated biotransformation, and oxygen serves as a substrate. The CYP superfamily is found in many organisms, with over 7700 known members across all species studied. At present, 57 human genes are known to encode CYP isoforms; of these, at least 15 are associated with xenobiotic metabolism. CYP isoenzymes are named according to sequence homology: amino acid sequence similarity > 40% assigns the numeric family (e.g., CYP1, CYP2); > 55% similarity determines the subfamily letter (e.g., CYP2C, CYP2D); isoforms with > 97% similarities are given an additional number (e.g., CYP2C9, CYP2C19) to distinguish them [23]. The major CYP isoforms responsible of metabolism of drugs include CYP1A2, CYP2B6, CYP2C9, CYP2C19, CYP2D6, CYP2E1, and CYP3A4/CYP3A5 (Table 1.5). However, CYP3A4 is the predominant isoform of CYP family (almost 30%) usually responsible for metabolism of approximately 37% of drugs followed by CYP2C9 (17% of drugs), CYP2D6 (15% of drugs), CYP2C19 (10% of drugs), CYP1A2 (9% of drugs), CYP2C8 (6% of drugs), and CYP2B6 (4%of drugs). The CYP2C9 isoform is mostly responsible for metabolism of nonsteroidal antiinflammatory drugs (NSAIDs), while proton pump inhibitors such as omeprazole, rabeprazole are metabolized by CYP2C19 and beta blockers as well as several antipsychotic and antidepressants are metabolized by CYP2D6 [24]. In addition to the liver, CYP3A4 isoenzyme is also present in significant amounts in the epithelium of the gut and orally administered drugs which are substrates of CYP3A4 may undergo significant metabolism before entering circulation.

These cytochrome enzymes show marked variations in different people. Some of these enzymes also exhibit genetic polymorphism (CYP2C19, CYP2D6) and a subset of the population may be deficient in enzyme activity (poor metabolizer). Therefore, if a drug is administered to a patient who is a poor metabolizer, drug toxicity may be observed even with a standard dose of the drug. Mutation of CYP2D6 affects analgesic effect of codeine and tramadol and polymorphism of CYP2C9 is potentially linked to an increase in adverse effects from therapy with NSAIDs [25]. Knowledge of polymorphism of various cytochrome P450 enzymes is important for management of patients receiving various anticancer drugs including tamoxifen, docetaxel, paclitaxel, cyclophosphamide, ifosfamide, imatinib, irinotecan, etoposide, teniposide, thalidomide, and vincristine [26]. Often the cytochrome P450 can be induced or inhibited by another drug or a herbal supplement. For example, St John's wort induces cytochrome P450 resulting in a lower plasma concentration of many drugs due to increased metabolism (see Chapter 22).

Phenotyping procedures commonly involve administration of a probe drug and calculating the urine or plasma metabolic ratio. Traditional therapeutic drug monitoring is useful for phenotyping and can be used to identify slow as well as fast metabolizers, the pharmacogenomics approach to personalized medicine is based on the utilization of genetic information data in pharmacotherapy and drug delivery thus ensuring better drug efficacy and safety in patient management. Currently, the concept of personalized medicine and pharmacogenetics are likely to improve the areas of pharmacokinetics and pharmacodynamics because genetic polymorphisms have already been detected and analyzed in genes coding drug metabolizing enzymes, transporters as well as target receptors. The potential of applying genotyping and haplotype analysis in future medical care could eventually lead to pharmacotyping referring to individualized drug delivery profiling based on genetic information [27]. The United States Federal Drug Administration (FDA) has granted market approval

TABLE 1.5
Isoforms of Cytochrome P450 Enzymes Involved in Metabolism of Commonly Monitored Drugs

Drug Class	Drug	Isoform of Cytochrome P450
Anticonvulsants	Phenytoin	CYP1A2, CYP2C9, CYP2C19, CYP3A4
	Carbamazepine	CYP1A2, CYP2B6, CYP2C8, CYP2C9, CYP3A4
	Phenobarbital	CYP1A2, CYP2A6, CYP2B6, CYP2C8, CYP2C9, CYP3A4
	Primidone	CYP3A4
	Valproic acid	CYP2A6, CYP2B6, CYP2C9, CYP3A4
Cardioactive drugs	Digoxin	CYP3A4
	Procainamide	CYP2B6
	Quinidine	CYP2D6, CYP3A4
	Lidocaine	CYP2B6, CYP3A4
	Mexiletine	CYP1A2, CYP2D6
	Propanolol	CYP1A2, CYP2D6
	Amiodarone	CYP1A2, CYP2C9, CYP3A4
	Verapamil	CYP1A2, CYP3A4
Antiasthmatic	Theophylline	CYP1A2, CYP2E1, CYP3A4
Antidepressants	Amitriptyline	CYP2C19, CYP2D6, CYP3A4
	Doxepin	CYP2C19, CYP2D6, CYP3A4
	Imipramine	CYP1A2, CYP2C19, CYP2D6, CYP3A4
	Clomipramine	CYP2C19, CYP2D6
	Haloperidol	CYP2D6, CYP3A4
	Paroxetine	CYP1A2, CYP2D6
	Sertraline	CYP2D6, CYP3A4
Immunosuppressants	Cyclosporine	CYP3A4
	Tacrolimus	CYP3A4
	Sirolimus	CYP3A4
Antiretroviral drugs	Amprenavir	CYP3A4
	Indinavir	CYP3A4
	Ritonavir	CYP3A4
	Saquinavir	CYP3A4

for the first pharmacogenetic testing using a DNA microarray, the AmpliChip CYP450, which genotypes cytochrome P450 (CYP2D6 and CYP2C19). The test uses software to predict phenotypes and tests for 27 CYP2D6 alleles [28].

1.6   GENDER DIFFERENCES IN DRUG RESPONSE

Biological differences between men and women result in both pharmacokinetic and pharmacodynamic differences in response to a drug therapy. In general, men have a larger body size than women that may result in larger distribution volumes and faster total clearance of many drugs in men compared to women while greater body fat in women may lead to increases in distribution of lipophilic drugs in females. Although absorption of a drug is not different between men and women, the absorption rate may be slightly slower in females. Hepatic metabolism of drugs by Phase I (via CYP1A2, CYP2D6, and CYP2E1) and Phase II (by glucuronyl transferase, methyltransferases, and dehydrogenases) reactions appear to be faster in males than females. However, metabolisms of drugs by CYP2C9, CYP2C19 and N-acetyltransferase or clearance of drugs which are substrates for P-glycoprotein appear to be similar in both males and females [29]. Although glucuronidation of a drug appears to be slower in women compared to men as well as activities of certain CYP enzymes, the activity of CYP3A4 the predominant isoform of CYP enzymes is usually increased in women (up to 40%) compared to men. In general, epidemiological studies dealing with pharmacological aspects of drug metabolism indicate that there are approximately 30% more adverse reaction reports on women compared to men. In addition, drug induced *torsades des pointes* occur twice as frequently in women than men [30].

Phenytoin and naproxen are mainly metabolized by CYP2C9. Rugstad et al. reported that there was an increase in plasma naproxen concentrations with age and females also had higher plasma concentrations of naproxen compared to males [31]. Clomipramine, which is metabolized by CYP2D6 and CYP2C19, has a higher clearance rate in males compared to females [32]. Propranolol metabolism is also faster in males than females [33]. In contrast, metabolism of methylprednisolone is mediated by CYP3A4 and in one report metabolism was higher in women than men [34]. Wolbold et al. found two fold higher CYP3A4 levels in women compared to men based on their analysis of 94 well characterized surgical liver samples. Higher expression in women was also observed in CYP3A4 messenger RNA (mRNA) transcripts, suggesting a pretranslational mechanism. Expression of pregnane X-receptor (PXR) which plays a major role in induction of CYP3A4 was also correlated with CYP3A4 in messenger RNA level, but no sex difference was observed in the expression of PXR messenger RNA. No sex difference was also observed in P-glycoprotein expression [35]. Metabolism of erythromycin, verapamil and cyclosporine is also greater in women than men [36]. Many drugs are metabolized by conjugation. In one study, acetaminophen clearance was 22% greater in young males compared to age adjusted young females due to higher rate of drug conjugation in males [37]. Temazepam is conjugated 50% faster in males than females [36].

Women also have high levels of sex hormones and may also take oral contraceptives. Managing women with antiepileptic drugs is a challenge because in general estrogen is a proconvulsant while progesterone is an anticonvulsant. Hormonal contraceptive agents usually contain progesterone alone or in combination with estrogen (natural or synthetic). Both natural and synthetic estrogens and progesterones (including common ethinyl estradiol) are metabolized by cytochrome P450, especially CYP3A4. The antiepileptic drugs such as phenobarbital, primidone, carbamazepine, oxcarbazepine and phenytoin induce cytochrome P450 system and may cause higher clearance of oral contraceptives resulting in lack of contraception. Hormonal contraceptives can also interact with antiepileptic drugs. Ethinyl estradiol in combination with other components of oral contraceptive preparation can reduce serum lamotrigine level by 50% [38].

There are also gender specific pharmacodynamic differences in drug response. Women are at increased risk of QT prolongation with ceratin antiarrhythmic drugs compared to men even at the same levels of serum drug concentrations. In contrast, certain psychotropic drugs such as chlorpromazine, fluspirilene, and various antipsychotic drugs appear to be more effective in women than men for the same dosage [36]. In general, women have a more difficult time with smoking cessation and nicotine therapy is less effective in women than men probably due to a number of pharmacokinetic and pharmacodynamic factors including alteration of nicotine pharmacokinetics mediated by estrogen and at the same time ovarian hormones may act as noncompetitive antagonists of nicotine receptors [39].

1.7   ABNORMAL DRUG DISPOSITION IN DISEASES: NEED FOR THERAPEUTIC DRUG MONITORING

Various pathophysiological states can significantly alter drug dispositions resulting in significant changes in drug levels in serum or plasma. Such changes can be easily recognized by therapeutic drug monitoring and proper dosage adjustments can be achieved. Without routine drug monitoring these patients may experience drug toxicity or may suffer from treatment failure due to subtherapeutic concentration of a drug in serum. It is well documented in the literature that diseases such as renal impairment, liver disease, thyroid disorders, and cardiovascular disease alter drug disposition and metabolism. Drug metabolism is also altered in pregnancy.

1.7.1 RENAL IMPAIRMENT AND DRUG CLEARANCE

Renal disease causes impairment in the clearance of many drugs by the kidney. Correlations have been established between creatinine clearance and clearance of digoxin, lithium, procainamide, aminoglycoside and many other drugs. The clearance of a drug is closely related to glomerular filtration rate (GFR) and creatinine clearance is considered as a valid way to determine GFR. Serum cystatin C is another marker of GFR. In clinical practice, the degree of renal impairment is widely assessed by using the serum creatinine concentration and creatinine clearance predicted using the Cockcroft–Gault formula [40]. However, under certain pathological conditions creatinine clearance may be a poor predictor of GFR. In addition, elderly patients may have unrecognized renal impairment and caution should be exercised when medications are prescribed to elderly patients. Serum creatinine remains normal until GFR has fallen by at least 50%. Nearly half of the older patients have normal serum creatinine but reduced creatinine clearance. Dose adjustments based on renal function is recommended for many medications in elderly patients even for medications that exhibit large therapeutic windows [41]. Renal disease also causes impairment of drug protein binding because uremic toxins compete with drugs for binding to albumin. Such interactions leads to increases in concentration of pharmacologically active free drug concentration which is clinically more important for strongly protein bound drugs. Measuring free drug concentrations of strongly protein bound anticonvulsant drugs such as phenytoin, carbamazepine and valproic acid is recommended in uremic patients in order to avoid drug toxicity [42].

Drug-induced renal failure is a frequent complication in critically ill patients, affecting 2–15% patients admitted to the hospital or intensive care units. The mechanism leading to drug induced renal failure includes hemodynamic effects, epithelial toxicity, and crystalline nephropathy. Many drugs may cause acute or chronic renal failure (with long term use such as immunosuppressants, NSAIDs, etc.) [43–45]. A list of common drugs that may cause renal impairment is given in Table 1.6. This list is a representative example of several drugs that may cause renal impairment and is not by any means complete.

TABLE 1.6
Common Drugs that may cause Renal Impairment

Acetaminophen	Acyclovir	ACE inhibitors
Adefovir	Allopurinol	Aminoglycosides
Aspirin	Barbiturates	Carbamazepin
Cephalosporins	Cidofovir	Cimetidine
Codeine	Cyclosporine	Diazepam
Dipivoxil	Diuretics	Foscarnet
5-Fluorouracil	Ifosfamide	Indinavir
Interferon	Lovastatin	Mithramycin
Methotrexate	NSAIDS*	Pentamidine
Penicillin	Phenytoin	Quinine
Quinidine	Quinolones	Radiocontrast agents
Sulfonamides	Tacrolimus	Tetracycline
Tenofovir	Vancomycin	

Note: Representative list of drugs, not a complete list.
* NSAID: nonsteroidal anti-inflammatory drugs.

1.7.2 HEPATIC DYSFUNCTION AND DRUG DISPOSITION

Liver dysfunction not only reduces clearance of a drug metabolized through hepatic enzymes or biliary mechanism but also affects plasma protein binding due to reduced production of albumin and other drug binding proteins, and thus affects distribution and elimination of drugs. Mild to moderate hepatic disease causes an unpredictable effect on drug clearance. Portal-systemic shunting which is commonly encountered in patients with advanced liver cirrhosis may significantly reduce first pass metabolism of high extraction drugs after oral administration leading to higher oral bioavailability [46].

Hepatic cytochrome P450 enzyme activities and gene expression can be profoundly altered in disease states. In general, the levels of affected cytochrome P450 enzymes are depressed by diseases causing potential and documented impairment of drug clearance causing drug toxicity [47]. The activities of several isoenzymes of cytochrome P450 enzymes (CYP1A1, CYP2C19, and CYP3A4/5) are reduced in liver dysfunction while activities of other isoenzymes such as CYP2D6, CYP2C9, and CYP2E1 are less affected. The patterns of cytochrome P450 isoenzyme alteration also vary depending on the etiology of liver disease [48]. Although, the Phase I reaction involving cytochrome P450 enzymes may be impaired in liver disease, the Phase II reaction (glucuronidation) seems to be affected to a lesser extent. However, both Phase I and Phase II reactions in drug metabolism are substantially impaired in patients with advanced cirrhosis. In addition, these patients may also experience significant renal impairment. Patients with liver cirrhosis are more susceptible to adverse effects of opioid analgesics and renal adverse effects of NSAIDs. In contrast, a reduced therapeutic effect of certain diuretics and beta-adrenoreceptor antagonists are observed in these patients. At this point there is no universally accepted endogenous marker to access hepatic impairment and the semiquantitative Child–Pugh score is frequently used to determine severity of hepatic dysfunction and thus dosage adjustments, although there are limitations to this approach [46]. Significant decreases in clearance and marked prolongation of half-lives of certain antiarrhythmic drugs (carvedilol, lidocaine, propafenone, and verapamil) have been observed in patients with hepatic impairment. Therefore, two to three fold reductions in dosage of these drugs are recommended for patients with moderate to severe liver cirrhosis. However, for drugs that are mostly eliminated through the renal route (sotalol, disopyramide, and procainamide) dosage adjustment may not be necessary in patients with hepatic dysfunction as long as renal function is normal [49].

Mild to moderate hepatitis infection may also alter clearance of drugs. Trotter et al. reported that total mean tacrolimus dose in year one after transplant was 39% lower in patients with hepatitis C compared to patients with no hepatitis C infection. The most likely explanation for these findings is decreased hepatic clearance of tacrolimus caused by mild hepatic injury from recurrent hepatitis C virus [50]. Zimmermann et al. reported that oral dose clearance of sirolimus (rapamycin) was significantly decreased in subjects with mild to moderate hepatic impairment compared to controls and authors stressed the need for careful monitoring of trough whole blood sirolimus concentrations in renal transplant recipients exhibiting mild to moderate hepatic impairment [51].

Hypoalbuminemia is often observed in patients with hepatic dysfunction thus impairing protein binding of many drugs. As free (unbound) drugs are responsible for pharmacological action, careful monitoring of free concentrations of strongly albumin bound antiepileptic drugs such as phenytoin, carbamazepine, and valproic acid is recommended in patients with hepatic dysfunction in order to avoid drug toxicity [42].

Many drugs are known to cause hepatotoxicity. Some drugs are metabolized to toxic metabolites by liver enzymes and may cause liver damage. Well documented examples of such drugs are acetaminophen and halothane. In addition covalent binding of toxic metabolite to cytochrome (CYP) enzymes lead to formation of anti-CYP antibodies and immune mediated hepatotoxicity (hydralazine, tienilic acid). Anti-CYP2D6 antibodies are encountered in patients with type II autoimmune hepatitis [48]. Common drugs that may result in drug induced liver injuries are given in Table 1.7 (the list is representative and not a complete list).

TABLE 1.7
Common Drugs that may cause Hepatotoxicity

Acetaminophen	Allopurinol	Amiodarone
Aspirin	Chlorpropamide	Diclofenac
Erythromycin	Halothane	Statins
Indomethacin	Isoniazid	Methotrexate
Methyldopa	Niacin	Phenothiazine
Propylthiouracil	Phenytoin	Quinidine
Tetracycline	Valproic acid	

Note: Representative list of drugs, not a complete list.

1.7.3 Altered Drug Disposition in Cardiovascular Disease

Cardiac failure is often associated with disturbances in cardiac output, influencing the extent and pattern of tissue perfusion, sodium and water metabolism as well as gastrointestinal motility. These factors may affect absorption and disposition of many drugs thus requiring proper dosage adjustment. For drugs which are metabolized by the liver, decreased blood flow in the liver may result in reduced clearance of drugs. Hepatic elimination of drugs via oxidative Phase I metabolism is generally impaired in patients with congestive heart failure which may be related to decreased hepatic oxygen supply as well as other factors such as reduced liver enzyme content, reduced enzyme activity, or direct physical effect of liver congestion on hepatocytes [52].

Theophylline metabolism which is largely independent of hepatic blood flow is reduced in patients with severe cardiac failure and dose reduction is needed. Digoxin clearance is also decreased. Quinidine plasma level may also be high in these patients due to lower volume of distribution [53]. Elimination half-life is directly related to the volume of distribution and inversely related to clearance. Pharmacokinetic changes are not always predictable in patients with congestive heart failure but it appears that the net effect of reduction in volume of distribution and impairment in metabolism usually results in higher plasma concentrations of a drug in a patient with congestive heart failure compared to healthy subjects. Therefore, therapeutic drug monitoring is crucial in avoiding drug toxicity in these patients. Physiological changes in critically ill patients can significantly affect the pharmacokinetics of many drugs. These changes include absorption, distribution, metabolism and excretion of drugs in critically ill patients. Understanding these changes in pharmacokinetic parameters is essential for optimizing drug therapy in critically ill patients [54]. Moreover, usually free fractions of strongly protein bound drugs are elevated in the critically ill patients due to low serum albumin concentrations.

1.7.4 Altered Drug Disposition in Thyroid Dysfunction

Patients with thyroid disease may have an altered response to drugs. Thyroxine is a potent activator of the cytochrome P450 enzyme system and hypothyroidism is associated with inhibition of hepatic oxidative metabolism of many drugs. Croxson et al. measured serum digoxin concentration using a radioimmunoassay in 17 hyperthyroid and 16 hypothyroid patients and observed significantly lower levels of digoxin in patients with hyperthyroidism and significantly higher levels of digoxin in patients with hypothyroidism [55]. Although there is a general conception that serum phenytoin clearance is not affected by thyroid function state, Sarich and Wright reported a case where a 63-year-old female, who developed decreased serum levels of free T_4 showed phenytoin toxicity which may be related to decreased cytochrome P450 mediated hydroxylation of phenytoin [56].

Hypothyroidism also affects the metabolism of immunosuppressants. Haas et al reported a case where a patient developed hypothyroidism six months after single lung transplantation and was admitted to the hospital for anuric renal failure. The patient showed a toxic blood level of tacrolimus which was resolved with the initiation of thyroxine replacement therapy and dose reduction of tacrolimus [57].

The iodine rich amiodarone affects the thyroid gland causing thyroid disorder which may affect warfarin sensitivity. Kurnik et al. described three cases where patients developed amiodarone induced thyrotoxicosis resulting in a significant decrease in warfarin requirement [58]. The mechanism of interaction of thyroid hormone with warfarin is complex. One proposed mechanism is the alteration of kinetics of the clotting factors with an increase in catabolism of vitamin K-dependent factors in patients with hyperthyroidism. This interaction increases sensitivity to warfarin in patients with hyperthyroidism but decreases sensitivity of warfarin in patients with hypothyroidism [59].

1.7.5 ALTERED DRUG DISPOSITION IN PREGNANCY

Epidemiologic surveys have indicated that between one third and two thirds of all pregnant women will take at least one medication during pregnancy. Drug therapy in pregnant women usually focuses on safety of the drug on the fetus (tetragonic effect of drug). However, pharmacokinetics of many drugs is also altered during pregnancy. Therapeutic drug monitoring during pregnancy aims to improve individual dosage improvement, taking into account pregnancy related changes in drug disposition [60]. Physiological changes that occur during pregnancy may significantly alter absorption, distribution, metabolism and elimination of drugs thus affecting efficacy and safety of the drugs towards pregnant women unless careful dosage adjustments are made. During the third trimester, gastrointestinal function may be prolonged. Moreover, the amount of total body water and fat increase throughout pregnancy results in increases in cardiac output as well as renal and hepatic blood flow. In addition, plasma protein concentrations are reduced, increasing the unbound fraction of a drug. Therefore, careful therapeutic drug monitoring of the free (unbound) concentration of strongly protein bound drugs, such as phenytoin, carbamazepine, and valproic acid is recommended in pregnant women. Moreover, changes occur in the drug metabolizing capacity of the hepatic enzymes in pregnancy. Renal absorption of sodium is increased. Placental transport of a drug, compartmentalization of a drug in the embryo/placenta as well as metabolism of a drug by the placenta and the fetus also play important roles in the pharmacokinetics of a drug during pregnancy [61].

In general, bioavailability of a drug is not significantly altered in pregnancy but increased plasma volume and changes in protein binding may alter volume of distribution of many drugs. Pregnancy may also cause increased or decreased clearance of a drug depending on whether a drug is excreted unchanged in urine or is subjected to hepatic metabolism. The renal excretion of unchanged drugs is increased in pregnancy. In addition, metabolism of drugs catalyzed by isoenzymes of cytochrome P450 (CYP3A4, CYP2D6, and CYP2C9) and uridine diphosphate glucuronosyltransferase (UGT1A4 and UFT2B7) are increased in pregnancy. Therefore dosages of drugs that are metabolized by these routes may need to be increased during pregnancy in order to avoid loss of efficacy. In contrast, activities of some isoenzymes (CYP1A2 and CYP2C19) are reduced in pregnancy. Therefore, dosage reduction may be needed for drugs that are metabolized via these isoenzymes [62].

The increased secretion of estrogen and progesterone in normal pregnancy affect hepatic drug metabolism depending on the specific drug. A higher rate of hepatic metabolism of certain drugs, for example phenytoin, can be observed due to the induction of the hepatic drug metabolizing enzymes by progesterone. On the other hand, the hepatic metabolism of theophylline and caffeine are reduced secondary to the competition of these drugs with progesterone and estradiol for enzymatic metabolism by the liver. The cholestatic effect of estrogen may interfere with the clearance of drugs for example, rifampin [60]. By the end of pregnancy, total and unbound phenobarbital concentrations are reduced up to 50% of the original concentration, but primidone concentrations are altered marginally. Total phenytoin concentrations may fall by 40% compared to serum phenytoin levels prior to pregnancy. Total and free carbamazepine values may also alter due to pregnancy but reports are conflicting [63]. Significant increases in clearance of lamotrigine have been reported in pregnancy. Apparent clearance seems to increase steadily during pregnancy until it peaks approximately at 32nd week when 330% increases in clearance from base line values can be observed [64]. Lower serum concentrations of lithium have been reported in pregnancy and this may be related to an increase in the GFR in pregnancy. Altered pharmacokinetics of ampicillin can be observed in pregnancy where serum concentrations may be lower by 50% in pregnant women compared to non-pregnant women. Faster elimination of phenoxymethylpenicillin (penicillin V) in pregnant women has also been demonstrated [60]. Combined antiretroviral therapy can significantly reduce transmission of the human immunodeficiency virus (HIV) from mother to fetus. However, pregnancy may alter the pharmacokinetics of the antiretroviral drugs. Available data indicate that pharmacokinetics of zidovudine, lamivudine, didanosine, and stavudine are not altered significantly during pregnancy. However, nevirapine half-life is significantly prolonged in pregnancy. For protease inhibitors, reduction of maximum plasma concentration of indinavir was observed in pregnancy. This may be due to induction of cytochrome P450. Standard adult doses of nelfinavir and saquinavir produced lower drug concentration in HIV-infected pregnant women compared to nonpregnant women [61].

During pregnancy the thyroid is hyper-stimulated resulting in changes in thyroid hormone concentrations. Gestational age-specific reference intervals are now available for thyroid function tests. Knowledge of expected normal changes in thyroid hormone concentrations during pregnancy allows individual supplementation when needed [65]. Hypothyroidism is common in pregnancy and therapeutic drug monitoring of antithyroid drugs is important. Consistently lower serum concentrations of propylthiouracil were observed in pregnant women compared to nonpregnant women [66].

In general dosage adjustments are required for anticonvulsants, lithium, digoxin, certain beta blockers, ampicillin, cefuroxime and certain antidepressants in pregnant women. In addition, certain drugs such as tetracycline, antithyroid medications, coumarin anticoagulants, aspirin, indomethacin, opioids, barbiturates, and phenothiazine may have unwanted effects in the fetus despite careful adjustment of maternal dosage [67,68].

1.8   ALTERED DRUG DISPOSITION IN NEONATES, CHILDREN, AND ELDERLY

In the fetus, CYP3A7 is the major hepatic cytochrome responsible for steroid metabolism. Variably expressed in the fetus, CYP3A5 is also present in significant levels in half of children. However, in adults CYP3A4 is the major functional hepatic enzyme responsible for metabolism of many drugs. CYP1A1 is also present during organogenesis while CYP2E1 may be present in some second trimester fetuses. After birth, hepatic CYP2D6, CYP2C8/9 and CYP2C18/19 are activated. CYP1A2 becomes active during the fourth to fifth months [69]. In general decreased capacity of neonatal liver to metabolize drugs may prolong action of drugs such as phenobarbital, theophylline, and phenytoin. In addition, reduced capacity of glucuronide conjugation of drugs in neonate's liver not only may cause neonatal jaundice but may also explain chloramphenicol induced gray infant syndrome. Age related sensitivity to drug may be related to differences of metabolism of drugs by the liver. Young children are more resistant to acetaminophen hepatotoxicity because in children sulfation predominates over glucuronidation of acetaminophen, thus, reducing, the formation of toxic metabolite. In addition, infants also have a greater capacity to synthesize glutathione that inactives toxic metabolite of acetaminophen. However, children are more susceptible to valproic acid toxicity compared to adults [70].

In general, age is not considered to have a major influence on the absorption of drugs from the gut except for the first few weeks of life when absorption steps may be less efficient. Neonates and infants demonstrate increased total body water to body fat ratio compared to adults whereas the reverse is observed in the elderly. These factors may affect volume of distribution of drugs depending on their lipophilic character in infants and elderly compared to adult population. Moreover, altered plasma binding of drugs may be observed in both neonates and some elderly due to low albumin, thus, increasing the fraction of free drug. In general, drug metabolizing capacity by the liver enzymes is reduced in newborns particularly in premature babies but increases rapidly during the first few weeks and months of life to reach values which are generally higher than adult metabolizing rates. In contrast, efficiency of cytochrome P450 enzymes declines with old age. Renal function at the time of birth is reduced by more than 50% of the adult value but then increases rapidly in the first two to three years of life. Renal function then starts declining with old age. Oral clearance of lamotrigine, topiramate, levetiracetam, oxcarbazepine, gabapentin, tiagabine, zonisamide, vigabatrin, and felbamate is significantly higher (20–120%) in children compared to adults depending on the drug and the age distribution of the population. On the other hand, clearance of these drugs is reduced (10–50%) in the elderly population compared to middle-aged adults [71].

Clearance of aminoglycoside is dependent on the GFR which is markedly decreased in neonates, especially in premature newborns. These drugs appear to be less nephrotoxic and ototoxic in neonates compared to the adult population. The volume of distribution of aminoglycoside increases in neonates which may also contribute to a longer half-life of aminoglycoside in neonates. Decreased renal clearance in neonates is responsible for decreased clearance of most beta-lactam antibiotics [72]. Higher volume of distribution and lower clearance of gentamicin was also observed in neonates [73]. Conversion of theophylline to caffeine in human fetuses has been reported [74].

1.9   EFFECT OF SMOKING ON DRUG DISPOSITION

Approximately 4800 compounds are found in tobacco smoke including nicotine and carcinogenic compounds, for example polycyclic aromatic hydrocarbons (PAHs) and N-nitroso amines. Compounds in tobacco smoke can induce certain cytochrome P450 enzymes responsible for metabolism of many drugs. PAHs induce CYP1A1, CYP1A2, and possibly CYP2E1. Smoking may also induce other drug metabolism pathways such as conjugation [75]. Cigarette smoke, not nicotine is responsible for pharmacokinetic drug interactions. Therefore, nicotine replacement therapy does not cause hepatic enzyme induction [76].

Theophylline is metabolized by CYP1A2. In one study, the half-life of theophylline was reduced by almost two fold in smokers compared to nonsmokers [75]. Lee et al. reported that theophylline clearance was increased by 51.1% and steady state serum concentrations were reduced by 24.5 % in children who were exposed to passive smoking [77]. Significant reductions in drug concentrations with smoking have been reported for caffeine, chlorpromazine, clozapine, flecainide, fluvoxamine, haloperidol, mexiletine, olanzapine, proprandol, and tacrine due to increased metabolism of these drugs. Smokers may therefore require higher doses than nonsmokers in order to achieve pharmacological responses [76]. Warfarin disposition in smokers is also different than nonsmokers. One case report described an increase in INR to 3.7 from a baseline of 2.7–2.8 in an 80-year-old man when he stopped smoking. Subsequently, his warfarin dose was reduced by 14% [78].

Pharmacodynamic drug interactions in smokers may be due to nicotine, which may counteract the pharmacological effects of a drug. Smokers taking benzodiazepines, such as diazepam and chlordiazepoxide experience less drowsiness than nonsmokers and this interaction appears to be pharmacodynamic in nature because several studies did not find any significant difference between metabolism of benzodiazepines between smokers and nonsmokers. Therefore, larger doses may be needed to sedate a smoker [76]. Smokers may also need higher doses of opioids (codeine, propoxyphene, and pentazocine) for pain relief [75]. In one study, to determine whether smokers require more opioid analgesic, it was found that 20 smokers (ten cigarettes a day or more for at least one year) required 23% more (when adjusted for body weight) and 33% more (when adjusted for body mass index) opioid analgesics compared to 69 nonsmoking patients [79].

1.10   ALCOHOL CONSUMPTION AND DRUG DISPOSITION

Fatal toxicity may occur from alcohol and drug overdoses. In many instances, in the presence of alcohol, a lower concentration of drug may cause fatality due to drug alcohol interactions. In a Finnish study, it was found that median amitriptyline and propoxyphene concentrations were lower in alcohol related fatal cases compared to cases where no alcohol was involved. The authors concluded that when alcohol is present, a relatively small overdose of a drug may cause fatality [80]. Although alcohol is mostly metabolized in the liver by hepatic alcohol dehydrogenase, long term intake of large amount of alcohol induces other pathways of metabolism, in particular, the microsomal alcohol oxidizing system involving CYP2E1. In contrast, acute ingestion of alcohol is likely to cause inhibition of this enzyme [81]. CYP2E1 also metabolizes and activates many toxicological substrates to more active products and induction of CYP2E1 plays an important role in oxidative stress and toxicity in ethanol induced liver injury [82].

There are two types of interactions between alcohol and a drug: pharmacokinetic and pharmacodynamic. Pharmacokinetic interactions occur when alcohol interferes with the hepatic metabolism of a drug. Pharmacodynamic interactions occur when alcohol enhances the effect of a drug, particularly in the central nervous system. In this type of interaction alcohol alters the effect of a drug without changing its concentration in the blood [83]. The package insert of many antibiotics states that the medication should not be taken with alcohol although only a few antibiotics have reported interactions with alcohol. Erythromycin may increase blood concentration of alcohol by accelerating gastric emptying [83]. Histamine H_2 receptor antagonists, such as cimetidine, ranitidine, nizatidine and famotidine reduce the activity of alcohol dehydrogenase [84].

Alcohol increases the sedative effect of tricyclic antidepressants through pharmacodynamic interactions. In addition, alcohol can also cause pharmacokinetic interactions. Alcohol appears to interfere with first pass metabolism of amitriptyline, thus, increasing serum levels of this drug. Alcohol demonstrates pharmacodynamic effects with antihistamines, increasing the sedative effects of these OTC and prescription drugs. Alcohol also increases the sedative effect of phenobarbital and may also increase its serum concentration through pharmacokinetic interactions. Interactions between benzodiazepines and alcohol have also been reported. Alcohol consumption may result in accumulation of toxic breakdown products of acetaminophen [83].

1.11   DRUG–FOOD AND DRUG–HERB INTERACTIONS: ROLE OF THERAPEUTIC DRUG MONITORING

Drug–food interactions may be pharmacokinetic or pharmacodynamic in nature. Certain foods alter activity of drug metabolic enzymes and especially CYP3A4 appears to be the key enzyme in food drug interaction [85]. It has also long been recognized that intake of food and fluid can alter the extent of drug absorption. This alteration may be related to alteration of physiological factors in the gut such as gastric pH, gastric emptying time, intestinal motility, and hepatic blood flow or bile flow rate. Moreover direct interaction of food with drug may also alter bioavailability such as adsorption of a drug in insoluble dietary component, complex formation of a drug with a metal ion or partitioning of a drug in dietary fat. Food may be able to alter performance of modified released oral formulation [86]. It has been documented that smoking, intake of charcoal broiled food or cruciferous vegetables induces the metabolism of multiple drugs whereas grapefruit juice increases bioavailability of many drugs. Energy deficiency and low intake of a protein may cause about 20–40% decrease in clearance of theophylline and phenazone while elimination of these drugs may be accelerated in the presence of a protein rich diet [87]. Fegan et al. reported increased clearance of propranolol and theophylline in the presence of a high protein/low carbohydrate diet compared to a low protein/high carbohydrate diet using six volunteers. When the diet was switched from a low protein/high carbohydrate to a high protein/low carbohydrate, the clearance of propranolol was increased by an average of 74% and clearance of theophylline was increased by an average of 32% [88].

The most important interaction between fruit juice and drug involves consumption of grapefruit juice. It was reported in 1991 that a single glass of grapefruit juice caused a two to three-fold increase in the plasma concentration of felodipine, a calcium channel blocker after oral intake of a 5-mg tablet but a similar amount of orange juice showed no effect [89]. Subsequent investigations demonstrated that pharmacokinetics of approximately 40 other drugs are also affected by intake of grapefruit juice [90]. The main mechanism for enhanced bioavailability of drugs after intake of grapefruit juice is the inhibition of CYP3A4 in the small intestine. Grapefruit juice causes significant increases in the bioavailability of drugs after oral dosing but does not alter pharmacokinetic parameters of the same drug after intravenous administration. Therefore, it appears that grapefruit juice inhibits intestinal CYP3A4 but has no significant effect on liver CYP3A4 [91,92]. Multiple drug resistant (MDR) transporters play an important role in the disposition of many drugs. P-glycoprotein is a major MDR transporter that decreases the fraction of drug absorbed by carrying the drug back to the intestinal lumen from enterocytes. Although few studies showed activation of P-glycoprotein by grapefruit juice, most studies reported significant inhibition of P-glycoprotein by components of grapefruit juice [91,92]. Furanocoumarins found in the grapefruit juice are probably responsible for interactions between grapefruit juice and drugs. The major furanocoumarin present in grapefruit juice is bergamottin which showed time and concentration dependent inactivation of cytochrome P450 enzymes in vitro [93]. Paine et al. reported that furanocoumarin free grapefruit juice showed no interaction with felodipine, thus, establishing that furanocoumarins are responsible for interactions between felodipine and grapefruit juice [94]. Common drugs that interact with grapefruit juice are listed in Table 1.8.

Although most reports indicate increased bioavailability of drugs in the presence of grapefruit juice or no clinically significant interaction, Dresser et al. reported significant reduction in bioavailability of fexofenadine, a nonsedating antihistamine. This drug does not undergo any significant intestinal or hepatic metabolism. Recent developments indicate that the family of drug uptake transporters known as organic anion transporting polypepetides (OATPs) plays an important role in disposition of certain drugs. In the small intestine OATPs facilitate absorption of certain medications and inhibition of this transport system may cause reduced bioavailability. Grapefruit juice (300 or 1200 ml) produced lower mean maximum plasma concentration and AUC of fexofenadine compared to when the drug was taken with the same volume of water. The mean maximum plasma concentration of fexofenadine was 436 ng/ml when the drug was taken with 300 ml of water compared to the mean maximum plasma concentration of 233 ng/ml when the medication was administered

TABLE 1.8

Increased Bioavailability/Elevated Serum Concentration of Drugs Due to Intake of Grapefruit Juice

Amiodarone	Alprazolam	Atorvastatin
Benzodiazepines	Budesonide	Buspirone
Carbamazepine	Carvedilol	Cerivastatin
Cilostazol	Codeine	Cyclosporine
Dapsone	Diazepam	Diltiazem
Erythromycin	Felodipine	Fexofenadine*
Haloperidol	Indinavir	Lovastatin
Midazolam	Methadone	Nelfinavir
Nifedipine	Nicardipine	Paclitaxel
Pitavastatin	Quinidine	Simvastatin
Saquinavir	Simvastatin-Ezetimibe	Tacrolimus
Trazodone	Triazolam	Zolpidem

* In contrast to other drugs, plasma level of fexofenadine is reduced significantly due to intake of grapefruit juice.

with 300 ml of grapefruit juice. The reduction of maximum plasma concentration was more striking in the presence of 1200 ml of grapefruit juice. Similar reductions were also observed in AUC of fexofenadine. Because fexofenadine is a zwitter ion it has high solubility in aqueous medium over a wide pH range and it is unlikely that the acidic pH of grapefruit juice could reduce the solubility significantly. Therefore authors postulated that ingredients of grapefruit juice have prolonged inhibitory effects on inherent activity of intestinal OATP-A activity thus causing a clinically significant effect of reduced bioavailability of fexofenadine [95].

Although interaction between grapefruit juice and many drugs has been well documented, drug interaction with Seville orange juice, cranberry juice, and pomegranate juice may also have clinical significance. In addition, drug–herb interaction has serious clinical consequences, for example treatment failure with many drugs due to induction of hepatic enzyme by St. John's wort, an herbal antidepressant (see Chapter 22). Therapeutic drug monitoring is very useful to recognize these important drug–food and drug–herb interactions.

1.12   METHODS FOR THERAPEUTIC DRUG MONITORING

Concentrations of drugs in serum, plasma, urine, or other biological fluids can be measured by using various chromatographic techniques and immunoassays. Chromatographic techniques were the first reported methods for determination of concentrations of various drugs in biological fluids. During the 1960s therapeutic drug monitoring of antiepileptic drugs was performed using gas chromatography (GC). Several bioassays were available for monitoring certain antibiotics. Later various assays for therapeutic drugs using high performance liquid chromatography (HPLC) were reported but in the 1970s immunoassays were available for determination of concentrations of various drugs in serum and plasma, thus revolutionizing the field of therapeutic drug monitoring. Immunoassays are widely used in clinical laboratories for routine drug monitoring due to ease of operation (adaption of immunoassays on automated analyzers), simplicity and speed. However, immunoassays are not commercially available for all drugs currently monitored in clinical practice and various sophisticated techniques such as HPLC combined with tandem mass spectrometry or GC combined with mass spectrometry are used for determination of concentrations of these drugs in biological matrix. There are also many limitations of immunoassays but the major limitations of immunoassays are interferences from drug metabolites, other drugs with similar structures, herbal supplements as well as various endogenous factors. In addition, the presence of high bilirubin in the serum or plasma, high lipid concentration, hemolysis and variety of other factors may significantly alter true concentration of a drug measured by immunoassays (see also Chapter 3 for detail). Therefore, despite advances in immunoassay techniques for therapeutic drug monitoring, chromatographic techniques play an important role in analytical measurement of concentrations of many drugs in clinical laboratories. Moreover, no immunoassay is commercially available for more recently approved drugs, also many other drugs require monitoring and for these drugs chromatographic techniques are the only choice.

1.13   HISTORY OF CHROMATOGRAPHIC TECHNIQUES

Chromatographic techniques are separation techniques by physical means where a complex mixture can be resolved into individual components or components of interest without physically altering the components. The word chromatography was derived from Greek "chroma" which means color and "graphein" which means writing. Therefore, chromatography means color writing. At the beginning of the twentieth century, chromatographic separation of compounds was primarily based on principles of adsorption as well as partition chromatography. The first known work on adsorption chromatography was done by Mikhail S. Tswett (1872–1919), starting around 1902. In a lecture at the meeting of the Warsaw Society of Natural Science in 1903, Tswett described the separation of plant pigments on a column packed with powdered calcium carbonate or alumina [96]. Because such a technique produced separation of colored plant product, the term chromatography (color writing) was appropriate to describe the process. At that time, the separation was assumed to be based on the difference in molecular interactions between the compounds and the adsorbents. This type of chromatography initiated a new era in separation of single compounds from a complex mixture, in contrast to very old methodology of purification by extraction and repeated crystallization. Later in 1952, Borgstrom introduced silicic acid to separate lipids from fats and fatty acids, thus initiating the modern era of chromatographic separation techniques [97].

1.14   VARIOUS TYPES OF CHROMATOGRAPHIC TECHNIQUES

In chromatographic techniques there is a stationary phase and a mobile phase and the separation takes place in the stationary phase when a mixture dissolved in the mobile phase is passed through the stationary phase due to differential partition of various components with the stationary and mobile phase. The chromatography may be preparative or analytical in nature. Analytical chromatographic techniques involving small amounts of specimens are used in clinical laboratories for the purpose of therapeutic drug monitoring. Chromatography may be either column chromatography (most common) where a column is packed with the desired stationary phase and mixture dissolved in mobile phase is passed through the column and the elution of various components from the column is detected by various physical or chemical means (postcolumn derivatization). Chromatography may also take place using open stationary phase (planar chromatography) such as paper chromatography (thin layer chromatography). Various types of chromatography are discussed in this chapter.

1.14.1   Thin-Layer Chromatography (TLC)/Paper Chromatography

The technique was first described by Izmailov and Shraiber in 1938 where the authors added a drop of belladonna extract on a glass plate with 2 mm film of alumina and developed it into cocentric zones by drop wise addition of methanol. The substances in the zones were visualized under ultraviolet (UV) lamp [98]. Application of the technique was difficult because the loosely bound adsorbent was not stable on the glass plate. Later this technique was further developed by Meinhard and Hall in 1949 and then by Kirchner et al. in 1951. In TLC separation, the migration of the compound on a specific absorbent under specific developing solvent(s) is the characteristic of the compound. This is expressed by comparing the migration of the compound to that of the solvent (ratio to front, retention factor, or retardation factor, R_f).

Separation of biological compounds using paper was reported as early as 1906 by a Hungarian scientist, Janos Plesch [99]. In this technique, the author used a drop of urine on a filter paper and then a drop of sulfanilic acid-hydrochloric acid to detect the bile pigment bilirubin as a circular colored ring. Migration of bilirubin from the center of the spot and detection by color reaction was the basis of circular paper chromatography. Later, in 1944, Consden et al. introduced paper chromatography for separation of amino-acids [100]. Typically, compounds are spotted on at the edge of a paper strip and a mixture of polar solvents is allowed to migrate through the paper as the mobile phase. Compounds are separated based on the principle of partition chromatography in which water from the solvent mixture is adsorbed and tightly held on the paper fibers, so the compounds partition between the migrating mobile phase and tightly held water. Various detection techniques can be used for detecting compound of interest after separation in TLC and paper chromatography. UV detection is a very popular method due to its simplicity. In addition, various reagents can be sprayed on the plate in order to visualize spots. Although use of paper chromatography for toxicological analysis has been reported, it is rarely used for the purpose of therapeutic drug monitoring. Alkaloids are generally detected by Dragendorff's reagent (potassium bismuth iodide prepared by dissolving bismuth hydroxide in concentrated hydrochloric acid followed by addition of aqueous potassium iodide and aqueous acetic acid. This reagent is also commercially available). There are many other reagents for visualization of spots on the TLC plates but none of them are specific for a particular compound. Therefore, the TLC method lacks specificity for compound identification and is rarely used in therapeutic drug monitoring, although ToxiLab technique (a type of paper chromatography) is used for qualitative analysis of drug of abuse in urine specimens in some clinical laboratories as a screening technique.

1.14.2 GAS-CHROMATOGRAPHY (GC)

In 1941, Martin and Synge in their original paper on liquid-liquid chromatography first predicted the use of a gas instead of a liquid as the mobile phase in a chromatographic process [101]. Later in 1952, James and Martin systemically separated volatile compounds based on the theory of GC [102]. In the method, the separations were achieved by using a linear glass column of 122 cm long × 4 mm internal diameter packed with kieselguhr (silica). The separations were essentially similar to those used by fractional distillation, but could be applied to a relatively smaller amount of compound. Foundations of this separation are based on differences in vapor pressure of the solutes and on the theory of Raoult's law. Originally, GC columns started with wide-bore coiled columns (6 mm I.D. × 200 mm long) packed with an inert support of high surface area. The support was coated with a low volatile liquid phase considered as the stationary phase. Currently, capillary columns are used for better resolution of compounds in GC and columns are coated with liquid phases such as methyl, methyl-phenyl, propylnitrile, and other functional groups chemically bonded to the silica support. Unlike the number of known plates used for fractional distillation of petroleum, the effectiveness of the GC columns is based on number of theoretical plates (n) as defined by the equation;

$$n = 16\left(\frac{t_r}{w_b}\right)^2$$

t_r: retention time of the solute and w_b: width of the peak at the baseline.

Because the GC separations are based on the differences in vapor pressures (boiling points), compounds with high vapor pressures (low boiling points) will elute faster than the compounds with low vapor pressures (high boiling points). Generally, boiling point increases with increasing polarity. This causes compounds with low polarity to elute faster than the compounds with high polarity. Compounds are typically identified by the retention time (RT) or travel time needed to pass through the GC column. After separation by GC, compounds can be detected by flame-ionization detector (FID), electron-capture detector (ECD), nitrogen–phosphorus detector (NPD), or other electrochemical detectors. Although ECD and NPD are specific to some of the functions of the compounds, none of the detectors are compound specific. Mass spectrometer (MS) is a specific detector for GC because mass spectral fragmentation patterns are specific for compounds except for optical isomers. GC combined with MS (GC-MS) is widely used in clinical laboratories for both therapeutic drug monitoring and drugs of abuse analysis. Despite the potential for application of GC-MS in the clinical laboratory, integration of these two instruments was a major problem. MS typically operates at a vacuum of 10^{-6}–10^{-5} torr whereas the gas flow through a wide-bore packed GC column was greater than 10 mL/min. This problem was alleviated by placing a separator between the GC and MS. In this separation, only a limited amount of effluents was directed to the MS. With the advantages of both sensitivity and selectivity, MS-detection significantly improved the confidence in confirmation.

One advantage of GC over the TLC and paper chromatography is that a suitable internal standard can be used to determine the amount of drug in the specimen. The quantification is better when the drug and internal standard have similar physical and chemical properties and separate well in the GC. With the introduction of capillary GC in the early 1980s, wide-bore packed GC is now rarely used in clinical laboratories.

1.14.3   HIGH-PRESSURE OR HIGH-PERFORMANCE LIQUID CHROMATOGRAPHY (HPLC OR LC)

With the advent of theory of separation in TLC and GC, Knox in 1966 studied the effects of fluid velocities and column diameters on the chromatographic behaviors of potassium permanganate eluted with 10% potassium chloride [103]. Almost at the same time, Horvath and his colleagues introduced a HPLC method for separation of nucleotides in a stainless steel column (1 mm internal diameter × 193 cm length) packed with glass beads (diameter 44–105 μm) coated with styrene-divinyl or polyethylene-imine polymers and under pressure of 2.7–20.5 atm [104,105]. The concept of using a reverse phase with nonpolar polymers as the stationary phase and polar hydroxy solvents as the mobile phase was the basis of this experiment. This is sharp contrast to the column chromatography where the stationary phase is polar silica and the mobile phase (eluting solvent) is relatively nonpolar. For an effective separation in HPLC, gradient elution technique is often used by gradually changing the composition of the eluting solvents. The stationary phase generally consists of packing materials with n-alkyl chains (C_8- or C_{18}-) covalently bonded to silica. Other packing materials are also available to meet specific need in analysis (cyano, amide, polyethylene glycol, mixed mode, and others). For some compounds where high or low pH is required for the analysis, the base materials are made of cross-linked polystyrene instead of silica. Silica is sensitive at pH > 9 when the Si–O–Si bond hydrolyses to silicate salt whereas at pH < 2 the bond breaks down to form silicic acid. HPLC technique is especially applicable to polar or ionic compounds that are difficult to analyze by GC.

Initially, most toxicologists detected LC separated compounds by UV and fluorescent detectors. However, over the course of time, these nonspecific detectors were slowly replaced by the MS detector. Similar to GC-MS, eliminating the excess solvents (mobile phase) before introducing the compound into the high vacuum MS is a problem. Several interfaces, such as moving belt, direct liquid insertion, continuous-flow fast atom bombardment, particle beam, thermospray, electrospray or atmospheric-pressure chemical ionization (APCI) were developed in order to be effective as detectors for compound eluting from the column (also see Chapter 4).

Liquid chromatography has some advantages over GC. Use of GC is limited only to compounds that are thermally stable and can be volatilized. Compounds with carboxylic (COOH), hydroxyl (OH), primary amino (NH_2) or secondary amino (NHR) as well as sulfhydryl (SH) functional groups are polar and are difficult to separate using GC and require derivatization before they can be analyzed. Because the partitions of these polar compounds are more in favor of the hydroxy solvents, HPLC is more suitable than GC for their separation and in most cases; derivatization is not required for HPLC analysis. Unlike GC, the polar compounds are eluted before the nonpolar compounds in the reverse-phase liquid chromatography.

1.15   APPLICATION OF GAS CHROMATOGRAPHY (GC) IN THERAPEUTIC DRUG MONITORING

Many therapeutic drugs are small molecules and can be determined by GC. In the 1970s therapeutic drug monitoring of anticonvulsants were exclusively performed using various GC methods. Roger et al. described simultaneous determination of carbamazepine, phenobarbital, phenytoin, primidone, and mephenytoin using GC. Plasma specimen was supplemented with 5-phenyl-5-(p-tolyl)-hydantoin as an internal standard, buffered with phosphate buffer and extracted with dichloromethane. After drying, the residue was treated with methanol and 0.5 M hydrochloric acid and acidic solution was washed twice with hexane and then extracted again with dichloromethane, organic phase evaporated to dryness and dry residue was reconstituted with trimethylphenyl-ammonium hydroxide for GC analysis where on column methylation of phenobarbital, primidone, mephobarbital, mephenytoin, and phenytoin took place. The limit of detection of each drug was 0.5 μg/ml in plasma [106]. Kuperberg described a GC method for quantitative analysis of phenytoin, phenobarbital, and primidone in plasma [107]. Another GC method for simultaneous analysis of phenobarbital, primidone, and phenytoin in patient's sera utilized N,N-dimethyl derivatives of these drugs and "on-column" derivatization technique [108]. Later many GC-MS methods were developed for therapeutic drug monitoring of various anticonvulsants. Speed et al. described analysis of six anticonvulsants carbamazepine, pheno-barbital, phenytoin, primidone, ethosuximide and valproic acid using GC-MS. The authors used deu-terated drugs were used as internal standards and drugs along with internal standards were extracted from whole blood or liver tissue samples using solid phase extraction. Butyl derivatives of drugs were prepared using n-iodobutane and tetramethyl ammonium hydroxide. Stable butyl derivatives (stable for many days) were formed for all anticonvulsants analyzed except for carbamazepine where the butyl derivative breaks down at the injection port producing iminostilbenes and 9-methyl acridine. Therefore, the authors optimized condition to maximize formation of iminostilbenes by using injec-tor port temperature of 280°C and glass wool packing in the injection port liner. Primidone formed both mono and di-substituted product and di-substituted product was selected for the analysis [109]. In Figure 1.1 sample chromatogram showing separation of six anticonvulsants drugs (as butyl deriva-tives) is given as reported by Speed et al. The authors spiked blank specimens with six anticonvulsants (carbamazepine, phenobarbital, phenytoin, primidone, ethosuximide, and valproic acid) and analyzed the specimen by GC-MS. The authors used selected ion monitoring for GC-MS analysis and in Figure 1.2 the chosen ions were labeled and the ions that produced the best CV (coefficient of variation) were marked with an asterisk [109]. In another report, Pocci et al. described analysis of barbiturates in human urine using GC-MS and solid phase extraction [110].

GC or GC-MS can be used for therapeutic drug monitoring of new generation of anticonvulsants, various cardioactive drugs, neoplastic drugs and other drugs which are relatively volatile or can be converted to relatively volatile derivatives. GC combined with nitrogen phosphorus detector or MS can also be used for determination of specific neoplastic drugs. Kerbusch et al. determined con-centration of ifosfamide, 2- and 3-dechloroethylifosfamide in human plasma by using GC coupled with nitrogen phosphorus detector or MS without any derivatization. Sample preparation involved liquid-liquid extraction with ethyl acetate after adding trofosfamide as the internal standard and making the serum alkaline. The authors concluded that GC with nitrogen phosphorus detector was more sensitive for analysis of these compounds compared to GC combined with positive ion elec-tron-impact ion trap MS [111]. Concentrations of cardioactive drug mexiletine in serum or plasma can be determined by GC-MS. Minnigh et al. used p-chlorophenylalanine as the internal standard.

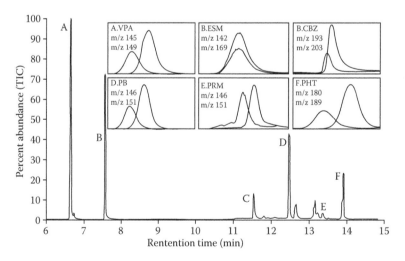

FIGURE 1.1 Sample chromatogram (TIC for all selected ions) for blank blood supplemented with six anticonvulsants, valproic acid (VPA), ethosuximide (ESM), carbamazepine (CBZ), phenobarbital (PB), primidone (PRM), and phenytoin (PHT). Peak shapes for the base ion and relevant internal standards are shown in the inserts. (Reprinted from Speed DJ, Dickinson SJ, Cairns ER, Kim ND, *J Anal Toxicol*, 24, 685–690, 2000. With permission.)

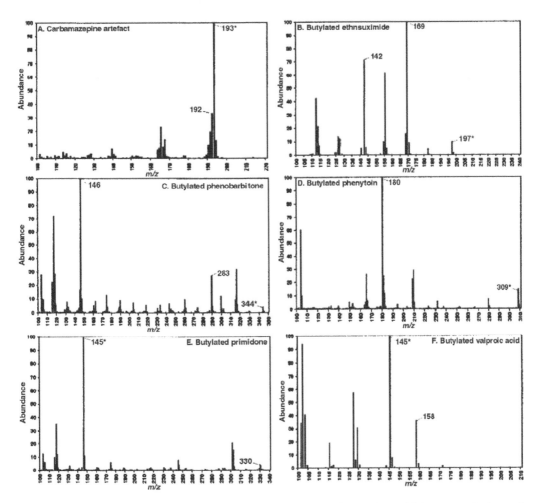

FIGURE 1.2 Mass spectra of the butyl derivatives. The labeled peaks are those which were routinely monitored; peaks given rise to the best CVs are marked with an asterisk. (Reprinted from Speed DJ, Dickinson SJ, Cairns ER, Kim ND, *J Anal Toxicol*, 24, 685–690, 2000. With permission.)

The drug and the internal standard were extracted from plasma by a combination of ethyl acetate, hexane and methanol (60:40:1 by volume) followed by evaporation of organic phase and derivatization to pentafluoropropyl derivatives. The MS was operated in a selected ion monitoring mode [112]. Other derivatization techniques for determination of mexiletine concentration in serum have been described. Mexiletine can be extracted from alkaline serum with dichloromethane followed by derivatization with 2,2,2-trichloroethyl chloroformate. The reaction was completed in 30 min at 70°C. N-propylamphetamine was used as the internal standard. The assay was linear for serum mexiletine concentrations between 0.2 and 2.5 mg/L [113]. GC-MS analysis of mexiletine in human serum after extraction and derivatization with perfluorooctanoyl chloride has also been reported [114]. Mexiletine was extracted along with the internal standard (N-propyl amphetamine) from alkaline plasma using dichloromethane and after evaporation of solvent dry residue was treated with perfluorooctanoyl chloride (at 80°C for 20 min) for derivatization. Baseline separation of both mexiletine and the internal standard was achieved using GC-MS. The MS can be operated in both electron ionization mode and chemical ionization mode for analysis of mexiletine. In Figure 1.3 total ion chromatogram of analysis of a patient specimen containing 1.4 μg/ml of mexiletine is shown. The MS was operated in electron impact mode with selected ion monitoring (*m/z* 122, 454, and 575 were monitored for derivatized mexiletine and *m/z* 91, 118, 440, and 452 were monitored for the derivatized internal standard). In Figure 1.4 full scan electron impact mass spectrum of derivatized mexiletine is given and in Figure 1.5 full scan chemical ionization mass spectrum of derivatized mexiletine is given (authors own data).

One of the major areas of therapeutic drug monitoring where GC-MS methods are widely used is the therapeutic drug monitoring of patients undergoing pain management therapy. Many narcotic analgesic drugs such as morphine, codeine, oxycodone, hydrocodone, oxymorphone, hydromorphone, etc. are used for treating patients with severe pain. Because of high abuse potential of these

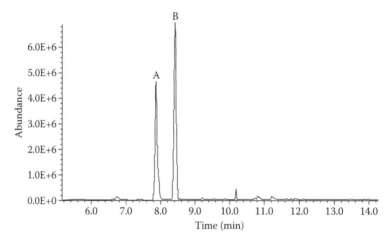

FIGURE 1.3 Total ion chromatogram of a patient specimen containing 1.4 mg/ml mexiletine (mexiletine and the internatal standard N-propyl amphetamine were analyzed after derivatization with perfluorooctanoyl chloride). Peak A is derivatized internal standard and peak b is the derivatized mexiletine. (Author's own data)

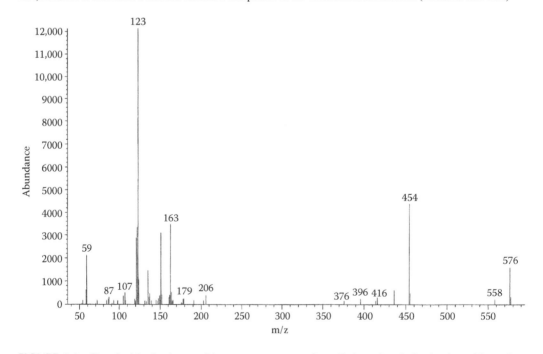

FIGURE 1.4 Chemical ionization total ion mass spectrum of mexiletine after derivatization with perfluorooctanoyl chloride.

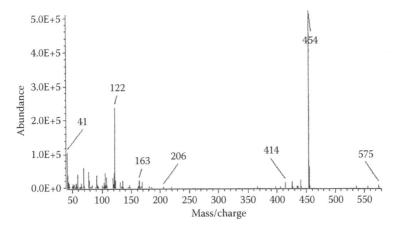

FIGURE 1.5 Chemical ionization total ion mass spectrum of mexiletine after derivatization with perfluorooctanoyl chloride.

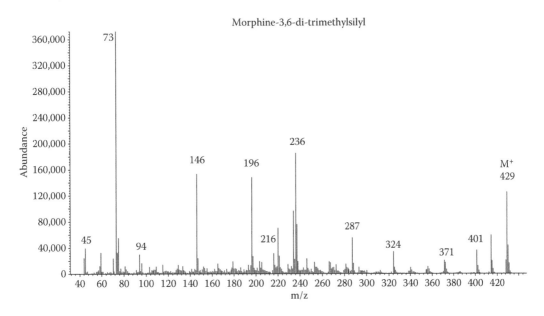

FIGURE 1.6 Full scan trimethylsilyl derivative of morphine. (Courtesy of Dr. Buddha D. Paul of Armed Forces Institute of Pathology, Rockville, MD.)

drugs routine monitoring is necessary in order to determine patient compliance as well as potential abuse of these drugs (see Chapter 21). More recently, LC/MS methods for monitoring these drugs have also been reported.

The most commonly prescribed opiates are codeine, hydrocodone, and oxycodone. When ingested, these compounds metabolize to morphine, hydromorphone, and oxymorphone, respectively, and to their conjugates. After hydrolysis of the conjugates, the solutions are treated with hydroxylamine to transform 6-keto-opiates to the corresponding 6-oximes and following extraction, the compounds are derivatized to the trimethylsilyl derivatives. Morphine and codeine (which lack keto group) are only converted to their corresponding trimethylsilyl derivatives. Full scan mass spectrum of trimethylsilyl derivative of morphine is given in Figure 1.6 while full scan trimethylsilyl derivative of codeine is given in Figure 1.7. Codeine, morphine along with related opiates (keto-opitates) can be analyzed by GC-MS after converting them to oxime derivative followed

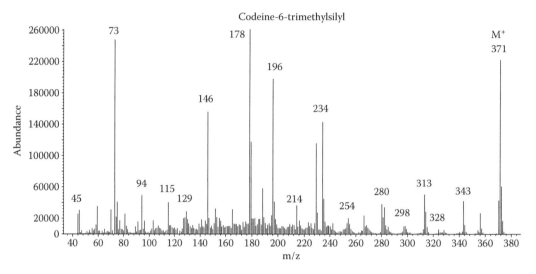

FIGURE 1.7   Full scan trimethylsilyl derivative of codeine. (Courtesy of Dr. Buddha D. Paul of Armed Forces Institute of Pathology, Rockville, MD.)

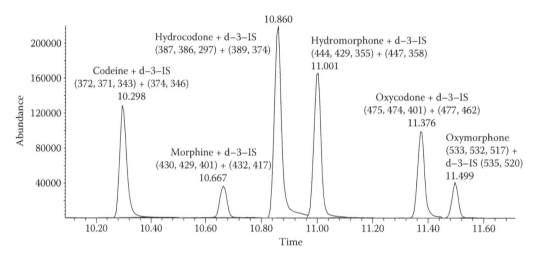

FIGURE 1.8   Total ion chromatogram showing baseline separation of codeine, hydrocodone, morphine, hydromorphone. Oxycodone and oxymorphone and their deuterated internal standards; codeine as 6-trimethylsilyl, morphine as 3,6-di-trimethylsilyl, hydrocodone as 6-(trimethylsilyl)oxime, hydromorphone as 3-(trimethylsilyl-6-(trimethylsilyl)oxime, hydromorphone as 3-trimethylsilyl-6-(trimethylsilyl)oxime, oxycodone as 14-trimethylsilyl-6-(trimethylsilyl)oxime and oxymorphone as 3,14-di-trimethylsilyl-6-(trimethylsilyl)oxime. (Courtesy of Dr. Buddha D. Paul of Armed Forces Institute of Pathology, Rockville, MD.)

converting them to the corresponding trimethylsilyl derivatives. Baseline separation between these compounds can be achieved by using selected ion monitoring for each derivatized opiates and their deuterated internal standards. The total ion chromatogram of such separation is given in Figure 1.8 and ions monitored for each compound as well as the corresponding internal standard are given with each peak corresponding to respected opiate.

Many other derivatization techniques for codeine and morphine have been described in the literature including acetylation, propionylation, and pentafluoropropionylation at the 6-hydroxy group of codeine. When codeine is derivatized, morphine is also simultaneously derivatized to the

3,6-diacetyl-, 3,6-dipropionyl-, or 3,6-dipentafluoropropionyl-morphine. The full scan mass spectrum of acetyl derivative of morphine is shown in Figure 1.9 while the full scan mass spectrum of acetyl derivative of codeine is given in Figure 1.10.

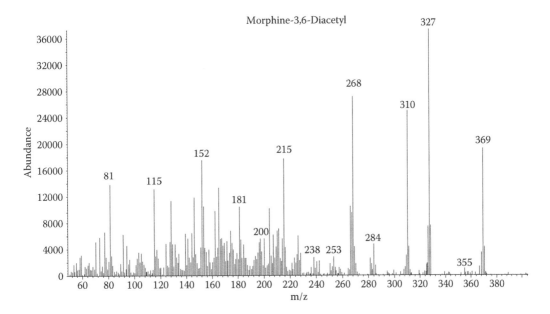

FIGURE 1.9 Full scan acetyl derivative of morphine. (Courtesy of Dr. Buddha D. Paul of Armed Forces Institute of Pathology, Rockville, MD.)

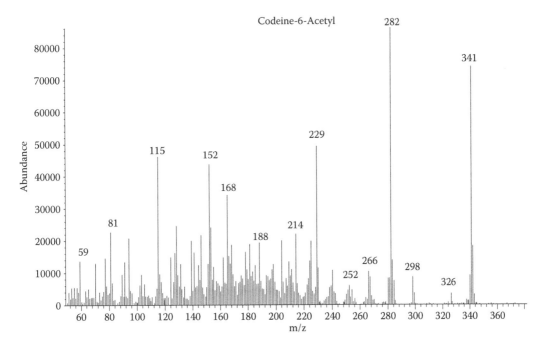

FIGURE 1.10 Full scan acetyl derivative of codeine. (Courtesy of Dr. Buddha D. Paul of Armed Forces Institute of Pathology, Rockville, MD.)

1.16   APPLICATION OF HIGH-PERFORMANCE LIQUID CHROMATOGRAPHY (HPLC) IN THERAPEUTIC DRUG MONITORING

Although only relatively volatile non polar compounds can be analyzed by GC, both polar and nonpolar compounds can be analyzed by liquid chromatography and as expected there are numerous reports of analysis of various classes of drugs using liquid chromatography in the literature. Both classical anticonvulsants and newer anticonvulsants can be analyzed by liquid chromatography. Recently, Subramanian et al. describes LC/MS analysis of nine anticonvulsants; zonisamide, lamotrigine, topiramate, phenobarbital, phenytoin, carbamazepine, carbamazepine, 10,11-diol, 10-hydroxycarbamazepine and carbamazepine 10,11-epoxide. Sample preparation included solid phase extraction for all anticonvulsants and HPLC separation was achieved by a reverse phase C-18 column (4.6 × 50 mm, 2.2 μm particle size) with a gradient mobile phase of acetate buffer, methanol, acetonitrile and tetrahydrofuran. Four internal standards were used. Detection of peaks was achieved by APCI MS in selected ion monitoring mode with constant polarity switching [115]. In Figure 1.11 mass spectral scans of all antiepileptic drugs (AEDs) analyzed by the authors; zonisamide (ZNS), phenobarbital (PB), phenytoin (PHT) and topiramate (TPM), carbamazepine (CBZ), lamotrigine (LTG), carbamazepine-10,11-diol (CBZ-Diol), 10-hydroxycarbazepine (MHD), carbamazepine-10,11-epoxide (CBZ-E) and levetiracetam (LEV) are shown. In Figure 1.12 mass spectral scans of commonly monitored AEDs; $^2H_{10}$-carbamazepine, $^{13}C_2$, ^{15}N-limotrigene, pregabalin, gabapentin, felbamate and oxcarbazepine (in positive mode), as well as $^2H_{10}$-phenytoin, $^2H_{12}$-topiramate, tiagabine and valproic acid (in negative mode) are shown. In Figure 1.13 an MS chromatogram of standards (A, B, and C) and a patient sample (D) are shown. In patient specimen D collected from a patient receiving carbamazepine, topiramate and lamotrigine, all three parent drugs as well as metabolites of carbamazepine (carbamazepine diol, carbamazepine epoxide) were detected [115].

Other than anticonvulsants, various cardioactive drugs, antidepressants, antibiotics, immunosuppressant, antineoplastic drugs, antiretroviral drugs, antifungal medications and variety of other drugs are routinely measured in clinical laboratories using various liquid chromatographic techniques. Verbesselt et al. described a rapid HPLC assay with solid phase extraction for analysis of 12 antiarrhythmic drugs in plasma; amiodarone, aprindine, disopyramide, flecainide, lidocaine, lorcainide, mexiletine, procainamide, propafenone, sotalol, tocainide and verapamil. Because most of these drugs are basic compounds, alkalinization of column produced good absorption of these drugs in the extraction column. However, for amiodarone, an acidic pH (3.5) was maintained and aprindine was eluted at neutral pH. After washing with water, the compounds were eluted with methanol except for amiodarone, which was eluted with acetonitrile and acetate buffer (8:5 by volume) at pH 5. Chromatographic separation was achieved by using a Spherisorb hexyl column (150 × 4.6 mm I.D. with particle size of 5 μm) and mobile phase was composed of a mixture of acetonitrile or methanol with phosphate or acetate buffer at a different pH. Detection of peaks was achieved by either a UV detector or a fluorescence detector [116]. Concentrations of encainide and its metabolites can be determined in human plasma by HPLC [117].

Kamberi et al. described a simple HPLC method for analysis of antibiotic ciprofloxacin in human serum or urine. Plasma proteins were removed using acetonitrile but urine does not require such treatment. HPLC separation of ciprofloxacin was achieved using reverse phase column and isocratic mobile phase of acetic acid, acetonitrile and water. The column was heated at 50°C and elution of peaks was monitored using UV. Lomefloxacin was used as an internal standard [118].

Chromatographic techniques are the only available method for therapeutic drug monitoring for many drugs including antiretroviral drugs, various antibiotics and several cardioactive drugs where there is no commercially available immunoassays. Although immunoassays are readily available for monitoring immunosuppressants, chromatographic techniques are still the method of choice because of the issue of metabolic cross-reactivity with various commercially available immunoassays for immunosuppressants.

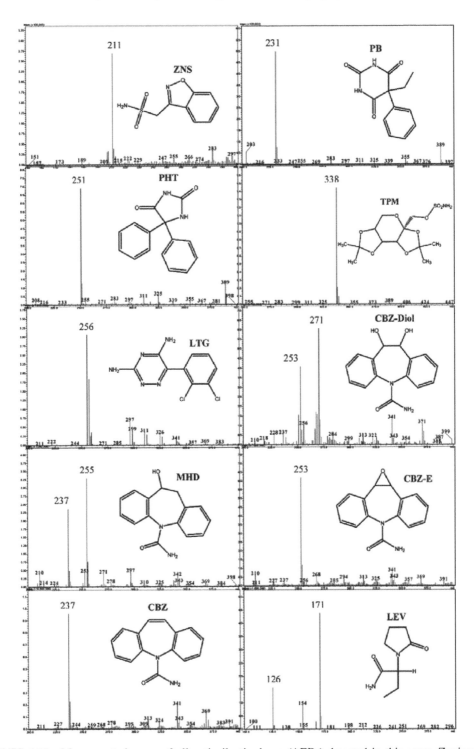

FIGURE 1.11 Mass spectral scans of all antiepileptic drugs (AEDs) detected in this assay. Zonisamide (ZNS), phenobarbital (PB), phenytoin (PHT) and topiramate (TPM) are in negative mode, while carbamazepine (CBZ), lamotrigine (LTG), carbamazepine-10,11-diol (CBZ-diol), 10-hydroxycarbazepine (MHD), carbamazepine-10,11-epoxide (CBZ-E) and levetiracetam (LEV) are in positive mode. (From Subramanian M, Birnbaum AK, Remmel RP, *Ther Drug Monit,* 30, 347–356, 2008. With permission from Wolters/Lippincott Williams and Wilkins.)

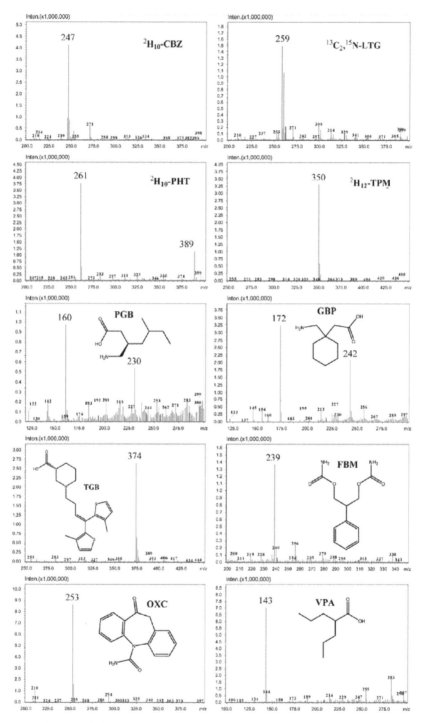

FIGURE 1.12 MS scans of all commonly monitored AEDs. 2H10-CBZ (carbamazepine), 13C2, 15N-LTG (lamotrigine), pregabalin (PGB), gabapentin (GBP), felbamate (FBM) and oxcarbazepine (OXC) are in positive mode, while 2H10-PHT (phenytoin), 2H12-TPM (topiramate), tiagabine (TGB) and valproic acid (VPA) are in negative mode. (From Subramanian M, Birnbaum AK, Remmel RP, *Ther Drug Monit,* 30, 347–356, 2008. With permission from Wolters/Lippincott Williams and Wilkins.)

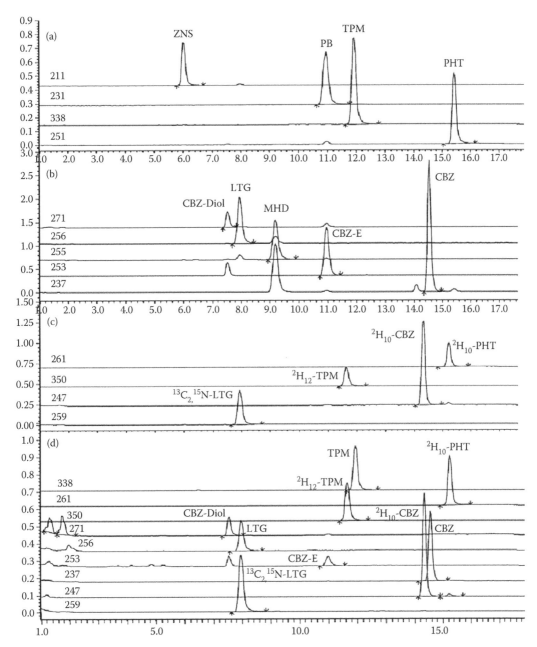

FIGURE 1.13 Mass spectrometry (MS) chromatogram of standards (A, B, and C) and a patient sample (D). A, negative-mode AEDs; B, positive-mode AEDs; C, four internal standards; D, plasma sample of a patient receiving lamotrigine (LTG), carbamazepine (CBZ), and topiramate (TPM). The metabolites carbamazepine-10,11-epoxide (CBZ-E) and carbamazepine-10,11-diol (CBZ-Diol) were also detected. Concentrations in A: 10, 8, 6, and 8 mg/mL for ZNS, PB, TPM, and PHT, respectively. Concentrations in B: 5, 5, 8, 5, and 5 mg/mL for CBZ-Diol, LTG, MHD, CBZ-E, and CBZ, respectively. Internal standard concentrations in (C) were all 10 mg/mL; concentrations of the detected AEDs and metabolites in (D) were 3.8, 2.5, 0.7, 2.7, and 4.5 mg/mL for CBZ-Diol, LTG, CBZ-E, TPM, and CBZ, respectively. (From Subramanian M, Birnbaum AK, Remmel RP, *Ther Drug Monit*, 30, 347–356, 2008. With permission from Wolters/Lippincott Williams and Wilkins.)

1.17   CONCLUSIONS

Although immunoassays are available for therapeutic drug monitoring of commonly monitored drugs for many drugs which require monitoring, chromatographic techniques are the only available methods. In addition, immunoassays suffer from many limitations including interferences from components of matrix, drug metabolites, structurally similar drugs as well as endogenous compounds. In general chromatographic techniques are analytically more robust techniques and are free from such interferences. In addition, for monitoring immunosuppressant drugs, chromatographic techniques are clearly superior because immunoassays suffer from significant cross-reactivity from metabolites. Moreover, there is no commercially available immunoassay for monitoring various antiretroviral drugs, some antineoplastic drugs, several new general anticonvulsants and different antibiotics. For these drugs, chromatographic techniques are used in clinical laboratories for therapeutic drug monitoring. Also for therapeutic drugs where immunoassays are commercially available, chromatographic techniques are still considered as the gold standard especially in resolving discordant results in specimens obtained by various immunoassays. Different immunoassays depending on antibody specificity may have significantly different cross-reactivity towards the drug metabolite as well as other endogenous and exogenous compounds.

REFERENCES

1. Hersh EV, Pinto A, Moore PA. 2007. Adverse drug interactions involving common prescription and over the counter analgesics. *Clin Ther* 29: 2477–2497.
2. Watson I, Potter J, Yatscoff R, Fraser A et al. 1997. Editorial. *Ther Drug Monit* 19: 125.
3. Peterson GM, Khoo BH, von Witt RJ. 1991. Clinical response in epilepsy in relation to total and free serum levels of phenytoin. *Ther Drug Monit* 13: 415–419.
4. Rajendran SD, Rao YM, Thanikachalam S, Muralidharan TR, Anbalagan M et al. 2005. Comparison of target concentration intervention strategy with conventional dosing of digoxin. *Indian Heart J* 57: 265–267.
5. Pawinski T, Pulik P, Gralak B, Horban A. 2008. Pharmacokinetic monitoring of HIV-1 protease inhibitors in the antiretroviral therapy. *Acta Pol Pharm* 65: 93–100.
6. Chugh SS, Socoteanu C, Reinier K, Waltz J et al. 2008. A community-based evaluation of sudden death associated with therapeutic levels of methadone. *Am J Med* 121: 66–71.
7. Gillisen A. 2007. Patient's adherence in asthma. *J Physiol Pharmacol* 58 (suppl 5, Pt 1): 205–222.
8. Patsalos PN, Berry DJ, Bourgeois BF, Cloyd JC et al. 2008. Antiepileptic drugs-best practice guidelines for therapeutic drug monitoring: a position paper by the sub commission on therapeutic drug monitoring, ILAE commission on therapeutic strategies. *Epilepsia* 49: 1239–1276.
9. Bigger JT, Leahey EB Jr. 1982. Quinidine and digoxin: an important interaction. *Drugs* 24: 229–239.
10. Black RE, Lau WK, Weinstein RJ, Young LS, Hewitt WL. 1976 Ototoxicity of amikacin. *Antimicrob Ag Chemother* 9: 956–961.
11. Duffull SB, Begg EJ. 1994. Vancomycin toxicity: what is the evidence for dose dependence? *Adverse Drug React Toxicol Rev* 13: 103–114.
12. Begg EJ, Barclay ML, Kirkpatrick C. 1999. The therapeutic monitoring of antimicrobial agents [review]. *J Clin Pharmacol* 47: 23–30.
13. Ryback MJ, Albrecht LM, Boike SC, Chandrasekar PH. 1990. Nephrotoxicity of vancomycin: alone or with an aminoglycoside. *J Antimicrob Chemother* 25: 679–687.
14. Cimino MA, Rotstein C, Slaughter RL, Emrich LJ. 1987. Relationship of serum antibiotic concentrations to nephrotoxicity in cancer patients receiving concurrent aminoglycoside and vancomycin therapy. *Am J Med* 83: 1091–1096.
15. Florence AT, Jani PU. 1994. Novel oral drug formulations: their potential in modulating adverse effects. *Drug Saf* 10: 233–266.
16. Tedesco-Silva H, Bastien MC, Choi L, Felipe C et al. 2005. Mycophenolic acid metabolite profile in renal transplant patients receiving enteric coated mycophenolate sodium or mycophenolate mofetil. *Transplant Proc* 37: 852–855.
17. van Hoogdalem E, de Boer AG, Breimer DD. 1991. Pharmacokinetics of rectal drug administration, Part I: General considerations and clinical applications of centrally active drugs. *Clin Pharmacokinet* 21: 11–26.

18. Fischer JH, Patel TV, Fischer PA. 2003. Fosphenytoin: clinical pharmacokinetics and comparative advantages in the acute treatment of seizures. *Clin Pharmacokinet* 42: 33–58.
19. Pajouhesh H, Lenz GR. 2005. Medicinal chemicals properties of successful central nervous system drugs. *NeuroRx* 2: 541–553.
20. Ningaraj NS. 2006. Drug delivery to brain tumors: challenges and progress. *Expert Opin Drug Deliv* 3: 499–509.
21. Morgan MM, Khan DA, Nathan RA. 2005. Treatment for allergic rhinitis and chronic idiopathic urticaria: focus on oral antihistamines. *Ann Pharmacother* 39: 2056–2064.
22. Rollins DE, Klaassen CD. 1979. Biliary excretion of drugs in man. *Clin Pharmacokinet* 4: 368–379.
23. Evans WE, Relling MV. 1999. Pharmacogenomics: translating functional genomics into rational therapeutics. *Science* 286: 487–491.
24. Zager UM, Turpeinen M, Klein K, Schwab M. 2008. Functional pharmacogenetics/genomics of human cytochrome P450 involved in drug biotransformation. *Anal Bioanal Chem* Aug 10 [E-pub ahead of print].
25. Rollason V, Samer C, Piguet V, Dayer P et al. 2008. Pharmacogenomics of analgesics: toward the individualization of prescription. *Pharmacogenomics* 9: 905–933.
26. van Schaik RH. 2008. CYP450 pharmacogenetics for personalized cancer therapy. *Drug Resist Updat* 11: 77–98.
27. Vizirianakis IS. 2004. Challenges in current drug delivery from the potential application of pharmacogenomics and personalized medicine in clinical practice. *Curr Drug Deliv* 1: 73–80.
28. de Leon J. 2006. Amplichip CYP450 test: personalized medicine has arrived in psychiatry. *Expert Rev Mol Diagn* 6: 277–286.
29. Schwartz JB. 2003. The influence of sex on pharmacokinetics. *Clin Pharmacokinet* 42; 107–121.
30. Brosen K. 2007. Sex differences in pharmacology [in Danish]. *Ugeskr Laeger* 169: 2408–2411.
31. Rugstad HE, Hundal O, Holme I, Herland OB et al. 1986. Piroxicam and naproxen plasma concentrations in patients with osteoarthritis: relation to age, sex, efficacy and adverse events. *Clin Rheumatol* 5: 389–398.
32. Gex-Fabry M, Balant-Georgia AE, Balant LP, Garrone G. 1990. Clomipramine metabolism: model based analysis of variability factors from drug monitoring data. *Clin Pharmacokinet* 19: 241–255.
33. Walle T, Walle UK, Cowart TD, Conradi EC. 1989. Pathway selective sex differences in the metabolic clearance of propranolol in human subjects. *Clin Pharmacol Ther* 46: 257–263.
34. Lew KH, Ludwig EA, Milad MA, Donovan K. 1993. Gender based effects on methylprednisolone pharmacokinetics and pharmacodynamics. *Clin Pharmacol Ther* 54: 402–414.
35. Wolbold R, Klein K, Burk O, Nussler AK et al. 2003. Sex is a major determinant of CYP3A4 expression in human liver. *Hepatology* 38: 978–988.
36. Rademaker M. 2001. Do women have more adverse drug reactions? *Am J Clin Dermatol* 2: 349–351.
37. Miners JO, Attwood J, Birkett DJ. 1983. Influence of sex and oral contraceptives on paracetamol metabolism. *Br J Clin Pharmacol* 16: 503–509.
38. Noe KH. 2007. Gender specific challenges in the management of epilepsy in women. *Semin Neurol* 27: 331–339.
39. Pauly JR. 2008. Gender specific differences in tobacco smoking dynamics and the neuropharmacological actions of nicotine. *Front Biosci* 13: 505–516.
40. Cockcroft DW, Gault MH. 1976. Prediction of creatinine clearance from serum creatinine. *Nephron* 16: 31–41.
41. Terrell KM, Heard K, Miller DK. 2006. Prescribing to older ED patients. *Ann J Emerg Med* 24: 468–478.
42. Dasgupta A. 2007. Usefulness of monitoring free (unbound) concentrations of therapeutic drugs in patient management. *Clin Chim Acta* 377: 1–13.
43. Joannidis M 2004. Drug-induced renal failure in the ICU. *Int J Artif Organs* 27: 1034–1042.
44. Izzedine H, Launay-Vacher V, Deray G. 2005. Antiviral drug induced nephrotoxicity. *Am J Kidney Dis* 45: 804–817.
45. Choudhury D, Ahmed Z. 1997. Drug-induced nephrotoxicity. *Med Clin North Am* 81: 705–717.
46. Verbeeck RK. 2008. Pharmacokinetics and dosage adjustment in patients with hepatic dysfunction. *Eur J Clin Phramacol* September 2 [E-pub ahead of print].
47. Cheng PY, Morgan ET. 2001. Hepatic cytochrome P 450 regulation in disease states. *Curr Drug Metab* 2: 165–183.
48. Villeneuve JP, Pichette V. 2004. Cytochrome P450 and liver disease. *Curr Drug Metab* 5: 273–282.
49. Klotz U. 2007. Antiarrhythmics: elimination and dosage considerations in hepatic impairment. *Clin Pharmacokinet* 46: 985–996.

50. Trotter JF, Osborne JC, Heller N, Christians U. 2005. Effect of hepatitis C infection on tacrolimus does and blood levels in liver transplant recipients. *Aliment Pharmacol Ther* 22: 37–44.

51. Zimmermann JJ, Lasseter KC, Lim HK, Harper D et al. 2005. Pharmacokinetics of sirolimus (rapamycin) in subjects with mild to moderate hepatic impairment. *J Clin Pharmacol* 45: 1368–1372.

52. Ng CY, Ghabrial H, Morgan DJ, Ching MS et al. 2000. Impaired elimination of propoanolol due to right heart failure: drug clearance in the isolated liver and its relationship to intrinsic metabolic capacity. *Drug Metab Dispo* 28: 1217–1221.

53. Benowitz NL, Meister W. 1976. Pharmacokinetics in patients with cardiac failure. *Clin Pharmacokinet* 1: 389–405.

54. Boucher BA, Wood GC, Swanson JM. 2006. Pharmacokinetic changes in critical illness. *Crit Care Clin* 22: 255–271.

55. Croxson MS, Ibbertson HK. 1975. Serum digoxin in patients with thyroid disease. *Br Med J* 3 (5983): 566–568.

56. Sarich TC, Wright JM. 1996. Hypothyroxinemia and phenytoin toxicity: a vicious circle. *Drug Metabol Drug Interact* 13: 155–160.

57. Haas M, Kletzmayer J, Staudinger T, Bohmig G et al. 2000. Hypothyroidism as a cause of tacrolimus intoxication and acute renal failure: a case report. *Wien Klin Wochenschr* 112: 939–941.

58. Kurnik D, Loebstein R, Farfel Z, Ezra D et al. 2004. Complex drug-drug disease interactions between amiodarone, warfarin and the thyroid gland. *Medicine* (Baltimore) 83: 107–113.

59. Kellett HA, Sawers JS, Boulton FE, Cholerton S et al. 1986. Problems of anticoagulation with warfarin in hyperthyroidism. *Q J Med* 58: 43–51.

60. Loebstein R, Koren G. 2002. Clinical relevance of therapeutic drug monitoring during pregnancy. *Ther Drug Monit* 24: 15–22.

61. Rakhmanina N, van den Anker, Soldin SJ. 2004. Safety and pharmacokinetics of antiretroviral therapy during pregnancy. *Ther Drug Monit* 26: 110–115.

62. Anderson GD. 2005. Pregnancy induced changes in pharmacokinetics: a mechanistic based approach. *Clin Pharmacokinet* 44: 989–1008.

63. Tomson T. 2005. Gender aspects of pharmacokinetics of new and old AEDs: pregnancy and breast feeding. *Ther Drug Monit* 27: 718–721.

64. Pennell PB, Newport DJ, Stowe ZN, Helmers SL et al. 2004. The impact of pregnancy and childbirth on the metabolism of lamotrigine. *Neurology* 27: 292–295.

65. Soldin OP. 2006. Thyroid function testing in pregnancy and thyroid diseases: trimester-specific reference intervals. *Ther Drug Monit* 28: 8–11.

66. Koren G, Soldin O. 2006. Therapeutic drug monitoring of antithyroid drugs during pregnancy. *Ther Drug Monit* 28: 12–13.

67. Hodge LS, Tracey TS 2007. Alterations in drug disposition during pregnancy: implications for drug therapy. *Expert Opin Drug Metab Toxicol* 3: 557–571.

68. Mucklow JC. 1986. The fate of drugs in pregnancy. *Clin Obstet Gynacecol* 13: 161–175.

69. Oesterheld JR. 1998. A review of developmental aspects of cytochrome P 450. *J Child Adolesc Psychopharmacol* 8: 161–174.

70. Oineiro-Carrero VM, Pineiro EO. 2004. Liver [Review]. *Pediatrics* 113 (4 Suppl) 1097–1106.

71. Perucca E. 2005. Pharmacokinetics variability of new antiepileptic drugs at different age. *Ther Drug Monit* 27: 714–717.

72. Paap CM, Nahata MC. 1990. Clinical pharmacokinetics of antibacterial drugs in neonates. *Clin Pharmacokinet* 19: 280–318.

73. Williams BS, Ransom JL, Gal P, Carlos RQ et al. 1997. Gentamicin pharmacokinetics in neonates with patent ductus arteriosus. *Crit Care Med* 25: 272–275.

74. Brazier JL, Salle B. 1981. Conversion of theophylline to caffeine by the human fetus. *Semin Perinatol* 5: 315–320.

75. Zevin S, Benowitz NL. 1999. Drug interactions with tobacco smoking: an update. *Clin Pharmacokinetic* 36: 425–438.

76. Kroon LA. 2006. Drug interactions and smoking: raising awareness for acute and critical care provider. *Crit Care Nurs Clin N Am* 18: 53–62.

77. Lee BL, Benowitz NL, Jacob P. 1987. Cigarette abstinence, nicotine gum and theophylline disposition. *Ann Intern Med* 106: 553–555.

78. Colucci VJ, Knapp JE. 2001. Increase in International normalization ratio associated with smoking cessation. *Ann Pharmacother* 35: 385–386.

79. Creekmore FM, Lugo RA, Weiland KJ. 2004. Postoperative opiate analgesic requirements for smokers and non smokers. *Ann Pharmacother* 38: 949–953.

80. Koski A, Vuori E, Ojanpera I. 2005. Relation of postmortem blood alcohol and drug concentrations in fetal poisonings involving amitriptyline, propoxyphene and promazine. *Hum Exp Toxicol* 24: 389–396.

81. Song BJ. 1996. Ethanol inducible cytochrome P450 (CYP2E1): biochemistry, molecular biology and clinical relevance-an update. *Alcoholism Clin Exp Res* 20 (Supply 8): 136A–146A.

82. Jimenez-Lopez JM, Cederbaum AI. 2005. CYP2E1 dependent oxidative stress and toxicity: role in ethanol induced liver injury. *Expert Opin Drug Metab Toxicol* 1: 671–685.

83. Weathermon R, Crabb DW. 1999. Alcohol and medication interactions. *Alcohol Res Health* 23: 40–54.

84. Caballeria J, Baraona E, Deulofeu R, Hernandez-Munoz R et al. 1991. Effect of H-32 receptor agonists on gastric alcohol dehydrogenase activity. *Diges Dis Sci* 36: 1673–1679.

85. Fujita K. 2004. Food drug interactions via human cytochrome P450 3A (CYP3A). *Drug Metabol Drug Interact* 20: 195–217.

86. Evans AM. 2000. Influence of dietary components on the gastrointestinal metabolism and transport of drugs. *Ther Drug Monit* 22: 131–136.

87. Walter-Sack I, Klotz U. 1996. Influence of diet and nutritional status on drug metabolism. *Clin Pharmacokinet* 31: 47–64.

88. Fegan TC, Walle T, Oexmann MJ, Walle UK et al. 1987. Increased clearance of propranolol and theophylline by high-protein compared with high carbohydrate diet. *Clin Pharmacol Ther* 41: 402–406.

89. Bailey DG, Spence JD, Munoz C, Arnold JM. 1991. Interaction of citrus juices with felodipine and nifedipine. *Lancet* 337: 268–269.

90. Saito M, Hirata-Koizumi M, Matsumoto M, Urano T, Hasegawa R. 2005. Undesirable effects of citrus juice on the pharmacokinetics of drugs: focus on recent studies. *Drug Saf* 28: 677–694.

91. Uno T, Ohkubo T, Sugawara K, Higashiyama A et al. 2000. Effects of grapefruit juice on the stereoselective disposition of nicardipine in humans: evidence for dominant presystematic elimination at the gut site. *Eur J Clin Pharmacol* 56: 643–649.

92. Dahan A, Altman H. 2004. Food-drug interaction: grapefruit juice augments drug bioavailability-mechanism, extent and relevance. *Eur J Clin Nutr* 58: 1–9.

93. Tian R, Koyabu N, Takanaga H, Matsuo H et al. 2002. Effects of grapefruit juice and orange juice on the intestinal efflux of P-glycoprotein substrates. *Pharm Res* 19: 802–809.

94. Paine MF, Widmer WW, Hart HL, Pusek SN. 2006. A furanocoumarin-free grapefruit juice establishes furanocoumarins as the mediators of the grapefruit juice-felodipine interaction. *Am J Clin Nutr* 83: 1097–1105.

95. Dresser GK, Kim RB, Bailey DG. 2005. Effect of grapefruit juice volume on the reduction of fexofenadine bioavailability: possible role of anion transporting polypeptides. *Clin Pharmacol Ther* 77: 170–177.

96. Berezkin VG Ed.1990. *Chromatographic Absorption Analysis: selected works of M.S. Tswett.* Ellis Horwood, New York.

97. Borgstrom B. 1952. Investigation on lipid separation methods. Separation of phospholipids from natural fat and fatty acids. *Acta Physiol Scand* 25: 101–110.

98. Izmailov NA, Shraiber MS. 1938. The application of analysis by drop-chromatography to pharmacy. *Farmazia* 3: 1–7 [in Russian]. (For English translation, *see* N Pelick, HR Bollinger, and HK Mangold 1966. In JC Giddings and RA Keller eds., *Advances in Chromatography.* Vol. 3. Mercel Dekker, New York, 85–118.)

99. Plesch J. 1906. About the diazobenzol reaction of bilirubin. *Zentrablatt fur Innere Medizin* 27: 1–3 [in German]. (For English translation *see* ED Morgan and ID Wilson. 2004. An early description of paper chromatography. *Chromatgraphia* 60: 135–136.)

100. Consden R, Gordon AH, Martin AJP. 1944. Qualitative analysis of proteins: a partition chromatographic method using paper. *Biochem J* 38: 224–232.

101. Martin AJP, Synge RLM. 1941. A new form of chromatogram employing two liquid phases. 1. A theory of chromatography, 2. Application to the micro-determination of the higher monoamino-acids in proteins. *Biochem J* 35: 1358–1368.

102. James AT, Martin AJP. 1952. Gas-liquid partition chromatography: the separation and micro-estimation of volatile fatty acids from formic acid to dodecanoic acid. *Biochem J* 50: 679–690.

103. Knox JH. 1966. Evidence for turbulence and coupling in chromatographic columns. *Anal Chem* 38: 253–261.

104. Horvath CG, Lipsky SR. 1966. Use of liquid ion exchange chromatography for the separation of organic compounds. *Nature* 211: 748–749.
105. Horvath CG, Preiss BA, Lipsky SR. 1967. Fast liquid chromatography: an investigation of operating parameters and the separation of nucleotides on pellicular ion exchangers. *Anal Chem* 39: 1422–1428.
106. Roger JC, Rodgers G, Soo A. 1973. Simultaneous determination of carbamazepine (Tegretol) and other anticonvulsants in human plasma by gas-liquid chromatography. *Clin Chem* 19: 590–592.
107. Kuperberg HJ. 1970. Quantitative estimation of diphenylhydantoin, primidone and Phenobarbital in plasma by gas liquid chromatography. *Clin Chim Acta* 29: 282–288.
108. Davis HL, Falk KJ, Bailey DG. 1975. Improved method for the simultaneous determinations of Phenobarbital, primidone and diphenylhydantoin in patients' serum by gas liquid chromatography. *J Chromatogr* 9: 61–66.
109. Speed DJ, Dickinson SJ, Cairns ER, Kim ND. 2000. Analysis of six anticonvulsant drugs using solid phase extraction deuterated internal standards and gas chromatography-mass spectrometry. *J Anal Toxicol* 24: 685–690.
110. Pocci R, Dixit V, Dixit VM. 1992. Solid phase extraction and GC/MS confirmation of barbiturates from human urine. *J Anal Toxicol* 16: 45–47.
111. Kerbusch T, Jeuken MJ, Derraz J, van Putten JW et al. 2000. Determination of ifosfamide, 2 and 3-dechloroethylifosfamide using gas chromatography with nitrogen-phosphorus or mass spectrometry detection. *Ther Drug Monit* 22: 613–620.
112. Minnigh MB, Alvin JD, Zemaitis MA. 1994. Determination of plasma mexiletine levels with gas chromatography-mass spectrometry and selected ion monitoring. *J Chromatogr B Biomed Appl* 662: 118–122.
113. Dasgupta A, Appenzeller P, Moore J. 1998. Gas chromatography-electron ionization mass spectrometric analysis of serum mexiletine concentration after derivatization with 2,2,2-trochloroethyl chloroformate: a novel derivative. *Ther Drug Monit* 20: 313–318.
114. Dasgupta A, Yousef O. 1998. Gas chromatographic-mass spectrometric determination of serum mexiletine concentration after derivatization with perfluorooctanoyl chloride, a new derivative. *J Chromatogr B Biomed Sci Appl* 705: 282–288.
115. Subramanian M, Birnbaum AK, Remmel RP. 2008. High speed simultaneous determination of nine antiepileptic drugs using liquid chromatography-mass spectrometry. *Ther Drug Monit* 30: 347–356.
116. Verbesselt R, Tjandramaga TB, de Schepper PJ. 1991. High performance liquid chromatographic determination of 12 antiarrhythmic drugs in plasma using solid phase extraction. *Ther Drug Monit* 13: 157–165.
117. Dasgupta A, Rosenzweig IB, Turgeon J, Raisys VA. 1990. Encainide and metabolites analysis in serum or plasma using a reversed- phase high performance liquid chromatographic technique. *J Chromatogr* 526: 260–265.
118. Kamberi M, Tsutsumi K, Kotegawa T, Nakamura K et al. 1998. Determination of ciprofloxacin in plasma and urine by HPLC with ultraviolet detection. *Clin Chem* 44: 1251–1255.

2 Preanalytical Variables and Therapeutic Drug Monitoring

Valerie Bush
Bassett Healthcare

CONTENTS

2.1 INTRODUCTION

The quality of specimen results is dependent on the quality of the sample analyzed [1]. The preanalytical phase consists of all steps from preparing the patient to specimen analysis. Preanalytical errors can occur in vivo or in vitro. Many of these artifacts can alter test results by producing changes that do not reflect the patient's physiological condition. The in vivo factors are more difficult for the laboratory to control, but some can be managed by enforcing specimen collection and handling requirements. Other preanalytical patient factors include: patient identification, time of dose versus collection, hemolysis/lipemia, drug interactions and degree of protein binding. The most common preanalytical variables associated with therapeutic drug monitoring occur after the blood is collected and relate to the drug's stability in blood collection tubes. In vitro drug stability is dependent upon several factors including the primary tube used, the fill volume in the tube, along with the time and temperature of storage. Another important preanalytical variable is the collection of hydrophobic antibiotics through intravenous lines. This chapter will focus on preanalytical variables during collection and processing and their impact on therapeutic drug values.

2.2 IN VIVO PREANALYTICAL FACTORS

Several physiological factors can affect blood levels of therapeutic drugs; many of which are influenced by bioavailability, volume of distribution, and clearance. Comprehensive reviews of these physiological fundamentals can be found elsewhere [2]. Common patient associated preanalytical factors include: patient compliance, age, diet, body weight changes, exercise, time of dose vs. time of collection, hemolysis or lipemia, drug interactions, and degree of protein binding. Patient compliance in geriatrics with degenerative mental capacity can be challenging for health care providers to manage. These patients frequently forget if they have taken their medication and may take extra doses or skip a dose. Some therapies, e.g., digoxin, are lifelong treatments. As an individual ages and body habitus changes drug dosages should be adjusted accordingly to avoid under or over-dosing the patient. Routine monitoring of these patients is important to maintaining therapeutic levels.

Recommended times of draw depend on the half-life of the drug of interest, but steady-state trough levels are customarily used. Approximately five half-lives are necessary before steady state (equilibrium) is reached in serum values. Trough levels should be obtained shortly before the next dose. Other sampling schedules may be desired depending on the properties of the drug and patient needs. For example, measurements of peak and trough concentrations of aminoglycosides and sulfonamides are common in early dosing regimens to achieve proper therapeutic levels. The time and date of the last dose should be noted, along with the time of collection, to aid in interpretation. Inaccurate specimen labeling is a common cause of patient identification error [3]. The Clinical Laboratory Standards Institute provides guidelines for specimen collection for therapeutic drug monitoring [4].

In addition, drug–drug interactions can influence the concentration of some drugs by interfering with the volume of distribution and metabolism. It is easier to determine if a coadministered drug may be responsible for discordant results than it is to identify an interfering substance from herbal medicines (e.g., ginseng, chan su, or dan shen) [5,6]. The use of traditional herbal medicines by non-traditional cultures has increased as populations immigrate into Western society. Herbal medicines compete in metabolic pathways, protein binding, and may interfere with the analytical measurement of traditional therapeutic drugs. Digibind is a therapeutic antibody consisting of the Fab fragment of digoxin antibody administered to neutralize digitalis toxicity. At high concentrations, Digibind causes false positive interference in many digoxin immunoassays. A blocking agent can be used to reduce interferences from Digibind [7]. Additionally, imaging agents or radiographic contrast agents have also been reported to interfere with fluorescence polarization immunoassays (FPIAs) for vancomycin [8]. A multidisciplinary approach between the laboratory, pharmacy, nursing and providers can help assure drug concentrations at specified collection times after dosing are meaningful.

The binding of some therapeutic drugs to protein has been shown to be pH dependent [9,10]. Some have shown that the free fraction of phenytoin, valproic acid, and phenobarbital decreased as pH decreased from 8.4 to 7.0, while the free fractions of theophylline and carbamazepine are elevated [10]. Acidic drugs (pKa <7.0) are nearly completely ionized at physiological pH as are basic drugs at pKa >8.4 [10]. A decrease in blood pH, as may be seen between serum and plasma, has affected the free fractions of these drugs.

The effect of hemolysis or lipemia on drug analyses is similar to those of other analytes where interferences with the detection method may be observed. Noticeable hemolysis and hyperlipidemia may interfere with antibody–antigen reactions of immunoassays and with some signal detection methods [11]. Depending on the instrument platform used, hemolysis, bilirubin and lipemia can demonstrate varying effects [12]. Ryder showed that fewer erroneous results from hemolyzed or lipemic specimens would be expected using EMIT (enzyme multiplied immunoassay technique, Syva, San Jose, CA) and FPIA (fluorescence polarization immunoassay, Abbott Laboratories, Abbott Park, IL) assays [12]. Most kit manufacturers provide the level of interfering substances for each assay in the package insert. The laboratory can then appropriately set hemolysis or lipemia indexes on the instrument or compare the specimen to visual charts for specimen acceptance or rejection.

2.2.1 Site of Collection

The site of specimen collection can also influence drug levels. It has been standard practice that blood should not be collected from the same arm in which drugs or other fluids are infused [4]. Doing so can lead to erroneous results by contamination from the infusion fluid. For example, cyclosporine is a hydrophobic, lipophilic drug. When cyclosporine is administered intravenously (IV), it tends to bind to the hydrophobic surface of some intravenous catheter tubing. When blood is collected from the indwelling line, cyclosporine concentrations are significantly higher than if collected by direct venipuncture [13]. Conversely, Ptachcinski et al. showed the stability of the oral dose form of cyclosporine in plastic syringes [14]. The plastic material used for flexible IV tubing (e.g., polyurethane, polyethylene, polyvinyl, Teflon®, or Vialon®) and rigid syringes (e.g., polypropylene polymer) differ, but may be contributing to the differences noted by these two studies. More study is warranted to understand the mechanisms of cyclosporine recovery from flexible IV tubing and plastic syringes. Some variables to consider are the type of plastic or additives used in the manufacture of the device and the exposed surface area.

A few studies have compared capillary and venous collections and the number of analytes tested [15,16], but little is known about whether drug levels by capillary collection differ from those by venipuncture. In some patient populations (e.g., pediatric, geriatrics, oncology), a capillary specimen is preferred because blood volume loss by venipuncture can be limited. However, drug concentrations measured in capillary blood may not necessarily correlate with venous measurements. The major concerns with skin puncture collections are contamination from interstitial fluid, intercellular fluid, hemolysis, and residual contaminates from the surface of the skin. Theoretically, for drugs with a high volume of distribution and a poor puncture necessitating "milking" with the finger that could alter the drug values by the presence of tissue fluid in the blood collected. Drugs that are highly protein-bound have low volumes of distribution because only a small portion of the drug is free and available to diffuse into extravascular spaces. To verify this concept we compared collection methods (fingerstick vs. venipuncture) for patients taking phenytoin (90–95% protein-bound) and salicylate (~50% protein-bound). We measured serum total phenytoin by EMIT and salicylate by colorimetric technique and found essentially no difference in collection methods for either drug (Bush et al., unpublished data). Capillary drug concentrations compared with venous values deserves further study, as only two drugs were examined and our sample size was small.

Some investigators have examined capillary drug values of the immunosuppressants cyclosporine and methotrexate. Whole blood measurements of the highly erythrocyte-bound cyclosporine were determined from ethylenediaminetetraacetic acid (EDTA) anticoagulated blood. Merton et al. as well as Pettersen et al. compared fingerstick, ear prick, and venipuncture cyclosporine values from organ transplant patients and showed a high degree of correlation among the different blood collection techniques [17,18]. These investigators also suggested that fingerstick collections were the preferred method to reduce blood loss and preserve venous integrity in this patient population. Ritzmo et al. examined capillary and venous methotrexate levels from nine cancer pediatric cancer patients during hospital stays [19]. Venous blood was obtained from a central venous catheter. The authors also showed a high correlation ($r^2 = 0.98$) between fingerstick and venous draws where the venous to capillary plasma concentration ratio was 1.00 for 85% of the data independent of drug concentration. These studies have shown very little differences between capillary collections and venous collections for whole blood measurements of the measurement of immunosuppressants. Laboratories should verify the use of collection tubes and methods as recommended by national and state accrediting agencies.

2.3 FACTORS AFFECTING PROTEIN BINDING

A brief overview of drug binding with plasma proteins is provided herein as it relates to preanalytical error. For more detailed review please see References 20 and 21. It is well known that drug binding to plasma proteins varies from near zero to over 90% depending upon the drug. The remaining free form is available to pass through cell membranes. Some drugs are capable of binding to blood cells, but a majority of drugs are bound to plasma proteins. The fraction of free versus bound drug in plasma is influenced by endogenous and exogenous compounds that compete with the drug for binding to albumin or other proteins. When the concentration of these proteins is altered through a pathological or physiological condition, alterations in the total to free drug are observed [23]. Because the free fraction is pharmacologically active, measurement of the free fraction is usually desirable. Several factors have been shown to influence protein binding or displacement of therapeutic drugs from proteins. The in vivo variables include: inflammatory conditions, malignancies, stress, pregnancy, liver disease, malnutrition, and competition of highly bound drugs with weaker binding drugs. In vitro factors include: the presence of drug-displacement agents present in blood collection tubes, heparin, and changes in pH. Shifts in plasma pH can change the equilibrium of free and bound drug in the specimen. In patients where the total drug level is within the therapeutic range, but the patient presents with indications of either toxic or nontherapeutic drug concentrations, altered protein binding may be responsible. For any drug with a pKa that is significantly different from the pH of plasma (e.g., phenytoin), measurement of free drug levels should be considered. For drugs that have a pKa similar to plasma pH (e.g., phenobarbital), total drug measurements are adequate to assess therapeutic levels.

Protein binding of some basic drugs was shown to be inhibited when blood was collected into Vacutainer® tubes in the late 1970s. Cotham and Shand demonstrated spuriously low plasma propranolol concentrations from the redistribution of propranolol between plasma and red blood cells when blood was collected in a specific brand of blood collection tubes [22]. They also found that this effect was similar to blood collected through indwelling polyvinyl catheters [22]. Since Tygon®, Teflon® or polyethylene catheters did not exhibit the same effect, the low plasma drug levels was attributed to a drug-displacing agent in the Vacutainer® tube. This drug-displacing agent was linked to tris (2-butoxyethyl) phosphate (TBEP) present in the rubber stoppers of the Vacutainer® tubes [24]. The displacement interaction was shown to have occurred between TBEP and one or more of the binding proteins (e.g., α1-acid glycoprotein, lipoproteins and albumin). The displacement effect of TBEP with albumin was less likely due to the low concentration of TBEP relative to plasma albumin [25], but the authors noted considerable variability among tubes and between individuals. Drug-displacement appeared to only affect highly bound basic drugs (e.g., tricyclic antidepressants). Lidocaine values were also influenced by stopper material yielding spuriously low concentrations in serum or plasma [26]. By 1983, the manufacturer of Vacutainer® tubes and catheters had removed the drug-displacing agent so this is rarely seen today. However, TBEP is a common ingredient in rubber stoppers that may be used in other products in the preanalytical, analytical or post-analytical steps. Shah et al. has outlined a procedure for testing possible interference from TBEP if this is suspected [27].

Another reported "contaminant" from blood collection tubes, IV lines and IV bags are the phthalate plasticizers, i.e., diethylphthalate or di(2-ethylhexyl) phthalate (DEHP), that act as a digoxin-like immunoreactive substance and lead to falsely elevated digoxin concentration [28,29]. Information of these compounds in specific products may be obtained from the manufacturer.

Anticoagulants, particularly heparin, have also been shown to affect protein binding of drugs. Heparin does not cause changes in pH, as do other anticoagulants, and would not displace protein bound drugs via this mechanism. Instead, heparin increases the concentration of free fatty acids that, in turn, affects binding of acidic drugs to albumin and basic drugs to α1-acid glycoprotein thus influencing the measurement of the free drug [30,31]. The in vivo heparin effects on free fatty acids and disopyramide have been reported in hemodialysis patients. Horiuchi et al. found an increase in the free fraction of disopyramide on dialysis days that was associated with elevated free fatty acid levels in the plasma [32]. Others have shown an approximate 24% increase in unbound quinidine in patients during cardiac catheterization due to the presence of heparin [33].

Not only can heparin interfere with protein binding preanalytically, but can also interfere analytically if present in the specimen at high enough concentrations. This interference can be method dependent as demonstrated with aminoglycoside assays. O'Connell et al. examined the accuracy of aminoglycoside determinations by three different immunoassays (EMIT, radio immunoassay and FPIA) in the presence of heparin [34]. The authors showed the interference was caused by heparin binding to detection enzymes in homogeneous enzyme immunoassays (EIA) while no effect was shown with the RIA or FPIA methods. Further, the in vitro interference appeared to be dose dependent from 2 to 1000 USP, depending on the drug assayed. Heparin interferences could occur at concentrations found in blood collection tubes or blood gas syringes, particularly if the tubes are under-filled. Blood collection tubes typically contain 10–30 IU/ml of liquid or dry heparin, while calcium-balanced blood gas syringes contain 40–60 IU/ml dry heparin. Determining the acceptability of blood collection products and enforcing specimen acceptance policies within a laboratory system will minimize errors due to heparin or blood collection tubes.

Several factors have been shown to influence the displacement of therapeutic drugs from proteins thereby increasing the free fraction of drugs. The type of displacement agent will affect basic drugs differently from acidic drugs.

2.3.1 SERUM VERSUS PLASMA

Today all plastic, evacuated tubes are composed of polyethylene teraphthalate (PET) and contain no additive (as a "discard" or specialty tube), an anticoagulant, or clotting agent. Incorrect filling of the collection tube will cause alterations in the blood to additive ratio. Blood to additive ratios are maintained by allowing the tube to fill naturally to its stated draw volume. Instrument sampling errors can occur if a collection tube is inadequately filled or if clotting of the specimen is incomplete and fibrin is aspirated into the sample probe. These issues can be avoided by following the manufacturer's recommendations for collection and clotting. Accepted laboratory practice for serum is to allow the specimen to clot prior to centrifugation to avoid fibrin contamination. Instrument sampling error can be avoided by ensuring the instrument probes are set appropriately or knowing the maximum depth a liquid-level sensing probe will travel.

Serum or plasma concentrations of analytes and therapeutic drugs are frequently used interchangeably but they are not necessarily synonymous. Morovat et al. showed significant biases (defined as >5%) in plasma specimens for several endocrine immunoassays on determined by using Centaur® instrument [35]. Many reagent manufacturers claim serum or plasma can be used for analysis of many therapeutic drugs, although some recommend only serum. The presence of heparin is not usually a factor with highly automated methods that measure total drug levels. For example, the Vitros®, Dimension®, and Centaur® suggest either serum or plasma for their drug assays, except digoxin on the Centaur® is restricted to serum (from respective package inserts). While serum or plasma can be used, plasma values may be 10% higher than serum values by other methods. Amiodarone and desethylamiodarone by high performance liquid chromatography (HPLC) were found to be approximately 11 and 9% higher in serum, respectively [36]. This may necessitate different therapeutic ranges depending upon the sample type and the drug.

Laboratory professionals should be cognizant of the specimen type recommended and validated for each drug assay on a particular platform. Plasma has the advantage of a faster turn-around-time, as the blood clotting is not necessary. Serum tends to be a cleaner specimen without potential interferences from particulates when sufficiently clotted or from anticoagulants. However, for many drugs, values are comparable between plasma and serum [37].

Most drug measurements are performed on serum samples. This is due to four reasons: (1) the drug is in equilibrium with serum proteins and is uniformly distributed in the serum portion of blood, (2) instrument manufacturer's have validated their methods using serum, (3) heparin has been shown to interfere with some therapeutic drug measurements, and (4) plasma is not a cell-free matrix as is serum. Drugs are present in the serum as free drug or bound to proteins. While some drugs are capable of binding to blood cells, the prominent and clinically significant binding occurs with plasma proteins. Once drugs are bound to plasma proteins, they form stable complexes [20,38]. At the time of blood collection into a closed blood collection tube, the drug concentration in the blood is constant and the ratio of free to protein-bound drug does not change. Heparin is, frequently, the preferred anticoagulant because it does not cause shifts in electrolytes and water between plasma and cells [39]. Heparin (in vitro) does not cause large changes in pH, as do other anticoagulants, and would not initiate changes in free versus protein-bound drug via this mechanism. For example, no differences in the total or free valproic acid concentrations between samples collected in serum or heparinized plasma have been found [40]. However, variations in protein binding in the presence of heparin have been shown for other drugs (e.g., carbamazepine, theophylline, and phenobarbital) [41]. This is not a pH effect, but a displacement effect from the release of free fatty acids due to heparin induced lipolysis. Heparin interferences with aminoglycoside assays are method dependent and documented [34,42]. The interference is caused by heparin binding to detection enzymes in homogenous EIA and radioenzymatic assays [42]. The interference appears to be dose dependent, but may occur at concentrations in blood collection tubes, particularly if the tubes are under filled, with some assays [34,43]. If anticoagulated blood for aminoglycoside testing is desired, potassium oxalate can be used [44]. Tricyclic antidepressant parent and metabolite concentrations in serum and heparinized plasma are comparable [45,46].

Measurement of lithium concentrations from blood collected in lithium heparin tubes will yield falsely elevated results that appear toxic. Wills et al. examined blood collected into lithium heparin tubes from individuals not taking lithium [47]. Baseline lithium levels were <0.2 mmol/L. Depending upon the volume of blood collected into the green top tubes (full draw, 2 ml or 1 ml), the lithium values ranged from 1.0 to 4.2 mmol/l.

Nyberg and Mårtensson conducted an extensive study to test the effects of ten types of blood collection tubes, including two plasma separator tubes, for the stability of tricyclic antidepressants: amitriptyline, imipramine, clomipramine and their monodemethylated metabolites [48]. The authors found that EDTA-containing (lavender top) tubes provided the most stable plasma and red top tubes the most stable serum samples due to specimen quality. They also showed that freshly sampled blood from heparin containing (green top) tubes could be stored at room temperature for 24 hours without significant losses. Freeze-thaw cycles at −20°C did not influence serum or plasma concentrations.

For cyclosporine, EDTA is preferred over heparin as the anticoagulant of choice. The stability of cyclosporine in EDTA has been demonstrated. The differences in cyclosporine concentrations collected in glass (K_3EDTA) and plastic (K_2EDTA) tubes is <10% [49]. The small differences observed could be attributed to dilution effects by the liquid K_3EDTA compared to the dry K_2EDTA.

It is important for laboratories to enforce specimen collection and rejection policies to avoid misinterpretation of results due to a preanalytical error.

2.3.2 Glass versus Plastic Collection Tubes

Correlation studies between glass and plastic blood collection tubes for common analytes and some hormones and tumor markers have been documented [50,51]. In addition, many laboratory professionals have performed their own evaluations of plastic tubes to document analyte compatibility before converting, but have not always published their findings. Dasgupta et al. examined the stability of 13 therapeutic drugs stored in plastic tubes compared to glass tubes using quality control material [52]. The authors found no significant reduction in concentrations of caffeine, primidone, procainamide, NAPA, acetaminophen, salicylate, amikacin, valproic acid, methotrexate, or cyclosporine. When comparing volume of serum in the tube, they observed significant reductions in concentration of phenytoin, phenobarbital, carbamazepine, quinidine and lidocaine after storage of 500 μl of serum versus 1 ml in both glass and plastic gel tubes. The poor recovery of these drugs was attributed to the gel in the tubes, rather than the tube material.

Faynor and Robinson examined the suitability of plastic blood collection tubes for cyclosporine measurement [49]. Specimens from renal transplant patients were collected into glass and plastic BD Vacutainer® EDTA tubes. Tubes were stored at room temperature and 4°C after collection and between testing intervals of 0, 1, 4 and 7 days. The drug levels in the plastic tubes were slightly higher than those from the glass tubes at both storage temperatures and did not appear to be time dependent. All of the differences for individual pairs of samples were within 10%. The authors concluded that cyclosporine levels are stable in plastic tubes over seven days at room temperature or refrigerated. Similarly, Ptachcinski et al showed stability of oral dosing solutions of cyclosporine stored in plastic syringes [14].

Boeynaems et al. compared Terumo's Venoject® glass tubes with Venosafe® PET tubes with clot activator and heparin for several therapeutic drugs at 2 and 24 hours post collection [53]. Blood was spiked with the parent drug to low, mid and high therapeutic levels. The investigators found no consistent, significant differences among the tube types for the panel of drugs tested. These data agree with other comparisons between Venoject® II and BD Vacutainer® plastic tubes [54].

The use of plastic collection tubes, manufactured from PET, has minimal impact on therapeutic drugs. These tubes can be used for therapeutic drug monitoring. However, transferring specimens to a secondary tube for analysis or transport to a reference laboratory is common practice. Secondary tubes are typically polypropylene or polystyrene. Serum proteins interact with various plastics differently due to differences in surface charges and protein or cellular binding characteristics [55]. Very little has been published on the time and temperature stability of therapeutic drugs when stored in secondary tubes, although these tubes are thought to be inert.

2.3.3 Serum Separator Collection Tubes

The use of serum separator tubes in clinical laboratories is common due to the capability of storing serum over time in the primary collection tube. If analysis of the serum is not performed shortly after processing, the laboratory may store the specimen under a variety of conditions. Serum separator tubes provide a closed system that allows for collection, transport, processing, sampling, and storage of specimens. Different barrier materials are available among tube manufacturers, but all are thixotropic materials that facilitate separation of serum or plasma from the cells and prevent hemolysis on prolonged storage. The base material in the gel is currently, either acrylic, silicone or a polyester polymer. The stability of various serum components in gel tubes has been studied and well documented. Errors in drug recovery from specimens collected in gel barrier tubes were first discovered in the early 1980s [56,57]. Although improvements have been made to the tubes from these early studies, the gel barrier materials have remained relatively unchanged.

An important limitation of gel barrier tubes is the absorption of specific drugs and some steroid hormones into the gel [48,58,59]. The stability, or instability, of several drugs in gel tubes has been widely studied where the instability of drugs in gel serum separator tubes is defined as a loss of recovery of the drug of interest. This occurs when a drug is absorbed into the gel barrier. The following five factors influence drug stability in gel tubes:

1. The chemical nature of the drug and the gel influence which drugs are absorbed by the gel. While the exact mechanism of this interaction is not well understood, in simple terms, the drugs will associate with the phase that they are most soluble. Thus, if the gel is hydrophobic in nature, then hydrophobic drugs will tend to be absorbed and hydrophilic drugs remain in the aqueous fraction. Those drugs that are susceptible to absorption (instability) are specific and few compared to all drugs that are monitored therapeutically [60–65].

2. Sample volume on the barrier, where greater relative absorption is observed with lower sample volumes [61,62,66]. When blood is collected into a gel tube, the total volume of blood is exposed to a constant surface area of gel. This volume to surface area ratio of whole blood to gel is approximately twice that of the serum on the gel. Drug absorption in whole blood is typically <1% of the total concentration as shown by comparing non-gel tube with gel tube drug levels at initial time after processing. Additionally, the surface area of the gel centrifuged in a fixed angle centrifuge is greater than that when centrifuged in swing bucket centrifuge. Higher gel surface area can lead to greater drug absorption into the gel.

3. The length of time the serum is in contact with the gel also influences drug stability for those drugs susceptible to absorption [61,62,65,66,68,69]. The longer the serum remains in contact with the gel, more drug is absorbed, until an equilibrium is reached. For those drugs susceptible to absorption, equilibrium is reached at approximately 24 hours.

4. The temperature of storage also influences drug stability. The rate of absorption increases with increasing temperatures, until equilibrium is achieved [70]. For example, the average losses in phenytoin were approximately 18% at 25°C and 25% at 32°C.
5. The test method(s) used is the last factor that may influence drug recovery in gel tubes. Highly sensitive assays will detect small differences in concentration than less sensitive assays [60,71–73]. As more drugs are developed and growth in more sensitive detection methods continues, this area may have greater importance in the future.

Table 2.1 summarizes the current literature of drug stability in gel tubes.

Some investigators have compared the stability of various drugs among different types of barrier tubes. Landt et al. showed when blood was processed and analyzed shortly after collection, none of the separator tubes had any effect on seven drugs studied (theophylline, digoxin, phenytoin, pheno-barbital, gentamicin, and ethanol) [74]. The authors also examined the impact under stressed conditions by partially filling the various barrier tubes on these seven drugs. Only phenytoin, at 1 ml fill volume in a 7-ml polyester separator tube, showed modestly lower recovery (92%). Interestingly, the authors also included cyclosporine because of its known avidity to polymeric materials. It is not surprising that they found no differences in recovery of cyclosporine when using corresponding heparinized versions of each tube type. The majority of the drug itself is protected from interacting with the barrier as most is bound intracellularly and measurements are performed on whole blood.

The most extensive study on suitability of gel barrier tubes for therapeutic drug monitoring was published by Karppi et al [63]. The authors studied the stability of 41 drugs, including: tricyclic antidepressants, benzodiazepines, antiepileptic, asthma drugs, aminoglycosides, other antibiotics and cardioactive drugs, when specimens were stored in three different gel tubes (BD SST™ tubes, Terumo Autosep and Sarstedt Microvette® gel tubes). After 24 hour storage time, absorbed drugs ranged 5–20% of the concentration at initial time for all analyzed drugs. The authors concluded that the studied gel tubes were satisfactory for blood collection for antidepressant drug measurements if separation step is performed within 3 hours after blood clotting.

The outcome of published studies on drug stability in gel tubes has varied significantly depending on the sample type used in the evaluation. Greater differences in stability are noted in studies using spiked serum or blood compared to patient serum or blood (Table 2.1). The use of spiked samples does not adequately represent true physiologic forms of the drug and should be avoided. This is likely due to the presence of free parent drug rather than physiologic protein-bound drug and its metabolites.

The data presented support the stability of hydrophilic drugs in gel tubes for several days when stored at 4°C. Ambient temperature storage may also be used for many hydrophilic drugs. Some differences may be observed with digoxin due to the magnitude of concentration measured. Concentrations of some hydrophobic drugs can be underestimated when specimens are stored on the gel over time. The rate of absorption by hydrophobic drugs is temperature and volume dependent. Laboratory policies should allow accurate testing of hydrophobic drugs through monitoring draw volume, time, and temperature of storage in gel tubes.

2.4 SAMPLE PREPARATION STEPS

Chromatographic techniques for drug analysis usually require sample preparation (liquid or solid phase extraction(s) and derivatization) in order to isolate the drug and its metabolites from a complex biological matrix. Sample preparation depends upon the number of compounds in the serum, their concentration, the presence of interfering substances, and the column used for separation. Ineffectual separation can occur from interactions of sample impurities with the stationary phase, increasing the noise level at the detector, interaction of the drug of interest with other matrix components and poor resolution. To minimize these effects, extraction step(s) are employed to isolate the drug(s) of interest from the specimen matrix. Purification of the sample with high yield of the drug

TABLE 2.1
Summary of Drug Stability in Gel Tubes

Drug Class	Drugs Tested	Literature Reference Number				Results
		Direct Draw	Spiked Blood	Spiked Serum	Patient Serum	
Cardioactive	Quinidine (hydrophobic)	50		69	62,67,68	Stable
	Procainamide/NAPA (hydrophilic)			61,69	62	Unstable*
				61		Stable
	Digoxin (hydrophilic)	63,75	60	61,69	67,68	Stable
			74			
Antiepileptic	Lidocaine (hydrophobic)			61,69	62	Unstable*
	Total Phenytoin (hydrophobic)	50	60,63,66,73,74		67,68	Stable
	Free Phenytoin (hydrophobic)	72,75	60,70	69	61,62	Unstable*
		72				Unstable*
	Phenobarbital (hydrophobic)	50,75	60,63	69	62,67,68	Stable
		75		61		Unstable*
	Pentobarbital (hydrophobic)			69		Stable
	Carbamazepine (hydrophobic)	50,75	73	69	67,68	Stable
		75,74		61	62	Unstable*
	Primidone (hydrophobic)	50		61,69		Stable
	Ethosuximide (hydrophilic)			61		Stable
	Valproic acid (hydrophilic)	63,75		61,69	67	Stable
Antidepressant	Amitriptyline/Nortriptyline or Imipramine/Desipramine (hydrophobic)	48,64,76	63		58,67	Unstable*
	Clomipramine/Desmethlclomipramine (hydrophobic)		63			
	Doxepin/Nordoxepin (hydrophobic)		63			Stable
	Lithium (hydrophilic)	75			68	Stable

(*Continued*)

TABLE 2.1 (Continued)

Drug Class	Drugs Tested	Literature Reference Number				Results
		Direct Draw	Spiked Blood	Spiked Serum	Patient Serum	
Antibiotics	Amikacin (hydrophilic)			61,69	67,68	Stable
	Gentamicin (hydrophilic)		60,74	69	67,68	Stable
	Tobramycin (hydrophilic)	63	60	61,69	67,68	Stable
	Vancomycin (hydrophilic)	63			67	Stable
	Chloramphenicol (hydrophilic)			69		Stable
	Netilmicin (hydrophilic)	63				Stable
Bronchodilator	Theophylline (hydrophilic)	63,66,75	60,74	61,69	62,67,68	Stable
	Caffeine (hydrophilic)			61		Stable
Analgesic	Acetaminophen (hydrophilic)			61	67	Stable
	Salicylate (hydrophilic)			61	62,67	Stable
Antineoplastic	Methotrexate (hydrophilic)			61,69		Stable
Benzodiazepine	Alprazolam/Clonazepam/ Nitrazepam (hydrophobic)		63			Unstable*
	Diazepam/Nordiazepam/Oxazepam (hydrophobic)		63			Stable

* Instability under stressed conditions due to volume and/or time effects.

of interest is the goal in sample preparation. By converting the drugs to derivatives, more efficient separation of the components may be achieved. Selecting the proper liquid or solid extraction phase, internal standard and derivatization agents should enhance the accuracy and resolution of the drugs of interest. The internal standard should behave chemically similar to the drug of interest so that it reflects losses in sample preparation and inconsistencies in injection volume, as well as chromatographic behavior. A more thorough discussion of sample preparation for specific drugs can be found elsewhere [77].

2.5 CONCLUSIONS

The quality of test results is dependent on the quality of the specimen analyzed. Several artifacts were discussed that could alter test results by producing changes that do not reflect the patient's physiological condition. There are many preanalytical variables that can influence test results. In vitro study designs vary and may not always represent true practice. Caution should be used in interpreting the outcome of such studies. The materials used in devices for collection, processing and storage may influence plasma or serum drug concentrations. Thorough medical device evaluations, premarket, should help minimize many of the preanalytical errors described herein. Understanding the limitations of blood collection tubes and possible mechanisms of interferences allows the laboratory to develop specimen collection and handling policies and procedures to minimize inaccuracies in reporting due to a preanalytical error. By minimizing errors in the preanalytical phase, the laboratory can improve the quality of analytical results.

ACKNOWLEDGMENT

The author expresses appreciation to Sol Green, PhD for his review and comments.

REFERENCES

1. Green S. 2008. Improving the preanalytical process. The focus on specimen quality. *J Med Biochem* 27(3):343–347.
2. Brunton L, Lazo J and Parker K (Eds). 2006. *Goodman and Gilman's The Pharmacological Basis of Therapeutics*. New York: McGraw-Hill.
3. Bonini P, Pleblani M, Ceriotti F and Rubboli F. 2002. Errors in laboratory medicine. *Clin Chem* 48:691–698.
4. Clinical and Laboratory Standards Institute. 2007. *Toxicology and Drug Testing in the Clinical Laboratory*. Wayne, PA: Clinical and Laboratory Standards Institute.
5. Dasgupta A, Wu S, Actor J, Olsen M, Wells A and Datta P. 2003. Effect of Asian and Siberian ginseng on serum digoxin measurement by five digoxin immunoassays. *Amer J Clin Path* 119:298–303.
6. Datta P, Dasgupta A. 2002. Effect of Chinese medicines Chan Su and Danshen in EMIT 2000 and Randox digoxin immunoassays: wide variation in digoxin-like immunoreactivity and magnitude of interference in digoxin measurement by different brands of the same product. *Ther Drug Monit* 24:637–644.
7. Datta P. 1995. A blocker reagent to reduce Digibind interference in a non-pretreatment digoxin assay [abstract]. *Ther Drug Monit* 17:407.
8. Wood FL, Earl JW, Nath C, Coakley JC. 2000. Falsely low vancomycin results using the Abbott TDx. *Ann Clin Biochem* 37:411–413.
9. Albani F, Riva R, Contin M, Baruzzi A. 1984. Valproic acid binding to human serum albumin and human plasma: effects of pH variation and buffer composition in equilibrium dialysis. *Ther Drug Monit* 6:31–33.
10. Ohshima T, Hasegawa T, Johno I, Kitazawa S. 1989. Variations in protein binding of drugs in plasma and serum. *Clin Chem* 35:1722–1725.
11. Wild D (Ed). 1994. *The Immunoassay Handbook*. New York: Stockton Press.
12. Ryder KW, Trundle DS, Bode MA, Cole RE, Moorehead WR, Glick MR. 1991. Effects of hemolysis, icterus and lipemia on automated immunoassays. *Clin Chem* 37:1134–1135.
13. Blifeld C and Ettenger RB. 1987. Measurement of cyclosporine levels in samples obtained from peripheral sites and indwelling lines. *New Eng J Med* 317:509.

14. Ptachcinski RJ, Walker S, Burckart GJ and Venkataramanan R. 1986. Stability and availability of cyclosporine stored in plastic syringes. *Am J Hosp Pharm* 43:692–694.
15. Meites S, Levitt MJ. 1979. Skin puncture and blood collection techniques in infants. *Clin Chem* 25:183–189.
16. Kupke IR, Kather B, Zeugner S. 1981. On the composition of capillary and venous blood serum. *Clin Chim Acta* 112:177–185.
17. Merton G, Jones K, Lee M, Johnston A, Holt DW. 2000. Accuracy of cyclosporine measurements made in capillary blood samples obtained by skin puncture. *Ther Drug Monit* 22(5):594–598.
18. Pettersen MD, Driscoll DJ, Moyer TP, Dearani JA, McGregor CG. 1999. Measurement of blood serum cyclosporine levels using capillary "fingerstick" sampling: a validation study. *Transpl Int* 12:429–432.
19. Ritzmo C, Albertioni F, Cosic K, Soderhall S, Eksborg S. 2007. Therapeutic drug monitoring of methotrexate on the pediatric oncology ward: can blood sampling from central venous accesses substitute for capillary finger punctures? *Ther Drug Monit* 29(4):447–451.
20. Vallner JJ. 1977. Binding of drugs by albumin and plasma proteins. *J Pharma Sci* 66:447–465.
21. Koch-Weser J and Sellers EM. 1976. Binding of drugs to serum albumin. *New Eng J Med* 294:311–316, 526–531.
22. Cotham RH and Shand D. 1975. Spuriously low plasma propranolol concentrations resulting from blood collection methods. *Clin Pharmacol Ther* 18(5 Pt 1):535–8.
23. Pike E, Shuterud B, Kiefulf P, Fremstad S, Abdel SM, Lunde PKM. 1981. Binding and displacement of basic, acidic and neutral drugs in normal and orosomucoid-deficient plasma. *Clin Pharmacokinet* 6:367–374.
24. Misson AW and Dickson SJ. 1974. Contamination of blood samples by plasticizer in evacuated tubes. *Clin Chem* 20:1247.
25. Borga O, Piafsky KM and Nilsen OG. 1977. Plasma protein binding of basic drugs. *Clin Pharmacol Ther* 22(5 Pt 1):539–544.
26. Stargel WW, Roe CR, Routledge PA, Shand DG. 1979. Importance of blood-collection tubes in plasma lidocaine determinations. *Clin Chem* 25(4):617–619.
27. Shah VP, Knapp G, Skelly JP, Cabana BE. 1982. Interference with measurements of certain drugs in plasma by a plasticizer in Vacutainer tubes. *Clin Chem* 28:2327–2328.
28. Malik S, Landicho D, Halverson K, Ahmad S and Kenny M. 1991. Digoxin like immunoreactivity and plasticizers in hemofiltrate of dialysis patients. *Clin Chem* 37:931.
29. Datta P, Hinz V, Klee G. 1996. Comparison of four digoxin immunoassays with respect to interference from digoxin-like immunoreactive factors. *Clin Biochem* 29:541–547.
30. Daniel R, Thomas JB, Alejandro EDR. 1971. Effect of free fatty acids on binding of drugs by bovine serum albumin, by human serum albumin and by rabbit serum. *J Pharmacol Exp Ther* 176:261–272.
31. Horiuchi T, Johno I, Kitazawa S, Goto M, Hata T. 1987. Plasma free fatty acids and protein binding of disopyramide during hemodialysis. *Eur J Clin Pharmacol* 33:327–329.
32. Horiuchi T, Johno I, Kitazawa S, Goto M, Hata T. 1989. Inhibitory effect of free fatty acids on plasma protein binding of disopyramide in haemodialysis patients. *Eur J Clin Pharmacol* 36(2):175–180.
33. Kessler KM, Leech RC and Spann JF. 1979. Blood collection techniques, heparin and quinidine protein binding. *Clin Pharmacol Ther* 25:204–210.
34. O'Connell ME, Heim KL, Halstenson CE, Matzke GR. 1984. Analytical accuracy of determinations of aminoglycoside concentrations by enzyme multiplied immunoassay, fluorescence polarization immunoassay and radioimmunoassay in the presence of heparin. *J Clin Microbiol* 20(6):1080–1082.
35. Morovat A, James TS, Cox SD, Norris SG, Rees MC, Gales MA and Taylor RP. 2006. Comparison of Bayer Advia Centaur® immunoassay results obtained on samples collected in four different Becton Dickinson Vacutainer® tubes. *Ann Clin Biochem* 43:481–487.
36. Siebers RWL, Chen CT, Ferguson FI, Maling TJB. 1988. Effect of blood sample tubes on amiodarone and desethylamiodarone concentrations. *Ther Drug Monit* 10:349–351.
37. Pasciolla P, Ince G, Fay A, Lin F, Narayanan S and Portney AL. 1980. An evaluation of selected enzyme immunoassay procedures using serum and plasma. *Clin Chem* 26:937.
38. Burtis CA and Ashwood ER (Eds). 1999. *Tietz Textbook of Clinical Chemistry.* Philadelphia, PA: Saunders.
39. Henry JB. 1979. *Clinical Diagnosis and Management by Laboratory Methods.* 16th Edition. Philadelphia, PA: Saunders, pp. 150–151.
40. Tarasidis CG, Garnett WR, Kline BJ and Pellock JM. 1986. Influence of tube type, storage time and temperature on the total and free concentration of valproic acid. *Ther Drug Monit* 8:373–376.
41. Godolphin W, Trepanier J and Farrell K. 1983. Serum and plasma for total and free anticonvulsant drug analyses: effects on EMIT assays and ultrafiltration devices. *Ther Drug Monit* 5:319–323.

42. Krogstad DJ, Granich GG, Murray PR, Pfaller MA and Valdes R. 1982. Heparin interferes with the radio-enzymatic and homogenous enzyme immunoassays for aminoglycosides. *Clin Chem* 28:1517–1521.

43. Nilsson L, Maller R, Ansehn S. 1981. Inhibition of aminoglycoside activity in heparin. *Antimicrob Agents Chemother* 20:155–158.

44. Ebert SC, Leroy M and Darcey B. 1989. Comparison of aminoglycoside concentrations measured in plasma versus serum. *Ther Drug Monit* 11:44–46.

45. Spina E, Ericsson O and Nordin C. 1985. Analysis of tricyclic antidepressants in serum and plasma yield similar results. *Ther Drug Monit* 7:242–243.

46. Levering SCM, Oostelbos, MCJM, Toll, PJM, Loonen, AJM. 1996. Influence of heparin on the assay of amitriptyline, clomipramine and their metabolites. *Ther Drug Monit* 18(3):304–305.

47. Wills BK, Mycyk MB, Mazor S, Zell-Kanter M, Brace L, Erickson T. 2006. Factitious lithium toxicity secondary to lithium heparin containing blood tubes. *J Med Toxicol* 2(2):61–63.

48. Nyberg G and Mårtensson E. 1986. Preparation of serum and plasma samples for determination of tricyclic antidepressants: effects of blood collection tubes and storage. *Ther Drug Monit* 8(4):478–482.

49. Faynor SM and Robinson R. 1998. Suitability of plastic collection tubes for cyclosporine measurements. *Clin Chem* 44:2220–2221.

50. Hill BM, Laessig RH, Koch DD, Hassemer DJ. 1992. Comparison of plastic vs glass evacuated serum-separator (SST) blood-drawing tubes for common clinical chemistry determinations. *Clin Chem* 38(8 pt1):1474–1478.

51. Smets EM, Dijkstra-Lagemaat JE, Blankenstein MA. 2004. Influence of blood collection in plastic vs glass evacuated serum-separator tubes on hormone and tumour marker levels. *Clin Chem Lab Med* 42(4):435–439.

52. Dasgupta A, Blackwell W, Bard D. 1996. Stability of therapeutic drug measurement in specimens collected in VACUTAINER plastic blood-collection tubes. *Ther Drug Monit* 18:306–309.

53. Boeynaems JM, De Leener A, Dessars B, Villa-Lobos HR, Abury JC, Cotton F and Thiry P. 2004. Evaluation of a new generation of plastic evacuated blood collection tubes in clinical chemistry, therapeutic drug monitoring, hormone and trace metal analysis. *Clin Chem Lab Med* 42:67–71.

54. Landt M, Wilhite TR, Smith CH. 1995. A new plastic evacuated tube with plasma separator. *J Clin Lab Anal* 9:101–106.

55. Brasch JL. 1991. Role of plasma protein adsorption in the response of blood to foreign surfaces. In *Blood Compatible Materials and Devices*, Sharma CP and Szycher M (Eds). Lancaster, PA: Technomic Publishing Co., 3–24.

56. Janknegt R, Lohman JJHM, Hooymans PM, Merkus FWHM. 1983. Do evacuated blood collection tubes interfere with therapeutic drug monitoring? *Pharm Week Scientific Ed* 5:287–290.

57. Quattrocchi F, Karnes HT, Robinson JD, Hendeles L. 1983. *Ther Drug Monitor* 5:359–362.

58. Bergqvist, Y. Eckerbom, S and Funding L. 1984. Effect of use of gel-barrier sampling tubes on determination of some antiepileptic drugs in serum. *Clin Chem* 30:465–466.

59. Smith, RL. 1985. Effect of serum-separator gels on progesterone assays. *Clin Chem* 31:1239.

60. Landt, M, Smith, CH and Hortin, GL. 1993. Evaluation of evacuated blood-collection tubes: Effects of three types of polymeric separators on therapeutic drug-monitoring specimens. *Clin Chem* 39:1712–1717.

61. Dasgupta, A, Blackwell, W and Bard, D. 1996. Stability of therapeutic drug measurement in specimens collected in VACUTAINER plastic blood-collection tubes. *Ther Drug Monitor* 18:306–309.

62. Dasgupta, A, Dean, R, Saldana, S, Kinnaman, G and McLawhon, RW. 1994. Absorption of therapeutic drugs by barrier gels in serum separator blood collection tubes. *Am J Clin Path* 101:456–461.

63. Karppi J, Akerman K, Parviainen M. 2000. Suitability of collection tubes with separator gels for collecting and storing blood samples for therapeutic drug monitoring. *Clin Chem Lab Med* 38: 313–320.

64. Orsulak PJ, Sink M, Weed J. 1984. Blood collection tubes for tricyclic antidepressant drugs: a reevaluation. *Ther Drug Monit* 6:444–448.

65. Bush V, Blennerhasset J, Wells A, Dasgupta A. 2001. Stability of therapeutic drugs in serum collected in Vacutainer serum separator tubes containing a new gel (SST II). *Ther Drug Monit* 23:259–262.

66. Devine JE. 1986. Assessment of the Corvac blood collection tube for drug specimen processing. *Ther Drug Monit* 8:241–243.

67. Dasgupta A, Yared MA and Wells A. 2000. Time-dependent absorption of therapeutic drugs by the gel of Greiner Vacuette blood collection tubes. *Ther Drug Monit.* 22:427–431.

68. Bailey DN, Coffee JJ and Briggs JR. 1988. Stability of drug concentrations in plasma stored in serum separator blood collection tubes. *Ther Drug Monitor.* 10:352–354.

69. Koch T, Platoff G. 1990. Suitability of collection tubes with separator gels for therapeutic drug monitoring. *Ther Drug Monit* 12: 277–280.

70. Parish, RC and Alexander, T. 1990. Stability of phenytoin in blood collected in vacuum blood collection tubes. *Ther Drug Monitor* 12:85–89.
71. Datta P. 1998. Stability of digoxin and digitoxin in specimens collected in blood collection tubes containing serum separator gels. *Clin Biochem* 31(4):273–275.
72. Cai W, Leader G, Porter W, Chandler M. 1993. Influence of serum separator tubes on total and free phenytoin concentrations and dosage. *Ther Drug Monit* 15: 427–430.
73. Mauro L, Mauro V. 1991. Effect of serum separator tubes on free and total phenytoin and carbamazepine serum concentrations. *Ther Drug Monit* 13: 240–243.
74. Landt M, Norling LL, Steelman M, Smith CH. 1986. Monoject samplette capillary blood container with serum separator evaluated for collection of specimens for therapeutic drug assays and common clinical tests. *Clin Chem* 32:523–526.
75. Wilson JM, Leonard KS and Posey YF. 2002. Evaluation of plastic blood collection tubes for therapeutic drug monitoring. *Clin Chem* 48:A43.
76. Levy AB, Walters M, Stern SL. 1987. Reduced serum tricyclic levels due to gel separators. *J Clin Pyschopharmacol* 7:423–4.
77. Gupta RN. 1988. *CRC Handbook of Chromatography*, Volume III. Boca Raton, FL: CRC Press.

3 Immunoassays for Therapeutic Drug Monitoring: Pitfalls and Limitations

Pradip Datta
Siemens Healthcare Diagnostics

Amitava Dasgupta
University of Texas Medical School

CONTENTS

3.1 INTRODUCTION

Currently, immunoassays are widely used for therapeutic drug monitoring (TDM) in clinical laboratories. Immunoassays measure the analyte concentration in a specimen by forming a complex with a specific binding molecule, which in most cases is an analyte-specific antibody (or a pair of specific antibodies). In the 1970s and 1980s immunoassays were introduced for TDM, replacing tedious chromatographic methods. Currently over 25 immunoassays are commercially available for analysis of various therapeutic drugs in clinical laboratories. Different formats are used for immunoassay design and more than one commercial vendor may use a similar format (Table 3.1). Most immunoassay methods use specimens without any pretreatment and assays can be performed on fully automated, continuous, random access analyzers. The assays use very small amounts of sample volume (< 100 μL), reagents can be stored in the analyzer and calibration curves can be electronically stored in the analyzer.

TABLE 3.1
Various Types of Commercial Immunoassay Kits

Assay Format	Immunoassay Types	Example	Assay Signal
Homogeneous	Competition (for small molecules)	1. FPIA (TDx® from Abbott, Abbott Park, IL)	Fluorescence polarization
		2. EMIT® (Siemens, IL)	Colorimetry (enzyme modulation)
		3. CEDIA® (Microgenics, Fremont, CA)	Colorimetry (enzyme modulation)
Homogeneous	Both competition and sandwich (both small and large molecule)	1. LOCI® on Dimension Vista (Siemens, IL)	Chemiluminescence
		2. ADVIA Chemistry (Siemens)	Turbidimetry, latex
		3. IMx, AxSym® (Abbott)	Microparticle assisted. or enzyme immunoassay (using fluorescence substrate)
Heterogeneous	Both competition and sandwich (both small and large molecule)	1. ADVIA Centaur® (Siemens)	Chemiluminescence (acridinium ester label)
		2. Architect (Abbott)	
		3. ACCESS® (Beckman, Fullerton, CA)	Enzyme immunoassay (using chemiluminescent substrate)
		4. Elecsys® (Roche, Diagnostics Indianapolis, IN)	Electrochemiluminescence

3.2 IMMUNOASSAY PRINCIPLES

The immunoassay technology is based on binding of the analyte of interest with a specific binding protein (antibody) and then measuring the signal generated due to such interaction. There are many different designs of the immunoassay, differing by assay formats and by the type of signal generated. Thus, by assay format, there are two types of immunoassays: competition and immunometric (commonly referred as "sandwich"). Competition immunoassays are mostly used for analysis of analytes with small molecular weight such as therapeutic drugs, requiring a single analyte specific antibody. In contrast, sandwich immunoassays are mostly used for large molecular weight analytes such as proteins or peptides and use two different antibodies for the analyte.

In the competition format the analyte molecules in the specimen compete with analyte (or, its analogs) labeled with a suitable tag and provided in the reagent for binding with limited number of analyte-specific antibody (also provided in the reagent). Thus, higher the analyte concentration in the sample, less of label can bind to the antibody to form the conjugate. If the bound label provides the signal, the analyte concentration in the specimen is inversely proportional to the signal produced. On the other hand, if the free label provides the signal then intensity of signal is proportional to the analyte concentration. The signals are mostly optical in nature; absorbance, fluorescence, or chemiluminescence.

An immunoassay may be homogeneous or heterogeneous. In the former, the bound label has different properties than the free label. For example, in fluorescent polarization immunoassay (FPIA), the free label (which has relatively low molecular weight) has different Brownian motion than when the label is complexed to a large antibody (140,000 D). This results in difference in the fluorescence polarization properties of the label and only the label bound to antibody can generate the signal [1]. In another type of homogeneous immunoassay, an enzyme is the label, whose activity is modulated differently in the free vs the complexed form with the antibody. Examples of this format include the enzyme multiplied immunoassay technique (EMIT®) and cloned enzyme donor immunoassay (CEDIA®) assays [2,3]. In the EMIT method the label enzyme, glucose 6-phosphodehydrogenase is in active unless in the antigen-antibody complex where enzymatic activity is restored. The active enzyme reduces nicotinamide adenine dinucleotide (NAD) to NADH, and the absorbance is monitored at 340 nm (NAD has no absorption at 340 nm but NADH absorbs at 340 nm). Similarly, in the CEDIA method, two genetically engineered inactive fragments of the enzyme beta-galactosidase are coupled to the antigen and the antibody reagents. When they combine, the active enzyme is produced and the substrate, a chromogenic galactoside derivative, produces the assay signal. In a third commonly used format of homogeneous immunoassay (turbidimetric immunoassay, or TIA), analytes (antigen) or its analogs are coupled to colloidal particles, e.g., of latex [4]. Since antibody is bivalent, the latex particles agglutinate in presence of the antibody. However, in presence of analytes in the specimen, there is less agglutination. In a spectrophotometer, the resulting turbidity can be monitored as end-point or as rate. Another example of homogeneous chemiluminescent immunoassay technology is the luminescent oxygen channeling assay (LOCI) in which the immunoassay reaction is irradiated with light, generating singlet oxygen molecules in microbeads ("Sensibead") coupled to the analyte. When bound to the respective antibody molecule, also coupled to another type of bead ("Chemibead") which reacts with singlet oxygen, chemiluminescence signals are generated, proportional to the concentration of the analyte-antibody complex. This technology is used in the Siemens Dimension Vista® automated assay system [5].

In heterogeneous immunoassays format the bound label is physically separated from the unbound labels followed by measuring the signal. The separation is often done magnetically, where the reagent analyte (or its analog) is provided as coupled to paramagnetic particles (PMP), and the antibody is labeled. Conversely, the antibody may also be provided as conjugated to the PMP, and the reagent analyte may carry the label. After separation and wash, the bound label is reacted with other reagents to generate the signal. In the chemiluminescent immunoassays (CLIA), the label may be a small molecule which generates chemiluminescent signal. Examples of immunoassay systems where the chemiluminescent labels generate signal by chemical reaction are assays for ADVIA Centaur® (Siemens, Tarrytown, NY) and Architect® (Abbott Laboratories, Abbott Park, IL) platforms [6]. An example where the small label is activated electrochemically is the ELECSYS® automated immunoassay system available from Roche Diagnostics (Indianapolis, IN) for application on the ELECSYS analyzer [7]. The label also may be an enzyme (enzyme-linked immunosorbent assay, or ELISA) which generates chemiluminescent, fluorimetric, or colorimetric signal. Examples of commercial automated assay systems using the ELISA technology and chemiluminescent labels are Immulite® (Siemens) and ACCESS® from Beckman–Coulter (Brea, CA) [8,9]. Another type of heterogeneous immunoassay uses polystyrene particles. If these are particles are microsizes, that type of assay is called microparticle enhanced immunoassay (MEIA) (Abbott Laboratories) [10]. In older immunoassay formats, the labels were radioactive: radio-immunoassay or RIA, but because of safety and waste disposal issues, RIA is rarely used today.

Several types of antibodies or their fragments are now used in immunoassays. There are polyclonal antibodies, which are raised in an animal when the analyte (as antigen) along with an adjuvant is injected into the animal. For a small molecular weight analyte, it is most commonly injected as a conjugate of a large protein. Appearance of analyte-specific antibodies in the animal's sera is monitored and when sufficient concentration of the antibody is reached, the animal is bled. The serum can directly be used as the analyte specific binder in the immunoassay. Most commonly, however, the antibodies are purified from serum and used in the assay. Since there are many clones of the antibodies specific for the analyte, these antibodies are called polyclonal. In newer technologies, a mast cell of the animal can be selected as producing the optimum antibody and then can be fused to an immortal cell. The resulting tumor cell grows uncontrollably producing only the single clone of desired antibody. Such antibodies, called monoclonal antibody may also be grown in live animals or cell-culture. There are several benefits of the monoclonal antibodies over polyclonal ones:

A. The characteristics of polyclonal antibodies are dependent on the animal producing the antibodies; if the source individual animal must be changed, the resultant antibody may be quite different.
B. In general, polyclonal antibodies are less analyte specific than monoclonal antibodies.

TABLE 3.2
Various Sources of Interferences in Immunoassays

Sources of Interference	Comments
Endogenous	
Bilirubin	High bilirubin makes a specimen appear icteric (greenish). Normal bilirubin concentrations in specimen (0.2–1.2 mg/dL, total; up to 0.2 mg/dL for direct (conjugated) bilirubin) does not interfere with immunoassays. Bilirubin concentrations above 15 mg/dL may interfere (both positive and negative interference). Bilirubin interferes with the assay sinal due to its photometric or fluorometric properties and may also participate in side reactions thus interfering with and assay.
Hemoglobin	Plasma free hemoglobin concentration is usually low and does not interfere with immunoassays. However, in significantly hemolyzed specimens, hemoglobin is present in much higher concentrations and may interfere due to photometric, fluorometric and chemiluminescent properties of hemoglobin.
High lipid	High lipid content of a specimen (lipemic) may cause the specimen appears turbid or milky. Lipids interfere with immunoassays due to their light scattering properties.
Proteins	Very high or low protein content of a serum or plasma may alter the ideal matrix of a specimen and may cause interference with an immunoassay.
Paraproteins	Paraproteins are known to interfere with certain immunoassays.
Digoxin-Like Immunoreactive	
Substances (DLIS)	Found in elevated concentrations in volume expanded patients and DLIS interfere (both positive and negative interference) with various digoxin immunoassays (see Chapter 8).
Exogenous	
Various drugs/metabolites	See Table 3.3 of this chapter.
Herbal supplements	See Chapter 22.

Sometimes, instead of using the whole antibody, fragments of the antibody, generated by digestion of the antibody by peptidases, e.g., Fab (or their dimeric complexes) are used. Another important reagent component of the immunoassay is the labeled antigen (or, its analog). There are many different kinds of labels, generating different kinds of signals.

Even though the immunoassay methods are widely used in clinical laboratories, there are many limitations of this method of analysis. Many of the endogenous metabolites of the analyte may have very similar structural recognition motif as the analyte itself and may interact with the antibody. There are also other molecules structurally different from the analyte but producing comparable recognition motif as the analyte. These molecules are generally called cross-reactants. When present in the sample they will produce falsely elevated or falsely lower results in the relevant immunoassay. Other components in a specimen, e.g., bilirubin, hemoglobin, or lipid, may interfere in the immunoassay by interfering with the assay signal, and thus produce incorrect assay results. A third type of immunoassay interference involves endogenous human antibodies in the specimen, which may interfere with the assay. Such interference includes that from heterophilic antibodies or various human anti-animal antibodies. These factors are summarized in Table 3.2.

3.3   SPECIMEN TYPES USED IN IMMUNOASSAY

Serum and plasma are the most common types of specimen used in TDM. Whole blood specimens must be used for most of the immunosuppressant drugs. For such samples, hematocrit percentage may also affect the assay results. Thus, false positive tacrolimus results were reported in an MEIA tacrolimus assay (Abbott Laboratories, Abbott Park, IL) for patients with low hematocrit values and high imprecision at tacrolimus concentration less than 9 ng/mL [11]. The EMIT (Syva, San Jose, CA) assay for tacrolimus was not affected. When the authors divided the study specimens in three groups by hematocrit percentage (<25%, 25–35%, and >35%), the difference between MEIA and EMIT assays increased as hematocrit percentage decreased. Moreover, false positive results were reported in 63% of specimens with MEIA where patients did not receive any tacrolimus, but only 2.2% of specimens demonstrated false positive results using EMIT. Such false positive values in the MEIA and EMIT methods ranged up to 3.7 ng/mL and 1.3 ng/mL, respectively [11].

Urine specimens are rarely used in TDM except for checking patient compliance with narcotic analgesic drugs. Saliva, sweat, tears, cerebrospinal and stomach fluids, or bronchial secretions are also used as specimens for analysis of therapeutic drugs and drugs of abuse [12–16] but these types of specimens are rarely used for TDM.

3.4 EXAMPLES OF IMMUNOASSAYS USED IN THERAPEUTIC DRUG MONITORING (TDM)

Immunoassays are commercially available for many drugs routinely analyzed in the clinical laboratory.

- Antiasthmatic drugs like theophylline and caffeine
- Antibiotics including amikacin, gentamicin, tobramycin, and vancomycin
- Anticonvulsant drugs like carbamazepine, phenobarbital, phenytoin, valproic acid, etc.
- Tricyclic antidepressants (TCAs)
- Analgesics, like, acetaminophen, salicylate
- Cardioactive drugs like digoxin, procainamide, lidocaine, quinidine, and disopyramide
- Antineoplastic drug like methotrexate

3.5 PITFALLS IN IMMUNOASSAY

Immunoassays suffer from different types of interference, rendering false negative or false positive results. The sources of interference may be an endogenous compound or a drug, drug metabolite, component of a herbal remedy or other exogenous factors (Table 3.2). It is important to recognize the sources of such discordant results and conduct follow-up studies to provide clinically useful and important results.

3.5.1 INTERFERENCE FROM ENDOGENOUS COMPONENTS

Immunoassays use various types of signals, the most common being colorimetry, fluorimetry, and chemiluminescence. Elevated concentrations of serum components: bilirubin (icterus), hemoglobin (hemolysis), lipids (turbidity), and proteins may interfere with the assay depending on the format or label used. Commercial assay kits report the result of such interference in the package inserts (up to levels of ≥20 mg/dL bilirubin, ≥500 mg/dL hemoglobin, and ≥1000 mg/dL lipids). The interference is caused by the optical, fluorescent, or chemiluminescent properties of these interferents. Thus, bilirubin interferes by its absorption and fluorescence properties, hemoglobin by its absorption, fluorescence, and chemiluminescence properties and lipids interfere mostly from its light scattering (turbidity) properties. Modern auto-analyzers can detect all three interfering substances and flag the results. In addition to these three common sources of interference, both hypo- and hyperproteinemia can affect assay results. Paraproteins when present in a sample in high concentrations, may interfere in many assays by precipitating out during sample blanking or immunoreaction steps, giving false results. If the results are suspected, the assay should be repeated either by removing the interferent from the sample or by using a different method which is known to suffer less from that type of interference. Additionally, collection tube additives for plasma or whole blood specimens, like ethylene diamino-tetra-acetate (EDTA), heparin, citrate, fluoride, and oxalate may chelate metal ions, and thus interfere with label enzymes used in immunoassays, like alkaline phosphatase, and thus generate false positive or negative results (see Chapter 2).

Bilirubin absorbs around 450–460 nm. Hemoglobin begins to absorb from about 340 nm to 560 nm with absorbance peak observed at 541 nm for oxyhemoglobin. Thus assays generating signal at or around these wavelengths will be affected by hemolytic or icteric conditions of a sample. Hemolysis may affect assays which use the absorbance properties of NADH or NADPH [17] at 340 nm, e.g., EMIT. Bilirubin and hemoglobin can also interfere in assays through unintended side reactions. Both participate in redox reactions, commonly used in TDM assays that are not immunoassays. Most manufacturers of these assays follow the EP7-P protocol from National Committee for Clinical Laboratory Standardization ("NCCLS," currently Clinical Laboratory Standards Institute or CLSI), where the interference is studied at two different steps [18]. In the "screening" protocol, serum pools containing a clinically important concentration of the analyte is supplemented with various concentrations of the interferent, and the assay results are compared with a suitable control sample (without supplemented interferent). Interference is judged significant when the results of a supplemented sample are statistically different from the control sample, and the difference between the two means is $\geq 10\%$. The protocol also recommends plotting analyte versus interferent concentrations to find the pattern of interference, if any [19].

Sample blanking and robust assay design can be used to minimize these interferences, including matrix effect arising from protein and other non-specific constituent in the specimen. When suspected, the interferents may be removed from the specimen by specific agents, ultrafiltration or centrifugation, before reanalysis. Alternatively the specimen may be analyzed by a different method which is known to be free from such interference.

3.5.2 Bilirubin Interference

Bilirubin is derived from hemoglobin of aged or damaged red blood cells (RBC). Bilirubin does not have iron but is rather a derivative of the heme group. Some part of serum bilirubin is conjugated as glucuronides ("direct" bilirubin); the unconjugated bilirubin is also referred to as indirect bilirubin. Normal adult bilirubin concentrations in serum are 0.3–1.2 mg/dL (total) and <0.2 mg/dL (conjugated) [20]. In different forms of jaundice, total bilirubin can rise to as high as 20 mg/dL, but the ratio of direct versus indirect bilirubin varies. In obstructive jaundice, the increase in total bilirubin is contributed mainly by direct bilirubin. In hemolytic and neonatal jaundice the increase is mostly in indirect bilirubin, while in hepatitis, both fractions of bilirubin increase. Elevated bilirubin may cause interference which may be proportional to its concentration. If the assay is enzymatic or colorimetric, bilirubin may also interfere by reacting chemically to the reagents [21].

In one case study a severely jaundiced 17-year-old male patient (total bilirubin 19.8 mg/dL) with abdominal pain and increased serum transaminase results was suspected of acetaminophen overdosing, though the patient himself denied using any medications containing acetaminophen within the previous week. The apparent plasma acetaminophen concentration by an enzyme method was found to be 3.4 mg/dL. In this method, acetaminophen is enzymatically (by arylacylamidase) hydrolyzed to p-aminophenol, which is condensed with o-cresol in the presence of periodate to form the blue indophenol chromophore. The assay was performed using a Roche analyzer (Indianapolis, IN), with absorbance measurement at 600 nm (2-point rate) and background correction at 800 nm [22]. When authors analyzed 12 hyperbilirubinemic plasma specimens (total bilirubin 15.9–33.8 mg/dL) from patients without any recent history of acetaminophen ingestion, the apparent acetaminophen concentrations ranged from 0.5 to 1.8 mg/dL. Serial dilution of these specimens with saline showed nonlinear decreases in apparent acetaminophen concentrations and values approaching zero when bilirubin concentrations were below 5 mg/dL. The authors concluded that their data are consistent with bilirubin interference in the enzymatic and or chromogenic reactions involved in acetaminophen methods [22]. Kellmeyer et al. also reported bilirubin interference in colorimetric assay for acetaminophen [23].

Wood et al. reported a case where increased bilirubin (22.6 mg/dL), mainly consisting of high percentage of conjugated fraction (82%), caused negative interference in a FPIA (Abbott Laboratories, Abbott Park, IL) vancomycin assay [24]. In their study, the authors first compared 28 plasma samples with total bilirubin <5.9 mg/dL, using the TDx and the AxSYM vancomycin assays (both available from Abbott Laboratories). Vancomycin, a glycopeptide antibiotic used in treating serious infections, is toxic with plasma concentration >20 μg/mL (trough) and >80 μg/mL (peak). The TDx method is a homogeneous FPIA, using a polyclonal sheep antibody and fluorescein-labeled antigen. The AxSYM assay also uses the same assay principle, but uses a different, monoclonal mouse antibody. The vancomycin results from these 28 samples, ranging from 2.0 to 34.5 μg/mL were in close agreement between the assays (Pearson's correlation coefficient of $r^2 = 0.996$). When plasma specimens containing abnormal bilirubin were analyzed, the authors observed falsely lower vancomycin values with TDx analyzer compared to vancomycin values obtained by using the AxSYM analyzer. For example, in one specimen containing 22.6 mg/dL of bilirubin, the vancomycin concentration observed using the TDx analyzer was 2.6 μg/mL but the vancomycin value in the same specimen was 8.0 μg/mL when AxSYM analyzer was used [24]. The negative interference in the TDx assay was probably caused by direct bilirubin generating falsely increased fluorescence blanks. The authors noted that the TDx assay's package insert reported interference of <5% for bilirubin concentrations of 15 mg/dL. However, authors observed more significant negative interference of bilirubin than reported in the package insert. This suggested a possibility that the package insert data was generated with unconjugated bilirubin, which as the authors' data show, does not interfere with this assay. The authors concluded that while the AxSYM assay somehow was not affected by high direct bilirubin (either because of the antibody difference, or from method), the TDx assay gave clinically significant false negative results for such samples [24].

3.5.3 Interference from Hemoglobin and Blood Substitutes

Hemoglobin is released from hemolysis of RBC. Hemolysis can occur in vivo, during venipuncture and blood collection or during processing of the sample. Serum appears hemolyzed when hemoglobin concentrations reach above 20 mg/dL. Icteric serum may contain higher concentration of hemoglobin before hemolysis can be noticed by visual inspection. Hemoglobin interference is caused not only by the spectrophotometric properties of hemoglobin but also by its possible chemical reaction with sample or reactant components as well [25]. The absorbance maxima of the heme moiety in hemoglobin are at 540–580 nm wave lengths. However, absorption may begin around 340 nm with absorbance increasing at 400–430 nm as well. The iron atom in the center of the heme group is the source of such absorbances. Methemoglobin (where the iron is in 3+ oxidation state) and cyanmethemoglobin (cyanide complex of hemoglobin) also absorb at 500 and 480 nm, respectively. However, methemoglobin shows poor absorption at 340 nm [25,26].

If the type of blood for a patient is in short supply hospitals may use blood substitutes, which are mostly derivatized or polymerized hemoglobin. The blood substitutes interfere in many analyses in the same way as hemoglobin. Thus, it was shown that O-raffinose cross-linked hemoglobin blood substitute, Hemolink® showed positive or negative interference in many routine chemistry and immunochemistry assays [27]. Another type of blood substitute is polyfluorocarbon, which may also interfere with immunoassays.

3.5.4 Lipid Interference

All lipids in plasma are present as lipoproteins although free fatty acids may also be found in plasma. Lipoproteins, consisting of various proportions of lipids, range from 10 to 1000 nm in size. The higher the percentage of the lipid, lower is the density of the lipoprotein, and larger is the particle size. Chylomicrons (diameter 70–1000 nm, density <0.95 g/mL) are present in plasma after an individual ingests a fatty meal. Chylomicrons originate in the intestinal epithelial cells and consist mostly of lipids. Chylomicrons are absorbed by the adipose tissue and liver. Liver secretes lipoprotein particles called very low-density lipoproteins (VLDL, density < 1.006 g/mL), low-density lipoproteins (LDL, density = 1.006–1.063 g/mL), and high-density lipoproteins (HDL, density = 1.063–1.21 g/mL), containing decreasing amounts of lipids in that order. The lipoprotein particles with high lipid contents are micellar and are the main source of interference. Unlike bilirubin and hemoglobin, lipids normally do not participate in side reactions and cause interference due to their turbidity. The micellar particles scatter light: lower the wavelength, higher is the amount of light scattered. Since scattered light do not follow Lambert–Beer law of absorbance, scattering normally reduces absorbance resulting in false positive or false negative results depending on assay design. Lipemic interference is most pronounced in spectrophotometric assays, less important in fluorimetric methods and rarely interferes with chemiluminescent methods. Thus, assays which use turbidimetry for signal are the ones most affected by lipid interference [28]. Lipemia may also interfere with assays for fat-soluble analytes, such as steroids and their derivatives. In such cases interference arises from solvent partitioning and solute exclusion of the analyte between the lipid and aqueous phases.

Like bilirubin and hemolysis, assay package inserts do report the extent of lipid interference in a commercial assay. Lipids, however, present a special problem: lack of readily available, standardized materials. Most manufacturers use IntraLipid, a synthetically produced emulsion containing soybean oil and egg phospholipids, and used for intravenous administration, to simulate lipemic samples. However, samples with IntraLipid do not exactly mimic lipemic samples [29]. Among the plasma lipoproteins, chylomicrons, and VLDL particles only scatter light. VLDL exists in three size classes: small (27–35 nm), intermediate (35–60 nm), and large (60–200 nm). Only the latter two sizes of VLDL scatter light. Chylomicron particles vary greatly among individuals, and even in the same individual, depending upon the time that the sample is collected after the meal [30]. Kazmierczak argues that interference studies need to be done with specimens from patients with hyper-lipidemia, or hyper-bilirubinemia because the subject to subject variation makes it impossible to guarantee that an assay will not be subject to interference from these lipids [31].

3.5.5 Interference from Proteins and Paraproteins

Interference from proteins is possible in patients with both hypo and hyper-proteinemia (normal serum protein concentration is about 6–8 g/dL; in plasma fibrinogen adds to total protein by about 0.2–0.4 g/dL). Plasma protein concentrations alter in older population as well as in various physiological states such as pregnancy. Ezan et al. attempted to estimate interferences of proteins in TDM assays using plasma samples and an experimental drug and concluded that recovery of the drug may be influenced by protein content of the specimens [32].

Plasma specimens, which have been refrigerated for prolonged periods or which have undergone freeze-thaw cycles demonstrate protein interference from fibrins which may precipitate under such conditions. These fibrin clots may block sample probe of an auto-analyzer, generating incorrect results. Such samples should be centrifuged to remove any precipitates prior to analysis. However, most modern auto-analyzers include clot-detection and alert systems to flag results suspected of interference from clot. Hyper-proteinemia may also increase the viscosity of the specimen, thus interfering with accurate sampling for the assay.

Paraproteins circulate as the result of multiple myeloma or similar diseases. The concentrations of a specific class and idiotype of immunoglobulins (Igs) are greatly increased. Paraproteins are known to interfere with many types of clinical chemistry assays including immunoassays. Hullin reported a case study, where a 77-year-old man whose plasma samples had 500 mg/dL of paraprotein (IgMκ monoclonal component), ingested high amount of acetaminophen 18 h prior to reporting to the hospital [33]. Serum acetaminophen concentration determined using a commercial enzyme assay kit was 5.3 mg/dL, but the blank reading was very high. Suspecting interference, the authors measured acetaminophen concentration using high performance liquid chromatography (HPLC) and the observed value was 8.6 mg/dL. The presence of paraprotein in the sample was also indicated by the formation of flocculant precipitate when a drop of serum was added to water (the Sia water test).

Recently Brauchili et al. reported significant interference of paraproteins in the particle-enhanced turbidimetric inhibition assay (PENTINA) assay of phenytoin (Dade Behring, Newark, NY). A 73-year-old female patient was admitted to the hospital and was treated with intravenous phenytoin but the phenytoin level was undetectable using the PENTINA phenytoin assay and Dimension analyzer. The patient was also receiving valproic acid and the valproic acid of 32.6 µg/mL was measured by the PENTINA valproic acid assay. However, when phenytoin levels were measured using HPLC or FPIA phenytoin assay, significant phenytoin levels were observed as expected. For example, on day 5 of admission, the phenytoin level measured by the PENTINA assay was <0.4 µg/mL. In contrast, phenytoin levels measured on day 5 using HPLC and FPIA were 11.0 µg/mL and 10.1 µg/mL, respectively. Serum protein electrophoresis of this patient revealed a monoclonal immunoglobulin (IGMλ). The authors concluded that Igs may cause negative interference in serum phenytoin measurement using PENTINA assay [34].

3.5.6 INTERFERENCES FROM HETEROPHILIC ANTIBODIES

Heterophilic antibodies are endogenous human antibodies found in a serum/plasma specimen. Heterophilic antibodies may interact with assay antibodies (raised in various animals) causing false positive or negative results. The heterophilic antibodies are polyclonal and heterogeneous in nature, consisting of four types: (a) heterophilic antibodies which interact poorly and non-specifically with the assay antibodies, (b) antianimal antibodies, which interact strongly and specifically (with respect to the animal species in which the assay antibodies have been raised), (c) auto-antibody, endogenous human antibody interacting with an analyte, and (d) therapeutic antibody, where antibody given therapeutically interferes with an assay. The heterophilic antibody may arise in a patient in response to exposure to certain animals or animal products (handling an animal, therapy) or to infection by bacterial or viral agents or even nonspecifically. Although many of the immunoglobulin (Ig) clones in normal human serum may display antianimal antibody properties, only those antibodies with sufficient titer and affinity toward the reagent antibody used in an assay may cause interference. Among the human antianimal antibodies (HAAA), the most common occurrence is of human antimouse antibody (HAMA), because of wide use of murine monoclonal antibody products in therapy or imaging. The HAAA can belong to IgG, IgA, IgM, and rarely, the IgE class. In addition, rheumatoid factors (IgG) which may be present in 10% of patients may interfere with immunoassays.

Heterophilic antibody and antianimal antibody interference are often lumped together as heterophilic antibody interference. Such interference has been mostly found with immunometric sandwich assays, less often with competition (the types most commonly used in TDM/DAU) assays. There are many reports of falsely elevated serum beta-hCG (human chorionic gonadotropin) values due to the presence of heterophilic antibodies in the serum or plasma specimens and inappropriate clinical decision may result from such falsely elevated values. Heterophilic antibodies due to large molecular weight are absent in urine and measuring of urinary beta-hCG eliminates such effects [35]. In one study the author investigated effect of heterophilic antibodies on immunoassay results by surveying results of 74 analytes (21 hormones, 18 tumor markers, eight therapeutic drugs, five cardiac markers, four proteins, two vitamins, and 16 miscellaneous other tests) in 10 donors (having rheumatoid factors in their sera) from 66 laboratories in seven countries. The author observed that overall approximately 8.7% of the 3445 results were considered false positive and 21% of all erroneous results (1.8% of all results) were potentially misleading. However, some of these false positive results could be resolved by treating sera with heterophilic blocking agents but 49% of those misleading results (4.2% of all results) could not be resolved by using blocking agents. Assays such as plasma beta-hCG, α–fetoprotein, myoglobin, CA 19-9, estradiol, erythropoietin, etc. were affected but no TDM assay was affected [36]. In another report, authors described falsely elevated calcitonin results due to the presence of heterophilic antibody in serum specimens [37].

Although most TDM assays are competitive immunoassay using only single analyte-specific antibody in the reagent and are rarely affected by heterophilic antibodies, Liendo et al. reported a case where high serum digoxin level (4.2 ng/mL, using Roche assay, a competition type immunoassay utilizing a monoclonal antibody) was observed in a patient 24 hours after his last digoxin dose. The patient was also taking spironolactone which interferes with certain digoxin assays. However, 29 days after discontinuation of digoxin and spironolactone the digoxin value was still 3.6 ng/mL. Interestingly, when authors measured digoxin value using a FPIA assay on the TDx analyzer (Abbott), the digoxin value was 0.2 ng/mL, a value at the detecting limit of the assay. When authors measured digoxin in the protein free ultrafiltrate, no interference was observed even with the Roche assay. Because heterophilic antibodies due to large molecular size are absent in the ultrafiltrate (prepared by using a filter with 30,000 Daltons molecular cut-off), the authors concluded that the interference in the digoxin immunoassay was due to the presence of heterophilic antibody [38].

3.5.7 PITFALLS OF IMMUNOASSAYS: CROSS-REACTIVITIES FROM DRUGS/METABOLITES

Immunoassays are also affected by the presence of drug metabolites and other molecules in the specimen which may be recognized by the antibody of the assay. This phenomenon is termed as "cross-reactivity." Manufacturers of commercial immunoassays strive to test and publish in the package insert cross-reactivities of suspected compounds for each analyte. However, by definition, it is impossible to test all possible cross-reactants. Digoxin immunoassays are affected by many endogenous and exogenous compounds and perhaps have the highest number of published papers in the literature describing such interferences compared to any other therapeutic drugs. Endogenous digoxin-like immunoreactive substances (DLIS), spironolactone, and potassium canrenoate and various herbal supplements are known to affect digoxin immunoassays (see Chapter 8). Digitoxin may cause bi-directional (false positive at low concentration and false negative at higher concentration) interference with serum digoxin measurement using MEIA digoxin assay [39].

False positive serum tricyclic antidepressant (TCA) screen using the FPIA (Abbott Laboratories) due to the presence of carbamazepine has been reported. Chattergoon et al. reported apparent TCA levels of 80 ng/mL and 130 ng/mL in two patients who never received any TCAs [40]. These values are significant because TCA has a narrow therapeutic range (90–130 ng/mL for nortriptyline). Although the manufacturer of FPIA (Abbott Laboratories) for TCA only recommends its use for the diagnosis of an overdose, the assay is sometimes used in TDM. Carbamazepine 10, 11-epoxide, the active metabolite of carbamazepine interferes much less than carbamazepine in the FPIA assay. HPLC is the best method for therapeutic drug monitoring of TCA [41].

Carbamazepine 10, 11-epoxide, the metabolite of carbamazepine is present in 15–20% of total carbamazepine concentration at the steady state. The concentration of metabolite may be significantly higher in carbamazepine overdose or in patients with renal failure. The cross-reactivity of carbamazepine 10, 11-epoxide with different immunoassays for carbamazepine may vary between 0% (Vitros) to 93.6% (PENTINA assay on Dade Dimension analyzer). Therefore, PENTINA assay equally measures carbamazepine and the epoxide metabolite as there is no clinically significant difference between values obtained by the immunoassay and carbamazepine + epoxide value obtained by HPLC. Nevertheless, cross-reactivity of inactive metabolite carbamazepine diol is another issue [42]. Oxcarbazepine and its main metabolite 10-hydroxy-carbamzepine have structural similarity with carbamazepine. However, both compounds demonstrate low cross-reactivity with PENTINA and EMIT carbamazepine immunoassays [43].

Hydroxyzine is a commonly prescribed first generation antihistamine with sedative properties and has a benzhydryl piperazine structure. Hydroxyzine is metabolized to cetirizine which has antihistamine properties but is devoid of sedative effect. Cetirizine is also used as a second generation H_1-antagonist and has a lesser tendency to cross the blood-brain barrier compared to hydroxyzine. Parant et al. reported that hydroxyzine interferes with PENTINA carbamazepine (structures of hydroxyzine, cetirizine and carbamazepine are given in Figure 3.1) assay marketed by Dade–Behring for application on the Dimension analyzer and concluded that such interference could significantly affect proper interpretation of serum carbamazepine concentrations [44]. A 22–year-old female with a hydroxyzine concentration of 1.8 μg/mL and cetirizine concentration of 2.1 μg/mL showed an apparent carbamazepine level of 5.3 μg/mL. Another patient with a hydroxyzine level of 520 ng/mL and cetirizine level of 2.2 μg/mL demonstrated a carbamazepine level of 25.4 μg/mL. However, EMIT 2000 assay showed no cross-reactivity [44]. In addition, FPIA (Abbott Laboratories), CEDIA immunoassays and turbidimetric carbamazepine immunoassay on ADVIA analyzers (Siemens, Tarrytown, NY) are free from interferences of both hydroxyzine and cetirizine [45,46].

Interestingly, although not structurally related, both hydroxyzine and cetirizine caused significant interference with the total TCA measurement using FPIA assay. When aliquots of drug free serum pool were supplemented with hydroxyzine or cetirizine, measurable apparent TCA concentrations were observed (see Figure 3.1 for structure of TCA imipramine). The observed apparent tricyclic concentrations were 27.5, 87.7, and 106.2 ng/mL when aliquots of drug free serum pool were supplemented with hydroxyzine to achieve final concentrations of 1, 10 and 20 μg/mL of hydroxyzine, respectively. Finally with a hydroxyzine concentration of 40 μg/mL the observed TCA concentration was 136.4 ng/mL. Similar results were obtained when aliquots of the same drug free serum pool were supplemented with various amounts of cetirizine. When serum pools prepared from patients receiving TCAs were further supplemented with hydroxyzine or cetirizine, falsely increased TCA levels were observed [46].

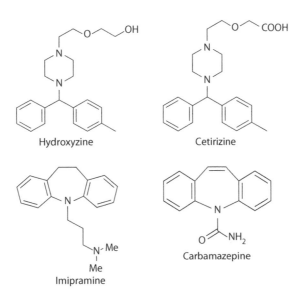

Hydroxyzine

Cetirizine

Imipramine

Carbamazepine

FIGURE 3.1   Chemical structures of hydroxyzine, cetirizine, imipramine, and carbamazepine.

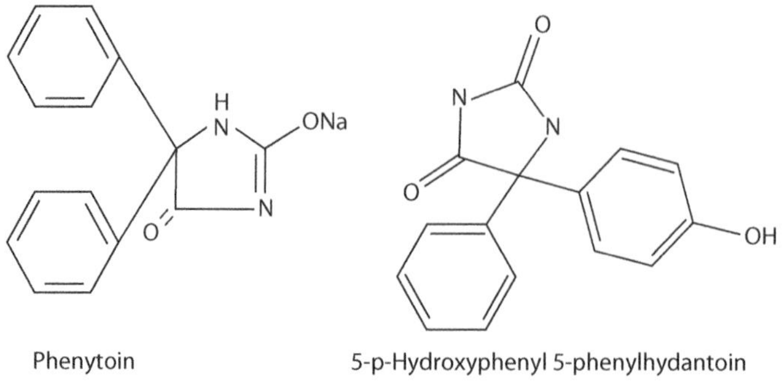

Phenytoin   5-p-Hydroxyphenyl 5-phenylhydantoin

FIGURE 3.2   Chemical structures of phenytoin and 5-p-hydroxyphenyl 5-phenylhydantoin (HPPH).

Phenytoin metabolite 5-p-hydroxyphenyl 5-phenylhydantoin (HPPH) (see Figure 3.2 for structures) and its glucuronide conjugate may accumulate in uremia. HPPH has 16% cross-reactivity and HPPH-glucuronide has 1.6% cross-reactivity with various immunoassays. Interference of metabolites may be significant in uremia. However, Roberts and Rainey disputed these findings and concluded that the accumulation of metabolites in uremia is mainly HPPH glucuronide, which due to minimal cross-reactivity should not cause clinically significant changes in phenytoin concentrations [47,48]. Datta et al. reported that a turbidimetric assay for phenytoin on the ADVIA analyzer has only 8.0% cross-reactivity with HPPH. In addition, a non-steroidal anti-inflammatory drug oxaprozin is known to interfere with the FPIA assay of phenytoin. However, the turbidimetric assay of phenytoin on the ADVIA analyzer is virtually free from such interference [49,50].

Fosphenytoin is a physiologically inactive phosphate ester prodrug of phenytoin that provides improved efficacy and safety when given intravenously or intramuscularly. After systemic administration, the phosphate moiety is rapidly cleaved to form an unstable intermediate that breaks down to yield phenytoin and formaldehyde. Fosphenytoin is known to cross-react with various phenytoin immunoassays. Highest cross-reactivity was observed with the FPIA assay (TDx analyzer, Abbott Laboratories), while the phenytoin immunoassay on the AxSYM analyzer showed lesser effect. The Chemiluminescent assay on the ACS: 180 analyzer (Chiron Diagnostics) was also affected [51]. Roberts et al. reported falsely elevated phenytoin values when measured by immunoassays compared to HPLC in uremic patients receiving fosphenytoin. For example, in one patient with renal failure, the phenytoin concentration measured by HPLC was 5.3 μg/mL. The corresponding phenytoin concentrations as measured by immunoassays were 22.0 (ACS: 180 analyzer), 12.7 (AxSYM analyzer), and 28.0 μg/mL (TDxII analyzer). The authors studied seven hospitalized patients receiving I.V fosphenytoin. All patients had renal failure. The authors observed falsely increased total and free phenytoin values in all patients using various immunoassays. HPLC measurement of phenytoin showed much lower values. A novel metabolite of fosphenytoin (oxymethylglucuronide) which has a very high cross reactivity with immunoassays for phenytoin was responsible for such interference (see also Chapter 5) [52,53].

Crystalline decomposition product (CDP-1) of vancomycin that accumulates in uremic patients may interfere with vancomycin immunoassays (FPIA). In one report interference in the FPIA vancomycin assay was also observed in a nonuremic patient. The authors were unable to conclude whether the interference was results from CDP-1 or not [54]. Clinically significant interferences of cyclosporine metabolites in cyclosporine immunoassays have been extensively documented in the literature (see Chapters 13 and 14). Soldin et al. reported significant interferences in cyclosporine immunoassays by cyclosporine metabolites and overall degree of interference decreased from Abbott TDx polyclonal > Abbott TDx monoclonal > DiaSorin Cyclo-sp-RIA > Syva EMIT cyclosporine [55]. Metabolites of another immunosuppressant, tacrolimus also interfere with tacrolimus immunoassays [56]. Common interferences encountered with immunoassays for various therapeutic drugs are summarized in Table 3.3.

TABLE 3.3

Common Drugs and Drug Metabolites that Interfere with various Immunoassays for Therapeutic Drug Monitoring

Drug/Drug Metabolite	Immunoassay Affected	Reference
Digitoxin	Digoxin, FPIA	39
Carbamazepine	Tricyclic antidepressant, FPIA	40,41
Carbamazepine, 10, 11-epoxide	Various carbamazepine assays	42
	PENTINA: 93.6% cross-reactivity	
	FPIA: 20.8% cross-reactivity (Abbott TDx analyzer)	
	FPIA: 10.4 % cross-reactivity (Roche Cobas Integra)	
	Beckman Synchron: 7.6% cross-reactivity	
	Vitros: 0% cross-reactivity (Johnson and Johnson)	
Oxcarbazepine	Low cross-reactivity with PENTINA and EMIT carbamazepine assay	43
10-Hydroxy-Carbazepine	Low cross-reactivity with PENTINA and EMIT carbamazepine assay	43
Hydroxyzine	PENTINA carbamazepine	44
Cetirizine	PENTINA carbamazepine	44
Hydroxyzine	Tricyclic antidepressant, FPIA (Abbott)	46
Cetirizine	Tricyclic antidepressant, FPIA (Abbott)	46
5-p-Hydroxyphenyl 5-Phenylhydantoin	Phenytoin, FPIA (Abbott)	49,50
Fosphenytoin	Various phenytoin immunoassays	51
Oxymethylglucuronide	A metabolite of fosphenytoin, present in uremic patients that cross-react with phenytoin immunoassays	52,53
Crystalline degradation product-1 of vancomycin (CDP-1)	FPIA vancomycin assay	54
Cyclosporine metabolites	Various cyclosporine assays	55
Tacrolimus metabolites	Various tacrolimus assays	56

3.6 FALSE RESULTS CAUSED BY SYSTEMS ISSUES

Today most of TDM assays are performed on automated systems, where the system pipette probe automatically picks up the required volume of a specimen, dispenses it into a reaction chamber (cuvette), adds reagents, separates and washes the bound label (if required), measures the signal, and converts it into reported results. Unless the system uses disposable pipette tips or the pipette probe is washed between successive specimens, errors may occur due to "carryover" phenomenon where an immunoassay result may be falsely elevated if analyzed after a specimen which has a high concentration of the analyte. However, carry-over phenomenon is rarely observed today because of improved technologies (disposable pipet of through washing protocol between specimens, etc.).

3.7 HOW TO DETECT AND ELIMINATE INTERFERENCES

Visual inspection of a serum or plasma specimen provides valuable information reading presence of endogenous interfering factors such as hemolysis, icterus (caused by increased bilirubin) and turbidity (caused by lipids), but in practice it is often impossible to inspect the specimen visually due to labels and barcodes present on the specimen. Many automated analyzers can measure the degree of hemolysis, icterus, and turbidity in the sample and alert the operator regarding such interferences by appropriate measures. The degree of interference, if any, is noted by an "index." Dahlin found a linear relationship between serum indices and interferent concentrations: hemoglobin, $R = 0.9976$ (range 0.0–9.9 g/dL), and bilirubin, $R = 0.9851$ (range < 1.0–10.6 mg/dL) [57]. However, because of the heterogenic nature of serum lipids, lipid indexes often do not correlate with the actual triglyceride levels of the specimens.

Sample blanking and robust assay design can be used to minimize these interferences. When suspected, the interferents may be removed from the specimen by specific techniques such as ultrafiltration or centrifugation before reanalysis. Since bilirubin in plasma is mostly bound to plasma proteins, wherever possible, assay with protein-free ultrafiltrate can avoid bilirubin interference. Ultrafiltration can also be used to remove interference of heterophilic antibodies and paraproteins in immunoassays. Hemoglobin and blood substitutes, however, are soluble, and can not be removed by ultrafiltration. The interfering triglyceride particles, chylomicron, and VLDL can be removed by ultra-centrifugation (lipids remain in the supernatant).

In certain assays which are affected by heterophilic antibodies, the manufacturers may also add various heterophilic antibody blocking agents to eliminate such interferences. Several blocking agents are commercially available including Ig Inhibiting Reagent, Heterophilic Blocking Reagent (HBR; Scantibodies), Heteroblock (Omega Biologicals), and MAB 33 (monoclonal mouse IgG1) and Poly MAB 33 (polymeric monoclonal IgG1/Fab; Boehringer Mannheim).

3.8   CONCLUSION

Immunoassays on automated systems are the principle methods of TDM in clinical laboratories. For such small molecular weight analytes, mostly the "competition" types of immunoassays are used. There are various assay formats, using photometric, luminometric, or fluorimetric signals, and homogeneous or heterogeneous reaction types. Serum or plasma is the main specimen types used for TDM immunoassays. Immunoassays suffer from various interferences both from endogenous and exogenous source and such interferences may cause medical errors. It is important for the laboratory scientist to be aware of such interferences and various techniques available for resolving such interferences.

REFERENCES

1. Jolley ME, Stroupe SD, Schwenzer KS, et al. 1981. Fluorescence polarization immunoassays III. An automated system for therapeutic drug determination. *Clin Chem* 27:1575–1579.
2. Hawks RL, Chian CN, Eds. 1986. *Urine testing for drugs of abuse*. Rockville, MD: National Institute of Drug Abuse (NIDA). Department of Health and Human Services, NIDA Research Monograph 73.
3. Jeon SI, Yang X, Andrade JD. 2004. Modeling of homogeneous cloned enzyme donor immunoassay. *Anal Biochem* 333:136–147.
4. Datta P, Dasgupta A. 2003. A new turbidimetric digoxin immunoassay on the ADVIA 1650 analyzer is free from interference by spironolactone, potassium canrenoate, and their common metabolite canrenone. *Ther Drug Monit* 25:478–482.
5. Snyder JT, Benson CM, Briggs C, et al. 2008. Development of NT-proBNP, Troponin, TSH, and FT4 LOCI(R) assays on the new Dimension (R) EXL with LM clinical chemistry system [Abstract]. *Clin Chem* 54:A92.
6. Dai JL, Sokoll LJ, Chan DW. 1998. Automated chemiluminescent immunoassay analyzers. *J Clin Ligand Assay* 21:377–385.
7. Forest J-C, Masse J, Lane A. 1998. Evaluation of the analytical performance of the Boehringer Mannheim Elecsys® 2010 Immunoanalyzer. *Clin Biochem* 31:81–88.
8. Babson AL, Olsen DR, Palmieri T, et al. 1991. The IMMULITE assay tube: a new approach to heterogeneous ligand assay. *Clin Chem* 37:1521–1522.
9. Christenson RH, Apple FS, Morgan DL. 1998. Cardiac troponin I measurement with the ACCESS® immunoassay system: analytical and clinical performance characteristics. *Clin Chem* 44:52–60.
10. Montagne P, Varcin P, Cuilliere ML, Duheille J. 1992. Microparticle-enhanced nephelometric immunoassay with microsphere-antigen conjugate. *Bioconjugate Chem.* 3:187–193.

11. Armedariz Y, Garcia S, Lopez R et al. 2005. Hematocrit influences immunoassay performance for the measurement of tacrolimus in whole blood. *Ther Drug Monit* 27:766–769.
12. Kidwell D, Holland J, Athanaselis S. 1998. Testing for drugs of abuse in saliva and sweat. *J Chromatogr B* 713:111–135.
13. Pichini S, Pacifici R, Altieri I, Pellegrini M, Zuccaro P. 1999. Determination of opiates and cocaine in hair as trimethylsilyl derivatives using gas chromatography-tandem mass spectrometry. *J Anal Toxicol* 5:343–348.
14. Van Haeringen NJ. 1985. Secretion of drugs in tears. *Curr Eye Res* 4:485–488.
15. Bonati M, Kanto J, Tognoni G. 1982. Clinical pharmacokinetics of cerebrospinal fluid. *Clin Pharmacokinet* 7:312–315.
16. Wong GA, Peierce TH, Goldstein E, Hoeprich PD. 1975. Penetration of antimicrobial agents into bronchial secretion. *Am J Med* 9:219–923.
17. Fonseca-Wolheim FD. 1993. Hemoglobin interference in the bichromatic spectrophotometry of NAD(P)H at 340/380 nm. *Eur J Clin Chem Clin Biochem* 31:595–601.
18. Clinical and Laboratory Standards Institute (formerly NCCLS) Recommendation. 1986. *Interference testing in Clinical Chemistry*. Wayne, PA: Clinical and Laboratory Standards Institute Document EP7-P. 6(13): 259–371.
19. Miller JM, Valdes R Jr. 1992. Methods for calculating cross reactivity in immunoassays. *J Clin Immunoassay* 15:97–102.
20. Tietz NW. 1985. *Clinical Guide to Laboratory Tests*. 3rd Edn. Philadelphia, PA: WB Saunders Company, 88–91.
21. Perlstein MT, Thibert RJ, Watkins RJ, Zak B. 1977. Spectrophotometric study of bilirubin and hemoglobin interactions in several hydrogen peroxide generating procedures [Abstract]. *Clin Chem* 23:1133.
22. Bertholf RL, Johannsen LM, Bazooband A, Mansouri V. 2003. False-positive acetaminophen results in a hyperbilirubinemic patient. *Clin Chem* 49:695–698.
23. Kellmeyer K, Yates C, Parker S, Hilligoss D. 1982. Bilirubin interference with kit determination of acetaminophen. *Clin Chem* 28:554–555.
24. Wood FL, Earl JW, Nath C, Coakley JC. 2000. Falsely low vancomycin results using the Abbott TDx. *Ann Clin Biochem* 37:411–413.
25. Sonntag O, Glick MR. 1989. Serum-index und interferogram-ein neuer weg zur prufung und darstellung von interferengen durch serumchromogene. *Lab Med* 13:77–82.
26. Wenk RE. 1994. Mechanism of interference by hemolysis in immunoassays and requirements for sample quality. *Clin Chem* 1998:2554.
27. Chance JJ, Norris EJ, Kroll MH. 2000. Mechanism of interference of a polymerized hemoglobin blood substitute in an alkaline phosphatase method. *Clin Chem* 46:1331–1337.
28. Kroll MH. 2004. Evaluating interference caused by lipemia. *Clin Chem* 50:1968–1969.
29. Weber TH, Kaoyho KI, Tanner P. 1990. Endogenous interference in immunoassays in clinical chemistry. *Scand J Clin Lab Invest Suppl* 201:77–82.
30. Bornhorst JA, Roberts RF, Roberts WL. 2004. Assay-specific differences in lipemic interference in native and Intralipid-supplemented samples. *Clin Chem* 50:2197–2201.
31. Kazmierczak SC, Catrou PG. 2000. Analytical interference, more than just a laboratory problem. *Amer J Clin Pathol* 113:9–11.
32. Ezan E, Emmanuel A, Valente D, Grognet J-M. 1997. Effect of variability of plasma interferentes on the accuracy of drug immunoassays. *Ther Drug Monit* 19:212–218.
33. Hullin DA. 1999. An IgM paraprotein causing a falsely low result in an enzymatic assay for acetaminophen. *Clin Chem* 45:155–156.
34. Brauchili YB, Scholer A, Schwietert M, Krahenbuhl S. 2008. Undetectable phenytoin serum levels by an automated particle-enhanced turbidimetric inhibition immunoassay in a patient with monoclonal IGMλ. *Clin Chimica Acta* 389:174–176.
35. ACOG Committee on Gynecologic Practice. 2003. Avoiding inappropriate clinical decisions based on false positive human chorionic gonadotropin test results. *Int J Gynaecol Obstet* 80:231–233.
36. Marks V. 2002. False-positive immunoassay results: a multicenter survey of erroneous immunoassay results from assays of 74 analytes in 10 donors from 66 laboratories in seven countries. *Clin Chem* 48:2008–2016.
37. Papapetrou PD, Polymeris A, Karga H, Vaiopoulos G. 2006. Heterophilic antibodies causing falsely high serum calcitonin values. *J Endocrinol Invest* 29:919–923.

38. Liendo C, Ghali JK, Graves SW. 1996. A new interference in some digoxin assays: anti-murine hetero-philic antibodies. *Clin Pharmacol Ther* 60:593–598.

39. Datta P, Dasgupta A. 1998. Bidirectional (Positive/negative) interference in a digoxin immunoassay: importance of antibody specificity. *Ther Drug Monit* 20:352–357.

40. Chattergoon DS, Verjee Z, Anderson M et al. 1998. Carbamazepine interferes with an immunoassay for tricyclic antidepressant in plasma. *J Toxicol Clin Toxicol* 36:109–113.

41. Dasgupta A, McNeese C, Wells A. 2004. Interference of carbamazepine and carbamazepine 10, 11-epox-ide in the fluorescence polarization immunoassay for tricyclic antidepressants: estimation of true tricyclic antidepressant concentration in the presence of carbamazepine using a mathematical equation. *Am J Clin Pathol* 121:418–425.

42. Hermida J, Tutor JC. 2003. How suitable are currently used carbamazepine immunoassays for quantify-ing carbamazepine 10, 11-epoxide in serum samples? *Ther Drug Monit* 25:384–388.

43. Parant F, Bossu H, Gagnieu MC, Lardet G et al. 2003. Cross-reactivity assessment of carbamazepine 10, 11-epoxide, oxcarbazepine, and 10-hydroxy-carbazepine in two automated carbamazepine immunoas-says: PENTINA and EMIT 2000. *Ther Drug Monit* 25:41–45.

44. Parant F, Moulsma M, Gagnieu MC, Lardet G. 2005. Hydroxyzine and metabolite as a source of interfer-ence in carbamazepine particle-enhanced turbidimetric inhibition immunoassay (PENTINA). *Ther Drug Monit* 27:457–462.

45. Datta P, Dasgupta A. 2007. Turbidimetric carbamazepine immunoassays on the ADVIA 1650 and 2400 analyzers is free from the interference of antihistamine drugs hydroxyzine and cetirizine. *J Clin Lab Anal* 21:188–192.

46. Dasgupta A, Wells A, Datta P. 2007. False positive tricyclic antidepressant concentrations using fluores-cence polarization immunoassay due to the presence of hydroxyzine and cetirizine. *Ther Drug Monit* 29:134–139.

47. Rainey PM, Rogers KE, Roberts WL. 1996. Metabolite and matrix interference in phenytoin immunoas-say. *Clin Chem* 42:1645–1653.

48. Roberts W, Rainey P. 2004. Phenytoin overview: metabolite interference in some immunoassays could be clinically important. *Arch Pathol Lab Med* 128:734.

49. Datta P. 1997. Oxaprozin and 5-(p-hydroxyphenyl)-5-phenylhydantoin interference in phenytoin immu-noassays. *Clin Chem* 43:1468–1469.

50. Datta P, Scurlock D, Dasgupta A. 2005. Analytical performance evaluation of a new turbidimetric immu-noassay for phenytoin on the ADVIA 1650 ® analyzer: effect of phenytoin metabolite and analogue. *Ther Drug Monit* 27:305–308.

51. Datta P, Dasgupta A. 1998. Cross-reactivity of fosphenytoin in four phenytoin immunoassays. *Clin Chem* 44:696–697.

52. Roberts W, De B, Coleman J, Annesley T. 1999. Falsely increased immunoassay measurement of total and unbound phenytoin in critically ill uremic patients receiving fosphenytoin. *Clin Chem* 45:829–837.

53. Annesley T, Kurzyniec S, Nordblom G et al. 2001. Glucuronidation of prodrug reactive site: isolation and characterization of oxymethylglucuronide metabolite of fosphenytoin. *Clin Chem* 46:910–918.

54. Bowhay S, Timms P. 1997. Interference with vancomycin fluorescence polarization immunoassay in a nonuremic patient. *Ther Drug Monit* 19:117–119.

55. Soldin SJ, Steele BW, Witte DL, Wang E et al. 2003. Lack of specificity of cyclosporine immunoassays: results of a College of American pathologists Study. *Arch Pathol Lab Med* 127:19–22.

56. Murthy JN, Davis DL, Yatscoff RW, Soldin SJ. 1998. Tacrolimus metabolite cross-reactivity in different tacrolimus assays. *Clin Biochem* 31:613–617.

57. Dahlin J, Omar A, Ng HT, et al. 2006. An evßaluation of automated serum indexing on the Roche Modular Serum Work Area [Abstract]. *Clin Chem* 52:A104.

4 Introduction to Tandem Mass Spectrometry

Glen L. Hortin
University of Florida College of Medicine

CONTENTS

4.1 INTRODUCTION

Tandem mass spectrometry (MS/MS) is a set of methodologies in which there is serial linkage of two MS separations. These separation steps can be performed either by linking two mass spectrometers in series or by performing two or more separation steps sequentially over time within a single instrument. There is an increasing diversity of mass spectrometers and options for introducing specimens into mass spectrometers that permit a wide range of applications from therapeutic drug monitoring, toxicology, endocrine testing, proteomics, and metabolomics as described in reviews [1–14]. Gas chromatography (GC) for many years has been linked to MS, with many applications of GC-MS/MS. The reader is referred to other publications for examples of GC-MS/MS applications [15,16]. Capillary electrophoresis (CE) also has been used as a separation technique linked to MS/MS [17]. The major focus of the present report, though, will be on liquid chromatography (LC) linked to MS/MS, as this has been the technique with most rapid growth in MS/MS applications [1–14]. There is a complex range of options for the latter technique based on different chromatographic methods, interfaces with mass spectrometers, types of mass spectrometers, and methods for molecular fragmentation. Another recent development has been growth in techniques for direct MS/MS analysis of specimens without any chromatographic separation [18–23]. These techniques, which show promise for applications such as forensic analysis and environment sampling, will also be discussed briefly in this chapter.

Just as the technology for LC-MS/MS has evolved rapidly in recent years, there has been corresponding expansion in the range of applications of this approach. It is increasingly apparent that LC-MS/MS can provide qualitative or quantitative analysis of most molecules with great specificity and sensitivity. Common targets of analysis by this technique include therapeutic drugs, metabolites, toxins, peptides, and proteins. Strengths of LC-MS/MS include its great versatility, high analytical sensitivity and specificity, the ability to analyze many molecules with minimal preparation and usually without derivatization, and the capacity to analyze many components in a single analysis. The latter capability has been of particular interest in fields such as proteomics and metabolomics, which attempt to analyze hundreds of components in a single run. The ability to analyze many molecules without derivatization distinguishes LC-MS/MS from GC-MS. In the clinical laboratory and the field of clinical pharmacology and toxicology, application of LC-MS/ MS has grown based on the ability to perform high-throughput analyses of multiple components. LC-MS/MS frequently has shown a better specificity for analysis of target molecules than immunoassay procedures and offers the ability to distinguish parent drugs from a series of drug metabolites in a single analysis.

Key elements of LC-MS/MS include not only the LC and ion separation systems, but also sample preparation and addition of internal standards before analysis, interface between LC and MS, and the process of ion fragmentation. There are a wide range of options for chromatographic separations, interfaces, and types of mass spectrometers. Some of the limitations and advantages of different options will be presented.

4.2   SAMPLE PREPARATION FOR LC-MS/MS ANALYSIS

Like most multistep separation processes, it is important to introduce some form of internal standard if quantitative results are desired. An internal standard should be added as the first step in sample preparation, and the internal standard should be selected to have physical properties similar to the analyte of interest. The ideal internal standards usually are the compound of interest modified by incorporation of stable isotopes of carbon, hydrogen, or nitrogen at two or more positions in the molecule. This yields a compound with nearly identical physical properties except for an increase in molecular mass of two or more daltons (Da). It is desirable for the internal standard to have a mass that is more than 1 Da higher because there is a natural abundance of about 1% of ^{13}C in natural compounds as well as some occurrence of heavier isotopes of nitrogen, hydrogen, and other atoms so that there is natural occurrence of heavy isotopic forms of drugs or other compounds that would overlap with internal standards just one mass unit higher than the analyte molecule. When compounds of interest are not available in isotopically labeled forms, such as for many therapeutic drugs, other compounds with similar physical properties are selected for use as internal standards. An alternative approach for assay standardization is to use isotopically labeled reagents to differentially label multiple specimens [24,25]. This provides relative quantification of compounds in different specimens. A variety of reagents are commercially available that allow the coding of up to eight or more specimens with different isotopic tags. This approach has been used widely in proteomic and metabolomic applications where there is interest in comparing the concentrations of many different components [8,25].

The high specificity of LC-MS/MS procedures often allows relatively simple sample preparation techniques to be used [26]. A protein precipitation step may be performed to remove the large amounts of protein that is present in blood, plasma, or other biological fluids. This avoids the fouling of chromatographic columns with protein. Protein precipitation can be achieved by addition of organic solvents such as acetonitrile or by addition of acids such as trichloroacetic acid or other precipitants. Solid phase extraction is another alternative for specimen cleanup [27]. Extraction steps may be coupled online with a later chromatography step to enhance the automation and reproducibility of analyses [5,28,29]. Turbulent flow chromatography has been identified as a technique well-suited as an initial extraction step that can be coupled to subsequent LC [28,29].

LC-MS/MS can analyze most molecules without derivatization, but for analyses of some polar compounds such as amino acids [11,12] and methylmalonic acid [30], derivatization step improves specimen preparation, chromatography, and/or ionization of compounds. Derivatization of nonpolar compounds, such as steroids, has been used to enhance their ionization for MS, thereby improving detection sensitivity [31].

4.3 LIQUID CHROMATOGRAPHY COMBINED WITH MS/MS (LC-MS/MS)

LC-MS/MS imposes some limitations on the chromatographic separations. There are constraints on the flow rate that is compatible with mass spectrometry. Most salts and buffers interfere with subsequent mass spectrometric analysis by suppressing ionization of other compounds, overloading interfaces, and building up as nonvolatile deposits in interfaces. Only salts with volatile components such as ammonium acetate and ammonium formate are compatible with the mass spectrometric analysis. When running under acidic conditions formic acid and acetic acid are common additives. Other acids such as trifluoroacetic acid, which is commonly used as an ion-pairing agent for chromatography, can interfere with ionization of compounds and mass spectrometric analysis. The chromatographic system usually must have a switching valve to divert the initial nonretained components in the specimen to waste. This avoids overloading the interface with salts and other nonvolatile components in the specimen. It also means that any components that are not significantly retained by the chromatographic column are not analyzed in the mass spectrometer. Reverse-phase (RP) chromatography has been the most widely used technique for coupling to mass spectrometry. It is well-suited as an initial step before mass spectrometry, because it usually is performed with volatile solvents or low ionic strength, and most salts in specimens are not retained and can be diverted to waste. Recent advances in LC, such as use of monolithic columns, columns packed with small particles less than 2 μm in diameter, capillary columns, and microfluidic systems are well-suited for coupling to tandem mass spectrometry [5,32,33]. These advances provide more rapid chromatographic separations that improve the throughput of LC-MS/MS, and the rapid detector response times of MS usually are well matched to the sharper peaks delivered by new LC techniques. There has been recent growth in application of normal phase or hydrophilic interaction chromatography (HILIC) in which specimens are eluted with a gradient of increasingly polar solvent and the most strongly retained molecules are highly polar compounds that do not bind to reverse-phase columns [5,34,35]. HILIC is an attractive approach for trying to analyze highly polar compounds that are not retained by reverse-phase columns.

4.4 INTERFACES AND ION SOURCES FOR LC-MS/MS

Mass spectrometers are designed to separate ions within a high vacuum. Moving molecules from a liquid solvent, ionizing the molecules as isolated particles, and transferring the ions into a high vacuum present challenges. Each milliliter of solvent emerging from LC represents about 1 L of gas at atmospheric pressure. This solvent must be evaporated and removed from the interface to avoid overwhelming the vacuum system within the MS. Solvent evaporation usually is achieved by heating and dispersing the solvent into small droplets with a nebulizing gas and an applied electrical potential. The neutral solvent and nebulizing gas molecules are removed through an exhaust port, while ions are conducted into a narrow capillary inlet to the mass spectrometer. The narrow capillary inlet hinders the flow of neutral gas molecules into the mass spectrometer, allowing maintenance of a high vacuum within the mass spectrometer, while serving as a gateway for the entry of ions. A flow of gas is commonly applied at the capillary inlet (the cone gas) to impede entry of neutral molecules into the capillary. Interfaces can be operated in either positive or negative ion modes that entail collecting either positively or negatively charged ions, by reversing the potential applied in the ion source. This serves as a means of improving specificity.

Several different approaches that can be used to ionize compounds of interest at the outlet of a liquid chromatograph are listed in Table 4.1.

TABLE 4.1
Types of Ionization Sources

Ionization Source	Application
Coupled to Separation Technique	
Electrospray ionization (ESI)	Readily ionizable molecules
Electrospray ionization (ESI) with ion pairing	Neutral molecules
Atmospheric pressure chemical ionization (APCI)	Nonpolar molecules
Atmospheric pressure photoionization (APPI)	Nonpolar and difficult to ionize molecules
Nanospray electrospray ionization	Readily ionizable molecules
	Low volume specimens
Uncoupled from Separation Techniques	
Matrix-assisted laser desorption/ionization (MALDI)	Ionizable molecules,
	High mw molecules
	Molecules in tissue
Desorption/ionization on silica (DIOS)	Low mw molecules
Desorption electrospray ionization (DESI)	Molecules on surfaces
Direct analysis in real time (DART)	Ionizable molecules in solution

1. Electrospray ionization is favorable for compounds that naturally acquire charge in solution. As the solvent is evaporated away, ions are left in a dispersed form and they can be directed by an electrical potential into the mass spectrometer [36–38].
2. Neutral molecules can be ionized during electrospray ionization by pairing with an ion. This has been used to enhance ionization of immunosuppressant drugs [39,40].
3. In atmospheric pressure chemical ionization (APCI) reactive molecules are generated and transfer charge to molecules of interest [41–43].
4. In atmospheric photoionization (APPI) a light source is used to ionize molecules [42–46]. A compound (dopant) with low ionization energy such as acetone, tetrahydrofuran, or toluene may assist with photoionization by transferring energy to other molecules. The dopant may be added to LC solvent or infused with the LC outflow into the APPI source.
5. Nanospray ionization represents a special case of electrospray ionization in which flow rates are less than 1 μL/min [47–50].

The type of ion source and optimization of parameters serve as important selectivity factors in analysis. Different compounds are preferentially ionized by different types of sources as shown by a comparison of analyses with multiple sources [14]. Electrospray ionization usually is applied to molecules that readily acquire charge, while APCI or APPI are required for efficient ionization of neutral nonpolar molecules such as steroids and hydrocarbons. The ability to analyze molecules by MS depends on the ability to generate ionized forms of the molecule, so that the ionization source is critical to the efficiency and selectivity of analysis. Nanospray ionization represents a special case in that the flow of liquid is so low that there is decreased need for a nebulizer gas and the efficiency of ion capture into MS is much higher—actually approaching 100% efficiency [48]. Nanospray interfaces therefore, offer extremely high detection sensitivity. The major drawbacks and limitations of nanospray applications have been the need for specialized chromatography equipment, capillary columns, and sources that are technically demanding and not as robust for routine applications. Recent applications of microfluidic LC or microfabricated electrospray sources may assist in making nanospray techniques more amenable for routine analytical applications [49,50].

Ionization of large molecules such as proteins and other polymers present some special challenges. Oftentimes, there may be other associated molecules or ligands attached. Use of low ionization potentials allows some noncovalent complexes to remain intact and provides a tool for studying molecular interactions [51–54]. Use of higher ionization and declustering potentials separates macromolecules from other bound components, but use of too high of a potential will start to fragment macromolecules or remove groups such as sulfates [55,56]. Finally, an additional complication in the analysis of macromolecules such as proteins is that they often form ions with multiple charge states during electrospray ionization. A single protein therefore will yield ions with multiple m/z values and yield multiple peaks in MS.

There are many factors and operating parameters that affect the efficiency of ion sources in complex ways: flow rate, surface tension and viscosity of solvent, polarity and volatility of solvent, ionic strength, ion-pairing between components, source temperature, gas flow rate, source potential, and geometry of the source and MS inlet. Use of gradient elution during LC introduces a complication in that the solvent and ionization efficiency in the ion source changes throughout the run. Some compounds may decompose in the source if the temperature is set too high or they may be fragmented if the source potential is set too high.

A fundamental problem of ion sources is ion suppression [57–61]. This is a lowering of the efficiency of ionization of molecules of interest by other components in a specimen or solvents. This may represent a change in factors that influence ionization of molecules of interest or competition of different molecules in the ionization process. Ion suppression can be unpredictable if it produced by compounds that have variable concentration in the specimen matrix. A recent report notes that even different batches of purified solvents exert variable suppression of ionization [59]. The incompletely understood and unpredictable occurrence of ion suppression in ion sources emphasizes the need for internal standards in mass spectrometric analyses. To correct for ion suppression that may vary during a chromatographic run, it is desirable for an internal standard to coelute with each compound that is being analyzed. Ion suppression is one of the major reasons that isotopically labeled forms of target analytes serve as ideal internal standards. Usually, they will have nearly identical LC retention and their ionization properties will be similar to the nonisotopic forms of the analyte.

4.5   ION SOURCES NOT COUPLED TO LIQUID CHROMATOGRAPHY

There are several other ionization sources that are used without direct coupling to LC. These include matrix-assisted laser desorption/ionization (MALDI) [62–67], desorption/ionization of silica (DIOS) [68,69], desorption electrospray ionization (DESI) [18–22,70,71], and direct analysis in real time (DART) [17–19]. These techniques for ionization can be applied to molecules separated by LC or by other techniques, but would require intermediate fraction collection rather than allowing direct coupling of LC to MS.

MALDI and DIOS are techniques in which molecules are vaporized and ionized by pulses of light energy from a laser. In MALDI the specimen is dried together with a light absorbing matrix molecule, while in DIOS the specimen is dried on a porous silica surface, which serves to capture and transfer energy from the laser. A major difference in these techniques versus direct interfaces with chromatography systems is that the specimen is dried before analysis and placed within the vacuum system of the mass spectrometer. These techniques can be coupled to chromatographic separations, but intermediate fraction collection, sample application and drying are required. For low molecular weight components, MALDI has the drawback of introducing background ions from the matrix, and this background can be minimized by use of DIOS. For large molecules such as proteins, MALDI has the unique characteristic of yielding predominantly singly charged ions and this simplifies the analysis versus the multiple charge states produced by electrospray ionization, but it also means that the upper limit of mass/charge (m/z) of the mass spectrometer must be higher. This usually necessitates coupling MALDI ionization to time-of-flight (TOF) mass analyzers [65]. Some attractive characteristics of MALDI and DIOS are the ability to perform high-throughput analyses and to analyze relatively complex specimens. Another application that sets MALDI apart from electrospray ionization is the ability to perform direct analyses of solid specimens, such as tissue, after application of matrix [66,67]. Direct tissue analysis has been applied to rapid analysis and localization of drugs and metabolites in different cell types and regions within a tissue such as brain. Data from MALDI MS/MS can be processed into images of tissue distribution of compounds.

DESI is another new technique which offers the ability to perform direct analysis of surfaces [18–22,70,71]. In this technique a fine spray of ionized droplets of a solvent such as a mixture of methanol and water is directed at a surface. Some molecules on the surface are displaced and ionized, and these ions are drawn into a vacuum interface to MS. This technique has been applied to forensic testing of surfaces, such as for detection of explosive residues, environmental testing, direct analysis of tissue, and analysis of fluids after transfer onto a surface such as paper. It is suitable for performing localized sampling of tissue sections such as used for MALDI imaging of tissue [71]. DESI may be useful as an ion source for small portable mass spectrometers for field applications such as explosives detection, toxin detection, or forensic applications. For some applications such as analysis of surfaces, it may be difficult to introduce an internal standard uniformly. In these cases, DESI may have a role primarily in qualitative analysis for detecting the presence or absence of a compound.

DART is a new ion source for direct injection of liquid specimens without chromatographic separation [18–20]. In this technique, a gas is energized by a glow discharge. Ionized gas molecules are removed, leaving a stream of energized neutral gas molecules that are passed over a liquid sample. Some of the molecules in the liquid are ionized and carried to the inlet of a mass spectrometer. This technique recently has been shown to offer efficient ionization of a large variety of pharmaceutical compounds that then could be detected with high sensitivity by MS/MS [18,19].

4.6 TYPES OF MASS SPECTROMETERS

There are multiple types of mass spectrometer used for separations of ions in tandem mass spectrometry. These include: quadrapole, ion trap, TOF, Fourier-transform ion cyclotron (FTICR), Orbitrap, accelerator, and magnetic sector mass spectrometers as well as ion mobility spectrometers. All of these mass analyzers separate ions in a vacuum based on m/z, except for ion mobility spectrometers. The latter type of instrument performs separations in a flight tube containing a gas, so that the mobility of the ion depends on the shape of the molecule as well as on m/z [72–74]. This can be quite useful in that it serves as a potential means of separating ions that have identical m/z and it is a complementary separation technique in series with other mass analyzers. In other mass analyzers performing separations in a vacuum, molecular shape has no influence on separations.

Each type of mass spectrometer has particular characteristics that contribute to or limit its suitability for particular types of analyses [8,9]. Quadrapole mass spectrometers are some of the most frequently used instruments for quantitative analysis. They consist of four parallel rods to which electrical and radiofrequency signals are applied and they serve as a filter, which selects ions of a particular m/z depending on the applied potentials. They are relatively compact and inexpensive and allow continuous analysis of a stream of ions. Ion traps serve as electromagnetic bottles, which collect ions for a period of time and then selectively retain or eject ions depending on their m/z. This provides a discontinuous cyclic analysis of ions. Traps usually have a capacity for only a few thousand ions, so that there is a need for gating of ion inputs to avoid overload and dynamic range for quantitative analysis can be limited. Recent development of linear ion traps has increased the ion capacity of this type instruments, however. TOF mass spectrometers separate ions based on acceleration down a flight tube and measuring how long it takes for ions to reach the end. These instruments tend to be larger in size, as flight tubes may be up to a meter or more in length for high-performance instruments. Analysis is discontinuous as ions must be injected as a brief pulse with all ions starting at the same time. FTICR, Orbitrap, magnetic sector, and accelerator instruments are massive,

TABLE 4.2
Types and Characteristics of Mass Spectrometers

Mass Spectrometer	Resolution	Mass Accuracy	Dynamic Range	Upper Limit of m/z	Ability to Scan All Ions
Quadrupole (Q)	Medium	Medium	High	Low	Low
Ion trap	Low	Low	Medium	Medium	High
Time-of-flight (TOF)	High	High	Medium	High	High
FTICR and Orbitrap	Very high	Very high	Medium	Medium	High

expensive instruments with very high resolution that usually are applied to complex research applications; readers are referred to other sources for discussion of these instruments [75–79].

Some of the characteristics of quadrupole, ion trap, and TOF mass spectrometers are listed in Table 4.2. Important characteristics include mass accuracy (how precisely and accurately mass can be determined, usually expressed in parts per million), resolution (the ability to separate ions that have very close m/z values, usually expressed as the peak width at half-height divided by m/z), detection sensitivity (limit of detection), upper limit of m/z that can be analyzed, and dynamic range. Each type of mass spectrometer has advantages and disadvantages, depending on the desired application. In general, quadrupole mass spectrometers offer moderate mass accuracy and mass resolution, and have an upper limit of m/z of about 1000–3000. The strengths of quadrupole mass spectrometers are a high dynamic range and sensitive detection based on continuous ion monitoring. Ion trap mass spectrometers have low mass accuracy, low resolution, upper mass limits of about 2000–5000, and low dynamic range. This technology offers good limits of detection and the ability to scan rapidly over a wide range of masses. TOF mass spectrometer come in a wide range of different forms from very small low performance instruments to massive instruments with flight tubes up to two meters or more in length. High-performance TOF instruments can achieve high mass accuracy of about 1 ppm and resolution about 10-fold higher than quadrapole instruments. Limits of detection and dynamic range have not been as good as for quadrupole instruments, but these have improved with recent advances. TOF instruments can analyze ions with very high m/z (>100,000) so that they are utilized in conjunction with MALDI sources for the analysis of proteins [65]. The limiting factor in the analysis of large ions often is the detector rather than the ability of the mass spectrometer to resolve the ions [80].

4.7 TANDEM MASS SPECTROMETRY (MS/MS)

MS/MS entails the sequential use of two or more MS separations with a fragmentation step interposed between the separations. MS/MS can be performed by linking two mass spectrometers in series or by performing sequential MS separations over time in an ion trap instruments. In an ion trap it is possible to retain a specific precursor ion, to fragment it, and then to analyze the resulting fragments all within a single mass spectrometer. In fact, it is possible to perform multiple sequential stages of mass selection and fragmentation MS^n, where n refers to the number of steps of mass spectrometric selection. This capability can be of value in identification of molecules or characterization of complex structures such as post-translationally modified peptides.

Various combinations of mass spectrometers have been used such as triple quadrupole (Q-Q-Q), Q-Q-TOF, Q-Q-ion trap, or TOF-TOF instruments [8,81,82]. In some of these tandem mass spectrometers, the second quadrupole is used as a collision cell, where a small amount of collision gas is added to induce fragmentation of precursor ions selected in the first stage MS. The third mass spectrometer is used to analyze the resulting fragment ions.

Triple quadrupole instruments have been the most widely used instruments for quantitative analysis of therapeutic drugs. This technology offers high detection sensitivity related to the ability to continuously monitor the stream of ions from the ion source and low background. The first quadrapole selects the precursor ion and the third quadrupole selects a specific fragment ion for analysis to perform so-called selected reaction monitoring (SRM). Multiple components, including an internal standard, can be analyzed by rapid switching of the selected precursor and/or fragment ions. This allows detection of up to 50 or more components and also has been termed multiple reaction monitoring (MRM) [83]. Accurate quantification can be achieved by ratioing signal intensities versus signals for an internal standard and relating the ratio to a calibration curve. The dynamic range of measurements often extends to as much as four orders of magnitude. The one major drawback of this form of analysis, however, is that only preselected components and a few of their fragment ions are detected.

For efforts at discovery of new molecular components or where extensive qualitative information is desired, ion trap and TOF instruments can be advantageous. Ion traps have been of great value in sequencing of peptides and identification of post-translational modifications, because they are facile at rapidly scanning a full spectrum of fragments derived from fragmentation of a single precursor ion. Q-Q-ion trap mass spectrometers combine some of the favorable characteristics of triple quadrapole and ion trap instruments. They have value in applications such as peptide sequencing and drug screening, where there is interest in rapid qualitative identification of components and analysis of complete fragment ion spectra rather than only one or two selected fragment ions [83–86]. High-performance Q-Q-TOF mass spectrometers are well-suited for identifying unknown components, because the high mass accuracy of TOF essentially yields the molecular formula for small molecules and narrows the search of unknowns to a much small number of compounds than for instruments with lower mass accuracy [82,83]. Q-Q-TOF mass spectrometers also can provide a full scan of precursor ions or fragments of a selected precursor ion. Therefore, they are well-suited for applications in metabolomics or proteomics where there is an interest in scanning the full complement of molecules in a specimen and to perform identifications of the components.

4.8 FRAGMENTATION OF IONS

Tandem mass spectrometry depends on the fragmentation of precursor ions selected in the first stage MS to yield fragment ions with different m/z. Precursor ions are selected within a m/z range of about ± 1, and, for complex specimens, there are likely to be ions representing multiple compounds within this range of m/z. Specificity for the ion of interest is improved by breaking it into characteristic fragment ions that will differ from most contaminants. Fragmentation is achieved most frequently by collision induced dissociation (CID), in which ions are collided with molecules of gases such as argon, helium, or nitrogen. The energy of collisions can be varied by adjusting the acceleration of ions within the collision cell. The optimal energy for fragmentation will vary for different ions, and this is another parameter requiring optimization to achieve maximal sensitivity and specificity. Fragmentation also can be achieved by other techniques that transfer energy to ions, such as electron transfer dissociation (ETD) [87]. In this technique, an electron donor is infused into the fragmentation cell and transfers electrons to ions. ETD has been used particularly for the analysis of peptide phosphorylation and other modifications, as it yields ions that retain the peptide modifications. CID tends to yield ions in which some peptide modifications are preferentially removed.

An example of the fragmentation of cortisol by CID in triple quadrapole MS is shown in Figure 4.1. In this example, cortisol, a molecule with mass of 362.47, forms singly charged positive ions by protonation with theoretical $m/z = 363.48$, and this ion is the major peak in components analyzed by the first quadrupole. When the peak at $m/z = 363$ is selected as the precursor ion by the first quadrupole and the fragment ion spectrum is analyzed by the third quadrupole, the major peak observed has $m/z = 121$ generated by fragmentation as diagramed in Figure 4.1. This type of analysis is performed in establishing a new method for a compound such as cortisol; favorable precursor and fragment ions are identified by continuous infusion of a standard solution. Once optimal precursor and fragment ions are identified, selected ion monitoring is

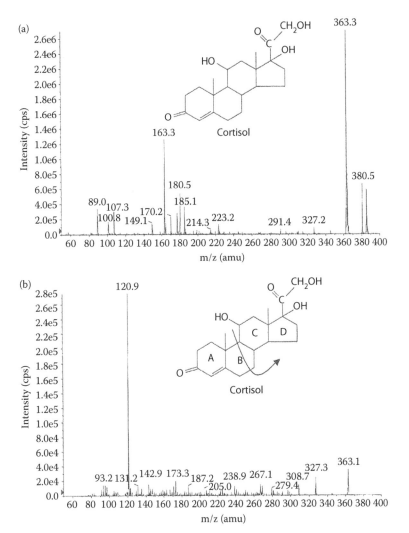

FIGURE 4.1 ESI spectrum of cortisol in positive ion mode analyzed by triple quadrapole MS. (a) Ions separated by the first quadrapole. The protonated ion of cortisol is at m/z = 363. (b) Fragment ion spectrum analyzed by the third quadrapole of the precursor ion at m/z = 363. (Reproduced from Taylor RL, Machacek D, Singh RJ, *Clin Chem,* 48, 1511–1519, 2002. With permission.)

performed in which the triple quadrapole mass spectrometer analyzes only the 363 precursor and 121 fragment ions rather than a complete scan of all ions generated. This allows rapid switching between different components such as cortisol, other steroids, and internal standards during a chromatographic run.

An alternative mode of fragmentation that can be used in MALDI TOF TOF tandem MS is laser-induced fragmentation. The initial desorption and ionization of molecules by MALDI imparts energy that leads to post-source decay of ions. MALDI TOF TOF serves as a rapid means of acquiring qualitative information about components observed in a complex mixture. This can be applied to rapid sequence identification of peptides as described in Figure 4.2 or to quantitative analysis by addition of appropriate internal standards. In the top panel of Figure 4.2, analysis of the mixture of peptides by a single stage of TOF is shown. In the middle panel, the selection of the precursor ion at *m/z* = 1046.55 is presented. The bottom panel shows the fragment spectrum derived from this precursor. The fragment spectrum derived from cleavages along the peptide chain can

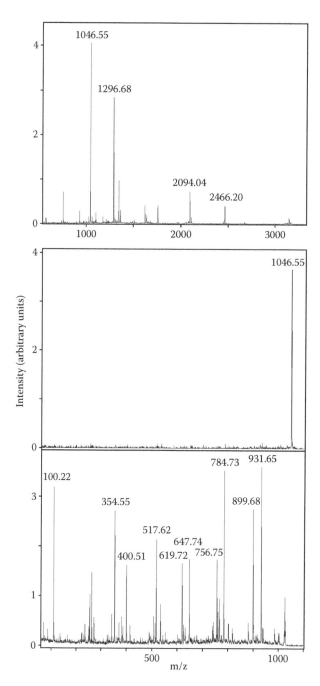

FIGURE 4.2 MALDI TOF TOF MS analysis of a peptide mixture. Top: Analysis of spectrum of ions by TOF MS analysis. Middle: Selection of a single precursor ion at m/z = 1046.55 in the first stage TOF. Bottom: Analysis by tandem TOF MS of fragment ions derived from the precursor with m/z = 1,046.55. (Courtesy of Dr. Steven Drake, Critical Care Medicine Department at the National Institutes of Health Clinical Center.)

be analyzed by computerized database searches to identify the peptide as angiotensin II with the sequence: AspArgValTyrIleHisProPhe which has calculated a mass of 1046.54 for a singly proto-nated ion. The TOF TOF MS analysis is better suited to examining complete spectra of fragments than is triple quadrapole MS. Other important characteristics of the TOF TOF MS analysis for qualitative analysis are its higher upper limit of *m/z* and its higher mass accuracy, which allows determining the mass of fragment ions accurate to two or three decimal places versus accuracy to about one decimal place for quadrapole analysis. The mass accuracy is important for molecular identification.

4.9   ION DETECTORS FOR MASS SPECTROMETERS

All mass spectrometric techniques, including MS/MS require some means of detecting the ions that are resolved in the instrument. Most instruments rely on colliding the ions with a detector at the outlet of the mass spectrometer. Usually, the detectors are some form of electron multiplier, such as a microchannel plate. As ions strike the surface of the detector, electrons are displaced, and the signal is amplified by an electron multiplier cascade. Signal intensity from the detector depends on the number of ions reaching the detector and the energy of the ions [65]. Microchannel plates offer very rapid response times that are necessary for TOF analysis. For high-resolution TOF analysis digitizers operate in the GHz range. Microchannel plate detectors tend to have diminished response with ions with high m/z and specialized superconducting detectors have been developed that allow detection of individual ions with high m/z [80].

An alternative means of detection is used in FTICR MS [75–77]. These instruments monitor the electromagnetic signals generated by moving ions. High sensitivity can be achieved by accumulating signals over a period of time.

4.10   APPLICATIONS OF TANDEM MASS SPECTROMETRY (MS/MS)

The range of potential applications of tandem mass spectrometry is virtually unlimited due to its high specificity, high sensitivity, high accuracy and precision of quantitative analysis, broad dynamic range, and capacity for simultaneous analysis of multiple components. Over the past decade, advances in instrumentation, have lowered the limits of detection of instruments by about two orders of magnitude and have substantially increased the range of molecules that can be analyzed. The linkage of serial separation technologies such as LC-MS/MS, provide high specificity for analysis that allow molecules to be analyzed with minimal sample preparation of complex matrices such as blood or plasma.

A sampling of some applications of tandem mass spectrometry is provided in Table 4.3. This table is meant to illustrate a sampling of diversity of techniques that can be used for sample preparation, internal standards, interfaces/ion sources, and MS techniques. These examples illustrate that there is no single approach for implementing MS/MS methods. Mass spectrometric methods cannot resolve stereoisomers, so resolution of stereoisomers requires chiral chromatography prior to MS/MS analysis [88]. In some analyses, it may be desirable to switch between negative and positive ion modes to provide optimal analyses of multiple components as in the case of a steroid profile [89]. A small sampling of the wide range of molecules analyzed by MS/MS include steroid hormones [89], amino acids [11,90], aminoglycosides [91], antidepressants [92], antiepileptic drugs [93], C-peptide [94], anabolic steroids [95], estrogens [96], thyroid hormones [97], and antiretroviral drugs [98].

Although LC-MS/MS delivers a high degree of specificity in analysis, a cautionary note is indicated by a number of observed examples where false-positive qualitative results or measurement errors in quantitative analyses can occur [99]. A number of measures were identified that help avoid these errors—use of stable isotope internal standards, checking of LC retention times, measurement of more than one fragment ion, and identifying narrow tolerances for the ratio between different fragment ions. Analysis of full scans of precursor and fragment ions also may help identify potential interferences as opposed to monitoring ions at only a few m/z values in selected ion monitoring. The findings in this report indicate the need to apply strict standards of data analysis and to remain vigilant for potential interferences.

TABLE 4.3
Examples of the Diversity of Methods used for MS/MS Applications

Compound/Internal Standard	Specimen	Separation Technique	Interface/Ion Source	MS/MS	Reference
Aminoglycosides/none	Serum	HILIC-HPLC	ESI (+)	Q-Q-Q	91
S/R-metoprolol/S/R propanolol	Plasma	Chiral-HPLC	ESI (+)	Ion trap	88
Amino acids/methionine sulfone	Tissue	CE	ESI (+)	Ion trap	90
Methylmalonic acid/ d$_3$-methylmalonic acid	Plasma	RP-HPLC of dibutyl derivative	ESI (−)	Q-Q-Q	30
Cyclosporine/Ritonavir	Blood	RP-HPLC with step elution	ESI (+ion pair)	Q-Q-Q	39
Steroids/deuterated cognates	Serum	RP-HPLC	APPI (+ and −) (polarity switching)	Q-Q-Q	89
L-235 (drug)/L-371 (drug)	Plasma	Solid phase extraction	MALDI (+)	Q-Q-Q	64

4.11 CONCLUSIONS

Rapid evolution of technology provides an increasingly broader range of options for performing MS/MS in routine clinical and analytical laboratories. For many routine quantitative applications triple quadrapole MS may continue to be the most popular option, but there are likely to be coupling of these instruments to microfluidic or other relatively new LC techniques or to new types of ion sources. Addition of ion mobility spectrometry ahead of MS/MS provides another potential tool for improving specificity of measurements as it serves as a complementary separation technique to MS. Availability of new hybrid tandem mass spectrometers that incorporate ion traps or TOF as the final separation offer more extensive qualitative analyses and better identification of unknown molecules.

ACKNOWLEDGMENT

The author thanks Dr. Steven Drake for suggestions.

REFERENCES

1. Yang Z, Wang S. 2008. Recent developments in application of high performance liquid chromatography-tandem mass spectrometry in therapeutic drug monitoring of immunosuppressants. *J Immunol Methods* 336:98–103.
2. Saint-Marcoux F, Sauvage FL, Marquet P. 2007. Current role of LC-MS in therapeutic drug monitoring. *Anal Bioanal Chem* 388:1327–1349.
3. Holcapek M, Kolarova L, Nobilis M. 2008. High-performance liquid chromatography-tandem mass spectrometry in the identification and determination of phase I and phase II drug metabolites. *Anal Bioanal Chem* 391:59–78.
4. Hsieh Y. 2008. HPLC-MS/MS in drug metabolism and pharmacokinetic screening. *Expert Opin Drug Metab Toxicol* 4:93–101.
5. Xu RN, Fan L, Rieser MJ, El-Shourbagy TA. 2007. Recent advances in high-throughput quantitative bioanalysis by LC-MS/MS. *J Pharm Biomed Anal* 44:342–355.
6. Maurer HH. 2007. Current role of liquid chromatography-mass spectrometry in clinical and forensic toxicology. *Anal Bioanal Chem* 388:1315–1325.

7. Politi L. Groppi A, Polettini A. 2005. Applications of liquid chromatography-mass spectrometry in doping control. *J Anal Toxicol* 29:1–14.

8. Domon B, Aebersold R. 2006. Mass spectrometry and protein analysis. *Science* 312:212–217.

9. Glish GL, Burinsky DJ. 2008. Hybrid mass spectrometers for tandem mass spectrometry. *J Am Soc Mass Spectrom* 19:161–172.

10. Vogeser M, Parthofer KG. 2007. Liquid chromatography tandem mass spectrometry (LC-MS/MS)—technique and applications in endocrinology. *Exp Clin Endocrinol Diabetes* 115:559–570.

11. Chace DH, Kalas TA. 2005. A biochemical perspective on the use of tandem mass spectrometry for newborn screening and clinical testing. *Clin Biochem* 38:296–309.

12. Turecek F, Sott CR, Gelb MH. 2007. Tandem mass spectrometry in the detection of inborn errors of metabolism for newborn screening. *Methods Mol Biol* 359:143–157.

13. Vogeser M, Seger C. 2008. A decade of HPLC-MS/MS in the routine clinical laboratory—goals for further developments. *Clin Biochem* 41:649–662.

14. Nordstrom A, Want E, Northen T, Lehtio J, Siuzdak G. 2008. Multiple ionization mass spectrometry strategy used to reveal the complexity of metabolomics. *Anal Chem* 80:421–429.

15. Garrido Frenich A, Plaza-Bolanos P, Martinez Vidal JL. 2008. Comparison of tandem-in-space and tandem-in-time mass spectrometry in gas chromatography determination of pesticides: application to simple and complex food samples. *J Chromatogr A* 1203:229–238.

16. Cognard E, Bouchonnet S, Staub C. 2006. Validation of a gas chromatography- ion trap tandem mass spectrometry for simultaneous analysis of cocaine and its metabolites in saliva. J *Pharm Biomed Anal* 41:925–934.

17. Elgstoen KB, Zhao JY, Anacleto JF, Jellum E. 2001. Potential of capillary electrophoresis, tandem mass spectrometry and coupled capillary electrophoresis-tandem mass spectrometry as diagnostic tools. *J Chromatogr A* 914:265–275.

18. Cooks RG, Ouyang Z, Takats Z, Wiseman JM. 2006. Ambient mass spectrometry. *Science* 311:1566–1570.

19. Zhao Y, Lam M, Wu D, Mak R. 2008. Quantification of small molecules in plasma with direct analysis in real time tandem mass spectrometry, without sample preparation and liquid chromatographic separation. *Rapid Commun Mass Spectrom* 22:3217–3224.

20. Wells JM, Roth MJ, Keil AD, Grossenbacher JW, Justes DR, Patterson GE, Barket DJ Jr. 2008. Implementation of DART and DESI ionization on a fieldable mass spectrometer. *J Am Soc Mass Spectrom* 19:1419–1424.

21. Zhao M, Zhang S, Yang C, Xu Y, Wen Y, Sun L, Zhang X. 2008. Desorption electrospray tandem MS (DESI-MSMS) analysis of methyl centralite and ethyl centralite as gunshot residues on skin and other surfaces. *J Forensic Sci* 53:807–811.

22. Lin Z, Zhang S, Zhao M, Yang C, Chen D, Zhang X. 2008. Rapid screening of clenbuterol in urine samples by desorption electrospray ionization tandem mass spectrometry. *Rapid Commun Mass Spectrom* 22:1882–1888.

23. Wiseman JM, Ifa DR, Zhu Y, Kissinger CB, Manicke NE, Kissinger PT, Cooks RG. 2008. Desorption electrospray ionization mass spectrometry: imaging drugs and metabolites in tissues. *Proc Natl Acad Sci USA* 105: 18120–18125.

24. Julka S, Regnier F. 2004. Quantification in proteomics through stable isotope coding: a review. *J Proteome Res* 3:644–652.

25. Griffin TJ, Xie H, Bandhakavi S, Popko J, Mohan A, Carlis JV, Higgins L. 2007. iTRAQ reagent-based quantitative proteomic analysis on a linear ion trap mass spectrometer. *J Proteome Res* 6:4200–4209.

26. Annesley TM. 2004. Simple extraction protocol for analysis of immunosuppressant drugs in whole blood. *Clin Chem* 50:1845–1848.

27. Gilar M, Bouvier ESP, Compton BJ. 2001. Advances in sample preparation in electromigration, chromatographic, and mass spectrometric separation methods. *J Chromatogr A* 909:111–135.

28. Mullett WM. 2007. Determination of drugs in biological fluids by direct injection of samples for liquid-chromatographic analysis. *J Biochem Biophys Methods* 70:263–273.

29. Zeng W, Musson DG, Fisher AL, Chen L, Schwartz MS, Woolf EJ, Wang AQ. 2008. Determination of sitagliptin in human urine and hemodialysate using turbulent flow online extraction and tandem mass spectrometry. *J Pharm Biomed Anal* 46:534–542.

30. Schmedes A, Brandslund I. 2006. Analysis of methylmalonic acid in plasma by liquid chromatography-tandem mass spectrometry. *Clin Chem* 52:754–757.

31. Higashi T, Shimada K. 2004. Derivatization of neutral steroids to enhance their detection characteristics in liquid chromatography-mass spectrometry. *Anal Bioanal Chem* 378:875–882.

32. Sung WC Makamba H, Chen SH. 2005. Chip-based microfluidic devices coupled with electrospray ionization-mass spectrometry. *Electrophoresis* 26:1783–1791.

33. Almeida R, Mosoarca C, Chirita M, Udrescu V, Dinca N, Vukelic Z, Allen M, Zamfir AD. 2008. Couple of fully automated chip-based electrospray ionization to high-capacity ion trap mass spectrometer for ganglioside analysis. *Anal Biochem* 378:43–52.

34. Hsieh Y. 2008. Potential of HILIC-MS in quantitative bioanalysis of drugs and drug metabolites. *J Sep Sci* 331:1481–1491.

35. Nguyen HP, Schug KA. 2008. The advantages of ESI MS detection in conjunction with HILIC mode separations: fundamentals and applications. *J Sep Sci* 31:1465–1480.

36. Cech NB, Enke CG. 2001. Practical implications of some recent studies in electrospray ionization fundamentals. *Mass Spectrom Rev* 20:362–387.

37. Leito I, Herodes K, Huopolainen M, Virro K, Kunnapas A, Kruve A, Tanner R. 2008. Towards the electrospray ionization mass spectrometry ionization efficiency scale of organic compounds. *Rapid Commun Mass Spectrom* 22:379–384.

38. Page JS, Kelly RT, Tang K, Smith RD. 2007. Ionization and transmission efficiency in an electrospray ionization-mass spectrometry interface. *J Am Soc Mass Spectrom* 18:1582–1590.

39. Volosov A, Napoli KL, Soldin SJ. 2001. Simultaneous simple and fast quantification of three major immunosuppressants by liquid chromatography-tandem mass-spectrometry. *Clin Biochem* 34:285–290.

40. Streit F, Armstrong VW, Oellerich M. 2002. Rapid liquid chromatography-tandem mass spectrometry routine method for simultaneous determination of sirolimus, everolimus, tacrolimus, and cyclosporine A in whole blood. *Clin Chem* 48:955–958.

41. Herrera LC, Grossert JS, Ramaley L. 2008. Quantitative aspects of and ionization mechanisms in positive-ion atmospheric pressure chemical ionization mass spectrometry. *J Am Soc Mass Spectrom* 19:1926–1941.

42. Van Berkel GJ. 2003. An overview of some recent developments in ionization methods for mass spectrometry. *Eur J Mass Spectrom* 9:539–562.

43. Hayen H, Karst U. 2003. Strategies for the liquid chromatographic-mass spectrometric analysis of nonpolar compounds. *J Chromatogr A* 1000:549–565.

44. Purcell JM, Hendrickson CL, Rodgers RP, Marshall AG. 2006. Atmospheric pressure photoionization fourier transform ion cyclotron resonance mass spectrometry for complex mixture analysis. *Anal Chem* 78:5906–5912.

45. Robb DB, Blades MW. 2008. State-of-the-art in atmospheric pressure photoionization for LC/MS. *Anal Chim Acta* 627:34–49.

46. Guo T, Taylor RL, Singh RJ, Soldin SJ. 2006. Simultaneous determination of 12 steroids by isotope dilution liquid chromatography-photospray ionization tandem mass spectrometry. *Clin Chim Acta* 372:76–82.

47. Wickremsinhe ER, Singh G, Ackermann BL, Gillespie TA, Chaudhary AK. 2006. A review of nanospray ionization applications for drug metabolism and pharmacokinetics. *Curr Drug Metab* 7:913–928.

48. Smith RD. 2006. Future directions for electrospray ionization for biological analysis using mass spectrometry. *Biotechniques* 41:147–148.

49. Yin H, Killeen K, Brennen R, Sobek D, Werlich M, van de Goor T. 2005. Microfluidic chip for peptide analysis of an integrated HPLC column, sample enrichment column, and nanoelectrospray tip. *Anal Chem* 77:527–533.

50. Zhang S, Van Pelt CK, Henion JD. 2003. Automated chip-based nanoelectrospray-mass spectrometry for rapid identification of proteins separated by two-dimensional gel electrophoresis. *Electrophoresis* 24:3620–3632.

51. Hewavitharana AK, Shaw PN. 2005. Enhancing the ratio of molecular ions to non-covalent compounds in the electrospray interface of LC-MS in quantitative analysis. *Anal Bioanal Chem* 382:1055–1059.

52. Hofstadler SA, Sannes-Lowery KA. 2006. Applications of ESI-MS in drug discovery: interrogation of noncovalent complexes. *Nat Rev Drug Discov* 5:585–595.

53. Burkitt WI, Derrick PJ, Lafitte D, Bronstein I. 2003. Protein-ligand and protein-protein interactions studied by electrospray ionization and mass spectrometry. *Biochem Soc Trans* 31:985–989.

54. Yin S, Xie Y, Loo J. 2008. A. Mass spectrometry of protein-ligand complexes: enhanced gas-phase stability of ribonuclease-nucleotide complexes. *J Am Soc Mass Spectrom* 19:1199–1208.

55. Singh R, Crow FW, Babic N, Lutz WH, Lieske JC, Larson TS, Kumar R. 2007. A liquid chromatographic-mass spectrometry method for the quantification of urinary albumin using a novel 15N-isotopically labeled albumin internal standard. *Clin Chem* 53:540–542.

56. Wolfender JL, Chu F, Ball H, Wolfender F, Fainzilber M, Baldwin MA, 1999. Burlingame AL. Identification of tyrosine sulfation in Conus pennaceus conotoxins a-PnIA and a-PnIB: further investigation of labile sulfo- and phosphopeptides by electrospray, matrix-assisted laser desorption/ionization (MALDI) ant atmospheric pressure MALDI mass spectrometry. *J. Mass Spectrom* 34:447–454.

57. Annesley TM. 2003. Ion suppression in mass spectrometry. *Clin Chem* 49:1041–1044.

58. Kostiainen R, Kauppila TJ. 2008. Effect of eluent on the ionization process in liquid chromatography-mass spectrometry. *J Chromatogr A* 1216: 685–699.

59. Annesley TM. 2007. Methanol-associated matrix effects in electrospray ionization tandem mass spectrometry. *Clin Chem* 53:1827–1834.

60. Taylor PJ. 2005. Matrix effects: the Achilles heel of quantitative high-performance liquid chromatography-electrospray-tandem mass spectrometry. *Clin Biochem* 38:328–334.

61. Leverence R, Avery MJ, Kavetskaia O, Bi H, Hop CE, Gusev AI. 2007. Signal suppression/enhancement in HPLC-ESI-MS/MS from concomitant medications. *Biomed Chromatogr* 21:1143–1150.

62. Gogichaeva NV, Williams T, Alterman MA. 2007. MALDI TOF/TOF tandem mass spectrometry as a new tool for amino acid analysis. *J Am Soc Mass Spectrom* 18:279–284.

63. Van Kampen JJ, Burgers PC, Gruters RA, Osterhaus AD, de Groot R, Luider TM, Volmer DA. 2008. Quantitative analysis of antiretroviral drugs in lysates of peripheral blood mononuclear cells using MALDI-triple quadrapole mass spectrometry. *Anal Chem* 80:4969–4975.

64. Volmer DA, Sleno L, Bateman K, Sturino C, Oballa R, MauialaT, Corr J. 2007. Comparison of MALDI to ESI on a triple quadrapole platform for pharmacokinetic analyses. *Anal Chem* 79:9000–9006.

65. Hortin GL. 2006. The MALDI TOF mass spectrometric view of the plasma proteome and peptidome. *Clin Chem* 52:1223–1237.

66. Cornett DS, Frappier SL, Caprioli RM. 2008. MALDI-FTICR imaging mass spectrometry of drugs and metabolites in tissue. *Anal Chem* 80:5648–5653.

67. Reyzer ML, Caprioli RM. 2007. MALDI-MS-based imaging of small molecules and proteins in tissues. *Curr Opin Chem Biol* 11:29–35.

68. Peterson DS. 2007. Matrix-free methods for laser desorption/ionization mass spectrometry. *Mass Spectrom Rev* 26:19–34.

69. Northen TR, Woo HK, Northen MT, Nordstrom A, Uritboonthail W, Turner KL, Siuzdak G. 2007. High surface area of porous silicon drives desorption of intact molecules. *J Am Soc Mass Spectrom* 18:1945–1949.

70. Kauppila TJ, Talaty N, Kuuranne T, Kotiaho T, Kostianinen R, Cooks RG. 2007. Rapid analysis of metabolites and drugs of abuse from urine samples by desorption electrospray ionization-mass spectrometry. *Analyst* 132:868–675.

71. Kertesz V, Ban berkel GJ, Vavrek M, Koeplinger KA, Schneider BB, Covey TR. 2008. Comparison of drug distribution images from whole-body thin sections obtained using desorption electrospray ionization tandem mass spectrometry and autoradiography. *Anal Chem* 80: 5168–5177.

72. Kanu AB, Dwivedi P, Tam M, Hill HH Jr. 2008. Ion-mobility-mass spectrometry. *J Mass Spectrom* 43:1–22.

73. Xia YQ, Wu ST, Jemal M. 2008. LC-FAIMS-MS/MS for quantification of a peptide in plasma and evaluation of FAIMS global selectivity from plasma components. *Anal Chem* 80:7137–7143.

74. McCullough BJ, Kalapothakis J, Eastwood H, Kemper P, MacMillan D, Taylor K, Dorin J, Barran PE. 2008. Development of an ion mobility quadrapole time of flight mass spectrometer. *Anal Chem* 80:6336–6344.

75. Brancia FL. 2006. Recent developments in ion-trap mass spectrometry and related technologies. *Expert Rev Proteomics* 3:143–151.

76. Rompp A, Taban IM, Mihalca R, Duursma MC, Mize TH, McDonnel LA, Heeren RM. 2005. Examples of Fourier transform ion cyclotron resonance mass spectrometry developments: from ion physics to remote access biochemical mass spectrometry. *Eur J Mass Spectrom* 11:443–456.

77. Perry RH, Cooks RG, Noll RJ. 2008. Orbitrap mass spectrometry: instrumentation, ion motion and applications. *Mass Spectrom Rev* 27:661–699.

78. Payne AH, Glish GL. 2005. Tandem mass spectrometry in quadrapole ion trap and ion cyclotron resonance mass spectrometers. *Methods Enzymol* 402:109–148.

79. Bereman MS, Lyndon MM, Dixon RB, Muddiman DC. 2008. Mass measurement accuracy comparisons between a double-focusing magnetic sector and a time-of-flight mass analyzer. *Rapid Commun Mass Spectrom* 22:1563–1566.

80. Twerenbold D, Gerber D, Gritti D, Gonin Y, Netuschill A, Rossel F, Schenker D, Vuilleumier JL. 2001. Single molecule detector for mass spectrometry with mass independent detection efficiency. *Proteomics* 1:66–69.

81. Spyridaki MH, Kiousi P, Vonaparti A, Valavani P, Zonaras V, Zahariou M, Sianos E, Tsoupras G, Georgakopoulos C. 2006. Doping control analysis in human urine by liquid chromatography-electro-spray ionization ion trap mass spectrometry for the Olympic Games Athens 2004: determination of corticosteroids and quantification of ephedrines, salbutamol, and morphine. *Anal Chim Acta* 573:242–249.

82. Bristow T, Constantine J, Harrison M, Cavoit F. 2008. Performance optimization of a new-generation orthogonal-acceleration quadrapole-time-of-flight mass spectrometer. *Rapid Commun Mass Spectrom* 22:1213–1222.

83. Chernushevich IV, Loboda AV, Thomson BA. 2001. An introduction to quadrapole-time-of-flight mass spectrometry. *J Mass Spectrom* 36:849–865.

84. Anderson L, Hunter CL. 2006. Quantitative mass spectrometric multiple reaction monitoring assays for major plasma proteins. *Mol Cell Proteomics* 5:573–588.

85. Sauvage FL, Saint-Marcoux F, Duretz B, Deporte D, Lachatre G, Marquet P. 2006. Screening of drugs and toxic compounds with liquid chromatography-linear ion trap tandem mass spectrometry. *Clin Chem* 52:1735–1742.

86. King R, Fernandez-Metzler C. 2006. The use of Qtrap technology in drug metabolism. *Curr Drug Metab* 7:541–545.

87. Cooper HJ, HakanssonK, Marshall AG. 2005. The role of electron capture dissociation in biomolecular analysis. *Mass Spectrom Rev* 24:201–222.

88. Jensen BP, Sharp CF, Gardiner SJ, Begg EJ. 2008. Development and validation of a stereoselective liquid chromatography-tandem mass spectrometry assay for quantification of S- and R-metoprolol in human plasma. *J Chromatogr B* 865:48–54.

89. Guo T, Taylor RL, Singh RJ, Soldin SJ. 2006. Simultaneous determination of 12 steroids by isotope dilution liquid chromatography-photospray ionization tandem mass spectrometry. *Clin Chem Acta* 372:76–82.

90. Shama N, Bai SW, Chung BC, Jung BH. 2008. Quantitative analysis of 17 amino acids in the connective tissue of patients with pelvic organ prolapse using capillary electrophoresis-tandem mass spectrometry. *J Chromatogr B* 865:18–24.

91. Oertel R, Neumeister V, Kirch W. 2004. Hydrophilic interaction chromatography combined with tandem-mass spectrometry to determine six aminoglycosides in serum. *J Chromatogr A* 1058:197–201.

92. Gutteck U, Rentsch KM. 2003. Therapeutic drug monitoring of 13 antidepressant and five neuroleptic drugs in serum with liquid chromatography-electrospray ionization mass spectrometry. *Clin Chem Lab Med* 41:1571–1579.

93. Subramanian M, Birnbaum AK, Remmel RP. 2008. High-speed simultaneous determination of nine anti-epileptic drugs using liquid chromatography-mass spectrometry. *Ther Drug Monit* 30:347–356.

94. Rodriguez-Cabaleiro D, Stockl D, Kaufman JM, Fiers T, Thienpont LM. 2006. Feasibility of standardization of serum C-peptide immunoassays with isotope-dilution liquid chromatography-tandem mass spectrometry. *Clin Chem* 52:1193–1196.

95. Huang G, Chen H, Zhang X, Cooks RG, Ouyang Z. 2007. Rapid screening of anabolic steroids in urine by reactive desorption electrospray ionization. *Anal Chem* 79:8327–8332.

96. Guo T, Gu J, Soldin OP, Singh RJ, Soldin SJ. 2008. Rapid measurement of estrogens and their metabolites in human serum by liquid chromatography-tandem mass spectrometry without derivatization. *Clin Biochem* 41:736–741.

97. Gu J, Soldin OP, Soldin SJ. 2007. Simultaneous quantification of free triiodothyronine and free thyroxine by isotope dilution tandem mass spectrometry. *Clin Biochem* 40:1386–1391.

98. Gu J, Soldin SJ. 2007. Modification of tandem mass spectrometric method to permit simultaneous quantification of 17 anti-HIV drugs which include atazanavir and tipranavir. *Clin Chim Acta* 378:222–224.

99. Sauvage FL, Gaulier JM, Lachatre G, Marquet P. 2008. Pitfalls and prevention strategies for liquid chromatography-tandem mass spectrometry in the selected reaction monitoring mode for drug analysis. *Clin Chem* 54:1519–1527.

100. Taylor RL, Machacek D, Singh RJ. 2002. Validation of a high-throughput liquid chromatography-tandem mass spectrometry method for urinary cortisol and cortisone. *Clin Chem* 48:1511–1519.

5 Analytical Support of Classical Anticonvulsant Drug Monitoring beyond Immunoassay: Application of Chromatographic Methods

JoEtta Juenke
Associated Regional and University Pathologists (ARUP)

Gwendolyn A. McMillin
University of Utah

CONTENTS

5.1   INTRODUCTION

Anticonvulsant drugs were among the first therapeutic drugs routinely monitored with blood concentrations to optimize dosing by evaluating individual pharmacokinetics. Such therapeutic drug monitoring (TDM) of anticonvulsant drugs also helps determine whether seizures and adverse effects occur due to noncompliance, resistance or refraction to drug response, drug–drug interactions, or excessive drug. TDM has been facilitated for classical anticonvulsant drugs by development and commercialization of automated, quantitative immunoassays.

Immunoassay reagents, in addition to commercially available quality control materials and proficiency testing challenges, are widely available for classical anticonvulsant drugs including phenytoin, carbamazepine, valproic acid (VPA), primidone, and ethosuximide. Commercial immunoassays and support materials are less commonly available, or are in development, for newer anticonvulsant drugs such as topiramate, lamotrigine and zonisamide. Class-based immunoassays are available for phenobarbital (barbiturates) and clonazepam (benzodiazepines), but they are not routinely used for TDM. No commercial immunoassays are currently available for some anticonvulsant drugs, such as oxcarbazepine and levetiracetam. The lack of immunoassay reagents for newer anticonvulsant drugs is a significant impediment to performing routine TDM in a time and cost-efficient manner, especially for smaller hospital laboratories.

Despite the wide availability of the immunoassay for some anticonvulsant drugs, this technology alone cannot meet all the needs of TDM for all drugs. In fact, immunoassays are inappropriate for TDM under circumstances such as the presence of cross-reacting compounds that contribute to falsely increased or falsely decreased results, the need to differentiate the concentrations of one or more active metabolite(s), the need to differentiate free drug concentrations (reflecting the proportion of drug that is not protein-bound) from total drug concentrations, or the need to resolve unknown sources of analytical interference. In these situations, chromatographic separation techniques are preferred.

This chapter describes briefly the history of TDM for classical anticonvulsant drugs, and describes specific situations for which chromatographic techniques are required to support TDM of classical anticonvulsants. Such scenarios in which chromatographic techniques are sought for both classical and newer anticonvulsant drugs are summarized in Table 5.1. Chromatographic methods to support TDM of anticonvulsant drugs are also discussed.

5.2 ANALYTICAL METHODS USED IN THERAPEUTIC DRUG MONITORING (TDM) OF ANTICONVULSANTS

The early analytical methods for TDM were based on chromatographic separation of components present in blood, coupled to various detection techniques. Perhaps the earliest description of chromatography from which TDM techniques were born is partition chromatography, published in 1941 [1]. Column chromatography is now the most common form of chromatography applied to TDM. Sensitivity and specificity of a chromatographic method depends on the physical process of separation, accomplished by understanding temporal distribution of the components between stationary (column) and mobile phases [2]. The components of a sample matrix will bind to the stationary phase and remain there, remain in the mobile phase and never bind to the stationary phase, or distribute between the two phases in a reversible, temporary manner. Components of the matrix will migrate through a column to a detector based on the affinity for the mobile phase versus the stationary phase. It is this mechanism that makes chromatography a useful tool in TDM. The most widely used forms of chromatography are gas chromatography (GC) and high performance (pressure) liquid chromatography (HPLC) in which the mobile phase is gas or liquid, respectively. Ultra-high performance (pressure) chromatography (UPLC) is a relatively recent and popular iteration of HPLC. Each chromatographic technique can be coupled to various detectors that are selected based on chemical properties of the analyte(s) of interest as well as required sensitivity and specificity.

GC was originally developed in 1952 to separate fatty acids [3]. A gaseous mobile phase was used to pass the volatile mixture through a stationary phase column. The gaseous mobile phase or carrier gas is generally an inert gas such as nitrogen, helium, hydrogen, or argon. The column materials vary but are frequently fused silica. The gas carries the separated parts of the mixture to the detector as they are eluted from the stationary phase over time by using a series of different temperatures. The height of peaks drawn by the integrator is proportional to the amount of that analytes present. Common detectors used with GC include universal detectors such as flame ionization detection (FID), thermal conductance (TCD) and mass spectrometers (MS) that detect most analytes, and more specialized detectors based on detection of nitrogen or phosphorus compounds (NPD), or electronegative groups by using electron capture detector (ECD).

TABLE 5.1

Scenarios for which Chromatographic Techniques may be most Appropriate to support TDM of Anticonvulsant Drugs Available in the USA in 2008

Generic Name	Common Trade Name	Proposed Therapeutic Range[a]	Active Metabolite	Metabolite Interference	Free Fraction Needed	No Commercial Immunoassay*
			Possible Reason for Chromatographic Assay			
Bromide		75–150 mg/dL				•
Carbamazepine	Tegretol	Total: 4–12 µg/mL Free: 1–3 µg/mL % Free: 8–35%	•	•	•	
Clonazepam	Klonopin	10–75 ng/mL				•
Ethosuximide	Zarontin	40–100 µg/mL				
Ethotoin	Peganone	5–50 µg/mL				•
Felbamate	Felbatol	30–60 µg/mL				•
Fosphenytoin	Cerebyx	See phenytoin	•	•	•	•
Gabapentin	Neurontin	2–10 µg/mL				•
Lamotrigine	Lamictal	3–14 µg/mL				•
Levetiracetam	Keppra	5–30 µg/mL				•
Methsuximide	Celontin	<1 µg/mL Normethsuximide metabolite: 10–40 µg/mL	•			•
Oxcarbazepine	Trileptal	Monohydroxy metabolite (MHD)=15–35 µg/mL	•			•
Phenobarbital	Luminal	>3 months: 15–40 µg/mL <3 months: 15–30 µg/mL				
Phenytoin	Dilantin	Adult total: 10–20 µg/mL Neonate: 6–14 µg/mL Free: 1–2 µg/mL % Free: 8–14%	•	•	•	

(Continued)

TABLE 5.1 (Continued)

Generic Name	Common Trade Name	Proposed Therapeutic Range[#]	Active Metabolite	Metabolite Interference	Free Fraction Needed	No Commercial Immunoassay*
					Possible Reason for Chromatographic Assay	
Primidone	Mysoline	5–12 µg/mL Phenobarbital metabolite: 15–40 µg/mL	•	•		
Topiramate	Topamax	5–20 µg/mL				
Valproic acid	Depakene Depakote	Total: 50–100 µg/mL Free: 6–22 µg/mL % Free: 5–18%			•	
Vigabitrin	Sabril	1–8 µg/mL				
Zonisamide	Zonegran	10–40 µg/mL				•

* Based on information available to the authors as of November, 2008 related to immunoassays designed for TDM.

Proposed therapeutic range based on monotherapy and as reported by several literature sources.

In the early 1970s, chromatography theory and application resulted in the development of HPLC [4]. With HPLC, the molecular distribution of matrix components is based on the interaction between a liquid mobile phase and a column (stationary phase) packed with small particles. Several different types of packing materials with affinity for specific molecules or chemical properties are available. The liquid mobile phase carries a sample mixture through the column wherein, like GC, the components are separated chemically and/or physically, and then the analytes of interest are eluted at specific times. The peak height and area that results is proportional to the amount of each component separated from the mixture. Common HPLC detectors are based on UV (ultraviolet) absorption, diode array (DAD, visible light), fluorescence, electrochemical, mass, or other physio-chemical properties of the analytes of interest.

While essentially all initial methods for TDM were originally based on chromatographic techniques, Federal Drug Administration (FDA) cleared immunoassays have been available commercially for classical anticonvulsants for more than thirty years. Immunoassays for TDM became popular in the 1980s and have remained popular because they are technically easy to perform, easily automated, and fast [5]. For a typical immunoassay, an antibody is raised with high affinity for a specific antigen (drug) to detect or "capture" that drug. Immunoassays used for TDM are typically based on competition of drug in the sample, with labeled drug included in the assay, which both bind to the antibody with known affinity. Thus, a known amount of labeled drug (antigen) is added to specimen containing an unknown amount of drug. The assay is usually homogenous, in that there are no wash steps, and the activity of the label attached to the antigen is directly modulated by antibody binding. The magnitude of the signal generated through the binding reaction is proportional to the concentration of the drug in the specimen. Sensitivity of the assay can be improved with different labels such as enzyme, fluorescent, chemiluminescent, or radioactive labels. However, sensitivity may not be adequate to measure concentrations of "free" drug, particularly when the assay is designed to quantify "total" drug concentrations and when the drug is >90% protein bound. Measurement of free drug concentrations may require a separate immunoassay designed specifically to measure low concentrations, or more sensitive chromatographic techniques.

Another limitation of immunoassays relates to antibody specificity. Falsely high or low results could be generated if antibodies on which an assay is based cross-react with metabolites (both active and inactive), structurally similar compounds, or other unrelated compounds. Naturally occurring immuno-globulins and other components of the specimen matrix also could falsely elevate or reduce results. In general, cross-reacting substances yield falsely elevated results and may contribute to inappropriate dose reductions or other changes to drug therapy. Overcoming these interferences may require an alternate antibody, or more specific chromatographic techniques.

5.3 WHEN CHROMATOGRAPHIC TECHNIQUES ARE PREFERRED FOR ANTICONVULSANT THERAPEUTIC DRUG MONITORING (TDM)

In this section limitations of immunoassays in TDM of classical anticonvulsants will be discussed along with chromatographic techniques available for each drug for more accurate measurements.

5.3.1 PHENYTOIN

Phenytoin (5,5-diphenylhydantoin) was first synthesized in 1908, was first reported as an anti-convulsant in 1938, and remains the drug of choice for many seizure types. Indeed, phenytoin is indicated for grand mal, focal and temporal lobe seizures. It is generally provided in oral doses, but a phosphorylated formulation (fosphenytoin) is administered intravenously (i.v.) or intramus-cularly (i.m.) for acute or emergency management of seizures. There are at least three scenarios when immunoassays are inappropriate for supporting TDM of phenytoin. First, when fospheny-toin is administered; second, when the protein status of the patient is unpredictable or drug-drug interactions due to competition of protein binding sites is suspected; and third, when the patient for which TDM is requested is uremic.

For the purposes of TDM for fosphenytoin, the active drug phenytoin is measured. Fosphenytoin is rapidly hydrolyzed to phenytoin [6,7], but will interfere with commercial immunoassays by producing falsely elevated plasma phenytoin levels when parent drug is present. The degree of cross-reactivity should be evaluated when immunoassays are used to measure phenytoin after fosphenytoin is administered. Furthermore, accurate documentation of the time of specimen collection relative to drug administration is critically important for accurate interpretation of drug concentrations in serum or plasma [8–10]. Alkaline phosphatase converts fosphenytoin into phenytoin. In one report, the authors added 10 μl of commercially available alkaline phosphatase solution to 1 mL of specimen and observed complete conversion of fosphenytoin into phenytoin after 5 min of incubation at room temperature. Such simple treatment eliminated interference of fosphenytoin in the phenytoin immunoassay but may not accurately reflect circulating phenytoin concentrations [11].

Dosing decisions for both fosphenytoin and phenytoin are routinely made based on total phenytoin concentrations. A well accepted therapeutic range for total phenytoin concentrations in an otherwise healthy patient is 10–20 μg/mL. Values greater than 30 μg/mL may cause signs of drug toxicity. This total concentration of the drug in the blood consists of the protein bound fraction and the free fraction, of which the free fraction is considered to be pharmacologically active. Due to the fact that phenytoin is highly bound to plasma proteins (>90%) in healthy patients, any alteration in the protein binding of phenytoin due to uremia, hypoalbuminemia, pregnancy, the ingestion of other drugs that compete for protein binding, or the natural aging process can result in significantly different composition of free (unbound) phenytoin concentration. For example, the amount of free phenytoin could double and only affect the total concentration by a small amount. This sort of clinically significant change in free phenytoin concentration cannot be adequately detected by measuring total phenytoin concentrations alone. With an at-risk patient, one in whom protein binding may change or be unpredictable, free phenytoin testing may be appropriate for optimizing phenytoin dose. Not surprisingly, commercial immunoassays for phenytoin may not be sensitive enough to measure free phenytoin concentrations accurately, and chromatographic techniques may be required.

Phenytoin is metabolized extensively. The primary metabolite is 5-(p-hydroxyphenyl-), 5-phenylhydantoin (HPPH), which may be further metabolized to a glucuronide conjugate, as well as a catechol that spontaneously oxidizes to semiquinone and quinone species. Many commercial immunoassays for phenytoin exhibit cross-reactivity with HPPH, yielding falsely elevated phenytoin values. The HPPH glucuronide is primarily eliminated in urine, and as such, accumulates in patients with compromised urine function. Thus, spuriously high values due to the cross-reactivity with accumulated HPPH are frequently observed in uremic patients [13–18].

If a uremic patient is receiving fosphenytoin, immunoassays usually demonstrate falsely elevated values due to the presence of a unique immunoreactive metabolite derived from fosphenytoin in sera of these patients. Roberts et al reported that phenytoin results may be falsely elevated up to 20 times if measured by certain immunoassays such as AxSYM phenytoin assay, TDx phenytoin assays (both from Abbott Laboratories, Abbott Park, IL), ACS:180 phenytoin assays (Chiron, now Siemens, Tarrytown, NY) and the Vitros phenytoin assay (Johnson and Johnson, Rochester, NY), when compared to the phenytoin concentration results generated by a specific HPLC method. The phenytoin concentration determined by aca star analyzer (Dade Behring aca phenytoin assay, Deerfield, IL) compared well with phenytoin value observed using the HPLC method [10]. Later Annesley et al. characterized this immunoreactive component using gradient reverse-phase HPLC-tandem mass spectrometry (HPLC-MS-MS) as a compound with a m/z 251 phenytoin ion and a parent m/z 457 ion. The authors then isolated and identified this metabolite by chemical derivatization, HPLC, MS-MS, exact mass analysis, isotope exchange, and nuclear magnetic resonance (NMR) spectroscopy as the N-3′-oxymethylglucuronide of phenytoin which was derived from fosphenytoin [12]. A copy of the comparison of immunoassay and HPLC-MS-MS integration responses, plotted against chromatographic time, for a serum specimen from a uremic patient

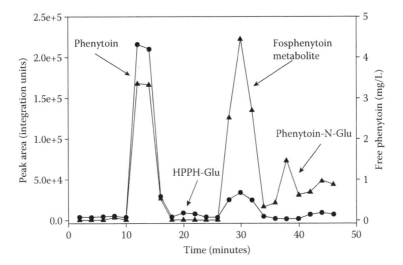

FIGURE 5.1 Immunoassay and MS-MS integration responses plotted against chromatographic time for a serum specimen from a uremic patient receiving fosphenytoin. Chromatography was performed on a Zorbax RX-C18 column (2.1 × 150 mm) in series with a Betamax Acid column (2.0 × 30 mm). Mobile phase: acetonitrile–1 mL/L acetic acid plus 6 mmol/L ammonium acetate in water (82:18 by volume). Flow rate, 0.3 mL/min. •, immunoassay. ▲, MS-MS integration. (From Annesley TM, Kurzyniec S, Nordblom GD, Buchanan N, et al. *Clin Chem,* 47, 910–918, 2001. Copyright ©2001 American Association for Clinical Chemistry. Reprinted with permission.)

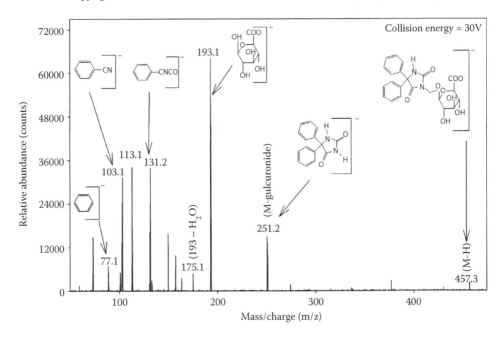

FIGURE 5.2 Fragmentation of parent ion at *m/z* 457 (*N*-3′-oxymethylglucuronide of phenytoin). From Annesley TM, Kurzyniec S, Nordblom GD, Buchanan N, et al., *Clin Chem,* 47, 910–918, 2001. Copyright ©2001 American Association for Clinical Chemistry. Reprinted with permission.)

receiving fosphenytoin is shown (with permission) in Figure 5.1 and mass fragmentation pattern (daughter ions) of *m/z* 457 (parent ion) is shown in Figure 5.2. Currently, the only way to resolve these glucuronide interferences observed commonly with immunoassays is to perform TDM with chromatographic techniques.

There are numerous chromatographic methods for supporting TDM of phenytoin, including GC of the underivatized drug with FID [19]. Other procedures incorporate methyl and trimethylsilyl dervitization techniques applied to sample preparation to improve sensitivity [20–22]. Additional methods include GC with NPD and MS detection [23,24] and HPLC with UV, DAD, and MS detection [25–28].

5.3.2 CARBAMAZEPINE

Carbamazepine is used to treat both generalized and partial seizures, due to its rapid control of excessive cerebral electrical discharges and low incidence of acute and chronic toxicity. Carbamazepine, an iminostilbene derivative, is therefore structurally related to many compounds that may produce positive interference in immunoassays.

Structurally similar compounds include carbamazepine metabolites, oxcarbazepine (and metabolites) and the tricyclic antidepressants (TCA) (see Figure 5.3 for structures). Although carbamazepine will interfere with immunoassays designed to detect TCA, interference of TCAs with carbamazepine assays is not observed clinically due to the much lower concentrations of TCAs in plasma (therapeutic range 100–250 ng/mL) compared to carbamazepine concentrations (therapeutic range 4–12 µg/mL). Although structurally unrelated, hydroxyzine and its metabolite cetirizine is known to interfere with the particle-enhanced turbidimetric inhibition immunoassays (PENTINA) for carbamazepine (Dade Behring, Deerfield, IL); EMIT carbamazepine immunoassay performance was not affected by hydroxyzine. The authors observed erroneous carbamazepine values in 35 out of 40 specimens collected from patients receiving hydroxyzine but no carbamazepine [29]. Structurally similar oxcarbazepine and its metabolite do not seem to be an issue with carbamazepine immunoassays [32,33].

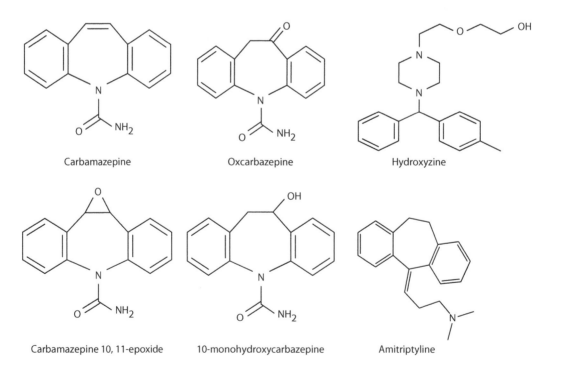

FIGURE 5.3 Chemical structures for carbamazepine, carbamazepine 10,11-epoxide, oxcarbazepine, 10-monohydroxyoxcarbazepine, amitriptyline, and hydroxyzine.

The primary metabolite of carbamazepine is carbamazepine 10,11-epoxide, which is pharmacologically active. The 10,11-epoxide is further metabolized and eliminated in the urine. One of the largest issues with immunoassays for carbamazepine is the cross-reactivity with the epoxide metabolite [30]. Hermida and Tutor observed widely different cross-reactivity of carbamazepine 10,11-epoxide with various carbamazepine immunoassays. While the PENTINA carbamazepine assay showed approximately 93.6% cross-reactivity with the carbamazepine 10,11-epoxide, the Cobas Integra immunoassay for carbamazepine (Roche Diagnostics, Indianapolis, IN) showed negligible cross-reactivity with the epoxide metabolite [31].

Carbamazepine immunoassays are very useful in the support of TDM for patients with normal renal function, but this is not the case for uremic patients. Thus, for patients with signs of renal failure, disproportionate increases in the epoxide concentration (relative to concentrations of parent drug) may be observed due to drug accumulation, a direct consequence of impaired elimination. In one report, the authors observed that the relative proportion of epoxide metabolite with respect to carbamazepine for patients with moderate to severe renal insufficiency is significantly increased and in these cases carbamazepine concentrations obtained using EMIT or other immunoassays having low cross-reactivity with epoxide may have been inadequate [34]. For uremic patients, measuring carbamazepine and the epoxide metabolite chromatographically may be required for dosage optimization.

Although protein binding with carbamazepine is not as extensive as was described above with phenytoin, between 65 and 80% of carbamazepine in plasma is protein-bound, mostly to albumin, over a total drug concentration range of 5–30 μg/mL. Changes to the protein binding of carbamazepine can affect the unbound fraction which varies from 8 to 35%. Because of this wide variation, adjustment of carbamazepine dosage may be better guided by monitoring the free concentration of the drug, which may require chromatographic methods with lower limits of quantification than routinely used immunoassays.

Carbamazepine and its metabolite are unstable under most GC conditions, but several GC methods that incorporate preanalytical derivitization have been successfully used for analysis of carbamazepine including dimethylformamide dimethylacetal [35,36] pentafluorobenzamide [37], N-cyano [38], and trimethylsilyl [39] derivatives. The only underivitized assays demonstrate variable decomposition to iminostilbene [40] or the use of MS detection [41]. Since the epoxide metabolite is so easily degraded by GC, the more popular approach for the simultaneous assay of parent and metabolite is HPLC [42–45]. A total ion chromatogram for a calibrator and a patient using an HPLC-MS-MS method that detects and quantifies carbamazepine, the 10,11-epoxide as well as oxcarbazepine and its monohydroxy metabolite is shown in Figure 5.4.

5.3.3 VALPROIC ACID (VPA)

VPA is a synthetic carboxylic acid derivative synthesized in 1881 that has been in use since 1967 as a broad spectrum anticonvulsant drug. This drug has demonstrated efficacy in the management of generalized tonic-clonic and myoclonic seizures as well as atypical absence, simple, and complex partial and mixed grand mal and petit mal seizures. The capability of treating many types of seizures with a single anticonvulsant has resulted in the wide use of VPA, particularly for children in whom tonic-clonic and myoclonic seizures are most prevalent, or for children that were refractory to other anticonvulsants.

VPA exhibits several peculiar pharmacokinetic characteristics including a nonlinear dose-concentration relationship and a variable (although dose-dependent) degree of plasma protein binding. The therapeutic plasma range is 50–100 μg/mL and protein binding may exceed 80%. The dose-concentration relationship for free VPA is linear, and as such, determination of the free fraction may be indicated, particularly for patients with renal disease, alcoholic cirrhosis, acute hepatitis, AIDS, and those being comedicated with drugs altering the protein binding of VPA. Although most commercial immunoassays could detect free VPA concentrations, chromatographic methods may be preferred to assure adequate specificity.

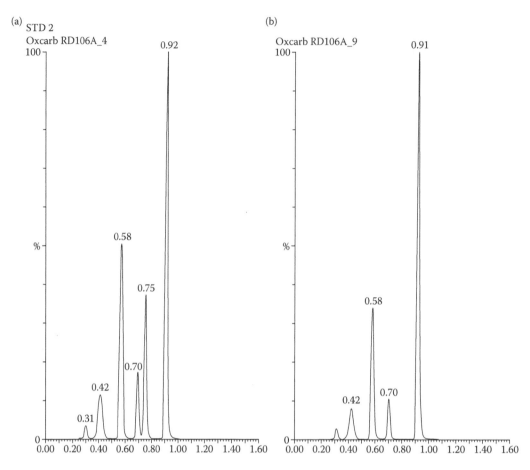

FIGURE 5.4 Sample total ion chromatogram from a UPLC-MS/MS method designed to detect and quantify five anticonvulsant drugs and metabolites in plasma by MRM (2 transitions per analyte), over 1 min for a calibrator (a) and a patient positive for oxcarbazepine, carbamazepine (and metabolite), and lamotrigine (b). The assay includes carbamazepine (0.92 min, 237.16 > 194.1, and 179.0) and the 10,11-epoxide metabolite of carbamazepine (0.70 min, 253.11 > 236.1, and 210.1); oxcarbazepine (0.76 min, 253.12 > 236.1, and 208.1) and the monohydroxy metabolite of oxcarbazepine (0.58 min, 237.1 > 194.0, and 179.0); lamotrigine (0.42 min, 256.08 > 211.1, and 165.7); and an internal standard (UCB17025, 0.31 min, 185.06 > 140.0, and 69.0). The method was performed with a Waters Acquity UPLC/TQD with a HSS T3 1.8 μm, 2.1×50 mm column, a gradient of 0.1% formic acid and acetonitrile, and a flow rate of 0.65 mL/min.

The most common chromatographic technique employed for VPA is GC, directly using FID [46–48] and an ester derivative [49–51], and by MS detection [52]. There are also several studies comparing immunoassay and GC methods [53,54]. Thus, Wohler and Poklis analyzed VPA concentrations in plasma using GC (wide-bore capillary column) without derivatization. The lower limit of detection was 5 μg/mL and the lower limit of quantitation was 10 μg/mL. The method was linear up to a plasma VPA concentration of 6,000 μg/mL [47]. Darius and Meyer described a sensitive capillary GC-MS determination of VPA and seven of its metabolites in human plasma. The method was based on selected ion monitoring of tert-butyldimethylsilyl derivative of VPA and metabolites prepared by using N-(tert-butyldimethylsilyl)-N-methyl-trifluoracetamide (MTBSTFA) as the derivatizing agent. The limit of detection of VPA and its metabolites were at low nanogram levels except for the 4-hydroxy metabolite, which had a detection limit of 100 ng/mL [52]. Leroux et al compared VPA concentrations obtained by GC and EMIT immunoassay and observed good correlation between results obtained by GC and EMIT for a range of VPA concentration of 16–139 μg/mL [54].

HPLC methods have also been reported [55,56] for determination of VPA in human plasma. For example, Hara et al. described a HPLC procedure for determination of VPA in human plasma. The method is based on direct derivatization of a plasma sample with 6,7-methylenedioxy-1-methyl-2-oxo-1,2-dihydroquinoxaline-3-ylpropionohydrazine. The derivatization can be carried out in aqueous medium in the presence of pyridine and 1-ethyl-3-(3-dimethylaminopropyl) carbodiimide at 37°C. The resultant derivative can be analyzed by using a reverse phase column with isocratic elution and peaks can be detected fluorometrically at 440 nm (using an excitation wavelength of 365 nm) [55]. Zhong et al. simultaneously analyzed VPA and mycophenolic acid (an immunosuppressant) using HPLC after precolumn derivatization of VPA with 4-bromomethyl-6,7-dimethoxycoumarin and online solvatochromism of mycophenolic acid by pH adjustment. Dichloromethane was used for simultaneous extraction of VPA and mycophenolic acid from human plasma [56].

5.3.4 PHENOBARBITAL

Phenobarbital is a barbiturate that has been used extensively as an anticonvulsant since 1912. Phenobarbital is also the major active metabolite of primidone (see below). Oral absorption of phenobarbital is complete but slow, with peak plasma levels being reached several hours after intake. Approximately 50% of the drug is bound to plasma proteins. After dosing, 25–50% is excreted unchanged in urine, and the remainder appears as inactive metabolites, mainly the parahydroxyphenyl and N-glucoside derivatives. Monitoring plasma concentrations of phenobarbital has been recommended for chronic therapy because of phenobarbital's narrow therapeutic index and wide interindividual variability in the rate of metabolism and clearance.

Phenobarbital is adequately detected by immunoassay, when this is the only barbiturate prescribed. Because of cross-reactivity of other barbiturates with commercially available immunoassays for barbiturates, chromatographic methods are advised when multiple barbiturates are used, and during times of transition between barbiturates. Chromatographically, phenobarbital is most often analyzed by GC generally using either a FID or NPD [24]. There are also many variations of HPLC assays [23,26,57].

5.3.5 PRIMIDONE

Primidone is effective against tonic-clonic seizures (grand mal seizures), simple partial seizure as well as complex partial seizure. Primidone is metabolized to phenobarbital and it is necessary to manage dosing by TDM of both primidone and phenobarbital. Primidone is metabolized in the liver by cytochrome P-450 (mainly CYP2C19) to phenobarbital and phenylethylmalonamide. Although parent drug primidone reaches steady state rapidly (30–40 h), phenobarbital may take 17–24 days to reach steady state. Immunoassays are available for TDM of primidone, as are GC and HPLC methods, however monitoring of phenobarbital is most critical.

5.3.6 METHSUXIMIDE, ETHOSUXIMIDE, AND ETHOTOIN

Both methsuximide and ethosuximide are effective in treating absence seizure. In addition, methsuximide is also effective in treating certain types of focal and refractory seizures. Ethosuximide undergoes extensive hepatic metabolism (CYP3A4) to inactive metabolites such as 2-hydroxyethyl-2-methylsuccinimide. Methsuximide is metabolized to desmethyl-methsuximide (normethsuximide) which is pharmacologically active [60].

Ethotoin is a hydantoin series drug used for the control of tonic-clonic and complex partial seizures. TDM of ethotoin is clinically useful to troubleshoot side effects and adverse reactions, and to evaluate compliance.

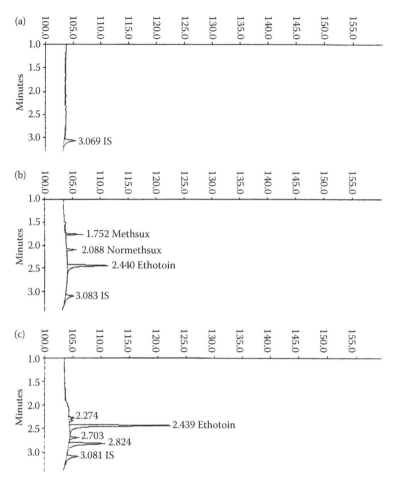

FIGURE 5.5 Chromatograms representing GC-NPD detection and quantification of ethotoin, methsuximide and normethsuximide metabolite for a drug-free patient blank (a) a calibrator, (b) and a patient positive for ethotoin (c). GC was performed adding an internal standard to an aliquot of the patient specimen, the aliquot is buffered to pH 3.0 with sodium phosphate buffer, and methsuximide, normethsuximide, ethotoin and the internal standard are extracted into ethyl acetate. The analytes are separated in the GC column (15 m×0.3 mm, film thickness 0.3 μm Alltech Drug 3 capillary) over a temperature gradient and detected with a nitrogen-phosphorous detector.

No commercial immunoassays for methsuximide or its active metabolite are commercially available, and they are typically monitored by GC methods. A simple GC-NPD assay for the analysis of methsuximide and metabolite and ethotoin can be performed with an aliquot of 500 μL of patient specimen, buffered to pH 3.0 with sodium phosphate buffer, internal standard added. Methsuximide, normethsuximide, ethotoin, and the internal standard are extracted into ethyl acetate. The tube is centrifuged, 100 μL is placed in an autosampler vial, and injected into the GC-NPD. The analytes are separated in the GC column (15 m × 0.3 mm, film thickness 0.3 μm Alltech Drug 3 capillary) over a temperature gradient and detected. The compounds are qualitatively identified by relative retention time, and quantitated from a calibration curve generated from calibrators included in the run. The acceptability of the run is evaluated by controls injected after the assay calibration. An example chromatogram of a calibrator, drug-free plasma, and a patient plasma specimen are shown in Figure 5.5.

5.4 MULTIDRUG THERAPEUTIC DRUG MONITORING (TDM): ANOTHER APPLICATION OF CHROMATOGRAPHIC TECHNIQUES

As mentioned earlier, there are many examples of chromatographic assays that allow for the concurrent measurement of both classic and newer anticonvulsants. This makes sense, since it is common that anticonvulsants are concurrently administered with other anticonvulsants. The use of a chromatographic assay allows for the measurement of all of these compounds in the same sample, which minimizes sample volume requirements (especially important relative to pediatric patients), is more cost- and time-efficient when compared to performing multiple TDM assays, and is useful in monitoring or identification of drug–drug interactions. Lamotrigine is commonly coadministered with both carbamazepine and oxcarbazepine. An UPLC-MS-MS assay that measures the classical anticonvulsant carbamazepine and it's active metabolite 10,11-epoxide as well as the newer anticonvulsant drugs of lamotrigine and oxcarbazepine and its monohydroxy metabolite is described here. By monitoring the five analytes together, processing and analytical time is saved. The assay consists of taking 60 μL of sample and precipitating that with methanol: acetonitrile solution containing an internal standard. The sample is then vortexed and centrifuged and the resulting supernatant is placed in a vial. 5 μL of this is injected into a UPLC-MS system using a Waters Acquity UPLC HSS T3 1.8 um, 2.1 × 50 mm for separation with an acetonitrile: water gradient. The assay serves as an important tool in monitoring patients on cotherapy. Total ion chromatographs appear in Figure 5.4a for a calibrator and Figure 5.4b for a patient comedicated with lamotrigine, carbamazepine, and oxcarbazepine. Table 5.2 lists the retention time and mass transitions used to detect and quantify the analytes.

Another example of a multianalyte panel is described by Queiroz et al., wherein a method for simultaneous determination of primidone, lamotrigine, carbamazepine (along with carbamazepine epoxide), phenytoin and phenobarbital in human plasma using solid phase microextraction and GC with thermionic specific detection is described [58]. Liu et al. reported simultaneous determination of primidone, carbamazepine, phenytoin and phenobarbital along with their principal metabolites in plasma, urine and saliva using HPLC-DAD. Acetonitrile was used for deproteinization of plasma and saliva samples while solid phase extraction technique was used for urine specimen. HPLC separation was carried out using a reverse phase column (C-18) and the column temperature was maintained at 40°C. Parent drugs and their metabolites were eluted from the column using a mobile phase comprised of phosphate buffer/acetonitrile/methanol (110:50:30 by vol) at a flow rate of 0.2 mL/min. Signals were monitored by DAD at a wavelength of 200 nm and bandwidth of 10 nm. Complete separation of drugs and metabolites was achieved within 15 min [59].

TABLE 5.2
Retention Times and Mass Transitions used to Detect and Quantify Anticonvulsant Drugs by LC-MS/MS (see Figure 5.3 for Example Total Ion Chromatograms)

	Retention Time (min)	Mass Transitions Monitored	
		Quantitative	Qualitative
Lamotrigine	0.42	256.08 > 211.1	256.08 > 165.7
Oxcarbazepine	0.76	253.12 > 236.1	253.12 > 208.1
Monohydroxy oxcarbazepine	0.58	237.1 > 194.0	237.1 > 179.0
Carbamazepine	0.92	237.16 > 194.1	237.16 > 179.0
Carbamazepine 10,11-epoxide	0.7	253.11 > 236.1	253.11 > 210.1
Internal standard (UBC17025)	0.31	185.06 > 140.00	185.06 > 69.0

Romanyshyn et al. used a reverse phase chromatographic column (Spherisorb ODS column with particle size of 3 μm) and isocratic mobile phase (phosphate buffer/acetonitrile/methanol; 70:16:14 by vol) for simultaneous analysis of felbamate, primidone, phenobarbital, carbamazepine (along with two metabolites; carbamazepine trans diol and carbamazepine 10,11-epoxide) and phenytoin (along with phenytoin metabolite 5-(4-hydroxyphenyl)-5-phenylhydatoin). The authors used UV detection at 210 nm [27]. Speed et al. analyzed six anticonvulsants ethosuximide, carbamazepine, phenobarbital, phenytoin, primidone, and VPA by GC-MS after converting these drugs to their corresponding butyl derivatives [61]. In another study, the authors reported a simple isocratic LC method for simultaneous analysis of ethosuximide, primidone, phenobarbital, phenytoin, carbamazepine and their bioactive metabolite using a C18 reverse phase HPLC column and mobile phase composition of acetone/methanol/acetonitrile/10 mmol/L phosphate buffer (10/21/8/61 by vol). The anticonvulsant drugs were extracted from 50 μl of plasma by adding 50 μl of acetonitrile containing the internal standard (tolylbarb 10 μg/mL) and after chromatographic analysis, elution of peaks was monitored at 200 nm. The chromatographic analysis was complete within 10 min [62]. Matar et al. also described a rapid sensitive HPLC protocol for simultaneous analysis of ethosuximide, primidone, lamotrigine, phenobarbital, phenytoin, and carbamazepine (along with carbamazepine metabolites) after extraction of these drugs from human plasma (100 μl) with ether using 9-hydroxymethyl-10-carbamyl acridan as the internal standard. The drugs and the metabolites were eluted from a Supelcosil C-18 column at ambient temperature with a mobile phase consisting of 0.01 M phosphate buffer/methanol/acetonitrile (65/18/17 by vol) adjusted to a pH of 7.5 with phosphoric acid and a flow rate of 1 mL/min. The effluents were monitored at 220 nm [63]. Thus, chromatographic methods provide significant potential for improved efficiency through multianalyte method development.

5.5 CONCLUSIONS

TDM of common classic anticonvulsant drugs is successfully accomplished using commercially available immunoassays for most patients. Special scenarios in which chromatographic methods should be used to provide TDM of these drugs include cross-reacting or otherwise interfering substances that lead to falsely elevated or reduced results, inadequate sensitivity to measure free drug concentrations, and when quantification of an active metabolite unique from the parent drug is desired. Possible scenarios for when chromatographic techniques may be preferred over immunoassays for these and other classical and newer anticonvulsant drugs are included in Table 5.1. A major advantage of recently described LC-MS/MS methods is the capability to detect and quantify multiple anticonvulsant drugs in the same sample. This approach minimizes sample requirements for patients managed with multiple drugs and has potential to improve efficiency in the laboratory. Additional experience with TDM for the newer anticonvulsant drugs as well as impending availability of immunoassays will reveal the most appropriate scenarios in which chromatographic versus immunoassay methodologies should be employed.

REFERENCES

1. Martin AJP, Synge RLM. 1941.A new form of chromatography employing two liquid phases: I. A theory of chromatography. II. Applications to the micro determination of the higher monoamino acids in proteins. *Biochem J*, 35: 1358–1368.
2. Ettre LS. 1993. Nomenclature for chromatography: IUPAC recommendations 1993. *Pure Appl Chem*, 65: 819–872.
3. James AT, Martin AJP. 1952. Separation and identification of methyl esters of saturated and unsaturated fatty acids from n-pentanoic to n-octadecanoic acids. *Analyst*, 77: 915–920.
4. Dorsey JG. 2000. Liquid chromatography: introduction. In Meyers, RA (ed), *Encyclopedia of Analytical Chemistry*. Chichester, UK: John Wiley & Sons, 1123–1133.
5. Johannessen SI, Battino D, Berry DJ, Bialer M, et al. 2003. Therapeutic drug monitoring of the newer antiepileptic drugs. *Ther Drug Monit* 25: 347–363.

6. Baselt R. 2004. *Phenytoin. Disposition of Toxic Drugs and Chemicals in Man*, 7th edition. Foster City, CA: Biomedical Publications, 901–903.

7. Baselt R. 2004. *Fosphenytoin. Disposition of Toxic Drugs and Chemicals in Man*, 7th edition. Foster City, CA: Biomedical Publications, 493.

8. Datta P, Dasgupta A.1998. Cross-reactivity of fosphenytoin in four phenytoin immunoassays. *Clin Chem*, 44: 696–697.

9. Kugler AR, Annesley TM, Nordblom GD, Koup JR, Olson SC. 1998. Cross-reactivity of fosphenytoin in two human plasma phenytoin immunoassays. *Clin Chem* 44(7): 1474–1480.

10. Roberts WL, De BK, Coleman JP, Annesley TM. 1999. Falsely increased immunoassay measurements of total and unbound phenytoin in critically ill uremic patients receiving fosphenytoin. *Clin Chem* 45: 829–837.

11. Dasgupta A, Handy BC, Datta P. 2000. Mathematical model to calculate fosphenytoin concentrations in the presence of phenytoin using phenytoin immunoassays and alkaline phosphatase. *Am J Clin Pathol* 113: 87–92.

12. Annesley TM, Kurzyniec S, Nordblom GD, Buchanan N, et al. 2001. Glucuronidation of prodrug reactive site: isolation and characterization of oxymethylglucuronide metabolite of fosphenytoin. *Clin Chem* 46: 910–918.

13. McDonald DM, Kabra PM. 1980. Renal disease may increase apparent phenytoin in serum as measured by enzyme-multiplied immunoassay. *Clin Chem* 26: 361–362.

14. Rainey PM, Rogers KE, Roberts WL. 1996. Metabolite and matrix interference in phenytoin immunoassays. *Clin Chem* 42: 1645–1653.

15. Reeves SE, Hanyok JJ, Amon SA, Godley PJ. 1985. Discrepancy in serum phenytoin concentrations determined by two immunoassay methods in uremic patients. *Am J Hosp Pharm* 42(2): 359–361.

16. Roberts WL, Annesley TM, De BK, Moulton L, et al. 2001. Performance characteristics of four free phenytoin immunoassays. *Ther Drug Monit* 23: 148–154.

17. Sirgo MA, Green PJ, Rocci ML Jr, Vlasses PH. 1984. Interpretation of serum phenytoin concentrations in uremia is assay-dependent. *Neurology* 34: 1250–1251.

18. Tutor-Crespo MJ, Hermida J, Tutor JC. 2007. Phenytoin immunoassay measurements in serum samples from patients with renal insufficiency: comparison with high-performance liquid chromatography. *J Clin Lab Anal* 21: 119–123.

19. Ritz DP. 1975. Single extraction GLC analysis of six commonly prescribed antiepileptic drugs. *Clin Toxicol* 8: 311–324.

20. Abraham CV, Joslin HD. 1976. Simultaneous gas chromatographic analysis for the four commonly used antiepileptic drugs in serum. *J Chromatogr* 128: 281–287.

21. Chang T, Glazko AJ. 1970. Quantitative assay of 5,5-diphenylhydantoin (Dilantin) and 5-(p-hydroxyphenyl)-5-phenylhydantoin by gas-liquid chromatography. *J Lab Clin Med* 75: 145–155.

22. Kupferberg HJ. 1970. Quantitative estimation of diphenylhydantoin, primidone and phenobarbital in plasma by gas-liquid chromatography. *Clin Chim Acta* 29: 282–288.

23. Nelson MH, Birnbaum AK, Nyhus PJ, Remmel RP. 1998. A capillary GC-MS method for analysis of phenytoin and [13C3]-phenytoin from plasma obtained from pulse dose pharmacokinetic studies. *J Pharm Biomed Anal* 17: 1311–1323.

24. Vandemark FL, Adams RF. 1976. Ultramicro gas-chromatographic analysis for anticonvulsants, with use of a nitrogen-selective detector. *Clin Chem* 22: 1062–1065.

25. Patil KM, Bodhankar, SL. 2005. Simultaneous determination of lamotrigine, phenobarbitone, carbamazepine and phenytoin in human serum by high-performance liquid chromatography. *J Pharm Biomed Anal* 39: 181–186.

26. Ramachandran S, Underhill S, Jones SR. 1994. Measurement of lamotrigine under conditions measuring phenobarbitone, phenytoin, and carbamazepine using reversed-phase high-performance liquid chromatography at dual wavelengths. *Ther Drug Monit* 16: 75–82.

27. Romanyshyn LA, Wichmann JK, Kucharczyk N, Shumaker RC et al. 1994. Simultaneous determination of felbamate, primidone, phenobarbital, carbamazepine, two carbamazepine metabolites, phenytoin, and one phenytoin metabolite in human plasma by high performance liquid chromatography. *Ther Drug Monit* 16: 90–99.

28. Subramanian M, Birnbaum AK, Remmel RP. 2008. High-speed simultaneous determination of nine antiepileptic drugs using liquid chromatography-mass spectrometry. *Ther Drug Monit* 30: 347–356.

29. Parant F, Moulsma M, Gagnieu MC, Lardet, G. 2005. Hydroxyzine and metabolites as a source of interference in carbamazepine particle enhanced turbidimetric immunoassays (PENTINA). *Ther Drug Monit* 27: 457–462.

30. Contin M, Riva R, Albani F, Perucca E, Baruzzi, A. 1985. Determination of total and free plasma carbamazepine concentrations by enzyme multiplied immunoassay: interference with the 10,11-epoxide metabolite. *Ther Drug Monit* 7: 46–50.

31. Hermida J, Tutor JC. 2003. How suitable are currently used carbamazepine immunoassays for quantifying carbamazepine 10, 11-epoxide in serum samples? *Ther Drug Monit* 25: 384–388.

32. Kumps A, Mardens Y. 1986. Cross-reactivity assessment of oxcarbazepine and its metabolites in the EMIT assay of carbamazepine plasma levels. *Ther Drug Monit* 8: 95–97.

33. Parant F, Bossu H, Gagnieu MC, Lardet G, Moulsma M. 2003. Cross-reactivity assessment of carbamazepine-10,11-epoxide, oxcarbazepine, and 10-hydroxy-carbazepine in two automated carbamazepine immunoassays: PETINIA and EMIT 2000. *Ther Drug Monit* 25: 41–45.

34. Tutor-Crespo MJ, Hermida J, Tutor JC. 2008. Relative proportion of serum carbamazepine and its pharmacologically active 10,11-epoxide derivative: effect of polytherapy and renal insufficiency. *Ups J Med Sci* 113: 171–180.

35. Millner SN, Taber CA. 1979. Rapid gas chromatographic determination of carbamazepine for routine therapeutic monitoring. *J Chromatogr* 163: 96–102.

36. Perchalski RJ, Wilder BJ. 1974. Rapid gas-liquid chromatographic determination of carbamazepine in plasma. *Clin Chem* 20: 492–493.

37. Schwertner HA, Hamilton HE,Wallace JE. 1978. Analysis for carbamazepine in serum by electron-capture gas chromatography. *Clin Chem* 24: 895–899.

38. Gerardin A, Abadie F, Laffont J.1975. GLC determination of carbamazepine suitable for pharmacokinetic studies. *J Pharm Sci* 64: 1940–1942.

39. Lensmeyer GL. 1977. Isothermal gas chromatographic method for the rapid determination of carbamazepine ("tegretol") as its TMS derivative. *Clin Toxicol* 11: 443–454.

40. Cocks DA, Dyer TF, Edgar K. 1981. Simple and rapid gas-liquid chromatographic method for estimating carbamazepine in serum. *J Chromatogr* 222: 496–500.

41. Hallbach J, Vogel H, Guder WG. 1997. Determination of lamotrigine, carbamazepine and carbamazepine epoxide in human serum by gas chromatography mass spectrometry. *Eur J Clin Chem Clin Biochem* 35: 755–759.

42. Babaei A, Eslamai MH. 2007. Evaluation of therapeutic drug level monitoring of phenobarbital, phenytoin and carbamazepine in Iranian epileptic patients. *Int J Clin Pharmacol Ther* 45: 121–125.

43. Bonato PS, Lanchote VL, deCarvalho D, Ache P. 1992. Measurement of carbamazepine and its main biotransformation products in plasma by HPLC. *J Anal Toxicol* 16: 88–92.

44. Elyas AA, Ratnaraj N, Goldberg VD, Lascelles PT. 1982. Routine monitoring of carbamazepine and carbamazepine-10,11-epoxide in plasma by high-performance liquid chromatography using 10-methoxycarbamazepine as internal standard. *J Chromatogr* 231: 93–101.

45. Paxton JW. 1982. Carbamazepine determination in saliva of children: enzyme immunoassay (EMIT) versus high pressure liquid chromatography. *Epilepsia* 23: 185–189.

46. Tosoni S, Signorini C, Albertini A. 1983. Gas-chromatographic determination of valproic acid in serum without derivatization. *Clin Chem* 29: 990.

47. Wohler AS, Poklis A. 1997. A simple, rapid gas-liquid chromatographic procedure for the determination of valproic acid in serum. *J Anal Toxicol* 21: 306–309.

48. Yu HY, Shih MC.1996. Determination of valproic acid in human plasma by capillary gas chromatography. *Ther Drug Monit* 18: 107–108.

49. Calendrillo BA, Reynoso G. 1980. A micromethod for the on-column methylation of valproic acid by gas-liquid chromatography. *J Anal Toxicol* 4: 272–274.

50. Morita Y, Ruo TI, Lee ML, Atkinson Jr AJ. 1981. On-column propylation method for measuring plasma valproate concentration by gas chromatography. *Ther Drug Monit* 3: 193–199.

51. Nishioka R, Kawai S, Toyoda S. 1983. New method for the gas chromatographic determination of valproic acid in serum. *J Chromatogr* 277: 356–360.

52. Darius J, Meyer FP. 1995. Sensitive capillary GC-MS method for the therapeutic drug monitoring of valproic acid and seven of it's metabolites in human serum. *J Chrom B* 656: 343–353.

53. Braun SL, Tausch A, Vogt W, Jacob K, Knedel M. 1981. Evaluation of a new valproic acid enzyme immunoassay and comparison with a capillary gas-chromatographic method. *Clin Chem* 27: 169–172.

54. Leroux M, Budnik D, Hall K, Irvine-Meek J, et al. 1981. Comparison of gas-liquid chromatography and EMIT assay for serum valproic acid. *Clin Biochem* 14: 87–90.

55. Hara S, Kamura M, Inoue K, Kukuzawa M, et al. 1999. Determination of valproic acid in human serum by high performance liquid chromatography with fluorescence detection. *Biol Pharm Bull* 22: 975–977.

56. Zhong Y, Jiao Y, Yu Y. 2006. Simultaneous determination of mycophenolic acid and valproic acid based on derivatization by high performance liquid chromatography with fluorescence detection. *Biomed Chromatogr* 20: 319–326.
57. Kabra PM, McDonald DM, Marton LJ. 1978. A simultaneous high-performance liquid chromatographic analysis of the most common anticonvulsants and their metabolites in the serum. *J Anal Toxicol* 2: 127–133.
58. Queiroz ME, Silva SM, Carvalho D, Lancas FM. 2002. Determination of lamotrigine simultaneously with carbamazepine, carbamazepine epoxide, phenytoin, phenobarbital and primidone in human plasma by SPME-GC-TSD. *J Chromatogr Sci* 40: 219–223.
59. Liu H, Delgado M, Forman LJ, Eggers CM, Montoy JL. 1999., Simultaneous determination of carbamazepine, phenytoin, phenobarbital, primidone and their principal metabolites by high-performance liquid chromatography with photodiode array detection. *J Chromatogr* 616: 105–115.
60. Wad N, Bourgeois B, Kramer G. 1999. Serum protein binding of desmethyl-methsuximide. *Clin Neuropharmacol* 22: 239–240.
61. Speed DJ, Dickinson SJ, Cairns ER, Kim, ND. 2000. Analysis of six anticonvulsant drugs using solid phase extraction, deuterated internal standard and gas chromatography-mass spectrometry. *J Anal Toxicol* 24: 685–690.
62. Ou CN, Rognerud, CL. 1984. Simultaneous measurement of ethosuximide, primidone, phenobarbital, phenytoin, carbamazepine and their bioactive metabolites by liquid chromatography. *Clin Chem* 30: 1667–1670.
63. Martar KM, Nicholls PJ, Tekle A, Bawazir SA, Al-Hassan, MI. 1999. Liquid chromatographic determination of six antiepileptic drugs and two metabolites in microsamples of human plasma. *Ther Drug Monit* 21: 559–566.

6 Clinical Practice of Therapeutic Drug Monitoring of New Anticonvulsants

Matthew D. Krasowski
University of Iowa Hospitals and Clinics

CONTENTS

6.1 INTRODUCTION

For many years, classical anticonvulsants such as phenytoin, phenobarbital, primidone, carbamazepine and valproic acid were the only drugs available to treat various seizure disorders. Although these classical anticonvulsants are still widely used in clinical practice, 10 new anticonvulsant drugs have been approved by the FDA (Food and Drug Administration of the United States Government). These drugs alone or in combination with classical anticonvulsants are used today in the management of patients with seizures. Although therapeutic drug monitoring (TDM) is essential for management of patients with classical anticonvulsants, the guidelines for TDM have not been clearly established for newer anticonvulsants. In addition, several newer anticonvulsants may not even require extensive TDM.

6.2 BACKGROUND ON THERAPEUTIC DRUG MONITORING (TDM) OF ANTICONVULSANT MEDICATIONS

Drugs used to treat and prevent seizures (antiepileptic drugs, AEDs) have been among the most common drugs for which TDM is performed [1,2]. Traditionally, TDM has been applied mainly to the "older" AEDs that have been on the market in the United States and many other countries for several decades, namely carbamazepine, phenobarbital, phenytoin, primidone, and valproic acid. These older AEDs in general have narrow therapeutic ranges and significant interindividual variability in their pharmacokinetics. Somewhat surprisingly, given the long history of TDM for AEDs, the evidence that TDM actually helps clinical management is mostly retrospective and anecdotal. Only two randomized, controlled studies of AED TDM have been performed and neither showed clear clinical benefits of TDM. Both studies did show, however, that physicians often apply information from TDM incorrectly, diminishing the clinical value of TDM [3,4]. This makes education regarding TDM a priority for the future.

TDM of AEDs faces several challenges [2]. Firstly, seizures by their nature occur irregularly, sometimes with long periods of time in between episodes. Therefore, long-term observation of any treatment of seizures (medication or otherwise) may be needed to determine clinical benefit. Secondly, for some drugs, the clinical symptoms of the underlying disease may be hard to differentiate from adverse effects of the medication(s) being used. Lastly, there are no simple tests that can assess clinical efficacy of anticonvulsants. Clinical observation and relatively time-consuming diagnostic tests such as the electroencephalogram (EEG) remain the mainstays of clinical assessment.

In applying TDM to any drug, the most basic assumption is that the concentration being measured (usually serum or plasma but occasionally some other fluid such as urine or cerebrospinal fluid) correlates with the concentration at the target site of action (e.g., ion channel in the brain). Factors that can affect negatively affect this correlation include tolerance to the drug, irreversibility of drug action, and active metabolites. In the cases of drugs with active metabolites, TDM can include measurement of the concentrations of both parent drug and metabolite(s) or just of the metabolite. As an example, TDM of oxcarbazepine often focuses on the major metabolite (10-hydroxycarbazepine), as will be discussed below.

6.3 REASONS FOR APPLYING THERAPEUTIC DRUG MONITORING (TDM)

There are multiple reasons why TDM may be applied to AEDs or other drugs. A common reason is that the pharmacokinetics (absorption, distribution, metabolism, and excretion) of the drug shows significant variability between individuals [5–7]. If the pharmacokinetics is very consistent and predictable, then dosing of the drug can often be done without monitoring serum/plasma concentrations. Metabolism is a major pharmacokinetic factor that can affect AEDs. Variability in metabolism may be due to genetic factors (pharmacogenetics), organ dysfunction (typically liver or kidney), or drug-drug or drug-food interactions. Several AEDs, namely carbamazepine, phenobarbital, and phenytoin, are well-known "inducers" of "drug-metabolizing" enzymes in the liver and other organs [8–12]. Therapy with these drugs causes an increase in expression of cytochrome P450 (CYP) and other enzymes (e.g., glucuronidation enzymes) that metabolize AEDs, leading to a decrease in the serum/plasma concentrations. Carbamazepine represents an example of a drug that shows "autoinduction," namely that the metabolism of carbamazepine increases as the drug is used over time [13]. This means that the dose needs to be increased over time to keep pace with the increases in metabolism, until the induction levels off. Other known enzymes inducers include rifampin (tuberculosis drug) and St. John's wort (herbal antidepressant) [14–17]. Some drugs may also inhibit metabolism of AEDs, potentially leading to excessively high concentrations of drug unless the dose is reduced appropriately. Valproic acid is a well-documented inhibitor of multiple liver enzymes that can cause drug-drug interactions with other AEDs [1]. Variability in pharmacokinetics may also occur due to alterations in drug absorption or distribution. AEDs that show substantial variability in pharmacokinetics are good candidates for TDM [2].

For some medications that are highly bound to serum proteins, monitoring of free (unbound) drug concentrations may be useful [18]. A number of factors may alter serum protein concentrations including liver disease, pregnancy, and old age. Concomitant medications (e.g., valproic acid) or endogenous substances may displace drugs from serum protein binding sites, leading to higher free drug concentrations. Uremia, as may occur in renal failure, may increase free anticonvulsant drug concentrations by displacement from serum protein binding sites. Free drug concentrations are typically measured by first creating an ultrafiltrate of serum/plasma and then analyzing the concentration of drug present in the ultrafiltrate. The technical challenge is that free drug concentrations may be substantially lower than total drug concentrations. Some analytical methods that may be adequate for measuring total drug concentrations may have insufficient limits of detection to measure the full range of clinically useful free drug concentrations [18].

TDM may also be used to assess compliance (adherence) to therapy [2]. Given that AEDs may be prescribed for months or years, even in the absence of seizures, it is understandable why some patients skip doses or stop taking the medication altogether. The presence of adverse effects can be another reason for noncompliance.

6.4   THE NEWER GENERATION OF ANTIEPILEPTIC DRUGS (AEDs)

In the last 15 years, ten new AEDs have entered the market in the United States [19–21]. These drugs are felbamate, gabapentin, lamotrigine, levetiracetam, oxcarbazepine, pregabalin, tiagabine, topiramate, vigabatrin and zonisamide (see Figure 6.1 for chemical structures). In comparison to the older AEDs, the newer agents often have wide therapeutic ranges and fewer serious adverse effects. Like some of the older AEDs, the newer agents may also be used for other conditions such as bipolar disorder, chronic pain, or migraine headaches [20–22]. This chapter focuses on TDM of the newer AEDs, emphasizing whether the pharmacokinetics and other properties of the drug make TDM potentially useful.

6.5   THE DIFFICULTY OF REFERENCE RANGES

There is considerable debate over the issue of reference ranges for the newer AEDs [2]. These drugs generally have been observed to be effective over a wide range of serum/plasma concentrations. Ideally, TDM would guide physicians toward serum/plasma concentrations that optimize seizure control/suppression while minimizing toxic effects. The "reference range" of an AED can be defined by two limits—a lower limit below which therapeutic effect is unlikely and an upper limit above which toxicity is likely [2]. However, it should be kept in mind that any particular individual may respond well at concentrations outside the reference range. A limitation of reference ranges is that they may not be generally applicable to patients with different types of seizures. For example, the range may be established in a clinical study of patients with refractory epilepsy, a group that may respond quite differently from patients with more responsive disease. Furthermore, many of the newer AEDs were originally studied as adjunctive therapy and not as monotherapy. Perucca has proposed the concept of "individual therapeutic concentrations" for AEDs [23]. In applying this concept, a patient is treated until good seizure control is achieved. The serum/plasma concentration is then determined and then serves as the patient's individual therapeutic concentration. TDM can then be applied periodically to determine whether the concentration is staying near the individual therapeutic concentration. This approach to TDM can be applied to new or old generation AEDs [23,24]. When changes that may alter the effects of AED are present, or will occur in the future (e.g., pregnancy, change in liver or kidney function, concomitant therapy with enzyme-inducing or inhibiting drugs), TDM can be applied to maintain the individual therapeutic concentration. One limitation of the individual therapeutic concentration is that clinical judgment may be needed to determine whether changes in the underlying seizure condition require establishment of a new individual therapeutic concentration.

With the background and theory on TDM above, each of the newer AEDs will be discussed in turn with regard to TDM. This chapter focuses on monitoring of serum or plasma, although it should be pointed out that there has been some research into monitoring AED concentrations in other fluids (e.g., saliva) [25]. Table 6.1 summarizes the pharmacokinetic parameters and reference

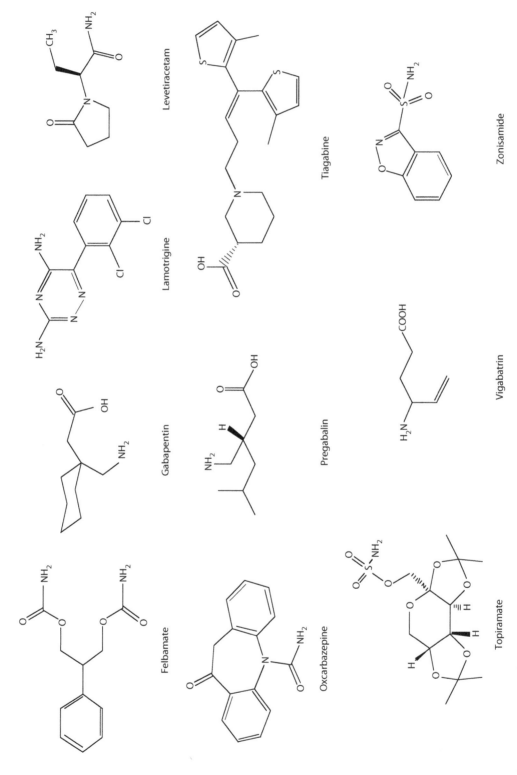

FIGURE 6.1 Structures of the 10 AEDs covered in this review.

TABLE 6.1
Pharmacokinetic Parameters and Reference Ranges for the AEDs

Drug	Oral Bioavailability (%)	Serum Protein Binding (%)	Time to Peak Concentration (hrs)	Half-Life in Absence of Concomitant Enzyme Inducers[a]	Half-Life in Patients on Concomitant Enzyme Inducers[a]	Reference Range in Serum (mg/L)	Comments
Felbamate	>90	25	2–6	16–22	10–18	30–60	
Gabapentin	<60	0	2–3	5–9	5–9	2–20	
Lamotrigine	≥95	55	1–3	15–35[b]	8–20	2.5–15	
Levetiracetam	≥95	0	1	6–8	5–7	12–46	
Oxcarbazepine	90	40	3–6	8–15	7–12	3–35	All parameters refer to active metabolite (10-hydroxycarbazepine)
Pregabalin	≥90	0	1–2	5–7	5–7	Not established	
Tiagabine	≥90	96	1–2	5–9	2–4	0.02–0.2	Free drug levels may be useful
Topiramate	≥80	15	2–4	20–30	10–15	5–20	
Vigabatrin	≥60	0	1–2	5–8	5–8	0.8–36	
Zonisamide	≥65	50	2–5	50–70	25–35	10–40	

[a] Enzyme inducers include carbamazepine, phenobarbital, phenytoin, rifampicin, and St. John's wort.
[b] Half-life increases to 30–90 hrs during concomitant therapy with valproic acid (enzyme inhibitor).

ranges for the AEDs, using data brought together by a consensus panel examining AED TDM and published in 2008 [2]. Table 6.2 summarizes the evidence for and against TDM of the ten AEDs discussed in this chapter.

6.6 FELBAMATE

Felbamate was approved in 1993 in the United States for the treatment of partial seizures (with and without secondary generalization) in adults and for Lennox–Gastaut syndrome, a type of childhood epilepsy that is often refractory to AED therapy [26–29]. However, by 1994, cases of aplastic anemia and later severe hepatic failure were identified and associated with felbamate therapy. The drug has remained on the market but with revised labeling and much restricted use [28,29]. In terms of pharmacokinetics, felbamate has high bioavailability (>90%) [30,31]. About 50% of the absorbed drug is metabolized by the liver to inactive metabolites [30,32]. It is suspected that one or more of the metabolites mediates the rare but serious adverse effects [30]. Inducers of liver metabolism (e.g., carbamazepine, phenytoin, phenobarbital) increase the metabolism of felbamate [33,34], while valproic acid inhibits the metabolism [35]. Felbamate does not have a clear reference range but typical doses result in serum/plasma concentrations of 30–60 mg/L [36,37]. The clearance of felbamate is 20-65% higher in children than in adults [6].

TABLE 6.2
Summary of Justifications for TDM of Newer AEDs

Drug	Evidence for use of TDM[a]	Indications for TDM	Reasons Against TDM
Felbamate	Medium	Variable metabolism	Unclear reference ranges, toxicity better monitored by complete blood counts and liver enzymes
Gabapentin	Low	Renal failure	Unclear reference range, low incidence of toxicity
Lamotrigine	High	Variable metabolism, differences in clearance across ages and during pregnancy	
Levetiracetam	Medium	Renal failure	Wide reference range, low incidence of toxicity
Oxcarbazepine	Medium to high	Variable metabolism, well-defined toxic concentrations	Complicated metabolism with active metabolites and parent drug
Pregabalin	Low	Renal failure	Unclear reference range, low incidence of toxicity
Tiagabine	Medium	High serum protein binding	Unclear reference range, trough levels need to be obtained
Topiramate	Medium to high	Variable metabolism	
Vigabatrin	Low		Irreversible mechanism of action, no clear reference range
Zonisamide	High	Variable metabolism, well-defined toxic concentrations	

[a] Low: TDM mainly useful only for assessing compliance to therapy and possibly to assess toxicity; medium: some additional indications for TDM but therapy can generally be managed without use of TDM; high: clear indications for TDM such as significant variation in drug metabolism that is difficult to predict without TDM.

The variable metabolism of felbamate and differences between children and adults in clearance suggest that TDM may be helpful in felbamate therapy. However, the serious nature of rare adverse effects of felbamate have severely limited the use of this drug [28,29]. Close monitoring of liver function and blood counts are advised during felbamate therapy.

6.7   GABAPENTIN

Gabapentin was originally approved in 1994 in the United States for the treatment in epilepsy but has achieved greater popularity as an adjunctive therapy for chronic pain [19,38]. Although structurally related to γ-aminobutyric acid (GABA; the major inhibitory neurotransmitter in the brain), gabapentin does not appear to interact with GABA receptors [19]. Gabapentin is rapidly absorbed by the L-amino acid transport system [39]. Gabapentin is not metabolized and not bound to any significant degree to serum proteins [39]. Nearly 100% is excreted renally and the half-life of the drug increases in renal failure [38]. A wide range of serum/plasma concentrations are associated with clinical effect [40] although effective control of seizures typically requires concentrations above 2 mg/L [41]. An approximate reference range of 2–20 mg/L has been proposed [42].

Other than to assess compliance or to adjust dosing during renal failure, gabapentin is not a good candidate for TDM. The lack of metabolism and unclear target serum/plasma concentrations make application of TDM difficult [2].

6.8   LAMOTRIGINE

Lamotrigine was approved by the FDA in late 1994 as an adjunctive therapy for partial seizures with or without secondary generalization [20]. Lamotrigine has since gained indications as monotherapy for partial seizures and also as a treatment for bipolar disorder ("manic depression") [1,2]. Lamotrigine is rapidly and completely absorbed from the gastrointestinal tract and is only 55% bound to serum proteins. The parent drug is extensively metabolized, mainly to an inactive glucuronide metabolite [43–45]. The metabolism of lamotrigine shows the phenomenon of "autoinduction," namely that the metabolism of the drug can increase over time. For most patients, autoinduction is complete within two weeks, with an approximately 17% reduction in steady-state serum/plasma concentrations if the dose is not changed [44]. The metabolism of lamotrigine is significantly affected by classic liver enzyme inducers (carbamazepine, phenobarbital, and phenytoin) [43–45]. The serum half-life of lamotrigine typically is 15–35 hr when used as monotherapy, 8–20 hr when use concomitantly with a liver enzyme inducer, and up to 60 hr when used together with valproic acid, a CYP enzyme inhibitor [43,45]. The clearance of lamotrigine is higher in children [6,46] and markedly higher (~300%) in pregnancy [6]. There is not a clear relationship between clinical response and serum/plasma concentrations [46], but a reference range of 3–14 mg/L has been suggested for refractory epilepsy therapy [47]. The incidence of toxicity increases significantly when concentrations exceed 15 mg/L [47,48].

The major adverse effect of lamotrigine is potentially severe skin reactions (including toxic epidermal necrolysis and Stevens–Johnson syndrome) [43,46,49]. The mechanism of this reaction is not well understood but dermatologic reactions typically occur within the first two to eight weeks of therapy. Cautious titration of dose and careful education of patients regarding the possibility of skin reactions has been effective in limiting serious reactions. Experience with lamotrigine over the last 15 years has shown a good safety profile during pregnancy when compared to traditional anticonvulsants such as carbamazepine and phenytoin and the anti-mania drug lithium that are clearly associated with teratogenic effects [50]. This has led to increasing use of lamotrigine in pregnant women with epilepsy and bipolar disorder.

Several factors favor application of TDM for lamotrigine. The drug shows significant interindividual variation in dose versus serum/plasma, in large part due to multiple factors that can affect liver metabolism of the drug. The clearance of lamotrigine varies substantially across age groups and also during pregnancy. TDM of lamotrigine during pregnancy is becoming more common as the drug gains increasing favor as a relatively safe option for treatment of epilepsy and bipolar disorder during pregnancy [50]. Lastly, although there is substantial overlap in serum/plasma concentrations between therapeutic responders and nonresponders, there is a fairly clear concentration threshold above which toxic side effects become more common [43–47,50]. There are numerous published chromatographic methods for lamotrigine (see Chapter 7). Recently, Microgenics introduced a homogenous turbidimetric immunoassay for determination of lamotrigine serum/plasma concentrations, making TDM of lamotrigine with fast turnaround time available to a range of clinical laboratories.

6.9   LEVETIRACETAM

Levetiracetam is a novel anticonvulsant whose mechanism of action is not well understood [51,52]. Levetiracetam is rapidly and nearly completely absorbed following oral administration [53]. The rate but not extent of oral absorption is slowed by coingestion with food [54]. Levetiracetam has low binding to serum proteins and linear pharmacokinetics. Nearly all of the absorbed drug is excreted by the kidneys [55], with approximately two-thirds as the parent drug and the remainder as the metabolite L057, formed by hydrolysis in the blood [56]. The serum half-life of levetiracetam is longer (16–18 hr) in neonates compared to adults (6–8 hr) [2]. An approximately 60% decrease in serum concentrations is observed in pregnancy [57]. Because levetiracetam is not metabolized by the liver, no significant drug–drug interactions have been noted. From evaluation of 470 patients in a specialty epilepsy clinic, a reference range of 12–46 mg/L has been proposed [58].

Other than to assess compliance or to evaluate possible toxicity, the value of TDM for levetiracetam is mostly in adjusting dosage for renal insufficiency or failure, as kidneys are the major elimination route [2,53,55,59]. In performing TDM, it is important to separate serum or plasma from whole blood rapidly, as artefactual hydrolysis of levetiracetam can occur in the blood tube [56].

6.10   OXCARBAZEPINE

Oxcarbazepine is structurally closely related to carbamazepine but does not produce nearly as much liver enzyme induction as carbamazepine and also shows a lower incidence of agranulocytosis [60–63]. Oxcarbazepine is rapidly and completely absorbed [63] and metabolized via presystemic 10-keto reduction to its monohydroxy derivative 10-hydroxycarbazepine. 10-Hydroxycarbazepine is equipotent to oxcarbazepine in anticonvulsant activity but accumulates to higher concentrations in serum than the parent drug [62]. 10-Hydroxycarbazepine is approximately 40% bound to serum proteins and further metabolized, primarily by glucuronidation. The clearance of 10-hydroxycarbazepine is reduced in the elderly [6] and also in the setting of renal insufficiency or failure [64]. The clearance of 10-hydroxycarbazepine is increased in pregnancy [65,66] and in patients taking liver enzyme-inducing drugs [63]. Young children require higher doses of oxcarbazepine per body weight than adults [67].

TDM of oxcarbazepine typically focuses on the metabolite 10-hydroxycarbazepine, although there are theoretically benefits to also monitoring the parent drug [2,60,68]. In a study of 947 patients, a wide range of serum concentrations (3–35 mg/L) were observed to be effective in seizure treatment [69]. Toxic side effects were more common at serum/plasma concentrations of 35 mg/L or higher [70]. For the purposes of TDM, oxcarbazepine is treated like a pro-drug, with monitoring focusing on the monohydroxy metabolite as the main mediator of the anticonvulsant effects [2]. TDM is justified when changes are expected that might alter 10-hydroxycarbazepine clearance including pregnancy, presence of liver enzyme-inducing drugs, and changes in renal function. Determination of 10-hydroxycarbazepine concentration is also helpful in evaluating possible drug toxicity [70].

6.11 PREGABALIN

Pregabalin was designed as a more potent analog of gabapentin [71]. Like gabapentin, pregabalin has shown effectiveness in treating chronic pain and additionally gained an indication in the United States for the treatment of fibromyalgia [20,72]. Pregabalin has predictable and favorable pharmacokinetics with excellent bioavailability [73], minimal binding to serum proteins, essentially no metabolism, and no reported drug–drug interactions. The majority of the absorbed dose (~98%) is excreted unchanged in the urine with a clearance that approximates glomerular filtration rate (GFR) [74]. Renal failure patients require reduced dosage [75]. No clear reference range has been established but an approximate range of 2.8–8.3 mg/L has been proposed [2]. The short half-life of pregabalin (4.6–6.8 hr) [76] means that care must be taken in drawing blood for TDM. If possible, trough levels should be obtained. Similar to gabapentin, other than to assess compliance or to adjust dosing during renal failure, pregabalin is not a good candidate for routine TDM. In patients being treated with pregabalin for chronic pain, assays for pregabalin may be used simply to verify compliance before trying other medications such as opioids that carry higher abuse liability.

6.12 TIAGABINE

Tiagabine is currently not widely used in the United States and Europe [20]. The mechanism of action is not clear although inhibition of GABA reuptake has been proposed [19]. Tiagabine is rapidly absorbed with bioavailability of more than 90% [77]. Unlike many of the other newer anticonvulsants that show low binding to serum proteins, tiagabine is highly bound to proteins (>96%). Valproic acid can displace tiagabine from plasma protein binding sites, leading to increased free concentrations of tiagabine [78]. Tiagabine is extensively metabolized with less than 1% of the absorbed parent drug excreted unchanged [77,79]. The metabolism of tiagabine is increased during concomitant therapy with classic liver enzyme inducers. The serum half-life is 2–4 hr in patients receiving enzyme inducers and 5–9 hr in those not receiving enzyme inducers [80]. Children have higher clearance than adults [81]. The serum half-life increases to 12–16 hr in severe liver failure [82].

The interindividual variation in liver metabolism, which can be affected by concomitant therapy with enzyme inducers or liver failure, makes tiagabine a candidate for TDM. The relatively short half-life of tiagabine under most conditions means that care must be taken in drawing blood for TDM, with trough levels obtained if feasible. The high binding to serum proteins further suggests that measurement of free drug concentrations may be useful [18]. However, there has been little investigation of the relationship between serum/plasma concentrations and therapeutic efficacy [2]. A broad reference range of 20–200 ng/mL has been proposed [79]. Analytical issues have been a difficult problem in measurement of tiagabine serum/plasma concentrations [83]. Limit of sensitivity is a problem in doing free drug concentrations. Research aimed at development of improved methodology for measurement of drug concentrations may be stimulated if the clinical popularity of tiagabine were to increase in the future.

6.13 TOPIRAMATE

Topiramate has approval for treatment of epilepsy of children and adults, and also more recently for treatment of migraine headaches [20]. Following oral administration, topiramate is absorbed rapidly with a bioavailability of 80% of higher [84] and also has low binding to serum proteins. Approximately 50% of the absorbed dose is metabolized by the liver, with an increase in metabolism seen in patients concomitantly receiving therapy with enzyme inducers. Enzyme inducers can decrease the serum half-life from 20–30 hr to approximately 12 hr [85–87]. Children generally eliminate topiramate faster than adults [6,88]. A reference range of 5–20 mg/L has been proposed for topiramate for epilepsy therapy [89].

The value of TDM of topiramate is mainly due to interindividual variation in metabolism. Polymedco and Microgenics both market homogeneous immunoassays for determination of serum/plasma concentrations of topiramate.

6.14 VIGABATRIN

Vigabatrin is an irreversible inhibitor of GABA transaminase, an enzyme that catalyzes the breakdown of GABA [90,91]. The drug is supplied as a racemic mixture, with the S(+) enantiomer being active and R(–) enantiomer being inactive therapeutically [91]. The drug has bioavailability of 60–80% [92], does not bind appreciably to serum proteins, and is primarily excreted unchanged in the urine [90]. Doses of vigabatrin generally need to be increased during renal failure [90].

The irreversible nature of the mechanism of action of vigabatrin undercuts one of the principle assumptions of TDM, namely that the concentration in serum/plasma correlates with that at the target site of action. This may be one reason why a wide range of trough serum/plasma concentrations (0.8–36 mg/L) have been found in patients treated with vigabatrin [21]. Other than to assess compliance, there is little justification for TDM of vigabatrin [21].

6.15 ZONISAMIDE

Zonisamide is approved in the United States for adjunctive treatment of partial seizures but is also used off-label for migraine headaches, chronic pain, and bipolar depression [20,93,94]. Zonisamide is rapidly absorbed after oral administration and is only 40–60% bound to serum proteins. Zonisamide displays linear pharmacokinetics but is extensively metabolized by oxidation, acetylation, and other pathways [95,96]. CYP3A4, the major liver drug-metabolizing enzyme in most people, is responsible for some of the metabolism of zonisamide. The metabolism of zonisamide can be significantly affected by enzyme inducers (e.g., carbamazepine, phenobarbital, and phenytoin). The serum half-life of zonisamide is approximately 50–70 hr for patients receiving zonisamide as monotherapy but decreases to 25–35 hr in patients also receiving enzyme inducers. Conversely, liver enzyme inhibitors such as valproic acid and ketoconazole may prolong zonisamide half-life [7]. Children require higher doses by weight than adults [6]. For treatment of partial seizures, the effective serum concentration range is 7–40 mg/L [94]. Toxic side effects are uncommon at serum concentrations below 30 mg/L [97,98]. A serum/plasma reference range of 10–40 mg/L has been proposed [94,99].

The interindividual variability in metabolism of zonisamide, especially seen in those receiving concomitant therapy with other drugs that can affect liver enzyme expression, makes zonisamide an attractive candidate for TDM. Recently, Microgenics introduced a homogeneous turbidimetric immunoassay for determination of zonisamide serum/plasma concentrations.

6.16 CONCLUSIONS

The newer generation of AEDs offers attractive pharmacological alternatives to the traditional AEDs for treatment of epilepsy and other disorders such as chronic pain, migraine headaches, and fibromyalgia. The newer AEDs generally have fewer adverse effects and wider therapeutic margins. The strongest cases for routine TDM can be made for lamotrigine, oxcarbazepine (mono-hydroxy metabolite), tiagabine, and zonisamide, mainly due to interindividual variation in metabolism and clearance. For other drugs, TDM may be clinically useful to assess adherence or to adjust dosing in organ failure. Future research is needed to better define reference ranges and to better document the value of TDM in clinical practice.

REFERENCES

1 Neels, H.M., A.C. Sierens, K. Naelerts, S.L. Scharpé, G.M. Hatfield, and W.E. Lambert. 2004. Therapeutic drug monitoring of old and newer anti-epileptic drugs. *Clin Chem Lab Med* 42 (11):1228–1255.

2. Patsalos, P.N., D.J. Berry, B.F.D. Bourgeois, J.C. Cloyd, T.A. Glauser, S.I. Johannessen, T. Tomson, and E. Perucca. 2008. Antiepileptic drugs—best practice guidelines for therapeutic drug monitoring: a position paper by the subcommission on therapeutic drug monitoring, ILAE Commission on Therapeutic Strategies. *Epilepsia* 49 (7):1239–1276.

3. Fröscher, W., M. Eichelbaum, R. Gugler, G. Hildebrand, and H. Penin. 1981. A prospective randomized trial on the effect of monitoring plasma anticonvulsant levels in epilepsy. *J Neurol* 224 (3):193–201.

4. Januzzi, G., P. Cian, C. Fattore, G. Gatti, A. Bartoli, F. Monaco, and E. Perucca. 2000. A multicenter randomized controlled trial on the clinical impact of therapeutic drug monitoring in patients with newly diagnosed epilepsy. *Epilepsia* 41 (2):222–230.

5. Bialer, M. 2005. The pharmacokinetics and interactions of new antiepileptic drugs: an overview. *Ther Drug Monit* 27 (6):722–726.

6. Perucca, E. 2006. Clinical pharmacokinetics of new-generation antiepileptic drugs at the extremes of age. *Clin Pharmacokinet* 45 (4):351–364.

7. Perucca, E., and M. Bialer. 1996. The clinical pharmacokinetics of the newer antiepileptic drugs. Focus on topiramate, zonisamide and tiagabine. *Clin Pharmacokinet* 31 (1):29–46.

8. Dickins, M. 2004. Induction of cytochromes P450. *Curr Topics Med Chem* 4:1745–1766.

9. Fuhr, U. 2000. Induction of drug metabolizing enzymes: pharmacokinetic and toxicological consequences in humans. *Clin Pharmacokinet* 38 (6):493–504.

10. Handschin, C., and U.A. Meyer. 2003. Induction of drug metabolism: the role of nuclear receptors. *Pharmacol Rev* 55 (4):649–673.

11. Luo, G., T. Guenthner, L-S. Gan, and W.G. Humphreys. 2004. CYP3A4 induction by xenobiotics: biochemistry, experimental methods and impact on drug discovery and development. *Curr Drug Metab* 5 (6):483–505.

12. Schuetz, E.G. 2001. Induction of cytochromes P450. *Curr Drug Metab* 2 (2):139–147.

13. Pitlick, W.H., and R.H. Levy. 1977. Time-dependent kinetics I: Exponential autoinduction of carbamazepine in monkeys. *J Pharmaceutical Sci* 66 (5):647–649.

14. Komoroski, B.J., S. Zhang, H. Cai, J.M. Hutzler, R. Frye, T.S. Tracy, S.C. Strom, T. Lehmann, C.Y.W. Ang, Y.Y. Cui, and R. Venkataramanan. 2004. Induction and inhibition of cytochromes P450 by the St. John's wort constituent hyperforin in human hepatocyte cultures. *Drug Metab Dispos* 32 (5):512–518.

15. Moore, L.B., B. Goodwin, S.A. Jones, G.B. Wisely, C.J. Serabjit-Singh, T.M. Willson, J.L. Collins, and S.A. Kliewer. 2000. St. John's wort induces hepatic drug metabolism through activation of the pregnane X receptor. *Proc Natl Acad Sci USA* 97 (13):7500–7502.

16. Skolnick, J.L., B.S. Stoler, D.B. Katz, and W.H. Anderston. 1976. Rifampin, oral contraceptives, and pregnancy. *JAMA* 236 (12):1382.

17. Van Buren, D., C.A. Wideman, M. Ried, S. Gibbons, C.T. Van Buren, M. Jarowenko, S.M. Flechner, O.H. Frazier, D.A. Cooley, and B.D. Kahan. 1984. The antagonistic effect of rifampin upon cyclosporine bioavailability. *Transplant Proc* 16 (6):1642–1645.

18. Dasgupta, A. 2007. Usefulness of monitoring free (unbound) concentrations of therapeutic drugs in patient management. *Clin Chim Acta* 377 (1–2):1–13.

19. LaRoche, S.M., and S.L. Helmers. 2004. The new antiepileptic drugs: scientific review. *JAMA* 291 (5):605–614.

20. LaRoche, S.M., and S.L. Helmers. 2004. The new antiepileptic drugs: clinical applications. *JAMA* 291 (5):615–620.

21. Patsalos, P.N. 1999. New antiepileptic drugs. *Ann Clin Biochem* 36 (1):10–19.

22. Iorio, M.L., U. Moretti, S. Colcera, L. Magro, I. Meneghelli, D. Motola, A.L. Rivolta, F. Salvo, and G.P. Velo. 2007. Use and safety profile of antiepileptic drugs in Italy. *Eur J Clin Pharmacol* 63 (4):409–415.

23. Perucca, E. 2000. Is there a role for therapeutic drug monitoring of new anticonvulsants? *Clin Pharmacokinet* 38 (3):191–204.

24. Johannessen, S.I., and T. Tomson. 2006. Pharmacokinetic variability of newer epileptic drugs? *Clin Pharmacokinet* 45 (11):1061–1075.

25. Liu, H., and M.R. Delgado. 1999. Therapeutic drug concentration monitoring using saliva samples. Focus on anticonvulsants. *Clin Pharmacokinet* 36 (6):453–470.
26. Bourgeois, B.F. 1997. Felbamate. *Semin Pediatr Neurol* 4 (1):3–8.
27. Leppik, I.E. 1995. Felbamate. *Epilepsia* 36 (Suppl 2):S66–S72.
28. Pellock, J.M. 1999. Felbamate in epilepsy therapy: evaluating the risks. *Drug Saf* 21 (3):225–239.
29. Pellock, J.M., E. Faught, I.E. Leppik, S. Shinnar, and M.L. Zupanc. 2006. Felbamate: consensus of current clinical experience. *Epilepsy Res* 71 (2–3):89–101.
30. Shumaker, R.C., C. Fantel, E. Kelton, K. Wong, and I. Weliky. 1990. Evaluation of the elimination of (^{14}C) felbamate in healthy men. *Epilepsia* 31 (Suppl):642.
31. Ward, D.L., and R.C. Shumaker. 1990. Comparative bioavailability of felbamate in healthy men. *Epilepsia* 31 (Suppl):642.
32. Thompson, C.D., M.T. Barthen, D.W. Hopper, T.A. Miller, M. Quigg, C. Hudspeth, G. Montouris, L. Marsh, J.L. Perhach, R.D. Sofia, and T.L. Macdonald. 1999. Quantification in patient urine samples of felbamate and three metabolites: acid carbamate and two mercapturic acids. *Epilepsia* 40 (6):769–776.
33. Kelley, M.T., P.D. Walson, S. Cox, and L.J. Dusci. 1997. Population pharmacokinetics of felbamate in children. *Ther Drug Monit* 19 (1):29–36.
34. Sachdeo, R.C., S.K. Howard, J.R. Narang-Sachdeo, R.K. Dix, R.C. Shumaker, J.L. Perhach, and A. Rosenberg. 1993. Steady-state pharmacokinetics and dose-proportionality of felbamate after oral administration of 1200, 2400, and 3600 mg/day of felbamate. *Epilepsia* 34 (Suppl 6):80.
35. Ward, D.L., M.L. Wagner, J.L. Perhach, L. Kramer, N. Graves, I. Leppik, and R.C. Shumaker. 1991. Felbamate steady-state pharmacokinetics during co-administration of valproate. *Epilepsia* 32 (Suppl 3):8.
36. Faught, E., R.C. Sachdeo, M.P. Remler, S. Chayasirisobhon, V.J. Iragui-Madoz, R.E. Ramsay, T.P. Sutula, A. Kanner, R.N. Harner, R. Kuzniecky, L.D. Kramer, M. Karmin, and A. Rosenberg. 1993. Felbamate monotherapy for partial-onset seizures: an active-controlled trial. *Neurology* 43 (4):688–692.
37. Sachdeo, R.C., L.D. Kramer, A. Rosenberg, and S. Sachdeo. 1992. Felbamate monotherapy: controlled trial in patients with partial onset seizures. *Ann Neurol* 32 (3):386–392.
38. McLean, M.J. 1995. Gabapentin. *Epilepsia* 36 (Suppl 2):S57–S86.
39. Vollmer, K.O., A. von Hodenberg, and E.U. Kölle. 1988. Pharmacokinetics and metabolism of gabapentin in rat, dog and man. *Arzneimittelforschung* 36 (5):830–839.
40. Armijo, J.A., M.A. Perna, J. Adin, and N. Vega-Gil. 2004. Association between patient age and gabapentin serum concentration-to-dose ratio: a preliminary multivariate analysis. *Ther Drug Monit* 26 (6):633–637.
41. Sivenius, J., R. Kälviäinen, A. Ylinen, and P. Riekkinen. 1991. A double-blind study of gabapentin in the treatment of partial seizures. *Epilepsia* 32 (4):539–542.
42. Lindberger, M., O. Luhr, S.I. Johannessen, S. Larsson, and T. Tomson. 2003. Serum concentrations and effects of gabapentin and vigabatrin: observations from a dose titration study. *Ther Drug Monit* 25 (4):457–462.
43. Biton, V. 2006. Pharmacokinetics, toxicology and safety of lamotrigine in epilepsy. *Expert Opin Drug Metab Toxicol* 2 (6):1009–1018.
44. Hussein, Z., and J. Posner. 1997. Population pharmacokinetics of lamotrigine monotherapy in patients with epilepsy: retrospective analysis of routine monitoring data. *Br J Clin Pharmacol* 43 (5):457–464.
45. Rambeck, B., and P. Wolf. 1993. Lamotrigine clinical pharmacokinetics. *Clin Pharmacokinet* 25 (6):433–443.
46. Bartoli, A., R. Guerrini, A. Belmonte, M.G. Alessandri, G. Gatti, and E. Perucca. 1997. The influence of dosage, age, and comedication on steady state plasma lamotrigine concentrations in epileptic children: a prospective study with preliminary assessments of correlations with clinical response. *Ther Drug Monit* 19 (3):252–260.
47. Morris, R.G., A.B. Black, A.L. Harris, A.B. Batty, and B.C. Sallustio. 1998. Lamotrigine and therapeutic drug monitoring: retrospective survey following the introduction of a routine service. *Br J Clin Pharmacol* 46 (6):547–551.
48. Besag, F.M., D.J. Berry, and F. Pool. 1998. Carbamazepine toxicity with lamotrigine: pharmacokinetic or pharmacodynamic interaction. *Epilepsia* 39 (2):183–187.
49. Wong, I.C., G.E. Mawer, and J.W. Sander. 2001. Adverse event monitoring in lamotrigine patients: a pharmacoepidemiologic study in the United Kingdom. *Epilepsia* 42 (2):237–244.
50. Pennell, P.B., L. Peng, D.J. Newport, J.C. Ritchie, A. Koganti, D.K. Holley, M. Newman, and Z.N. Stowe. 2008. Lamotrigine in pregnancy: clearance, therapeutic drug monitoring, and seizure frequency. *Neurology* 70 (22 Pt 2):2130–2136.

51. Klitgaard, H. 2001. Levetiracetam: the preclinical profile of a new class of antiseizure drugs? *Epilepsia* 42 (Suppl 4):S13–S18.
52. Leppik, I.E. 2001. The place of levetiracetam in the treatment of epilepsy. *Epilepsia* 42 (Suppl 4):S44–S45.
53. Patsalos, P.N. 2000. Pharmacokinetic profile of levetiracetam: toward ideal characteristics. *Pharmacol Ther* 85 (2):77–85.
54. Fay, M.A., R.D. Sheth, and B.E. Gidal. 2005. Oral absorption kinetics of levetiracetam: the effect of mixing with food or enteral nutrition formulas. *Clin Ther* 27 (5):594–598.
55. Patsalos, P.N. 2004. Clinical pharmacokinetics of levetiracetam. *Clin Pharmacokinet* 43 (11):707–724.
56. Patsalos, P.N., S. Ghattaura, N. Ratnaraj, and J.W. Sander. 2006. In situ metabolism of levetiracetam in blood of patients with epilepsy. *Epilepsia* 47 (11):1818–1821.
57. Tomson, T., and D. Battino. 2007. Pharmacokinetics and therapeutic drug monitoring of newer antiepileptic drugs during pregnancy and the puerperium. *Clin Pharmacokinet* 46 (3):209–219.
58. Leppik, I.E., J.O. Rarick, T.S. Walczak, T.A. Tran, J.R. White, and R.J. Gumnit. 2002. Effective levetiracetam doses and serum concentrations: age effects. *Epilepsia* 43 (Suppl 7):240.
59. Radtke, R.A. 2001. Pharmacokinetics of levetiracetam. *Epilepsia* 42 (Suppl):24–27.
60. Flesch, G. 2004. Overview of the clinical pharmacokinetics of oxcarbazepine. *Clin Drug Investig* 24 (4):185–203.
61. Larkin, J.G., P.J. McKee, G. Forrest, G.H. Beastall, B.K. Park, J.I. Lowrie, P. Lloyd, and M.J. Brodie. 1991. Lack of enzyme induction with oxcarbazepine (600 mg daily) in healthy subjects. *Br J Clin Pharmacol* 31 (1):65–71.
62. Lloyd, P., G. Flesch, and W. Dieterle. 1994. Clinical pharmacology and pharmacokinetics of oxcarbazepine. *Epilepsia* 3 (Suppl): 10–13.
63. May, T.W., E. Korn-Merker, and B. Rambeck. 2003. Clinical pharmacokinetics of oxcarbazepine. *Clin Pharmacokinet* 42 (12):1023–1042.
64. Rouan, M.C., J.B. Lecaillon, J. Godbillon, F. Menard, T. Darragon, P. Meyer, O. Kourilsky, D. Hillion, J.C. Aldigier, and P. Jungers. 1994. The effect of renal impairment on the pharmacokinetics of oxcarbazepine and its metabolites. *Eur J Clin Pharmacol* 47 (2):161–167.
65. Christensen, J., A. Sabers, and P. Sidenius. 2006. Oxcarbazepine concentrations during pregnancy: a retrospective study in patients with epilepsy. *Neurology* 24 (8):1497–1499.
66. Mazzucchelli, I., F.Y. Onat, C. Ozkara, D. Atakli, L.M. Specchio, A.L. Neve, G. Gatti, and E. Perucca. 2006. Changes in the disposition of oxcarbazepine and its metabolites during pregnancy and the puerperium. *Epilepsia* 47 (3):504–509.
67. Battino, D., M. Estienne, and G. Avanzini. 1995. Clinical pharmacokinetics of antiepileptic drugs in pediatric patients. Part II. Phenytoin, carbamazepine, sulthiame, lamotrigine, vigabatrin, oxcarbazepine and felbamate. *Clin Pharmacokinet* 29 (5):341–369.
68. Armijo, J.A., N. Vega-Gil, M. Shushtarian, J. Adin, and J.L. Herranz. 2005. 10-Hydroxycarbazepine serum concentration-to-oxcarbazepine dose ratio: influence of age and concomitant antiepileptic drugs. *Ther Drug Monit* 27 (2):199–204.
69. Friis, M.L., O. Kristensen, J. Boas, M. Dalby, S.H. Deth, L. Gram, M. Mikkelsen, B. Pedersen, A. Sabers, and J. Worm-Petersen. 1993. Therapeutic experiences with 947 epileptic out-patients in oxcarbazepine treatment. *Acta Neurol Scand* 87 (3):224–227.
70. Striano, S., P. Striano, P. Di Nocera, D. Italiano, C. Fasiello, P. Ruosi, L. Bilo, and F. Pisani. 2006. Relationship between serum mono-hydroxy-carbazepine concentrations and adverse effects in patients with epilepsy on high-dose oxcarbazepine therapy. *Epilepsy Res* 69 (2):170–176.
71. Selak, I. 2001. Pregabalin (Pfizer). *Curr Opin Investig Drugs* 2 (6):828–834.
72. Acharya, N.V., R.M. Pickering, L.W. Wilton, and S.A. Shakir. 2005. The safety and effectiveness of newer antiepileptics: a comparative post-marketing cohort study. *J Clin Pharmacol* 45 (4):385–393.
73. Busch, J.A., J.C. Strand, E.L. Posvar, H.N. Bockbrader, and L.L. Radulovic. 1998. Pregabalin (CI-1008) single-dose pharmacokinetics and safety/tolerance in healthy subjects after oral administration of pregabalin solution or capsule doses. *Epilepsia* 39 (Suppl 6):58.
74. Corrigan, B.W., W.F. Poole, E.L. Posvar, J.C. Strand, C.W. Alvey, and L.L. Radulovic. 2001. Metabolic disposition of pregabalin in healthy volunteers. *Clin Pharmacol Ther* 69 (Suppl):P18.
75. Randinitis, E.J., E.L. Posvar, C.W. Alvey, A.J. Sedman, J.A. Cook, and H.N. Bockbrader. 2003. Pharmacokinetics of pregabalin in subjects with various degrees of renal functions. *J Clin Pharmacol* 43 (3):277–283.
76. Bockbrader, H.N., T. Hunt, J. Strand, E.L. Posvar, and A. Sedman. 2000. Pregabalin pharmacokinetics and safety in health volunteers: results from two phase I studies. *Neurology* 11 (Suppl 3):412.

77. Gustavson, L.E., and H.B. Mengel. 1995. Pharmacokinetics of tiagabine, a γ-aminobutyric acid-uptake inhibitor, in healthy subjects after single and multiple doses. *Epilepsia* 36 (6):605–611.

78. Patsalos, P.N., A.A. Elyas, N. Ratnaraj, and J. Iley. 2002. Concentration-dependent displacement of tiagabine by valproic acid. *Epilepsia* 43 (Suppl 8):143.

79. Uthman, B.M., A.J. Rowan, P.A. Ahmann, I.E. Leppik, S.C. Schachter, K.W. Sommerville, and V. Shu. 1998. Tiagabine for complex partial seizures: a randomized, add-on, dose-response trial. *Arch Neurol* 55 (1):56–62.

80. So, E.L., D. Wolff, N.M. Graves, I.E. Leppik, G.D. Cascino, G.C. Pixton, and L.E. Gustavson. 1995. Pharmacokinetics of tiagabine as add-on therapy in patients taking enzyme-inducing antiepilepsy drugs. *Epilepsy Res* 22 (3):221–226.

81. Gustavson, L.E., S.W. Boellner, G.R. Granneman, J.X. Qian, H.J. Guenther, T. el-Shourbagy, and K.W. Sommerville. 1997. A single-dose study to define tiagabine pharmacokinetics in pediatric patients with complex partial seizures. *Neurology* 48 (4):1032–1037.

82. Lau, A.H., L.E. Gustavson, R. Sperelakis, N.P. Lam, T. El-Shourbagy, J.X. Qian, and T. Layden. 1997. Pharmacokinetics and safety of tiagabine in subjects with various degrees of hepatic function. *Epilepsia* 38 (4):445–451.

83. Williams, J., M. Bialer, S.I. Johannessen, G. Krämer, R. Levy, R.H. Mattson, E. Perucca, P.N. Patsalos, and J.F. Wilson. 2003. Interlaboratory variability in the quantification of new generation antiepileptic drugs based on external quality assessment data. *Epilepsia* 44 (1):40–45.

84. Easterling, D.E., T. Zakszewski, M.D. Moyer, B.L. Margul, T.B. Marriott, and R.K. Nayak. 1988. Plasma pharmacokinetics of topiramate, a new anticonvulsants in humans. *Epilepsia* 29 (Suppl):662.

85. Britzi, M., E. Perucca, S. Soback, R.H. Levy, C. Fattore, F. Crema, G. Gatti, D.R. Doose, B.E. Maryanoff, and M. Bialer. 2005. Pharmacokinetic and metabolic investigation of topiramate disposition in healthy subjects in the absence and in the presence of enzyme induction by carbamazepine. *Epilepsia* 46 (3):378–384.

86. Mimrod, D., L.M. Specchio, M. Britzi, E. Perucca, N. Specchio, A. La Neve, S. Soback, R.H. Levy, G. Gatti, D.R. Doose, B.E. Maryanoff, and M. Bialer. 2005. A comparative study of the effect of carbamazepine and valproic acid on the pharmacokinetics and metabolic profile of topiramate at steady state in patients with epilepsy. *Epilepsia* 46 (7):1046–1054.

87. Sachdeo, R.C., S.K. Sachdeo, S.A. Walker, L.D. Kramer, R.K. Nayak, and D.R. Doose. 1996. Steady-state pharmacokinetics of topiramate and carbamazepine in patients with epilepsy during monotherapy and concomitant therapy. *Epilepsia* 37 (8):774–480.

88. Rosenfeld, W.E., D.R. Doose, S.A. Walker, J.S. Baldassarre, and R.A. Reifer. 1999. A study of topiramate pharmacokinetics and tolerability in children with epilepsy. *Pediatr Neurol* 20 (5):339–344.

89. Johannessen, S.I., D. Battino, D.J. Berry, M. Bialer, G. Kramer, T. Tomson, and P.N. Patsalos. 2003. Therapeutic drug monitoring of the newer antiepileptic drugs. *Ther Drug Monit* 25 (3):347–363.

90. Rey, E., G. Pons, and G. Olive. 1992. Vigabatrin. Clinical pharmacokinetics. *Clin Pharmacokinet* 23 (4):267–278.

91. Schechter, P.J. 1989. Clinical pharmacology of vigabatrin. *Br J Clin Pharmacol* 27 (Suppl 1):19S–22S.

92. Durham, S.L., J.F. Hoke, and T.M. Chen. 1993. Pharmacokinetics and metabolism of vigabatrin following a single oral dose of [^{14}C]vigabatrin in healthy male volunteers. *Drug Metab Dispos* 21 (3):480–484.

93. Leppik, I.E. 1999. Zonisamide. *Epilepsia* 40 (Suppl 5):S23–S29.

94. Mimaki, T. 1998. Clinical pharmacology and therapeutic drug monitoring of zonisamide. *Ther Drug Monit* 20 (6):593–597.

95. Buchanan, R., H.N. Bockbrader, T. Chang, and A.J. Sedman. 1996. Single- and multiple-dose pharmacokinetics of zonisamide. *Epilepsia* 37 (Suppl 5):172.

96. Ito, T., T. Yamaguchi, H. Miyazaki, Y. Sekine, M. Shimizu, S. Ishida, K. Yagi, N. Kakegawa, M. Seino, and T. Wada. 1982. Pharmacokinetic studies of AD-180, a new antiepileptic compound. Phase I trials. *Arzneimittelforschung* 32 (12):1581–1586.

97. Berent, S., J.C. Sackellares, B. Giordani, J.G. Wagner, P.D. Donofrio, and B. Abou-Khalil. 1987. Zonisamide (CI-912) and cognition: results from preliminary study. *Epilepsia* 28 (1):61–67.

98. Miura, H. 1993. Developmental and therapeutic pharmacology of antiepileptic drugs. *Jpn J Psychiatry Neurol* 47 (2):169–174.

99. Glauser, T.A., and C.E. Pippenger. 2000. Controversies in blood-level monitoring: re-examining its role in the treatment of epilepsy. *Epilepsia* 41 (Suppl 8):S6–S15.

7 Chromatographic Techniques in the Therapeutic Drug Monitoring of New Anticonvulsants

Christine L.H. Snozek and Loralie J. Langman
Mayo Clinic College of Medicine

CONTENTS

7.1 INTRODUCTION

Anticonvulsants, also termed antiepileptics (AEDs), are used to treat a variety of neurological and psychiatric disorders. The classic indication is of course epilepsy, but AEDs have also been used with success in nonseizure conditions such as bipolar disorder and anxiety disorders including post-traumatic stress [1,2]. Several commonly prescribed AEDs, such as phenytoin and valproic acid, are in clinical use for decades. However, since the early 1990s a second generation of compounds has been approved; these "new" AEDs are rapidly increasing in popularity as long-term therapeutic agents for both neurological and psychological conditions. Drugs considered new anticonvulsants include: felbamate, gabapentin, lamotrigine, levetiracetam, oxcarbazepine, pregabalin, topiramate, tiagabine, vigabatrin (outside of the United States), and zonisamide. Most have proven to be effective against a broad spectrum of epileptic disorders, with selective activity in psychiatric illnesses [1,2].

Like phenytoin, valproic acid, and other classic anticonvulsants, newer AEDs function by reducing neuronal excitability through a variety of mechanisms [3,4]. However, there are a number of differences between the new and the old generation drugs. Although each drug has unique characteristics (discussed below), some generalizations can be made for illustrative purposes. Newer AEDs have similar efficacy to their older counterparts, but typically display fewer or milder side effects and have a larger therapeutic index [5,6]. In this vein, certain older AEDs increase the likelihood of teratogenesis when taken by a woman in the first two trimesters of pregnancy; it is thought that the newer AEDs have lower risk of causing fetal malformation, but there are as yet insufficient data to confirm this [3,5,7–9]. Such issues are especially important given the long-term—often lifelong—nature of therapy with AEDs. The cost of the newer drugs is typically higher, although some are approaching or past patent expiration, allowing generic formulations. Finally, most new anticonvulsants are less subject to pharmacokinetic variability than older AEDs, alleviating in part some of the concerns that necessitate rigorous therapeutic drug monitoring (TDM) for these compounds [3,9].

7.2   DISTRIBUTION AND METABOLISM

The older anticonvulsants were notorious for a slew of undesirable phenomena, including modulation of enzymatic metabolism and competition for protein binding [4,10]. In general, the newer AEDs exhibit a far more favorable pharmacokinetic profile: the majorities are not extensively protein-bound, do not strongly induce or inhibit metabolic enzymes, and do not display dose-dependent absorption [4,9,10]. Older AEDs were heavily reliant upon Phase I cytochrome p450 (CYP)-mediated biotransformation for elimination, and several were strong inducers or inhibitors of various CYP enzymes [4,10]. In contrast, several newer anticonvulsants (gabapentin, pregabalin, levetiracetam, and vigabatrin) rely only minimally upon hepatic mechanisms, while others are metabolized by hepatic glucuronidation (UGT enzyme family) in addition to cytochrome (CYP)-mediated transformations [11,12]. Thus, although the CYP enzymes are involved, they tend to represent minor pathways of metabolism for the second-generation anticonvulsants rather than the predominant means of elimination. Accordingly, the new AEDs are less prone to affecting CYP activity, although several are comparatively weak inducers or inhibitors of CYP enzymes [11,12].

Other pharmacokinetic parameters are similarly improved in most new AEDs compared to their older counterparts. Bioavailability of oral formulations is generally high, with dose-independent absorption. Plasma transport does not rely upon binding to albumin or other proteins, thus, largely eliminating a major mechanism of drug interactions. Finally, the majority of new AEDs do not have active metabolites, which simplifies interpretation of TDM results [9].

Elimination of many drugs involves both the liver and kidney; however, some of the newer AEDs are excreted almost entirely via renal clearance. This provides better options for patients with hepatic disease or concomitant medications, though lower doses may be required for patients with renal dysfunction. Children typically display decreased half-life and enhanced clearance that necessitates increasing dosage; AED dose requirements for children of any age are often unpredictable, thus, TDM is essential [5]. However, the need for dose adjustments diminishes gradually as young patients approach adulthood [5]. Similarly, enhanced renal clearance in pregnancy may affect serum levels. Treatment of pregnant women with AEDs is not uncommon, and requires balancing the risks to the fetus of harm from exposure to medication versus injury from relapse of the mother's condition; pregnancy is thus one of the clearest indications for TDM of newer anticonvulsants [5,13].

7.3   CONCERNS IN THERAPEUTIC DRUG MONITORING (TDM) OF NEW ANTICONVULSANTS

In contrast to older AEDs, whose multifactorial pharmacokinetic variability provides clear rationale for TDM, newer anticonvulsant therapy has not seen the same degree of benefit from routine measurement of serum levels [9]. Although there are published recommendations for reference ranges for each of the new AEDs (Table 7.1), there are fewer large, prospective studies available for the newer anticonvulsants, in contrast to the older drugs [9]. Many of the studies that do exist are confounded by the prevalence of polytherapy in the study cohorts; many patients receive multiple AEDs, often resulting in drug–drug interactions that complicate interpretation of serum drug concentrations. In addition, population-based ranges are frequently not useful in managing individual patients: a given person may show toxicity within the recommended range, while another may respond well at apparently subtherapeutic levels [4,9]. These interindividual differences are often provided as reasons for disregarding TDM with newer AEDs.

However, given the lifelong nature of many of the conditions treated with anticonvulsants, TDM can be of great use in managing intraindividual variability over time [5,9,14]. Interpretation of a single serum value relative to population-based therapeutic ranges should be flexible; therapy

TABLE 7.1
Structure and Therapeutic Range of New Anticonvulsants

Compound and Therapeutic Range	Chemical Structure	Compound and Therapeutic Range	Chemical Structure
Felbamate 125–250 umol/L 30–60 ug/mL		Pregabalin 18–52 umol/L 2.8–8.2 ug/mL	
Gabapentin 70–120 umol/L 12–20 ug/mL		Tiagabine 5–250 nmol/L 20–100 ng/mL	
Lamotrigine 10–60 umol/L 2.5–15 ug/mL		Topiramate 15–60 umol/L 5–20 ug/mL	
Levetiracetam 35–120 umol/L 8–26 ug/mL		Vigabatrin No therapeutic range established.	
Oxcarbazepine 50–140 umol/L (as metabolite) 12–35 ug/mL (as metabolite)		Zonisamide 45–180 ug/mL 10–38 ug/mlL	

Sources: Tomson T, Battino D, *Clin Pharmacokinet,* 46, 209–19, 2007; Johannessen SI, Tomson T, *Clin Pharmacokinet,* 45, 1061–75, 2006; and Johannessen SI, Battino D, Berry DJ, Bialer M, Kramer G, Tomson T, Patsalos PN, *Ther Drug Monit,* 25, 347–63, 2003.

must be guided by the individual patient's clinical response. Once a desirable response has been achieved, serum concentrations help to ascertain a preferred baseline for a given patient and to monitor long-term compliance. In addition, TDM of newer AEDs is useful in managing physiological changes such as aging, pregnancy, and alterations in concomitant medications and comorbid conditions [5,9].

Long-term AED therapy in women has a number of specific issues that must be taken into consideration. Anticonvulsants can alter steroid hormone metabolism and disturb steroidogenesis, potentially affecting fertility [13]; AED metabolism can in turn be disrupted by coadministration of hormone-containing contraceptives [5]. In pregnancy, changes in drug disposition and clearance can lead to substantial fluctuations from previous steady-state levels. This greatly complicates the task of preventing harm to the fetus: early exposure to AEDs can increase risk of fetal malformation, but breakthrough seizures from under-medication can cause hypoxia and fetal distress, which may pose a greater risk to the fetus than the anticonvulsant itself [5,7]. Finally, postpartum re-equilibration can lead to rapid changes in serum drug levels and may result in additional exposure of nursing infants to AEDs [7]. For all these reasons, TDM is indicated in women of childbearing age to successfully manage patients dealing with contraception, preconception, pregnancy, and nursing.

Rapid physiological change, as with childhood or pregnancy, is the clearest situation calling for TDM of newer anticonvulsants. However, despite suggestions that population-based therapeutic indices are less definitive for the new AEDs compared to the older anticonvulsants, routine TDM is still important for patient management, though it may require determination of each individual's optimal serum drug level. Long-term therapy with anticonvulsants requires establishing a baseline of desirable clinical response, ensuring compliance to maintain that steady-state, and managing physiological changes over time; TDM can assist in all of these aspects of patient care [9].

7.4   NEW ANTICONVULSANTS

In this section, each of the commonly measured new AEDs will be discussed in greater detail, with emphasis on the features that distinguish each compound from the group as a whole.

7.4.1   FELBAMATE

Approved for monotherapy, pediatric treatment, and most types of seizures, felbamate acts via a poorly understood mechanism that may involve the N-methyl-D-aspartate (NMDA) receptor [9,15]. Despite its approval for a wide range of uses, felbamate is one of the few newer AEDs with potentially lethal side effects, namely hepatotoxicity and aplastic anemia [14]. It is metabolized by oxidation or hydrolysis to a variety of metabolites [9], and felbamate clearance can be affected by enzyme inducers, including several traditional AEDs [16]. Hepatic or renal dysfunction can raise serum felbamate levels and are indications for TDM-based dose adjustment [14].

7.4.2   GABAPENTIN

Despite being a structural analog of γ-aminobutyric acid (GABA), gabapentin appears to act at least in part through GABA receptor-independent mechanisms [9,14]. Interestingly, gabapentin modulates serotonin release from platelets and can affect platelet aggregation [17]. Unlike most new anticonvulsants, gabapentin exhibits nonlinear kinetics due to dose-dependent absorption, possibly due to saturation of an active transport system [9]. Its half-life of 5–7 hr [9,18] is notably shorter than other new AEDs and necessitates frequent dosing. However, purely renal clearance of gabapentin with minimal metabolism makes this drug useful for treating patients with severe hepatic disease [9]. There are few data available regarding the utility of gabapentin TDM, but its dose-dependent kinetics suggest that TDM would be helpful in establishing an individual baseline and after altering dosage.

7.4.3 LAMOTRIGINE

An inhibitor of voltage-gated sodium channels, lamotrigine is used clinically for a wide variety of seizures and bipolar disorder; some studies also suggest efficacy in treating anxiety [14]. Limited data indicate lamotrigine treatment in pregnancy confers a risk of major congenital malformations that is comparable to some older AEDs, though lower than that seen with valproic acid [13]. Clearance of lamotrigine is significantly increased in pregnancy, in some studies by >300%, providing strong indication for TDM for managing women of childbearing age [13]. Metabolism occurs primarily via UGT1A4-mediated glucuronidation; though lamotrigine has minimal effect on the pharmacokinetics of other drugs, its own metabolism is affected by UGT induction or inhibition, as seen with older AEDs such as phenytoin or valproic acid, respectively [9]. Drug interactions may in part explain why therapeutic ranges for lamotrigine have shifted over time, while early studies proposed a much lower range than most current recommendations, possibly due to greater inclusion of patients on combination therapy.

7.4.4 LEVETIRACETAM

Although levetiracetam affects several aspects of neuronal function, its primary mechanism of action appears to be regulation of a vesicle protein involved in exocytosis [9,19,20]. Levetiracetam is notable for several highly favorable pharmacokinetic parameters, including efficient, dose-independent absorption and minimal protein binding [21]. Hepatic metabolism is almost entirely bypassed and over half of levetiracetam is excreted unchanged in urine, while its major, inactive metabolite is formed via extrahepatic hydrolysis [21]. Thus, levetiracetam has little effect on the metabolism of other compounds, though serum levels can be mildly affected by coadministration of enzyme-inducing AEDs [21]. Levetiracetam is available as a parenteral formulation for acute clinical situations.

7.4.5 OXCARBAZEPINE

Oxcarbazepine is the 10-keto analog of carbamazepine, and shows similar therapeutic effects to the older compound. Oxcarbazepine is rapidly reduced by cytosolic arylketone reductases to its major active metabolite 10-hydroxy-10,11-dihydrocarbamazepine (licarbazepine or 10-hydroxycarbazepine), also called MHD for monohydroxy derivative [9,22]. The MHD is primarily responsible for drug activity and, therefore, TDM analysis generally targets this metabolite [22,23]. MHD is a chiral compound; *in vivo* conversion results in preferential (~80%) formation of the S-enantiomer, but R- and S-MHD are approximately equal in activity [24]. Both the parent drug and MHD undergo additional inactivating metabolism including glucuronidation, but unlike its close relative carbamazepine, oxcarbazepine does not substantially induce expression of metabolic enzymes [22]. Thus, oxcarbazepine exhibits fewer drug interactions than older anticonvulsants, although at high doses it can inhibit CYP2C19 and weakly induce UGT family members [22]. Intriguingly, oxcarbazepine therapy can reduce serum levels of oral contraceptives to the point of contraceptive failure, despite being only a weak inducer of CYP3A4 [22]. Renal failure will prolong oxcarbazepine exposure [25], but little clinical effect is seen with mild or moderate hepatic disease [9].

7.4.6 PREGABALIN

Approved in the United States in 2005, pregabalin is a structural analog of GABA that apparently lacks GABAergic activity [26,27]. Like gabapentin, pregabalin exhibits dose-dependent absorption, minimal protein binding and negligible hepatic metabolism. Pregabalin is excreted fairly rapidly and almost entirely unchanged in urine. To date, there are few TDM studies with pregabalin; dose adjustments may be required with renal dysfunction [26,27].

7.4.7 TIAGABINE

Structurally distinct from other new anticonvulsants, tiagabine appears to act by inhibition of GABA reuptake [9,28]. It resembles the older AEDs in that it exhibits a number of unfavorable pharmacokinetic parameters. Tiagabine is the only new AED to exhibit extensive protein binding, making it subject to alterations in protein levels (e.g., pregnancy) and to displacement by competitors (e.g., valproic acid) for the same binding sites [9]. The half-life of tiagabine is relatively short, though comparable to gabapentin and pregabalin; however, it is also quite variable between individuals. Tiagabine does not appear to affect the activity of most metabolic enzymes, but its own metabolism can be greatly influenced by hepatic insufficiency or by comedication with enzyme inducers [9,29]. Absorption of tiagabine is not dose-dependent though extremely rapid; administration with a meal slows absorption sufficiently to reduce fluctuations in serum concentration without affecting bioavailability [9].

7.4.8 TOPIRAMATE

With several mechanisms of action including modulation of voltage-dependent sodium channels, the $GABA_A$ receptor, and possibly the non-NMDA receptor [9,30], topiramate is approved as a single-agent therapy for various types of seizures. Topiramate is preferred in some settings for its ability to cause weight loss; however, it is also associated with kidney stones and adverse cognitive effects [31]. The pharmacokinetics of topiramate are largely favorable: it is rapidly and extensively absorbed, exhibits little protein binding, and is cleared slowly enough to allow daily or twice-daily dosing [9,30]. However, at high doses, topiramate induces CYP3A4 and may cause therapeutic failure of oral contraceptives; similarly, topiramate metabolism is affected by coadministration of enzyme-inducing medications [31].

7.4.9 VIGABATRIN

Not approved for use in the United States, vigabatrin is an irreversible inhibitor of GABA transaminase [32]. This enzyme is responsible for downregulation of GABA-mediated inhibitory signaling, thus treatment with vigabatrin potentiates GABAergic effects. Because enzyme inhibition by vigabatrin is irreversible, the duration of anti-seizure activity depends on the recovery rate of the transaminase rather than continued presence of the drug; vigabatrin efficacy is therefore somewhat independent of its concentration in serum. Since vigabatrin acts by irreversible inhibition of the enzyme GABA transaminase, there is a clear dissociation between its concentration profile in serum and the duration of pharmacological effect; the effect being related to the regeneration time of the enzyme [9]. For this reason, TDM is not particularly useful in long-term vigabatrin therapy except to ascertain compliance [9,14]. However, serum vigabatrin concentration as a check on recent compliance may be useful.

7.4.10 ZONISAMIDE

With the longest half-life of the newer AEDs, zonisamide is more amenable to infrequent dosing than most other anticonvulsants [33]. It exhibits some protein binding and accumulates in red blood cells in a concentration-dependent manner, thus serum levels do not correlate well with dose [33]. Zonisamide is metabolized by both oxidation and conjugation, and its serum levels can be affected by comedication with enzyme inducers [9,34]. As yet there is no clear relationship between zonisamide concentrations and clinical response; TDM is largely limited to ascertaining baseline levels, managing medication changes, and monitoring compliance [35].

7.5   ANALYTICAL CONSIDERATIONS

7.5.1   MATRIX

As with most therapeutic drugs, the matrix of choice for monitoring new AEDs is serum or plasma. However, alternate matrices have been examined as well, with variable success. Oral fluid (saliva) is an acceptable matrix for some compounds, such as phenytoin and carbamazepine [36]. It is important to note that, in the case of newer AEDs, the use of oral fluid is not well studied. Cerebrospinal fluid is also an acceptable matrix analytically; however, CSF drug levels at autopsy do not necessarily correlate well to blood for the newer AEDs. Finally, breast milk is a relatively common atypical specimen source, since AED therapy often must be maintained throughout pregnancy and in nursing mothers. Most new anticonvulsants will enter breast milk and be passed to the infant [37], but in general, cessation of breast feeding is not required [37].

7.5.2   IMMUNOASSAYS

TDM immunoassays for the traditional AEDs have been available for many years, from multiple companies, and are often compatible with high-throughput chemistry analyzers. In contrast, development of similar assays for the newer anticonvulsants has been slow, likely due at least in part to the relative lack of toxicity associated with the second-generation drugs. Some in-house radioimmunoassays were developed [38], however, since most laboratories have moved away from the use of radioisotopes, assays such as these have not been widely utilized. Thus, unfortunately, most of the newer AEDs do not have readily available immunoassays for TDM, although several are in development. The few compounds that currently have a commercial immunoassay available include topiramate, lamotrigine, and zonisamide [39,40]. However, these assays tend to be designed for a limited number of specialized platforms, and are not compatible with most common, high-throughput analyzers. This situation has therefore necessitated the development of robust and straightforward chromatographic assays.

7.5.3   CHROMATOGRAPHY

Most new AEDs can be measured successfully using gas chromatography (GC), though some require derivatization before analysis to maximize sensitivity. An exception to this latter point is felbamate (Figure 7.1), which can be isolated from serum using either solid-phase (SPE) or liquid-liquid extraction, followed by analysis on GC using flame ionization (FID) or nitrogen-phosphorous (NPD) detection without prior derivatization [41,42]. Like felbamate, gabapentin can be extracted by SPE followed by quantitation on GC with either FID [43] or mass spectrometric (MS) detection [44]. However, to consistently achieve the sensitivity necessary for measurement within the gabapentin therapeutic range, derivatization may be required. A method using tert-butyldimethylsilyl (t-BDMS) to derivatize both the carboxylic and amine moieties of the molecule has been described [43,44]. Other drugs such as lamotrigine can also be detected by GC-NPD [45] or GC-MS [46], either underivatized (Figure 7.1) [45] or using t-BDMS as a derivatizing agent [46]. For several of the new AEDs, however, derivatization is required for GC analysis, as is the case with tiagabine analysis by GC-MS [47].

Frequently, the detection method associated with a GC-based protocol is a critical component of achieving adequate sensitivity for routine use. For example, levetiracetam can be quantitated by GC, but it is poorly detected using FID [48]; however, GC-NPD or GC-MS methodologies provide

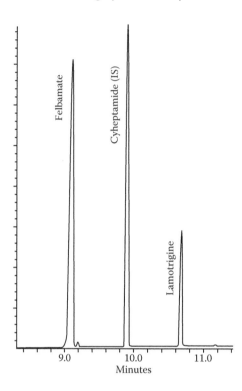

FIGURE 7.1   A total ion chromatogram of (TIC) of lamotrigine and felbamate and cyheptamide (IS, internal standard) by GC/MS. (From Langman LJ, Snozek CLH, unpublished data.)

sufficient sensitivity for clinical applications [48–50]. Conversely, topiramate can be detected readily by GC-FID [51] or GC-NPD [52–54], but it appears that the drug degrades at high injection port temperatures [55], making the GC conditions critical to successful measurement. Oxcarbazepine is also temperature-labile and decomposes under GC conditions, even when injected into a cooled, inert, fused-silica capillary column. In contrast, the trimethylsilyl (TMS) derivative of oxcarbazepine is heat-stable and amenable to analysis by GC-FID [56] or GC-NPD [57]. However, since measurement of the active MHD metabolite (which can be detected underivatized) is of greater utility for TDM, derivatization to detect oxcarbazepine may not be required for a clinically useful assay.

Although many of the newer AEDs can be quantitated by GC, liquid chromatography (LC)-based methods predominate; indeed, for some second-generation compounds such as vigabatrin, pregabalin and zonisamide, only LC-based assays have been described. Several newer anticonvulsants, e.g., felbamate, can be readily measured using high-performance liquid chromatography (HPLC) (Figure 7.2a) with ultraviolet (UV) detection [42,58–60], thus allowing TDM based on a relatively inexpensive and commonly available platform. Some, like gabapentin, lack a chromophore in the native molecule and therefore require derivatization to facilitate HPLC-UV analysis [61]. Derivatization with 1-fluoro-2,4-dinitrobenzene [62,63], phenylisothiocyanate [64], or 2,4,6-trinitrobenzene sulfonic acid has been for gabapentin assays [65]; additionally, trinitrobenzene derivatives of pregabalin can be analyzed by HPLC-UV [66]. Several methods have been used to determine other new AEDs by HPLC-UV including: oxcarbazepine and MHD [67–74], zonisamide [48,75–81], and lamotrigine (Figure 7.1a) [48,67,82–89]. Most of these assays are very similar in principle, with only minor variations in choice of column, mobile phase, or other details.

Unfortunately, not all new AEDs are easily detected with HPLC-UV, although several methods have been described using other common HPLC detectors. Tiagabine, for example, can be measured on HPLC with coulometric electrochemical (ECD) detection [90]. Fluorescence detection (FD) is another option; though few new AEDs have natural fluorescence, derivatization can

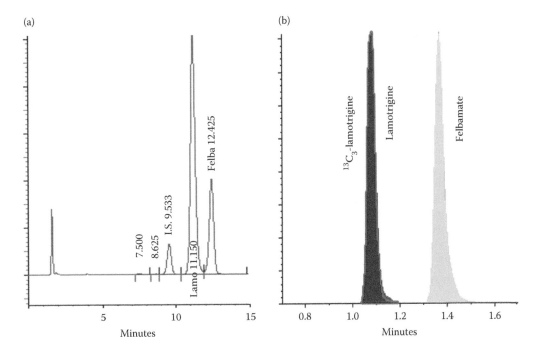

FIGURE 7.2   (a) Chromatogram of lamotrigine (50 ug/mL) and felbamate (150 ug/mL) by HPLC UV detection. (b) Chromatogram of lamotrigine (50 ug/mL) and felbamate (50 ug/mL) by LC-MS/MS. (From Langman LJ, Snozek CLH, unpublished data.)

generate compounds that are suitable for this detection system. Numerous methods for gabapentin [91–94] and pregabalin [95] have been described using o-phthalaldehyde-3-mercaptopropionic acid to provide a fluorophore. In addition, there are several other derivatizing agents available for HPLC-FD assays. Vigabatrin, for example, can be readily analyzed by FD after derivatization with o-phthaldialdehyde [93,94,96] or 4-chloro-7-nitrobenzofurazan [97].

Levetiracetam presents some unique analytical challenges. Unlike the other new AEDs, this compound is available in a parenteral formulation that allows intravenous dosing in urgent clinical situations such as status epilepticus. In these circumstances, very rapid turnaround time for plasma levetiracetam concentrations may be needed clinically [48]. Although this drug can be assayed by HPLC-UV [49,98–101], levetiracetam can cause analytical difficulties: its high polarity complicates extraction, while the lack of a good native chromophore hinders UV detection [48,75,102]. HPLC analysis of levetiracetam thus, frequently requires either derivatization, which extends turnaround time, or use of shorter UV wavelengths, which other biological compounds can absorb nonspecifically [48].

Nonspecificity of HPLC methods is a concern with anticonvulsants, since many patients are treated with combinations of two or more of these medications. Integration of as many AEDs as possible into multicomponent analytical methods is a useful approach to dealing with this issue. However, the chemical structures (Table 7.1) and chromatographic features of these drugs are quite diverse, so it can be difficult (though not impossible) to combine several into the same assay. HPLC methods that measure multiple anticonvulsants simultaneously have been reported [60,103–108]. However, most of these methods either focus primarily on analysis of classical AEDs or use liquid-liquid extraction, which is difficult to automate.

Other HPLC methods exist to analyze combinations of the classical and newer AEDs [60,67,68,71,72,83,109,110]. Unfortunately, the use of HPLC-UV requires chromatographic separation of each compound, typically leading to longer analysis times. Generally speaking, if HPLC can chromatographically resolve the drugs of interest, then LC-MS or LC-MS/MS platforms are also an option for analysis [111,112]. In fact, some drugs like topiramate are best measured by LC-MS/MS [112–115]. Most of the newer AEDs have LC-MS or LC-MS/MS assays published, including levetiracetam [116], felbamate [117], gabapentin [118,119], and lamotrigine [112], among others.

The use of MS or tandem MS detectors improves specificity and shortens run times, by allowing coeluting compounds to be distinguished according to their mass spectra or transitions rather than relying on chromatographic separation. Several methods for simultaneous measurement of carbamazepine and oxcarbazepine have been developed; for example, Breton et al. developed an LC-MS assay that quantitates carbamazepine, oxcarbazepine, and eight of their metabolites and precursors [120], and lamotrigine and felbamate (Figure 7.2b). However, it is important to note that carbamazepine and oxcarbazepine are structurally very similar, and are therefore simpler to combine into a single assay than most new AEDs. Another method describes simultaneous analysis of the structurally and chemically distinct compounds topiramate, gabapentin, and vigabatrin, in a single LC-MS method [121]. Of note, the liquid-liquid extractions used in these procedures are not readily amenable to automation. In contrast, SPE is generally able to be automated, thus methods that combine SPE and LC-MS/MS [112] have the potential to provide the best of all possible worlds in a multianalyte assay: automated extraction, rapid analysis, and high compound specificity.

7.6 CONCLUSIONS

In summary, few immunoassays are available for measurement of the newer AEDs. Although the risk of toxicity with these medications is less severe than with traditional anticonvulsants, clinical demands nonetheless necessitate providing accurate drug levels while minimizing turnaround time. GC and HPLC assays are available for many of the new AEDs, typically requiring less technical expertise while still providing drug levels within a clinically acceptable timeframe. However when laboratory resources and expertise permit, current method development trends are shifting towards measurement of these drugs using LC-MS or LC-MS/MS platforms. Until rapid, accurate immunoassays become commercially available for the new AEDs, chromatographic techniques will remain the cornerstone for analysis of these drugs.

REFERENCES

1. Mula M, Pini S, Cassano GB. 2007. The role of anticonvulsant drugs in anxiety disorders: a critical review of the evidence. *J Clin Psychopharmacol* 27:263–72.
2. Marken PA, Pies RW. 2006. Emerging treatments for bipolar disorder: safety and adverse effect profiles. *Ann Pharmacother* 40:276–85.
3. Perucca E. 2005. An introduction to antiepileptic drugs. *Epilepsia* 46 Suppl 4:31–37.
4. McNamara JO. 2001. Drugs effective in the therapy of the epiliepsies. In: Harman J, Limbird L, Gilman A, eds., *Goodman and Gilman's: The Pharmacological Basis of Therapeutics*. 10th edn. New York, NY: McGraw-Hill Professional, 521–47.
5. Johannessen SI, Landmark CJ. 2008. Value of therapeutic drug monitoring in epilepsy. *Exp Rev Neurother* 8:929–39.
6. LaRoche SM. 2007. A new look at the second-generation antiepileptic drugs: a decade of experience. *Neurologist* 13:133–39.
7. Tomson T, Battino D. 2007. Pharmacokinetics and therapeutic drug monitoring of newer antiepileptic drugs during pregnancy and the puerperium. *Clin Pharmacokinet* 46:209–19.
8. Patsalos PN, Berry DJ, Bourgeois BF, Cloyd JC, Glauser TA, Johannessen SI, et al. 2008. Antiepileptic drugs—best practice guidelines for therapeutic drug monitoring: a position paper by the subcommission on therapeutic drug monitoring, ILAE Commission on Therapeutic Strategies. *Epilepsia* 49:1239–76.
9. Johannessen SI, Tomson T. 2006. Pharmacokinetic variability of newer antiepileptic drugs: when is monitoring needed? *Clin Pharmacokinet* 45:1061–75.
10. Moyer TP, Shaw LM. 2006. Therapeutic drugs and their management. In: Burtis CA, Ashwood ER, Bruns DE, eds., *Tietz Textbook of Clinical Chemistry*. 4th edn. St. Louis, MO: Elsevier Saunders, 1237–85.

11. Ben-Menachem E. 2008. Strategy for utilization of new antiepileptic drugs. *Curr Opin Neurol* 21:167–72.
12. Patsalos PN, Perucca E. 2003. Clinically important drug interactions in epilepsy: general features and interactions between antiepileptic drugs. *Lancet Neurol* 2:347–56.
13. Pack AM. 2006. Therapy insight: clinical management of pregnant women with epilepsy. *Nature Clin Pract* 2:190–200.
14. Johannessen SI, Battino D, Berry DJ, Bialer M, Kramer G, Tomson T, Patsalos PN. 2003. Therapeutic drug monitoring of the newer antiepileptic drugs. *Ther Drug Monit* 25:347–63.
15. Kleckner NW, Glazewski JC, Chen CC, Moscrip TD. 1999. Subtype-selective antagonism of N-methyl-D-aspartate receptors by felbamate: insights into the mechanism of action. *J Pharmacol Exp Ther* 289:886–94.
16. Perucca E. 2006. Clinically relevant drug interactions with antiepileptic drugs. *Br J Clin Pharmacol* 61:246–55.
17. Pan CF, Shen MY, Wu CJ, Hsiao G, Chou DS, Sheu JR. 2007. Inhibitory mechanisms of gabapentin, an antiseizure drug, on platelet aggregation. *J Pharm Pharmacol* 59:1255–61.
18. Vollmer KO, von Hodenberg A, Kolle EU. 1986. Pharmacokinetics and metabolism of gabapentin in rat, dog and man. *Arzneimittel-Forschung* 36:830–39.
19. Noyer M, Gillard M, Matagne A, Henichart JP, Wulfert E. 1995. The novel antiepileptic drug levetiracetam (ucb L059) appears to act via a specific binding site in CNS membranes. *Eur J Pharmacol* 286:137–46.
20. Klitgaard H. 2001. Levetiracetam: the preclinical profile of a new class of antiepileptic drugs? *Epilepsia* 42 Suppl 4:13–18.
21. Perucca E, Johannessen SI. 2003. The ideal pharmacokinetic properties of an antiepileptic drug: how close does levetiracetam come? *Epileptic Disord* 5 Suppl 1:S17–26.
22. Flesch G. 2004. Overview of the clinical pharmacokinetics of oxcarbazepine. *Clin Drug Invest* 24:185–203.
23. Bialer M. 2005. The pharmacokinetics and interactions of new antiepileptic drugs: an overview. *Ther Drug Monit* 27:722–26.
24. May TW, Korn-Merker E, Rambeck B. 2003. Clinical pharmacokinetics of oxcarbazepine. *Clin Pharmacokinet* 42:1023–42.
25. Rouan MC, Lecaillon JB, Godbillon J, Menard F, Darragon T, Meyer P, et al. 1994. The effect of renal impairment on the pharmacokinetics of oxcarbazepine and its metabolites. *Eur J Clin Pharmacol* 47:161–67.
26. Ben-Menachem E. 2004. Pregabalin pharmacology and its relevance to clinical practice. *Epilepsia* 45 Suppl 6:13–18.
27. Warner G, Figgitt DP. 2005. Pregabalin: as adjunctive treatment of partial seizures. *CNS Drugs* 19:265–72; discussion 73–74.
28. Czuczwar SJ, Patsalos PN. 2001. The new generation of GABA enhancers. Potential in the treatment of epilepsy. *CNS Drugs* 15:339–50.
29. Adkins JC, Noble S. 1998. Tiagabine. A review of its pharmacodynamic and pharmacokinetic properties and therapeutic potential in the management of epilepsy. *Drugs* 55:437–60.
30. Langtry HD, Gillis JC, Davis R. 1997. Topiramate. A review of its pharmacodynamic and pharmacokinetic properties and clinical efficacy in the management of epilepsy. *Drugs* 54:752–73.
31. Landmark CJ, Rytter E, Johannessen SI. 2007. Clinical use of antiepileptic drugs at a referral centre for epilepsy. *Seizure* 16:356–64.
32. Schechter PJ. 1989. Clinical pharmacology of vigabatrin. *Br J Clin Pharmacol* 27 Suppl 1:19S–22S.
33. Perucca E, Bialer M. 1996. The clinical pharmacokinetics of the newer antiepileptic drugs. Focus on topiramate, zonisamide and tiagabine. *Clin Pharmacokinet* 31:29–46.
34. Levy RH, Ragueneau-Majlessi I, Brodie MJ, Smith DF, Shah J, Pan WJ. 2005. Lack of clinically significant pharmacokinetic interactions between zonisamide and lamotrigine at steady state in patients with epilepsy. *Ther Drug Monit* 27:193–98.
35. Mimaki T. 1998. Clinical pharmacology and therapeutic drug monitoring of zonisamide. *Ther Drug Monit* 20:593–97.
36. Langman LJ. 2007. The use of oral fluid for therapeutic drug management: clinical and forensic toxicology. *Ann NY Acad Sci* 1098:145–66.
37. Committee on D. 2001. The transfer of drugs and other chemicals into human milk. *Pediatrics* 108:776–89.

38. Biddlecombe RA, Dean KL, Smith CD, Jeal SC. 1990. Validation of a radioimmunoassay for the deter-mination of human plasma concentrations of lamotrigine. *J Pharm Biomed Anal* 8:691–64.
39. http://www.seradyn.com/oem/innofluor.aspx?id = 68. Accessed 8/12/2008.
40. http://www.thermo.com/com/cda/product/detail/0,1055,10141032,00.html. Accessed 8/12/2008.
41. Rifai N, Fuller D, Law T, Mikati M. 1994. Measurement of felbamate by wide-bore capillary gas chro-matography and flame ionization detection. *Clin Chem* 40:745–48.
42. Gur P, Poklis A, Saady J, Costantino A. 1995. Chromatographic procedures for the determination of felbamate in serum. *J Anal Toxicol* 19:499–503.
43. Wolf CE, Saady JJ, Poklis A. 1996. Determination of gabapentin in serum using solid-phase extraction and gas-liquid chromatography. *J Anal Toxicol* 20:498–501.
44. Kushnir MM, Crossett J, Brown PI, Urry FM. 1999. Analysis of gabapentin in serum and plasma by solid-phase extraction and gas chromatography-mass spectrometry for therapeutic drug monitoring. *J Anal Toxicol* 23:1–6.
45. Watelle M, Demedts P, Franck F, De Deyn PP, Wauters A, Neels H. 1997. Analysis of the antiepileptic phenyltriazine compound lamotrigine using gas chromatography with nitrogen phosphorus detection. *Ther Drug Monit* 19:460–64.
46. Dasgupta A, Hart AP. 1997. Lamotrigine analysis in plasma by gas chromatography-mass spec-trometry after conversion to a tert.-butyldimethylsilyl derivative. *J Chromatogr B Biomed Sci Appl* 693:101–17.
47. Chollet DF, Castella E, Goumaz L, Anderegg G. 1999. Gas chromatography-mass spectrometry assay method for the therapeutic drug monitoring of the antiepileptic drug tiagabine. *J Pharm Biomed Anal* 21:641–46.
48. Greiner-Sosanko E, Giannoutsos S, Lower DR, Virji MA, Krasowski MD. 2007. Drug monitoring: simul-taneous analysis of lamotrigine, oxcarbazepine, 10-hydroxycarbazepine, and zonisamide by HPLC-UV and a rapid GC method using a nitrogen-phosphorus detector for levetiracetam. *J Chromatogr Sci* 45:616–22.
49. Vermeij TA, Edelbroek PM. 1994. High-performance liquid chromatographic and megabore gas-liquid chromatographic determination of levetiracetam (ucb L059) in human serum after solid-phase extraction. *J Chromatogr B Biomed Appl* 662:134–39.
50. Isoherranen N, Roeder M, Soback S, Yagen B, Schurig V, Bialer M 2000. Enantioselective analysis of levetiracetam and its enantiomer R-alpha-ethyl-2-oxo-pyrrolidine acetamide using gas chromatography and ion trap mass spectrometric detection. *J Chromatogr B Biomed Sci Appl* 745:325–32.
51. Holland ML, Uetz JA, Ng KT. 1988. Automated capillary gas chromatographic assay using flame ioniza-tion detection for the determination of topiramate in plasma. *J Chromatogr* 433:276–81.
52. Riffitts JM, Gisclon LG, Stubbs RJ, Palmer ME. 1999. A capillary gas chromatographic assay with nitro-gen phosphorus detection for the quantification of topiramate in human plasma, urine and whole blood. *J Pharm Biomed Anal* 19:363–71.
53. Tang PH, Miles MV, Glauser TA, Coletta L, Doughman N, Doose D, et al. 2000. An improved gas chro-matography assay for topiramate monitoring in pediatric patients. *Ther Drug Monit* 22:195–201.
54. Wolf CE, Crooks CR, Poklis A. 2000. Rapid gas chromatographic procedure for the determination of topiramate in serum. *J Anal Toxicol* 24:661–63.
55. Gidal BE, Lensmeyer GL. 1999. Therapeutic monitoring of topiramate: evaluation of the saturable dis-tribution between erythrocytes and plasma of whole blood using an optimized high-pressure liquid chro-matography method. *Ther Drug Monit* 21:567–76.
56. von Unruh GE, Paar WD. 1985. Gas chromatographic assay for oxcarbazepine and its main metabolites in plasma. *J Chromatogr* 345:67–76.
57. Levine B, Green-Johnson D, Moore KA, Fowler DR. 2004. Hydroxycarbazepine distribution in three postmortem cases. *J Anal Toxicol* 28:509–11.
58. Clark LA, Wichmann JK, Kucharczyk N, Sofia RD. 1992. Determination of the anticonvulsant felbamate in beagle dog plasma by high-performance liquid chromatography. *J Chromatogr* 573:113–19.
59. Romanyshyn LA, Wichmann JK, Kucharczyk N, Sofia RD. 1994. Simultaneous determination of fel-bamate and three metabolites in human plasma by high-performance liquid chromatography. *Ther Drug Monit* 16:83–89.
60. Remmel RP, Miller SA, Graves NM. 1990. Simultaneous assay of felbamate plus carbamazepine, pheny-toin, and their metabolites by liquid chromatography with mobile phase optimization. *Ther Drug Monit* 12:90–96.
61. Hengy H, Kolle EU. 1985. Determination of gabapentin in plasma and urine by high-performance liquid chromatography and pre-column labelling for ultraviolet detection. *J Chromatogr* 341:473–78.

62. Souri E, Jalalizadeh H, Shafiee A. 2007. Optimization of an HPLC method for determination of gabapentin in dosage forms through derivatization with 1-fluoro-2,4-dinitrobenzene. *Chem Pharm Bull* 55:1427–30.

63. Jalalizadeh H, Souri E, Tehrani MB, Jahangiri A. 2007. Validated HPLC method for the determination of gabapentin in human plasma using pre-column derivatization with 1-fluoro-2,4-dinitrobenzene and its application to a pharmacokinetic study. *J Chromatogr B Analyt Technol Biomed Life Sci* 854:43–47.

64. Zhu Z, Neirinck L. 2002. High-performance liquid chromatographic method for the determination of gabapentin in human plasma. *J Chromatogr B Analyt Technol Biomed Life Sci* 779:307–12.

65. Lensmeyer GL, Kempf T, Gidal BE, Wiebe DA. 1995. Optimized method for determination of gabapentin in serum by high-performance liquid chromatography. *Ther Drug Monit* 17:251–58.

66. Windsor BL, Radulovic LL. 1995. Measurement of a new anticonvulsant, (S)-3-(aminomethyl)-5-methylhexanoic acid, in plasma and milk by high-performance liquid chromatography. *J Chromatogr B Biomed Appl* 674:143–48.

67. Contin M, Balboni M, Callegati E, Candela C, Albani F, Riva R, Baruzzi A. 2005. Simultaneous liquid chromatographic determination of lamotrigine, oxcarbazepine monohydroxy derivative and felbamate in plasma of patients with epilepsy. *J Chromatogr B Analyt Technol Biomed Life Sci* 828:113–17.

68. Franceschi L, Furlanut M. 2005. A simple method to monitor plasma concentrations of oxcarbazepine, carbamazepine, their main metabolites and lamotrigine in epileptic patients. *Pharmacol Res* 51:297–302.

69. Juenke JM, Brown PI, Urry FM, McMillin GA. 2006. Drug monitoring and toxicology: a procedure for the monitoring of oxcarbazepine metabolite by HPLC-UV. *J Chromatogr Sci* 44:45–48.

70. Kimiskidis V, Spanakis M, Niopas I, Kazis D, Gabrieli C, Kanaze FI, Divanoglou D. 2007. Development and validation of a high performance liquid chromatographic method for the determination of oxcarbazepine and its main metabolites in human plasma and cerebrospinal fluid and its application to pharmacokinetic study. *J Pharm Biomed Anal* 43:763–68.

71. Levert H, Odou P, Robert H. 2002. LC determination of oxcarbazepine and its active metabolite in human serum. *J Pharm Biomed Anal* 28:517–25.

72. Mandrioli R, Ghedini N, Albani F, Kenndler E, Raggi MA. 2003. Liquid chromatographic determination of oxcarbazepine and its metabolites in plasma of epileptic patients after solid-phase extraction. *J Chromatogr B Analyt Technol Biomed Life Sci* 783:253–63.

73. Matar KM, Nicholls PJ, al-Hassan MI, Tekle A. 1995. Rapid micromethod for simultaneous measurement of oxcarbazepine and its active metabolite in plasma by high-performance liquid chromatography. *J Clin Pharm Ther* 20:229–34.

74. Pienimaki P, Fuchs S, Isojarvi J, Vahakangas K. 1995. Improved detection and determination of carbamazepine and oxcarbazepine and their metabolites by high-performance liquid chromatography. *J Chromatogr B Biomed Appl* 673:97–105.

75. Juenke J, Brown PI, Urry FM, McMillin GA. 2006. Drug monitoring and toxicology: a procedure for the monitoring of levetiracetam and zonisamide by HPLC-UV. *J Anal Toxicol* 30:27–30.

76. Nakamura M, Hirade K, Sugiyama T, Katagiri Y. 2001. High-performance liquid chromatographic assay of zonisamide in human plasma using a non-porous silica column. *J Chromatogr B Biomed Sci Appl* 755:337–41.

77. Shimoyama R, Ohkubo T, Sugawara K. 1999. Monitoring of zonisamide in human breast milk and maternal plasma by solid-phase extraction HPLC method. *Biomed Chromatogr* 13:370–72.

78. Ito T, Yamaguchi T, Miyazaki H, Sekine Y, Shimizu M, Ishida S, et al.1982. Pharmacokinetic studies of AD-810, a new antiepileptic compound. Phase I trials. *Arzneimittel-Forschung* 32:1581–86.

79. Wagner JG, Sackellares JC, Donofrio PD, Berent S, Sakmar E. 1984. Nonlinear pharmacokinetics of CI-912 in adult epileptic patients. *Ther Drug Monit* 6:277–83.

80. Berry DJ. 1990. Determination of zonisamide (3-sulphamoylmethyl-1,2-benzisoxazole) in plasma at therapeutic concentrations by high-performance liquid chromatography. *J Chromatogr* 534:173–81.

81. Furuno K, Oishi R, Gomita Y, Eto K. 1994. Simple and sensitive assay of zonisamide in human serum by high-performance liquid chromatography using a solid-phase extraction technique. *J Chromatogr B Biomed Appl* 656:456–59.

82. Fraser AD, MacNeil W, Isner AF, Camfield PR. 1995. Lamotrigine analysis in serum by high-performance liquid chromatography. *Ther Drug Monit* 17:174–78.

83. Lensmeyer GL, Gidal BE, Wiebe DA. 1997. Optimized high-performance liquid chromatographic method for determination of lamotrigine in serum with concomitant determination of phenytoin, carbamazepine, and carbamazepine epoxide. *Ther Drug Monit* 19:292–300.

84. Torra M, Rodamilans M, Arroyo S, Corbella J. 2000. Optimized procedure for lamotrigine analysis in serum by high-performance liquid chromatography without interferences from other frequently coadministered anticonvulsants. *Ther Drug Monit* 22:621–25.

85. Forssblad E, Eriksson AS, Beck O. 1996. Liquid chromatographic determination of plasma lamotrigine in pediatric samples. *J Pharm Biomed Anal* 14:755–58.

86. Londero D, Lo Greco P. 1997. New micromethod for the determination of lamotrigine in human plasma by high-performance liquid chromatography. *J Chromatogr B Biomed Sci Appl* 691:139–44.

87. Vidal E, Pascual C, Pou L. 1999. Determination of lamotrigine in human serum by liquid chromatography. *J Chromatogr B Biomed Sci Appl* 736:295–98.

88. Barbosa NR, Midio AF. 2000. Validated high-performance liquid chromatographic method for the determination of lamotrigine in human plasma. *J Chromatogr B Biomed Sci Appl* 741:289–93.

89. Croci D, Salmaggi A, de Grazia U, Bernardi G. 2001. New high-performance liquid chromatographic method for plasma/serum analysis of lamotrigine. *Ther Drug Monit* 23:665–68.

90. Gustavson LE, Chu SY. 1992. High-performance liquid chromatographic procedure for the determination of tiagabine concentrations in human plasma using electrochemical detection. *J Chromatogr* 574:313–18.

91. Forrest G, Sills GJ, Leach JP, Brodie MJ. 1996. Determination of gabapentin in plasma by high-performance liquid chromatography. *J Chromatogr B Biomed Appl* 681:421–25.

92. Jiang Q, Li S. 1999. Rapid high-performance liquid chromatographic determination of serum gabapentin. *J Chromatogr B Biomed Sci Appl* 727:119–23.

93. Loscher W, Fassbender CP, Gram L, Gramer M, Horstermann D, Zahner B, Stefan H. 1993. Determination of GABA and vigabatrin in human plasma by a rapid and simple HPLC method: correlation between clinical response to vigabatrin and increase in plasma GABA. *Epilepsy Res* 14:245–55.

94. Wad N, Kramer G. 1998. Sensitive high-performance liquid chromatographic method with fluorometric detection for the simultaneous determination of gabapentin and vigabatrin in serum and urine. *J Chromatogr B Biomed Sci Appl* 705:154–58.

95. May TW, Rambeck B, Neb R, Jurgens U. 2007. Serum concentrations of pregabalin in patients with epilepsy: the influence of dose, age, and comedication. *Ther Drug Monit* 29:789–94.

96. Tsanaclis LM, Wicks J, Williams J, Richens A. 1991. Determination of vigabatrin in plasma by reversed-phase high-performance liquid chromatography. *Ther Drug Monit* 13:251–53.

97. Erturk S, Aktas ES, Atmaca S. 2001. Determination of vigabatrin in human plasma and urine by high-performance liquid chromatography with fluorescence detection. *J Chromatogr B Biomed Sci Appl* 760:207–12.

98. Grim SA, Ryan M, Miles MV, Tang PH, Strawsburg RH, deGrauw TJ, et al. 2003. Correlation of levetiracetam concentrations between serum and saliva. *Ther Drug Monit* 25:61–66.

99. Rao BM, Ravi R, Shyam Sundar Reddy B, Sivakumar S, Gopi Chand I, Praveen Kumar K, et al. 2004. A validated chiral LC method for the enantioselective analysis of Levetiracetam and its enantiomer R-alpha-ethyl-2-oxo-pyrrolidine acetamide on amylose-based stationary phase. *J Pharm Biomed Anal* 35:1017–26.

100. Pucci V, Bugamelli F, Mandrioli R, Ferranti A, Kenndler E, Raggi MA. 2004. High-performance liquid chromatographic determination of Levetiracetam in human plasma: comparison of different sample clean-up procedures. *Biomed Chromatogr* 18:37–44.

101. Ratnaraj N, Doheny HC, Patsalos PN. 1996. A micromethod for the determination of the new antiepileptic drug levetiracetam (ucb L059) in serum or plasma by high performance liquid chromatography. *Ther Drug Monit* 18:154–57.

102. Martens-Lobenhoffer J, Bode-Boger SM. 2005. Determination of levetiracetam in human plasma with minimal sample pretreatment. *J Chromatogr B Analyt Technol Biomed Life Sci* 819:197–200.

103. Chan K, Lok S, Teoh R. 1984. The simultaneous determination of five anti-epileptic drugs in plasma by high performance liquid chromatography. *Methods Find Exp Clin Pharmacol* 6:701–4.

104. Matar KM, Nicholls PJ, Tekle A, Bawazir SA, Al-Hassan MI. 1999. Liquid chromatographic determination of six antiepileptic drugs and two metabolites in microsamples of human plasma. *Ther Drug Monit* 21:559–66.

105. Juergens U. 1987. Simultaneous determination of Zonisamide and nine other anti-epileptic drugs and metabolites in serum. A comparison of microbore and conventional high-performance liquid chromatography. *J Chromatogr* 385:233–40.

106. Yoshida T, Imai K, Motohashi S, Hamano S, Sato M. 2006. Simultaneous determination of zonisamide, carbamazepine and carbamazepine-10,11-epoxide in infant serum by high-performance liquid chromatography. *J Pharm Biomed Anal* 41:1386–90.

107. Wad N. 1984. Simultaneous determination of eleven antiepileptic compounds in serum by high-performance liquid chromatography. *J Chromatogr* 305:127–33.
108. Meijer JW. 1991. Knowledge, attitude and practice in antiepileptic drug monitoring. *Acta Neurologica Scandinavica* 134:1–128.
109. Levert H, Odou P, Robert H. 2002. Simultaneous determination of four antiepileptic drugs in serum by high-performance liquid chromatography. *Biomed Chromatogr* 16:19–24.
110. Mandrioli R, Albani F, Casamenti G, Sabbioni C, Raggia MA. 2001. Simultaneous high-performance liquid chromatography determination of carbamazepine and five of its metabolites in plasma of epileptic patients. *J Chromatogr B Biomed Sci Appl* 762:109–16.
111. Maurer HH, Kratzsch C, Weber AA, Peters FT, Kraemer T. 2002. Validated assay for quantification of oxcarbazepine and its active dihydro metabolite 10-hydroxycarbazepine in plasma by atmospheric pressure chemical ionization liquid chromatography/mass spectrometry. *J Mass Spectrom* 37:687–92.
112. Subramanian M, Birnbaum AK, Remmel RP. 2008. High-speed simultaneous determination of nine antiepileptic drugs using liquid chromatography-mass spectrometry. *Ther Drug Monit* 30:347–56.
113. Park JH, Park YS, Lee MH, Rhim SY, Song JC, Lee SJ, et al. 2008. Determination of plasma topiramate concentration using LC-MS/MS for pharmacokinetic and bioequivalence studies in healthy Korean volunteers. *Biomed Chromatogr* 22:822–29.
114. Contin M, Riva R, Albani F, Baruzzi A. 2001. Simple and rapid liquid chromatographic-turbo ion spray mass spectrometric determination of topiramate in human plasma. *J Chromatogr B Biomed Sci Appl* 761:133–37.
115. Britzi M, Soback S, Isoherranen N, Levy RH, Perucca E, Doose DR, et al. 2003. Analysis of topiramate and its metabolites in plasma and urine of healthy subjects and patients with epilepsy by use of a novel liquid chromatography-mass spectrometry assay. *Ther Drug Monit* 25:314–22.
116. Guo T, Oswald LM, Mendu DR, Soldin SJ. 2007. Determination of levetiracetam in human plasma/serum/saliva by liquid chromatography-electrospray tandem mass spectrometry. *Clin Chim Acta* 375:115–18.
117. Thompson CD, Barthen MT, Hopper DW, Miller TA, Quigg M, Hudspeth C, et al. 1999. Quantification in patient urine samples of felbamate and three metabolites: acid carbamate and two mercapturic acids. *Epilepsia* 40:769–76.
118. Park JH, Jhee OH, Park SH, Lee JS, Lee MH, Shaw LM, et al. 2007. Validated LC-MS/MS method for quantification of gabapentin in human plasma: application to pharmacokinetic and bioequivalence studies in Korean volunteers. *Biomed Chromatogr* 21:829–35.
119. Ramakrishna NV, Vishwottam KN, Koteshwara M, Manoj S, Santosh M, Chidambara J, et al. 2006. Rapid quantification of gabapentin in human plasma by liquid chromatography/tandem mass spectrometry. *J Pharm Biomed Anal* 40:360–68.
120. Breton H, Cociglio M, Bressolle F, Peyriere H, Blayac JP, Hillaire-Buys D. 2005. Liquid chromatography-electrospray mass spectrometry determination of carbamazepine, oxcarbazepine and eight of their metabolites in human plasma. *J Chromatogr B Analyt Technol Biomed Life Sci* 828:80–90.
121. Langman LJ, Kaliciak HA, Boone SA. 2003. Fatal acute topiramate toxicity. *J Anal Toxicol* 27:323–4.

8 Problems with Digoxin Immunoassays

Amitava Dasgupta
University of Texas Medical School

CONTENTS

8.1 DIGOXIN: AN INTRODUCTION

Digoxin, a cardiac glycoside is an important drug found in foxglove plant (*Digitalis lantana*). Medicinal properties of cardiac glycosides were recorded in history as early as 1000 BC. Digoxin is widely used in clinical practice to treat various heart conditions including atrial fibrillation, atrial flutter and heart failure. Digoxin is the most commonly used drug for treatment of congestive heart failure in pediatric patients [1]. Digoxin is also used in treating adult patients with heart failure [2].

The main pharmacological effects of digoxin include a dose dependent increase in myocardial contractility and a negative chronotropic action. Digitalis also increases the refractory period and decreases impulse velocity in certain myocardial tissue (such as the AV node). The electrophysiological properties of digitalis are reflected in the ECG by shortening of the QT interval. Na, K-ATPase which actively transport Na^+ out and K^+ into the myocyte, is the receptor for cardiac glycosides exerting their positive inotropic effect by inhibiting Na, K-ATPase. This process eventually increases cellular content of calcium and also release of calcium during depolarization [3]. A recent article indicates that digitoxin; a cardiac glycoside mediates calcium entry directly into cells. Multimer of digitoxin molecules also can form calcium channels in pure planar phospholipid bilayer [4].

8.2 WHY THERAPEUTIC DRUG MONITORING OF DIGOXIN?

Digoxin has a narrow therapeutic index, thus therapeutic drug monitoring is essential for achieving optimal efficacy as well as to avoid digoxin toxicity. Despite the need for therapeutic drug monitoring of digoxin, Raebel et al. reported that 50% or more of ambulatory patients receiving digoxin were not monitored for serum digoxin concentrations [5]. The therapeutic range of digoxin usually is considered as 0.8–1.8 ng/mL, but there is a substantial overlap between therapeutic and toxic concentrations. Moreover, mild to moderate renal failure may also significantly increase the risk with digoxin therapy [6]. Digoxin toxicity may occur with a lower digoxin level, if hypokalemia, hypomagnesemia, or hypothyroidism coexists. Likewise, the concomitant use of drugs such as quinidine, verapamil, spironolactone, flecainide, and amiodarone can increase serum digoxin levels and increase the risk of digoxin toxicity. One clinical trial indicated that a beneficial effect of digoxin was observed at serum concentrations from 0.5 to 0.9 ng/mL whereas serum concentrations at or over 1.2 ng/mL appeared harmful [7].

8.3 DIGOXIN IMMUNOASSAYS VERSUS LIQUID CHROMATOGRAPHY/MASS SPECTROMETRY

The concentration of digoxin in serum or plasma can be detected accurately by sophisticated analytical techniques such as high performance liquid chromatography (HPLC) combined with tandem mass spectrometry. Mitamura et al. described a method for accurate determination of digoxin in human serum using stable isotope dilution liquid chromatography combined with electrospray ionization tandem mass spectrometry (LC/ESI-MS/MS). Digoxin and the internal standard [21,21,22-(2)H(3)] digoxin were extracted from 250 µL of serum using solid phase extraction cartridge and analyzed by LC/ESI-MS/MS in selected reaction monitoring mode. The reported range of assay was from 0.20 to 3.20 ng/mL. The authors clearly showed that this very specific assay for determination of digoxin concentrations in human serum is free from interferences of digoxin metabolites and endogenous digoxin-like immunoreactive substances (DLIS). When authors compared results obtained by LC/ESI-MS/MS and a specific RIA assay (radioimmunoassay) which is free from cross-reactivity of digoxin metabolites but not from DLIS, five out of 19 (26.3%) specimens showed more than 2.5 times higher values obtained by RIA when compared to values obtained by LC/ESI-MS/MS. For example, in one patient the digoxin value was 0.46 ng/mL by LC/ESI-MS/MS and 2.44 ng/mL by the RIA , a 4.3 fold increase in concentration when measured by the RIA. [8].

8.4 FACTORS AFFECTING DIGOXIN IMMUNOASSAYS

The liquid chromatography combined with mass spectrometry is a complex technique. Therefore, in clinical laboratories digoxin immunoassays are the preferred method due to automation and rapid turn around time. Immunoassays are subjected to interference by both exogenous and endogenous factors. Digoxin metabolites also cross-react with digoxin immunoassays and the magnitude of interference depends on antibody specificity of the immunoassay. Spironolactone, potassium canrenoate, and their common metabolite canrenone also interfere with serum digoxin measurements by immunoassays. Moreover, various Chinese medicines, oleander containing herbal products, Digibind as well as DLIS cross-react with digoxin immunoassays [9].

8.4.1 CROSS-REACTIVITY OF DIGOXIN METABOLITES WITH DIGOXIN IMMUNOASSAYS

Digoxin metabolites show different cross-reactivities with digoxin immunoassays because various assays differ in specificity of antibody used against digoxin in assay design. In general digoxin concentrations in serum obtained by more specific technique such as HPLC tend to be lower than the corresponding digoxin concentrations obtained by immunoassay because digoxin metabolites cross-react with digoxin immunoassays. Miller et al. reported that digoxigenin has 0.7% cross-reactivity with ACS assay (Ciba-Corning Diagnostics now Siemens Medical Diagnostic Solution), 103% cross-reactivity with fluorescence polarization immunoassay (FPIA on TDx Analyzer; Abbott Laboratories, Abbott Park, IL), 103% cross-reactivity with Stratus assay (Baxter Corporation, now Dade-Behring, Deerfield, IL) and 153% cross-reactivity with Magic digoxin assay (Ciba-Corning) [10].

Solnica compared performance of FPIA digoxin assay (Abbott Laboratories) and dry chemistry enzyme assay (EIA) on the Vitros 950 analyzer (Johnson & Johnson, Rochester, NY). The authors observed that the EIA showed a significantly higher analytical digoxin concentrations bias than the FPIA assay. The mean value of digoxin in sera of 88 patients as measured by the EIA was 1.342 ng/mL compared to the mean value of 1.196 ng/mL as obtained by the FPIA. The number of subtherapeutic digoxin values observed in the patients were higher with FPIA than EIA (29.7% vs. 21.8%) while values over 1.2 ng/mL in patients were lower using the FPIA compared with EIA (25.7% vs. 35.6%) further demonstrating the bias. The author speculated that the cause of bias is probably related to antibody specificity. The dry chemistry slides in the EIA assay uses a mouse monoclonal antibody while the FPIA assay utilizes a rabbit polyclonal antibody against digoxin. The mouse antibody of the EIA assay may be affected by the presence of heterophilic anti-mouse antibody present in the serum causing falsely elevated results. Another reason could be the interference of DLIS. The author also commented that HPLC combined with mass spectrometry is the reference method [11]. Cross-reactivity of some digoxin metabolites with various commercially available digoxin immunoassays are given in Table 8.1.

8.4.2 DIGIBIND AND DIGOXIN IMMUNOASSAYS

Digibind is a mixture of digoxin specific Fab fragment prepared by papain digestion of anti-digoxin antibody raised in sheep against a digoxin-human albumin conjugate [12]. The Fab fragments are purified by affinity chromatography. Digibind is used in life threatening overdose from digoxin but is also effective in treating digitoxin overdose. Digibind demonstrates the ability to neutralize cardenolides that are glycosylated in position 3 (digitoxin, ouabain, and neriifolin) with a similar potency to also neutralize digoxin regardless of substitutions in the steroid part of the molecule. Moreover, Digibind is capable of neutralizing both cardiac glycosides and respective aglycons. Digibind can also bind endogenous DLIS in rats and human and lowers blood pressure [13]. Digibind can neutralize oleandrin, the active component of oleander extract due to structural similarity between oleandrin and digoxin. Digibind may be effective in treating life threatening oleander toxicity [14]. Moreover, Digibind may be effective in treating mice poisoned with Chan Su, a Chinese medicine prepared from toad (*Bufo gargarizans*) and containing bufalin, cinobufotolin, cinobufagin, and other cardioactive steroids from bufadienolide class, but the efficacy of Digibind in treating Chan Su poisoning is poor compared to the efficacy in treating digoxin overdose. This is due to the poor specificity of Digibind to neutralize cinobufagin and cinobufatolin which are also the constituents of Chan Su as well as toad venom [15].

TABLE 8.1
Cross-reactivity of Digitoxin, Digoxin Metabolites, and Related Steroids with Selected Commercially Available Digoxin Immunoassays

Assay	Platform/Company	Metabolite	%Cross-Reactivity
Digoxin (PETIA)*	Architect/Abbott	Digitoxigenin	0.5%
		Digitoxin	3.1%
		Digoxigenin	4.0%
		Digoxigenin-bis-digitoxoside	112.0%
		Digoxigenin-mono-digitoxoside	78.2%
Vitros digoxin (dry slides)	Vitro Johnson & Johnson	Digitoxigenin	8%
		Digitoxin	18%
		Dihydrodigoxin	2%
		Digoxigenin	< 1%
		Digoxigenin-bis-digitoxoside	108%
		Digoxigenin-mono-digitoxoside	76%
		Lanatoside C	196%
		Ouabain	105%
Digoxin	ADVIA/SIEMENS	Digitoxigenin	8%
		Dihydrodigoxin	3.5%
		Digoxigenin-bis-digitoxoside	173%
		Digoxigenin-mono-digitoxoside	109%
TinaQuant digoxin	Roche	Lanatoside C	136%
		Digoxigenin-bis-digitoxoside	120%
		Digoxigenin-mono-digitoxoside	111%
		Deslanoside	93%
		β-Methyldigoxin	93%
		b-Acetyldigoxin	74%
		Digoxigenin	6.4%
		Digitoxigenin-bis-digitoxoside	5.1%
		Digitoxin	4.1%
		Gitoxin	1.9%
		Dihydrodigoxin	1.8%

* PETIA: Particle enhanced turbidimetric immunoassay.
Data based on package inserts.
This list is incomplete. There are many other commercially available digoxin assays. These manufacturers were chosen randomly to illustrate the point that digoxin metabolites and related steroids cross-react with digoxin immunoassays.

Digibind has been available in the United States since 1986 (Glaxo Wellcome Inc) and more recently in 2001 the Food and Drug Administration of the United States approved DigiFab for treating potentially life threatening digoxin toxicity or overdose. Digibind is produced by immunizing sheep with digoxin followed by the purification of the FAB fragment from blood, while the DigiFab is prepared by injecting sheep with digoxindicarboxymethylamine followed by the purification of Fab fragment. The molecular weight of DigiFab (46,000 Daltons) and Digibind

(46,200 Daltons) is also similar. Usually Digibind dosage is 80 times the digoxin body burden (in mg) or if neither the dose ingested nor the plasma digoxin concentration is known, then 380 mg of Digibind is usually injected into the patient. Neither Digibind not DigiFab can be given orally. The half-life of the Fab fragment in humans is 12–20 hours but this may be prolonged in patients with renal failure [16].

The Fab fragment is known to interfere with serum digoxin measurements using immunoassays and the magnitude of interference depends on the assay design and the specificity of the antibody used. The microparticle enzyme immunoassay of digoxin (MEIA on the AxSYM analyzer, Abbott Laboratories, Abbott Park, IL) as well as the Stratus digoxin assay show digoxin values which are higher than measured free digoxin concentration in the presence of Fab fragment [17]. McMillin et al. studied the effect of Digibind and DigiFab on 13 different digoxin immunoassays. Positive interference in the presence and absence of digoxin was observed with Digibind and DigiFab, although the magnitude of interference was somewhat less with DigiFab. The magnitude of interference varied significantly with each method while IMMULITE, Vitros, Dimension, and Access digoxin methods showed highest interference. The magnitudes of interference were in the order of Elecsys, TinaQuant, Integra, EMIT, and Centaur method while minimal interferences were observed with FPIA, MEIA, Synchron and CEDIA methods [18].

8.4.3 Elimination of Fab Interference by Ultrafiltration

The molecular weight of the Fab fragment (46,000 or 46,200 Daltons) is much higher than the cut-off of the Amicon Centrifree filters (30,000) used for the preparation of protein free ultrafiltrate in order to measure free digoxin concentrations. Therefore, Fab fragment is absent in the protein free ultrafiltrate and monitoring free digoxin concentration is not subjected to the interference by both Digibind and DigiFab. Jortani et al. reported that analysis of serum ultrafiltrate for digoxin concentration remains the most accurate approach in monitoring unbound digoxin in the presence of the Fab fragment. Moreover, no matrix bias was observed in measuring digoxin concentrations in protein free ultrafiltrates using immunoassays [19]. McMillin et al. commented that patients treated with Digibind can be monitored reasonably by using either MEIA (on AxSYM analyzer) or the Stratus. Another alternative is to measure free digoxin concentration in the protein free ultrafiltrate. The immunoassays for direct measurement of digoxin in serum in the presence of Digibind however will overestimate free digoxin concentration [18].

8.4.4 Interference of Spironolactone and Related Compounds in Digoxin Immunoassays

Spironolactone is a competitive aldosterone antagonist which blocks the binding of aldosterone to the renal receptor, causing sodium loss and potassium retention. Spironolactone is used clinically in treating primary aldosteronism, essential hypertension, congestive heart failure, and edema. After oral administration, spironolactone is rapidly and extensively metabolized to several metabolites and one of the metabolites, canrenone is also pharmacologically active. Although not in formulary in the United States, potassium canrenoate is used in Europe and other countries. Potassium canrenoate is also metabolized to canrenone. Spironolactone potassium canrenoate and canrenone have structural similarity with digoxin (Figure 8.1).

Spironolactone and digoxin are sometimes used concurrently in the management of patients. Therefore, significant interference of spironolactone and canrenone in therapeutic drug monitoring of digoxin is troublesome. Positive interference of spironolactone and its active metabolite canrenone in the radio-immunoassay for digoxin has been reported as early as 1974 [20]. Potassium canrenoate also showed significant positive interference with serum digoxin monitoring using radioimmunoassay and enzyme immunoassay [21,22]. Morris et al. reported positive interference of spironolactone

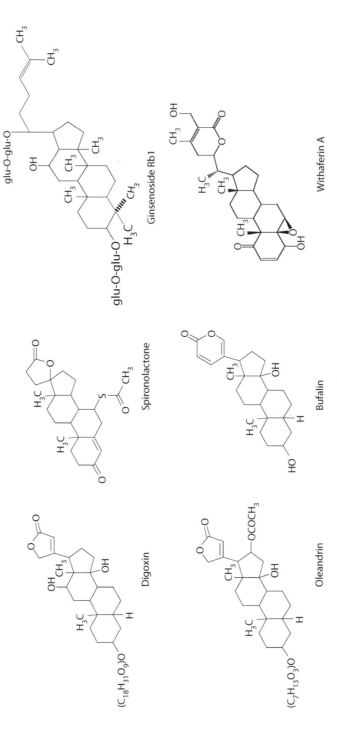

FIGURE 8.1 Chemical structures of digoxin, spironolactone, bufalin (active component of Chan Su), oleandrin (active component of oleander), ginsenoside Rb1 (active component of Asian ginseng), and withaferin A (active component of Ashwagandha).

in digoxin measurement using the FPIA (Abbott Laboratories) [23]. Subsequently, other authors verified the interference of spironolactone and canrenone in the FPIA and other commonly used digoxin immunoassays [24,25]. Okazaki et al. also reported falsely elevated digoxin concentrations in patients receiving digoxin and potassium canrenoate. The authors reported two cases where cross-reactivity of the assay system caused clinical problem and recommended use of the OPUS digoxin assay which showed minimum cross-reactivity with potassium canrenoate [26].

Steimer et al. reported for the first time the negative interference of canrenone in serum digoxin measurement when a microparticle enzyme immunoassay (MEIA, Abbott Laboratories) for digoxin was used. Misleading subtherapeutic concentrations of digoxin as measured on several occasions led to falsely guided digoxin dosing resulting in serious digoxin toxicity in the patients [27].

Interference of spironolactone, potassium canrenoate and their common metabolite canrenone may be positive or negative in serum digoxin measurement using immunoassays depending on the assay design and antibody specificity. Spironolactone and its metabolite canrenone can falsely elevate serum digoxin levels (positive interference) if measured by FPIA (Abbott Laboratories), aca (Dade Behring, Deerfield, IL) or Elecsys (Roche Diagnostics, Indianapolis, IN). Digoxin values are falsely lower (negative interference) if measured by MEIA, IMx (both from Abbott Laboratories) and Dimension digoxin assays (Dade Behring, Deerfield, IL). The magnitude of interference is more significant with potassium canrenoate where concentration of its metabolite canrenone can be significantly higher compared to spironolactone therapy where the concentration of the metabolite, canrenone is relatively low. In one report authors observed a 42% decline in expected value of serum digoxin in the presence of 3125 ng/mL of canrenoate using MEIA, 78% decline in using Dimension and 51% decrease using IMx. A positive bias was observed with the aca (0.7 ng/mL), TDx (0.62 ng/mL) and Elessys (0.58 ng/mL). EMIT 2000, TinaQuant (Roche Diagnostics, Indianapolis, IN) and the Vitros digoxin assay are free from such interference [28].

In our experience, Bayer's (now Siemens, Tarrytown, NY) chemiluminescent digoxin assay is relatively free from interferences of spironolactone, potassium canrenoate and their common metabolite canrenone. Another turbidimetric digoxin assay on the ADVIA 1650 analyzer (Tarrytown, NY) is also relatively free from such interferences. Moreover, interference of spironolactone and its metabolite canrenone can be mostly eliminated by ultrafiltration because both compounds are strongly bound to serum proteins (> 90%). However, in the case of therapy with K-canrenoate (not used in the United States), complete elimination of this interference in certain digoxin assays can not be achieved due to higher concentrations of K-canrenoate and relatively higher concentrations of its metabolite canrenone in plasma [29,30]. Howard et al. demonstrated that low dose spironolactone (up to 25 mg per day) as used for oral therapy does not cause clinically significant negative interference in the MEIA digoxin assay on the AxSYM analyzer by comparing results with the EMIT assay which is free from spironolactone interference [31]. However, with a higher spironolactone dose, such as 200 mg per day, a significant interference may be observed with the MEIA assay [32].

Therapeutic drug monitoring of spironolactone is not a standard practice in medicine. Nevertheless in a case of suspected overdose, determination of concentrations of both spironolactone and its active metabolite canrenone may be useful. Currently, there is no commercially available immunoassay in the market for determining concentrations of spironolactone or canrenone. Usually HPLC is the preferred analytical technique for measuring concentrations of these drugs in human serum or plasma. Dong et al. described a sensitive and specific technique for simultaneous determination of spironolactone and canrenone in human plasma by HPLC combined with atmospheric pressure chemical ionization mass spectrometry (APCI-MS). The authors used estazolam as the internal standard. Spironolactone, canrenone along with the internal standard were extracted from human plasma using methylene chloride/ethyl acetate (20:80 by vol) followed by separation using a reverse phase C-18 column with a mobile phase composition of methanol/water (57:43 by vol). Mass spectrometric analyses were performed in selected ion monitoring mode using target ions at m/z 341.25 for spironolactone and canrenone and m/z at 295.05 for the internal standard. The assay was linear for both spironolactone and canrenone concentrations between 2 ng/mL to 300 ng/mL [33].

8.5 INTERFERENCE OF HERBAL AND CHINESE MEDICINES IN DIGOXIN MEASUREMENT

The United States Food and Drug Administration (FDA) regulate drugs and require that drugs should be both safe and effective. Most complementary and alternative medicines are classified as dietary supplements or foods and are marketed pursuant to the Dietary Supplement Health and Education of act of 1994. FDA does not require documentation of efficacy of herbal supplements as long as these products do not claim any treatment benefit. Complementary and alternative medicines including Ayurvedic medicines are becoming increasingly popular in the United States, Europe and other parts of the world. Herbal medicines are readily available in the United States from stores without prescriptions. Chinese medicines are an important component of herbal medicines available today. In developing countries, as much as 80% of the indigenous populations depend on local traditional system of medicines. Within the European market, herbal medicines represent an important pharmaceutical market. Several Chinese medicines interfere with serum digoxin measurements by immunoassays. Herbal medicines in the European markets represent an important pharmaceutical market with annual sales of seven billion U.S. dollars. In the United States, the sale of herbal medicine increased from $200 million in 1988 to over $3.3 billion in 1997. The majorities of population who use herbal medicines in the United States have a college degree and fall in the age group of 25–49 years. In one study, 65% of people thought that herbal medicines are safe [34]. Most people consider herbal medicines safe and do not report to their physicians regarding use of herbal supplements. Abnormal test results can be observed in individuals taking herbal supplements including unexpected test results in therapeutic drug monitoring in patients who demonstrated therapeutic concentrations of a drug before [35].

Several Chinese medicines and herbal supplements interfere with serum digoxin measurements using immunoassays. The magnitude of interference depends on the antibody specificity of the assay. In general polyclonal antibody based digoxin immunoassays are more affected by these remedies than more specific monoclonal antibody based digoxin immunoassays. Significant interferences of Chinese medicines Chan Su and Lu-Shen-wan (LSW) with digoxin immunoassays have been reported. Oleander containing herbal products also has significant effect on digoxin assays while herbal supplements such as DanShen, Asian ginseng, Siberian ginseng, and Indian Ayurvedic medicine Ashwagandha have modest effects on digoxin immunoassays that utilize polyclonal antibody against digoxin in the assay design.

8.5.1 CHAN SU AND LU-SHEN-WAN (LSW)

Chan Su, is prepared from the dried white secretion of the auricular glands and the skin glands of Chinese toads (Bufo melanostictus Schneider or Bufo bufo gargarzinas Gantor). Chan Su is also a major component of other traditional Chinese medicines such as LSW and Kyushin [36,37]. These medicines are used for the treatment of such disorders as tonsillitis, sore throat and palpitation. Traditional use of Chan Su given in small doses also includes stimulation of myocardial contraction, anti-inflammatory effect and analgesia [38]. The cardiotonic effect of Chan Su is due to its major bufadienolides such as bufalin (Figure 8.1) [39]. Bufalin is known to block vasodilatation and increases vasoconstriction, vascular resistance and blood pressure by inhibiting Na, K-ATPase [40]. Xu et al. reported that Chan Su contains five major bufadienolides; bufalin, cinobufagin, resibufogenin, bufotalin and arenobufagin [41]. The structure of bufalin, the active component of Chan Su is given in Figure 8.1.

In 1995, Fushimi and Amino reported a serum digoxin concentration of 0.51 nmol/L (0.4 ng/mL) in a healthy volunteer after ingestion of Kyushin tablets containing Chan Su as the major component [42]. Then Panesar reported an apparent digoxin concentration of 1124 pmol/L (0.88 ng/mL) in a healthy volunteer who ingested LSW pills. The author used the FPIA and TDX analyzer (Abbott Laboratories) for the study [43]. Later, in another article Panesar commented that the digoxin measured by the FPIA assay in 2004 showed less sensitivity compared to the FPIA assay the authors used in their earlier report to demonstrate apparent digoxin concentrations in volunteers after taking Chan Su containing Chinese medicines [44]. An apparent digoxin concentration of 4.9 ng/mL (FPIA assay) was reported in one woman who died from ingestion of Chinese herbal tea containing Chan Su [45].

The interference of Chan Su and LSW to serum digoxin measurement can be positive (falsely elevated digoxin concentrations) or negative (falsely lower digoxin concentration) depending on the assay design. The FPIA assay, Beckman assay (Synchron LX system, Beckman Coulter) and Roche assay (TinaQuant) all showed positive interference in the presence of Chan Su. However, the magnitude of interference was almost 50% less compared to the FPIA assay. This may be related to the use of a more specific monoclonal antibody against digoxin in the assay design of both TinaQuant and the Beckman assay while the FPIA assay utilizes a rabbit polyclonal antibody against digoxin [46].

Falsely lowered digoxin concentrations (negative interference) were observed due to the presence of Chan Su extract in the serum specimen when the MEIA assay (Abbott Laboratories) and AxSYM analyzer were used for serum digoxin measurement. However, the components of Chan Su responsible for digoxin-like immunoreactivity are significantly bound to serum proteins (> 90%) and are virtually absent in the protein free ultrafiltrate. Therefore measuring free digoxin concentration in the protein free ultrafiltrate maybe used to mostly eliminate the interference of Chan Su in serum digoxin measurements. A chemiluminescent digoxin assay marketed by Bayer Diagnostics is also virtually free from interference of Chan Su [47]. Recently Abbott Diagnostics released a new digoxin assay for therapeutic drug monitoring of digoxin on the AxSYM analyzer. Chan Su and LSW also interfere with this assay but in contrast to the MEIA assay (on the AxSYM analyzer) both Chan Su and LSW demonstrate significant positive interference with the Digoxin III assay. When mice were fed with Chan Su, significant apparent digoxin concentrations were also observed in sera both one and two hours after feeding using the Digoxin III assay, indicating that this assay can be used for rapid detection of Chan Su poisoning. The half-life of digoxin-like immunoreactive components due to ingestion of Chan Su in mice was short (approximately 1.1 h) [48].

Taking advantage of high cross-reactivity of Chan Su and LSW with both the FPIA and Digoxin III assay, it is possible to further verify a suspected overdose with these Chinese medicines in a patient not taking digoxin. However, such approach is inadequate in medical-legal scenario. The presence of bufalin and related compound in the biological fluid must be confirmed by a specific analytical technique such as HPLC. Liang et al. recently reported a method for simultaneous determination of bufadienolides in rat plasma after oral administration of Chan Su extract by solid phase extraction and HPLC with photodiode array detection. The authors used a reverse phase C-18 column for the analysis [49]. Xu et al. used caudatin as the internal standard for analysis of five major bufadienolides in rat plasma following exposure to Chan Su. Bufadienolides along the internal standard were extracted from plasma using liquid–liquid extraction using ethyl acetate and HPLC analysis was carried out using a ZORBAX SB-18 column (2.1 mm × 100 mm, particle size 3.5 µm; Agilent Corporation, MA) and a C-18 guard column (4.0 mm × 2.0 mm, particle size 3.5 µm, Phenomenex, CA) with an isocratic mobile phase consisted of acetonitrile, water and formic acid (50:50:0.05 by vol). The detection of peaks was achieved by triple quadripole OLC/MS system which was operated under multiple reaction monitoring mode [41].

8.5.2 OLEANDER CONTAINING HERBS AND DIGOXIN IMMUNOASSAYS

The oleanders are evergreen ornamental shrubs with various colors of flowers that belong to the Dogbane family and grow in the Southern parts of the United States from Florida to California, Australia, India, Sri Lanka, China, and other parts of the world. There are two major varieties of oleander tree. The pink oleander plant (*Nerium oleander*) grows widely in the Southern parts of the United States with beautiful pink flowers and the yellow oleander tree (*Thevetia peruviana*) is common through much of the tropics and subtropics. All parts of both types of oleander plants are toxic. Human exposure to oleander includes accidental exposure, ingestion by children, administration in food or drink, medicinal preparations from oleander (herbal products) and criminal poisoning [50–53]. Despite toxicity, oleander is used in folk medicines [54]. The fatality rate from oleander toxicity is around 10% in Sri Lanka while approximately 40% of patients require specialized management in a tertiary care hospital. Deliberate ingestion of oleander seeds is also a popular method of suicide in Sri Lanka [55]. The toxic effect of oleander can occur with exposure from a small amount of the plant and even ingestion of a single leaf may be fatal especially in children. Boiling or drying the plant does not inactivate the toxins. Death from drinking a herbal tea containing oleander has been reported [56]. Oleander toxicity has been studied in a Tunisian toxicology intensive care unit from 1983 to 1998 in connection with plant poisoning and use of herbal medicines. The authors reported that 7% of all poisoning from the use of herbal medicines was due to oleander [57]. The American Association of Poison Control Centers received 3873 reports of oleander exposure between 1991 and 1995.

Many cardenolides have been isolated from yellow oleander including thevetin A, thevetin B (major components), peruvoside, neriifolin, thevetoxin, ruvoside and theveridoside. These cardenolides have structural similarity with digoxin and cross-react with antidigoxin antibodies utilized in digoxin immunoassays. Oleandrin, the active component of pink oleander also has structural similarity with digoxin and thus interferes with digoxin immunoassays. The structure of oleandrin is given in Figure 8.1.

In 1989, Cheung et al. reported detection of poisoning by plant origin (including oleander) using the FPIA digoxin assay on the TDx analyzer [58]. Later, Jortani et al. reported rapid detection of oleandrin and oleandrigenin using FPIA, fluorometric enzyme assay on Stratus analyzer, RIA, ACS:180 and On-Line digoxin assays [59]. Osterloh et al. reported an apparent digoxin level of 5.8 ng/mL after suicidal ingestion of oleander tea in a patient with no history of taking any cardioactive drug. The person eventually died from oleander toxicity [60]. Eddleston et al. reported a mean apparent serum digoxin concentration of 1.49 nmol/L (1.16 ng/mL) in patients who were poisoned with yellow oleander but eventually discharged from the hospital. Severe toxicity from oleander resulted in a mean apparent serum digoxin concentration of 2.83 nmol/L (2.21 ng/mL) as measured by the FPIA digoxin assay [61]. Roberts et al. studied pharmacokinetics of digoxin-cross reacting substances in patients with acute yellow oleander poisoning using the FPIA digoxin assay on the TDx analyzer (Abbott Laboratories) [62].

Most investigators used the FPIA assay for detection of plant poisoning including oleander poisoning because of the high cross-reactivity of this assay with components of both yellow and pink oleander. In our experience, the FPIA has the highest cross-reactivity with pink oleander extract as well as oleandrin, an active component of oleander extract. The Beckman digoxin assay on Synchron LX as well as the turbidimetric assay on the ADVIA 1650 analyzer (Bayer Diagnostics) also showed significant interference with oleander although the magnitude of interference was approximately 65% less with both the Beckman assay and the turbidimetric assay. The chemiluminescent assay, marketed by Bayer Diagnostics (now Siemens), is virtually free from interference of oleander [63]. More recently, Abbott Laboratories has released a new digoxin assay, Digoxin III for application on the AxSYM analyzer. This assay has high cross-reactivity with oleandrin and the magnitude of cross-reactivity is comparable to the FPIA assay. Therefore this new assay is also useful for rapid detection of oleander poisoning (author's data). However, in the case of medical legal situation, a suspected oleander poisoning, must be confirmed by demonstrating the presence of toxic glycoside of oleander in biological using HPLC and mass spectrometry (HPLC/MS), a direct analytical technique for detection of oleandrin in blood [64]. Tor et al. also reported a liquid chromatography-electrospray tandem mass spectrometric method for analysis of oleandrin in serum, urine and tissue samples. Oleandrin was extracted from serum and urine specimens using methylene chloride and from tissue samples using acetonitrile [65].

Although oleander extract caused positive interference with most digoxin immunoassays, negative interference of oleander extract in the MEIA digoxin assay (Abbott Laboratories) has been reported. Oleandrin is strongly bound to serum protein and is mostly absent in the protein free ultrafiltrate. Therefore, monitoring free digoxin in the protein free ultrafiltrate may eliminate some interference of oleander in serum digoxin assay provided that the oleandrin concentration is low to moderate [63]. For total elimination of interference, a specific analytical technique such as HPLC combined with mass spectrometry should be used for measurement of digoxin concentration.

8.5.3 Effects of Siberian Ginseng, Asian Ginseng and Ashwagandha on Digoxin Immunoassays

The ginseng that grows in Manchuria is *Panax ginseng*, which is commonly marketed as "Asian ginseng". It is used as an antioxidant, anti-inflammatory agent, anticancer remedy as well as a cardio protective agent in traditional Chinese medicines but its pharmacological properties has not been established by rigorous research. Although Asian ginseng (Panax ginseng) is commonly used, there are other types of ginseng such as Siberian ginseng, which is derived from the roots of Eleutherococcus senticosus. Siberian ginseng is different from Asian ginseng in that Panax-type ginsenosides are not found in Siberian ginseng although glycans and ligand glycoside such as eleutheroside found in Siberian ginseng and ginsenosides found in Asian ginseng have some structural similarity with digoxin. Structure of a major ginsenoside (ginsenoside Rb1) is given in Figure 8.1. Ashwagandha (*Withania somnifera*), also known as winter cherry, grows in India, Africa, some parts of Europe as well as North America. Ashwagandha is considered as a wonder shrub of India and has been used in Ayurvedic medicine for over 3,000 years for treating various conditions including cardiac dysfunction. Withaferin A, a major biochemical constituent of Ashwagandha also has structural similarity with digoxin (Figure 8.1).

There is one case report of interference of Siberian ginseng in serum digoxin measurement in the literature. A 74-year-old man had a steady serum digoxin level of 0.9–2.2 ng/mL for 10 years. His serum digoxin increased to 5.2 ng/mL on one occasion after taking Siberian ginseng. Although the level was toxic, the patient did not experience any signs or symptoms of digoxin toxicity. The patient stopped taking Siberian ginseng and his digoxin level returned to normal [66]. However, in our experience Siberian ginseng only has a very modest interference with FPIA and most digoxin assays we tested had no effect at all [67]. We also reported that Asian ginseng and Ashwagandha have only modest effect on serum digoxin measurements using the FPIA assay which utilizes a rabbit polyclonal antibody in the assay designs. Other digoxin immunoassays we tested utilize a more specific monoclonal antibody against digoxin (Roche, Bayer, and Beckmann) and such assays are not affected by Asian ginseng as well as Ashwagandha [67,68]. Interestingly, Ashwagandha does not interfere with any other immunoassays used for monitoring various therapeutic drugs [69].

8.5.4 DanShen and Digoxin Immunoassays

DanShen is another Chinese herb prepared from the root of the Chinese medicinal plant *Salvia miltiorrhiza*. This drug has been used in China for many years in the treatment of various cardiovascular diseases including angina pectoris and is readily available in the United States through Chinese herbal stores. More than 20 diterpene quinones known as tanshinones have been isolated from DanShen [70]. These compounds have structural similarity with digoxin. Feeding DanShen to mice caused digoxin-like immunoreactivity in sera when measured by the FPIA assay [71]. However more specific digoxin assays that utilize monoclonal antibody in the assay design such as TinaQuant (Roche) and Beckman assay (on Synchron LX analyzer) are completely free from the interference of DanShen. The digoxin-like immunoreactive components of DanShen are strongly protein bound

TABLE 8.2
Effects of Herbal Products on Digoxin Immunoassays

Herbal Product	Interference	Comments
Chan Su	High	Chan Su has active components like bufalin that cross-react with digoxin immunoassays. Most assays are affected. FPIA showed high interference.
Oleander	High	Active components of both Yellow oleander and pink oleander cross-react with both polyclonal and monoclonal antibody based digoxin immunoassays.
Uzara root (diuretic)	High	Additive effect with digoxin, also interferes with digoxin immunoassays.
Siberian ginseng	Low-moderate	May falsely increase digoxin level measured by FPIA and falsely lower digoxin level using MEIA. Other digoxin assays such as Roche, Beckman, and Bayer show no interference.
Asian ginseng	Low-moderate	May falsely increase digoxin level measured by FPIA and falsely lower digoxin level using MEIA. Other digoxin assays such as Roche, Beckman, and Bayer show no interference.
Ashwagandha	Low-moderate	May falsely increase digoxin level measured by FPIA and falsely lower digoxin level using MEIA. Other digoxin assays such as Roche, Beckman, and Bayer show no interference.
DanShen	Low	May interfere with FPIA assay for digoxin. Other immunoassays not affected.

and monitoring free digoxin eliminates interference of DanShen in digoxin measurement by FPIA [72]. The effects of different complementary and alternative medicines in serum digoxin measurements using immunoassays are given in Table 8.2.

8.5.5 UZARA ROOTS AND DIGOXIN IMMUNOASSAYS

Uzara (*Xysmalobium undulatum* (L.) R.Br) is a perennial plant which is widespread in South Africa's grassland. The Uzara roots which are prepared from two- to three-year-old plants has medicinal value and is used in treating non specific diarrhea because the Uzara slows bowl movement. Although popular in Germany, Uzara is not readily available in the US market. Four major cardenolide glycosides; uzarin, xysmalorin, allouzarin, and alloxysmlorin have been isolated from Uzara which have structural similarity with both digoxin and digitoxin [73]. Thurmann et al. reported that glycosides from Uzara roots may interfere with serum digoxin measurement by immunoassays. The authors investigated digoxin and digitoxin concentrations after four healthy volunteers ingested 1.5 mL (approximately 22 drops) of Uzara. Maximum digoxin concentrations of 1.4–6.34 μg/L (1.1–4.9 ng/mL) were observed six hours postdosing. Maximal apparent serum digitoxin concentrations between 198.0 and 919.8 μg/L (151.1–702.1 ng/mL) were also observed 4–8 hours after ingestion of Uzara roots. These values are elevated considering the reference range of digoxin (0.9–2.0 μg/L) and digitoxin (10–25 μg/L). The terminal half-life of glycosides was 8.87 ± 2.2 hours [74].

8.5.6 HERBAL CLEANSING AGENT AND DIGOXIN IMMUNOASSAY

There is a case report of a 36-year-old woman with no past medical history and taking no medicine ingested an herbal cleansing agent and reported to the emergency department. Her serum digoxin concentration was 1.7 ng/mL as measured by the FPIA and 0.34 ng/mL as measured by the more specific TinaQuant assay (Roche Diagnostics). The analysis of serum by HPLC revealed the presence of digitoxin metabolite but no parent drug was found. The patient responded well to Digibind therapy. This case indicated the possibility of cardioactive steroid poisoning following ingestion of an herbal cleansing agent [75].

8.6 ENDOGENOUS DIGOXIN-LIKE IMMUNOREACTIVE SUBSTANCES (DLIS) AND DIGOXIN IMMUNOASSAYS

After the discovery of endorphins, scientist hypothesize that there should be an endogenous equivalent of a digoxin, a cardiac glycoside. It was further hypothesized that antidigoxin antibody may be able to detect the presence of DLIS in body fluids. Gruber et al. first demonstrated the presence of endogenous DLIS in 1980, in volume expanded dogs [76]. Then Craver and Valdes reported an unexpected increase in serum digoxin concentration in a renal failure patient who was taking digoxin. Apparent serum digoxin level was still present after discontinuation of digoxin therapy [77]. DLIS were found in various human body fluids and tissues including cord blood, placenta, amniotic fluid, bile meconium, cerebrospinal fluid, and saliva [78,79].

DLIS can be divided into two groups. One class of DLIS interferes only with digoxin immunoassays due to their cross-reactivity with antidigoxin antibody and the other class of compounds inhibits or binds with Na, K-ATPase. These compounds may also cross-react with antidigoxin antibody. Because of the ability of DLIS to inhibit Na, K-ATPase, it was hypothesized that DLIS is a natriuretic hormone [80,81].

8.6.1 DIGOXIN–LIKE IMMUNOREACTIVE SUBSTANCES (DLIS) CONCENTRATIONS: HEALTHY INDIVIDUALS VERSUS DISEASE

8.6.1.1 Healthy Individuals

Usually concentrations of DLIS are undetectable in sera of normal individuals. In general, polyclonal antibody based digoxin immunoassay such as FPIA has higher sensitivity to detect the presence of DLIS in human sera. Monoclonal antibody based digoxin assays are minimally affected due to the presence of DLIS.

8.6.1.2 Volume Expanded Patients

Volume expansion is a major cause of elevated DLIS in blood. Elevated concentrations of DLIS have been reported in uremia, essential hypertension, hypertension of water volume expansion, liver disease, preeclampsia, transplant recipients, congestive heart failure, patients after myocardial infarction, premature babies and many other conditions [82–102]. Conditions that cause abnormality or change in DLIS concentrations are summarized in Table 8.3.

Howarth et al. reported elevated DLIS in plasma of intensive care unit patients using the FPIA digoxin assay for measuring DLIS concentration as apparent digoxin concentrations. Although some patients showed either hepatic or renal dysfunction, 42 patients who showed elevated DLIS had neither hepatic nor renal dysfunction. The DLIS concentrations ranged from 0.0 to1.69 nmol/L in 16 patients with coexisting hepatic and renal dysfunction, while 38 patients with hepatic dysfunction but normal renal function showed a range of DLIS concentration of 0.0–0.77 nmol/L (0.0–0.48 ng/mL) [103]. Berendes et al. reported that different types of endogenous glycosides are elevated in significant proportions in critically ill patients. The authors used FPIA assay for digoxin and digitoxin for measuring DLIS in patients not treated with cardiac glycosides. Out of 401 critically ill patients 343 (85.5%) patients demonstrated no measurable concentration of DLIS but the remaining 58 patients (14.5%) had measurable DLIS. Out of these 58 patients, 18 patients showed significant digoxin levels (0.54 ± 0.36 ng/mL) and 34 patients showed measurable digitoxin levels (2.28 ± 1.7 ng/mL) [104].

Concentration of DLIS may be significantly increased in cord blood as well as in sera of neonates. Chicella et al. measured DLIS concentrations in 80 pediatric patients never exposed to digoxin by using both FPIA and MEIA (both from Abbott Laboratories). The authors reported that 48% of the specimens showed measurable DLIS using the MEIA and 79% of the specimens showed measurable DLIS using FPIA, while values obtained by the FPIA assay were higher than the corresponding values obtained by the MEIA. The highest apparent digoxin concentration was 0.38 ng/mL [105]. Concentrations of DLIS in cord blood may be significantly elevated compared to maternal blood. In

TABLE 8.3
Conditions that may Significantly Increase DLIS Concentrations

Disease	Method for Measurement	Reference
Essential hypertension	RIA, Ouabain binding	82,89,90
Hypertension/volume expansion	Rubidium uptake	82,91
Uremic syndrome	RIA, FPIA, ACA	77,83,85
Liver disease, liver failure	EMIT, FPIA	84,85
Transplant recipients	FPIA, RIA, ACA	92
Premature babies/new born	FPIA	82,91
Cord blood	FPIA	106
Pediatric population	FPIA	105
Pregnancy and preeclampsia	RIA, FPIA, Na, K-ATP inhibition	82,86,91
Congestive heart failure	FPIA	93
Hypertropic cardiomyopathy	FPIA	93
Myocardial infarction	RIA, FIA, Na, K-ATP inhibition	95–97
Intensive care unit patients	FPIA	103
Critically ill patients	FPIA	104
Diabetes	RIA, FPIA	98,99
Mucocutaneous lymph node syndrome	RIA	100
Aneurysmal subarachnoid hemorrhage	FPIA	101
CSF of patients with fever	FPIA	78
Postmortem blood (adults and children)	RIA	102

Notes: RIA; radioimmunoassay, FPIA: fluorescence polarization immunoassay, ACA: Digoxin
assay marketed by Dade Behring, FIA: fluoroimmunoassay, CSF: cerebrospinal fluid.

one study, the mean DLIS concentration in umbilical cord plasma was 0.55 ng/mL while the average DLIS concentration in maternal plasma was 0.23 ng/mL (measured by FPIA). Moreover, dehydroepiandrosterone sulfate in maternal plasma and progesterone in maternal and umbilical cord plasma may be measured as digoxin by the FPIA [106].

8.6.2 POSITIVE AND NEGATIVE INTERFERENCE OF DLIS IN SERUM DIGOXIN MEASUREMENT: IMPACT ON MONITORING OF DIGOXIN

Positive interference of DLIS in the FPIA digoxin assay (Abbott Laboratories) is very well documented in literature. Many investigators used this assay to measure DLIS levels in a variety of patients not receiving digoxin. Miller et al. studied analytical performance of the CLIA digoxin assay on the ACS:180 analyzer (Ciba-Corning currently marketed by Bayer Diagnostics) by comparing this assay with the FPIA (Digoxin II), Stratus II digoxin assay and a RIA digoxin assay (Magic RIA, Ciba-Corning). The authors detected no DLIS in sera using CLIA, but measurable concentrations of DLIS were observed with the FPIA, Stratus II digoxin assay and the RIA method [107]. Way et al. compared three digoxin (Vitros, Johnson & Johnson; OnLine Digoxin assay, Roche; and MEIA, Abbott) assays using 26 adult patients receiving digoxin and observed mean digoxin concentrations of 1.30 ± 0.69 ng/mL (SD) by Roche assay, 1.34 ± 0.58 ng/mL by the Abbott assay and 1.46 ± 0.68 ng/mL by the Vitros digoxin assay. The authors concluded that the positive bias in the Vitros assay compared to Roche OnLine assay was probably due to DLIS [108].

Bonagura et al. reported high specificity of the Roche OnLine assay for digoxin, which had no cross reactivity with DLIS and negligible cross-reactivity with non cardioactive metabolites of digoxin [109]. Marzullo et al. reported that the EMIT 2000 digoxin immunoassay and the Roche OnLine digoxin immunoassay were least affected by DLIS compared to other digoxin assays [110].

More recently marketed digoxin immunoassays such as a turbidimetric assay on ADVIA 1650 analyzer and a enzyme-linked immunosorbent digoxin assay on the ADVIA IMS 800 I system (both marketed by Bayer Diagnostics) are virtually free from DLIS interference [111,112]. This may be related to the use of specific monoclonal antibodies targeted against digoxin in this new assay compared to rabbit polyclonal antibody targeted against digoxin in the FPIA assay.

Although most investigators reported positive interference of DLIS with serum digoxin measurement, negative interference (falsely lower digoxin values) of DLIS in the MEIA for digoxin has been reported. This may result in digoxin toxicity because a clinician may increase a digoxin dose based on a falsely low digoxin concentration due to elevated DLIS [113,114].

8.6.3 ELIMINATION OF DLIS INTERFERENCE IN DIGOXIN IMMUNOASSAY BY ULTRAFILTRATION

Valdes and Graves first reported strong serum protein binding of DLIS [115]. Therefore, DLIS is usually absent in the protein free ultrafiltrate. Taking advantage of high protein binding of DLIS and poor protein binding of digoxin (25%), both positive and negative interference of DLIS in serum digoxin measurement can be completely eliminated by measuring digoxin concentration in the protein free ultrafiltrate [116,117]. Protein free ultrafiltrate of digoxin can be easily prepared by centrifuging the specimen at $1,500-200 \times g$ in a Centrifree Micropartition System (Ultrafiltration device, Amicon, distributed by Millipore Corporation; Molecular weight cutoff 30,000 Daltons) for 20–30 min at room temperature. The immunoassay kits used for monitoring total digoxin concentration have adequate sensitivity to measure free digoxin concentration in the protein free ultrafiltrate.

8.7 CONCLUSIONS

Both endogenous and exogenous DLIS can cause significant interference in serum digoxin measurement. DLIS causes low to moderate false increases in serum digoxin value in most digoxin immunoassays. However, FPIA (Digoxin II) showed significant interference from DLIS. Negative interference of DLIS in the MEIA digoxin assay may also be problematic because the clinician may increase the digoxin dose based on falsely low serum digoxin concentrations. Both positive and negative interference in serum digoxin measurement can be eliminated by monitoring free digoxin concentration.

Interference in digoxin assays due to ingestion of Chinese medicines can cause more confusion. Most patients do not inform their physicians when they use alternative medicines. Present studies indicate that components of those Chinese medicines causing DLIS activity are strongly protein bound. Monitoring free digoxin may eliminate such interferences due to certain herbal supplements.

REFERENCES

1. El Desoky EA, Madabushi R, El Din S, Venkatesh A, et al. 2005. Application of two point assay of digoxin serum concentration in studying population pharmacokinetics in Egyptian pediatric patients with heart failure: does it make sense. *Am J Ther* 12: 320–327.
2. McMurray JJ, Carson PE, Komajda M, McKelvie R, et al. 2008. Heart failure with preserved ejection fraction: clinical characteristics of 4133 patients enrolled in the 1-PRESERVE trial. *Eur J Heart Fail* 10: 149–156.
3. Schwinger RH, Bundagaard H, Muller-Ehmsen J, and Kjeldsen K. 2003. The Na-K-ATPase in the failing human heart. *Cardiovasc Res* 57: 913–920.
4. Arispe N, Diaz JC, Simakova O and Pollard HB. 2008 Heart failure drug digitoxin induces calcium intake into cells by forming transmembrane calcium channels. *Proc Natl Acad Sci USA.* 105: 2610–2615.
5. Raebel MA, Carroll NM, Andrade SE, Chester EA, Lafata JE, Feldstein A, et al. 2006. Monitoring drugs with a narrow therapeutic range in ambulatory care. *Am J Manag Care* 12: 268–274.

6. Rea TD, Siscovick DS, Psaty BM, Pearce RM, et al. 2003. Digoxin therapy and risk of primary cardiac arrest in patients with congestive heart failure: effect of mild-moderate renal impairment. *J Clin Epidemol* 56: 646–650.

7. Adams KF, Patterson JH, Gattis WA, O'Connor CM, et al. 2005. Relationship of serum digoxin concentrations to mortality and morbidity in women in the digitalis investigation group trial: a retrospective study. *J Am Coll Cardiol* 46: 497–504.

8. Mitamura K, Horikawa A, Yamane Y, Ikeda Y, Fujii Y and Shimada K. 2007. Determination of digoxin in human serum using stable isotope dilution liquid chromatography/electrospray ionization tandem mass spectrometry. *Biol Pharm Bull* 30: 1653–1656.

9. Dasgupta A. 2006. Therapeutic drug monitoring of digoxin: impact of endogenous and exogenous digoxin-like immunoreactive substances. *Toxicol Rev* 25: 273–281.

10. Miller JJ, Straub RW and Valdes R. 1994. Digoxin immunoassays with cross-reactivity of digoxin metabolites proportional to their biological activities. *Clin Chem* 40: 1898–1903.

11. Solnica B. 2004. Comparison of serum digoxin concentration monitored by fluorescence polarization immunoassay on the TDxFLx and dry chemistry enzyme immunoassay on the Vitros 950. *Clin Chem Lab Med* 42: 958–964.

12. Curd J, Smith TW, Jaton JC and Haber E. 1971. The isolation of digoxin-specific antibody and its use in reversing the effects of digoxin. *Proc Natl Acad Sci USA* 68: 2401–2406.

13. Pullen MA, Brooks DP and Edwards RM. 2004. Characterization of neutralizing activity of digoxin specific Fab towards ouabain like steroids. *J Pharmacol Exp Ther* 310: 319–325.

14. Camphausen C, Hass NA and Mattke AC. 2005. Successful treatment of oleander intoxication (cardiac glycoside) with digoxin specific Fab antibody fragment in a 7 year old child: case report and review of literature. *Z Kardiol* 94: 817–823.

15. Brubacher JR, Lachmanen D, Ravikumar PR, Hoffman RS. 1999. Efficacy of digoxin specific Fab fragments (Digibind) in the treatment of toad venom poisoning. *Toxicon* 37: 931–942.

16. Flanagan RJ and Jones AL. 2004. Fab antibody fragments: some applications in clinical toxicology. *Drug Saf* 27: 1115–1133.

17. Rainey P. 1999. Digibind and free digoxin [Letter]. *Clin Chem* 45: 719–720.

18. McMillin GA, Qwen W, Lambert TL, De B, et al. 2002. Comparable effects of DIGIBIND and DigiFab in thirteen digoxin immunoassays. *Clin Chem* 48: 1580–1584.

19. Jortani SA, Pinar A, Johnson NA and Valdes R. 1999. Validity of unbound digoxin measurements by immunoassays in presence of antidote (Digibind). *Clin Chim Acta* 283: 159–169.

20. Huffman DH. 1974. The effects of spironolactone and canrenone in digoxin radioimmunoassay. *Res Comm Chem Pathol Pharmacol* 9: 787–790.

21. Lichey J, Rietbrock N and Borner K. 1979. The influence of intravenous canrenoate on the determination of digoxin in serum by radio and enzyme immunoassay. *Int J Clin Pharmacol Biopharm* 17: 61–63.

22. Silber B, Sheiner LB, Powers JL, Winter ME and Sadee W. 1979. Spironolactone-associated digoxin radioimmunoassay interference. *Clin Chem* 25: 48–50.

23. Morris RG, Frewin DB, Taylor WB, Glistak ML and Lehmann DR. 1988. The effect of renal and hepatic impairment and of spironolactone on serum digoxin assay. *Eur J Clin Pharmacol* 34: 233–239.

24. Pleasants RA, Williams DM, Porter RS and Gadsden RH. 1989. Reassessment of cross-reactivity of spironolactone metabolites with four digoxin assays. *Ther Drug Monit* 1989; 11: 200–204.

25. Foukaridis GN. 1990. Influence of spironolactone and its metabolite canrenone on serum digoxin assays. *Ther Drug Monit* 12: 82–84.

26. Okazaki M, Tanigawara Y, Kita T, Komada F and Okumura K. 1997. Cross-reactivity of TDX and OPUS immunoassay system for serum digoxin determination. *Ther Drug Monit* 19: 657–662.

27. Steimer W, Muller C, Eber B and Emmanuilidis K. 1999. Intoxication due to negative canrenone interference in digoxin drug monitoring [Letter]. *Lancet* 354: 1176–1177.

28. Steimer W, Muller C and Eber B 2002. Digoxin assays: frequent, substantial and potentially dangerous interference by spironolactone, canrenone and other steroids. *Clin Chem* 48: 507–516.

29. Dasgupta A, Saffer H, Wells A and Datta P. 2002. Bidirectional (Positive/Negative) interference of spironolactone, canrenone and potassium canrenoate on serum digoxin measurement: elimination of interference by measuring free digoxin or using a chemiluminescent assay. *J Clin Lab Anal* 16: 172–177.

30. Datta P and Dasgupta A. 2003. A new turbidimetric digoxin immunoassay on the ADVIA 1650 analyzer is free from interference by spironolactone, potassium canrenoate and their common metabolite canrenone. *Ther Drug Monit* 25: 478–482.

31. Howard G, Barclay M, Florkowski C, Moore G and Roche A. 2003. Lack of clinically significant interference by spironolactone with the AxSYM digoxin II assay. *Ther Drug Monit* 25: 112–113.

32. Steimer W. 2003.Lack of critically significant interference by spironolactone with the AxSYM digoxin II assay only applies to low dose therapy with spironolactone [Letter]. *Ther Drug Monit* 25: 484–485.
33. Dong H, Xu F, Zhang Z, Tian Y and Chen Y. 2006. Simultaneous determination of spironolactone and its active metabolite canrenone in human plasma by HPLC-APCI-MS. *J Mass Spectrom* 41: 477–486.
34. Mahady GB. 2001. Global harmonization of herbal health claims. *J Nutr* 131: 1120S–1123S.
35. Dasgupta A and Bernard DW. 2006. Complementary and alternative medicines: effects on clinical laboratory tests. *Arch Pathol Lab Med* 130: 521–528.
36. Hong Z, Chan K and Yeung HW. 1992. Simultaneous determination of bufadienolides in the traditional Chinese medicine preparations, Liu-Shen-Wan by liquid chromatography. *J Pharm Pharmacol* 44: 1023–1026.
37. Chan WY, Ng TB and Yeung HW. 1995. Examination for toxicity of a Chinese drug, the total glandular secretion product Chan SU in pregnant mice and embryos. *Biol Neonate* 67: 376–380.
38. Chen KK and Kovarikove A. 1967. Pharmacology and toxicology of toad venom. *J Pharm Sci* 56: 1535–1541.
39. Morishita S, Shoji M, Oguni Y, Ito C, et al. 1992. Pharmacological actions of "Kyushin" a drug containing toad venom: Cardiotonic and arrhythmogenic effects and excitatory effect on respiration. *Am J Chin Med* 20: 245–256.
40. Pamnani MB, Chen S, Bryant HJ and Schooley JF. 1991. Effect of three sodium-potassium adenosine triphosphate inhibitors. *Hypertension* 18: 316–324.
41. Xu W, Luo H, Zhang Y, Shan L et al. 2007. Simultaneous determination of five Main active bufadienolides of Chan Su in rat plasma by liquid chromatography tandem mass spectrometry. *J Chromatogr B Analyt Technol Biomed Life Sci* 859: 157–163.
42. Fushimi R and Amino N. 1995. Digoxin concentration in blood. *Rinsho Byori* 43: 34–40 [article in Japanese, abstract in English].
43. Panesar NS. 1992. Bufalin and unidentified substances in traditional Chinese medicine cross-react in commercial digoxin assay. *Clin Chem* 38: 2155–2156.
44. Panesar NS, Chan KW and Law LK. 2005. Changing characteristics of the TDx digoxin II assay in detecting bufadienolides in a traditional Chinese medicine: for better or worse? *Ther Drug Monit* 27: 677–679.
45. Ko R, Greenwald M, Loscutoff S, Au A, et al. 1996. Lethal ingestion of Chinese tea containing Chan SU. *Western J Med* 164; 71–75.
46. Chow L, Johnson M, Wells A and Dasgupta A. 2003. Effect of the traditional Chinese medicine Chan Su, Lu-Shen-Wan, DanShen and Asian ginseng on serum digoxin measurement by Tina-Quant (Roche) and Synchron LX system (Beckman) digoxin immunoassays. *J Clin lab Anal* 17: 22–27.
47. Dasgupta A, Biddle D, Wells A and Datta P. 2000. Positive and negative interference of Chinese medicine Chan SU in serum digoxin measurement: elimination of interference using a monoclonal chemiluminescent digoxin assay or monitoring free digoxin concentrations. *Am J Clin Pathol* 114: 174–179.
48. Reyes M, Actor JK, Risin SA and Dasgupta A. 2008. Effect of Chinese medicines Chan Su and Lu-Shen-wan on serum digoxin measurement by Digoxin III, a new digoxin immunoassay. *Ther Drug Monit* 30: 95–99.
49. Liang Y, Liu AH, Qin S, Sun JH, et al. 2008. Simultaneous determination and pharmacokinetics of five bufadienolides in rat plasma after oral administration of Chan Su extract by SPE-HPLC method. *J Pharm Biomed Anal* 46: 442–448.
50. Blum LM and Reiders F. 1987. Oleander distribution in a fatality from rectal and oral Nerium oleander extracts administration. *J Anal Toxicol* 82: 121–122.
51. Saravanapavananthan N and Ganeshamoorthy J. 1988. Yellow oleander poisoning: a case study of 170 cases. *Forensic Sci Int* 36: 247–250.
52. Brewster D. 1986. Herbal poisoning: a case report of fetal yellow oleander poisoning from the Solomon Island. *Ann Trop Paediatr* 6: 289–291.
53. Langford S and Boor PJ. 1999. Oleander toxicity: an examination of human and animal toxic exposure. *Toxicology* 109: 1–13.
54. Erdemoglu N, Kupeli E and Yesilada E. 2003. Anti-inflammatory and antinociceptive activity assessment of plants used as remedy in Turkish folk medicine. *J Ethnopharmacol* 89: 123–139.
55. Eddleston M, Ariaratnam CA, Meyer PW, Perera G, et al. 1999. Epidemic of self poisoning with seeds of yellow oleander tree (Thevetia peruviana) in north Sri Lanka. *Trop Med Int Health* 4: 266–273.
56. Haynes BE, Bessen HA, and Wightman WD. 1985. Oleander tea: herbal draught of death. *Ann Emerg Med* 14: 350–353.

57. Hamouda C, Amamou M, Thabet H, Yacoub M, et al. 2000. Plant poisonings from herbal medication admitted to a Tunisian toxicological intensive care unit, 1983–1998. *Vet Human Toxicol* 42: 137–141.

58. Cheung K, Hinds JA and Duffy P. 1989. Detection of poisoning by plant origin cardiac glycosides with the Abbott TDx analyzer. *Clin Chem* 1989: 295–297.

59. Jortani S, Helm A and Valdes R. 1996. Inhibition of Na,K-ATPase by oleandrin and oleandrigenin and their detection by digoxin immunoassays. *Clin Chem* 42: 1654–1658.

60. Osterloh J. 1988. Cross-reactivity of oleander glycosides [Letter]. *J Anal Toxicol* 12: 53.

61. Eddleston M, Ariaratnam CA, Sjostrom L, Jayalath S, et al. 2000. Acute yellow oleander (*Thevetia peruvica*) poisoning: cardiac arrhythmias, electrolyte disturbances, and serum cardiac glycoside concentrations on presentation to hospital. *Heart* 83: 310–306.

62. Roberts DM, Southcott E, Potter J, Roberts MS, et al. 2006. Pharmacokinetics of digoxin cross-reacting substances in patients with acute yellow oleander (*Thevetia peruviana*) poisoning, including the effect of activated charcoal. *Ther Drug Monit* 28: 784–792.

63. Dasgupta A and Datta P. 2004. Rapid detection of oleander poisoning by using digoxin immunoassays: comparison of five assays. *Ther Drug Monit* 26: 658–663.

64. Tracqui A, Kintz P, Branche F, and Ludes B. 1998. Confirmation of oleander poisoning by HPLC/MS. *Int J Legal Med* 111: 32–34.

65. Tor ER, Filigenzi MS and Puschner B. 2005. Determination of oleandrin in tissues and biological fluids by liquid chromatography-electrospray tandem mass spectrometry. *J Agri Food Chem* 53: 4322–4325.

66. McRae S. 1996. Elevated serum digoxin levels in a patient taking digoxin and Siberian ginseng. *Can Med Assoc J* 155: 293–295.

67. Dasgupta A, Wu S, Actor J, Olsen M, Wells A and Datta P. 2003. Effect of Asian and Siberian ginseng on serum digoxin measurement by five digoxin immunoassays: significant variation in digoxin-like immunoreactivity among commercial ginsengs. *Am J Clin Pathol* 119: 298–303.

68. Dasgupta A and Reyer M. 2005. Effect of Brazilian, Indian, Siberian, Asian and North American ginseng on serum digoxin measurement by immunoassays and binding of digoxin-like immunoreactive components of ginseng with Fab fragment of antidigoxin antibody (Digibind). *Am J Clin Pathol* 124: 229–236.

69. Dasgupta, Peterson A, Wells A and Actor JK. 2007. Effect of Indian Ayurvedic medicine Ashwagandha on measurement of serum digoxin and 11 commonly monitored drugs using immunoassays: study of protein binding and interaction with Digibind. *Arch Pathol Lab Med* 131: 1298–1303.

70. Lee AR, Wu WL, Chang WL, Lin HC, and King ML. 1987. Isolation and bioactivity of new tanshinones. *J Nat Prod* 50: 157–160.

71. Dasgupta A, Actor JK, Olsen M, Wells A, and Datta P. 2002. In vivo digoxin-like immunoreactivity in mice and interference of Chinese medicine Danshen in serum digoxin measurement: elimination of interference by using a chemiluminescent assay. *Clinica Chimica Acta* 317: 231–234.

72. Wahed A, and Dasgupta A. 2001. Positive and negative in vitro interference of Chinese medicine Danshen in serum digoxin measurement: elimination of interference by monitoring free digoxin concentrations. *Am J Clin Pathol* 116: 403–408.

73. Ghorbani M, Kaloga M, Frey HH, Mayer G and Eich E. 1997. Phytochemical reinvestigation of Xysmalobium undulatum roots (Uzara). *Planta Med* 63: 343–346.

74. Thurmann PA, Neff A and Fleisch J. 2004. Interference of Uzara glycosides in assays of digitalis glycosides. *Int J Clin Pharmacol Ther* 42: 281–284.

75. Barrueto F Jr., Jortani SA, Valdes R Jr., Hoffman RS and Nelson LS. 2003. Cardioactive steroid poisoning from an herbal cleansing preparation. *Ann Emerg Med* 41: 396–399.

76. Gruber KA, Whitaker JM and Buckalew VM. 1980. Endogenous digitalis-like substances in plasma of volume expanded dogs. *Nature* 287: 743–745.

77. Craver JL, Valdes R. 1983. Anomalous serum digoxin concentration in uremia. *Ann Intern Med* 98: 483–484.

78. Krivoy N, Lalkin A and Jakobi P. 1990. Digoxin-like immunoreactivity detected in cerebrospinal fluid of humans with fever. *Clin Chem* 36: 703–704.

79. Dasgupta A. 2006. Therapeutic drug monitoring of digoxin: impact of endogenous and exogenous digoxin-like immunoreactive factors. *Toxicol Rev* 25: 273–281.

80. Dasgupta A, Yeo K, Malik S, Sandu P, et al. 1987. Two novel endogenous digoxin-like immunoreactive substances isolated from human plasma ultrafiltrate. *Biochem Biophys Res Comm* 148: 623–628.

81. Qazzaz HM, and Valdes R. 1996. Simultaneous isolation of endogenous digoxin-like immunoreactive factor, ouabain-like factor, and deglycosylated congeners from mammalian tissue. *Arch Biochem Biophys* 328: 193–200.

82. Jortani SA and Valdes R Jr. 1997. Digoxin and its related endogenous factors. *Crit Rev Clin Lab Sci* 34: 225–274.
83. Graves SW, Brown BA and Valdes R. 1983. Digoxin-like immunoreactive substances in a patient with renal impairment. *Ann Intern Med* 99: 604–608.
84. Nanja AA and Greenway DC. 1985. Falsely raised plasma digoxin concentrations in liver disease. *BMJ* 290: 432–435.
85. Sault MH, Vasdev SC and Longerich LL. 1984. Endogenous digoxin –like substances in patients with combined hepatic and renal failure. *Ann Intern Med* 58: 748–751.
86. Graves SW. 1987. The possible role of digitalis-like factors in pregnancy induced hypertension. *Hypertension* 10 (Supply I): 184–186.
87. Cloix JF. 1987. Endogenous digitalis like compounds. *Hypertension* 10 (Supply I): 67–70.
88. Shilo L., Adwani A, Solomon G and Shenkman L. 1987. Endogenous digoxin –like immunoreactivity in congestive heart failure. *BMJ* 295: 415–416.
89. Ahmad S, Kenny M and Scribner BH. 1986. Hypertension and a digoxin-like substance in the plasma of dialysis patients; possible marker for a natriuretic hormone. *Clin Physiol Biochem* 4: 210–216.
90. Seccombe DW, Purdek, Nowaczynski W and Humphries KH. 1989. Digoxin-like immunoreactivity, displacement of ouabain and inhibition of Na+ /K+ ATPase by four steroids known to be increased in essential hypertension. *Clin Biochem* 22: 17–21.
91. Clerico A, Balzan S, Del Chicca MG, Paci A, et al. 1988. Endogenous cardiac glycoside-like substances in newborns, adults, pregnant women and patients with hypertension or renal insufficiency. *Drugs Exp Clin Res* 4: 603–607.
92. Schrader BJ, Maddux MS, Veremis SA and Mozes MF. 1991. Digoxin-like immunoreactive substance in renal transplant patients. *J Clin Pharmacol* 31: 1126–1131.
93. Hayashi T, Ijiri Y, Toko H, Shimomura H, et al. 2000. Increased digitalis like immunoreactivity in patients with hypertropic cardiomyopathy. *Eur Heart J* 21: 296–305.
94. Dasgupta A, Saldana S and Heimann P. 1990. Monitoring free digoxin instead of total digoxin in patients with congestive heart failure and high concentrations of digoxin-like immunoreactive substances. *Clin Chem* 36: 2121–2123.
95. Bagrov AYa, Fedorova OV, Maslova MN, Roukoyatkina NI, et al. 1991. Endogenous plasma Na,K-ATPase inhibitory activity and digoxin like immunoreactivity after acute myocardial infarction. *Cardiovas Res* 25: 371–377.
96. Kohn R, Lichardus B and Rusnak M. 1992. Endogenous digitalis-like factors in patients with acute myocardial infarction. *Cor Vasa* 34: 227–237.
97. Bargov AY, Kuznetsova EA and Fedorova OV. 1994. Endogenous digoxin-like factor in acute myocardial infarction. *J Intern Med* 235: 63–67.
98. Giampietro O, Clerico A, Gregori G, Bertoli S, et al. 1988. Increased urinary excretion of digoxin-like immunoreactive substances by insulin-dependent diabetic patients: a linkage with hypertension? *Clin Chem* 34: 2418–2422.
99. Strub RH, Elbracht R, Kramer BK, Roth M, et al. 1994. Influence of digoxin-like immunoreactive factor on late complications in patients with diabetes mellitus. *Eur J Clin Invest* 24: 482–487.
100. Tamura H, Shimoyama S, Sunaga Y, Sakaguchi M, et al. 1992. Digoxin-like immunoreactive substance in urine of patients with mucocutaneous lymph node syndrome (MCLS). *Angiology* 43: 856–865.
101. Lusic I, Ljutic D, Maskovic J and Jankovic S. 1999. Plasma and cerebrospinal fluid endogenous digoxin-like immunoreactivity in patients with aneurysmal subarachnoid haemorrhage. *Acta Neurochir (Wien)* 141: 691–697.
102. Spiehler VR, Fischer WR and Richards RG. 1985. Digoxin like immunoreactive substance in postmortem blood of infants and children. *J Forensic Sci* 30: 86–91.
103. Howarth DM, Sampson DC, Hawker FH and Young A. 1990. Digoxin-like immunoreactive substances in the plasma of intensive care unit patients: relationship to organ dysfunction. *Anaesth Intensive Care* 18: 45–52.
104. Berendes E, Cullen P, van Aken H, Zidek W, et al. 2003. Endogenous glycosides in critically ill patients. *Crit Care Med* 31: 1331–1337.
105. Chicella M, Branim B, Lee KR and Phelps SJ. 1998. Comparison of microparticle enzyme and fluorescence polarization immunoassays in pediatric patients not receiving digoxin. *Ther Drug Monit* 20: 347–351.
106. Ijiri Y, Hayashi T, Kamegai H, Ohi K, et al. 2003. Digitalis-like immunoreactive substances in maternal and umbilical cord plasma: a comparative sensitivity study of fluorescence polarization immunoassay and microparticle enzyme immunoassay. *Ther Drug Monit* 25: 234–239.

107. Miller JJ, Straub RW and Valdes R. 1996. Analytical performance of a monoclonal digoxin assay with increased specificity on the ACS:180. *Ther Drug Monit* 18: 65–72.
108. Way BA, Wilhite TR, Miller R, Smith CH and Landt M. 1998. Vitros digoxin immunoassay evaluated for interference by digoxin-like immunoreactive factors. *Clin Chem* 44: 1339–1440.
109. Bonagura E, Law T and Rifai N. 1995. Assessment of the immunoreactivity of digoxin metabolites and the cross-reactivity with digoxin-like immunoreactive factors in the Roche-TDM online digoxin assay. *Ther Drug Monit* 17: 532–537.
110. Marzullo C, Bourderont D and Dorr R. 1996. Interference of digoxin-like immunoreactive substances with four recent reagents for digoxin determination. *Ann Biol Chem (Paris)* 54: 91–96.
111. Datta P and Dasgupta A. 2004. Interference of endogenous digoxin-like immunoreactive factors in serum digoxin measurement is minimized in a new turbidimetric digoxin immunoassay on ADVIA 1650 analyzer. *Ther Drug Monit* 26: 85–89.
112. Dasgupta A, Kang E and Datta P. 2005. New enzyme-linked immunosorbent digoxin assay on the ADVIA IMS 800i system is virtually free from interference of endogenous digoxin-like immunoreactive factor. *Ther Drug Monit* 27: 139–143.
113. Valdes R, Jortani SA and Gheorghiade M. 1998. Standards of laboratory practice: cardiac drug monitoring. *Natl Acad Clin Biochem Clin Chem* 44: 1096–1109.
114. Dasgupta A and Trejo O. 1999. Suppression of total digoxin concentration by digoxin-like immunoreactive substances in the MEIA digoxin assay: elimination of interference by monitoring free digoxin concentrations. *Am J Clin Pathol* 111: 406–410.
115. Valdes R and Graves SW. 1985. Protein binding of endogenous digoxin-like immunoreactive factors in human serum and its variation with clinical condition. *J Clin Endocrinol Metab* 60: 1135–1143.
116. Christenson RH, Studenberg SD, Beck-Davis SS and Sedor FA. 1987. Digoxin-like immunoreactivity eliminated from serum by centrifugal ultrafiltration before fluorescence polarization immunoassay of digoxin. *Clin Chem* 33: 606–608.
117. Dasgupta A, Schammel D, Limmany A and Datta P. 1996. Estimating concentration of total digoxin and digoxin-like immunoreactive substances in volume expanded patients being treated with digoxin. *Ther Drug Monit* 18: 34–39.

9 Liquid Chromatography Combined with Immunoassay as a Reference Method for Analysis of Digitalis

Edward Peters Womack, Roland Valdes, and Saeed A. Jortani
University of Louisville School of Medicine

CONTENTS

9.1 INTRODUCTION

Therapeutic monitoring of digitalis compounds has been challenging, despite improvements made in immunochemistry assays over the past several decades. Commercial immunoassays that have been introduced have been plagued with bias and interference caused by exogenous and endogenous substances. Resolving individual cases has lead to the development of a method composed of an initial separation of immunoreactive components by high performance liquid chromatography (HPLC), the collection of eluted fractions, and the measurement of immunoreactive components by immunoassay. We refer to this approach as HPLC-immunoassay (HPLC-IA) technique–a reference method that effectively identifies the desired compound as well as interfering substance(s). This reference method also provides a means of generating purified compounds to confirm observed interference or

153

discrepancy between immunoassay results and better characterize the immunochemistry detection. This chapter will outline the challenges in clinical monitoring of digoxin, describe the HPLC-IA and present several examples in which this approach was used to resolve discrepant immunoassay results.

9.2 CHALLENGES IN CLINICAL MONITORING OF DIGOXIN

Although digoxin is the first drug to be therapeutically monitored using the immunoassay approach [1], it is still considered to be one of the most challenging analytes measured in the clinical laboratory. Digoxin is assessed at low nanomolar concentrations (1–2.60 nmol/L; 0.8–2.0 ng/mL) [2], has a narrow therapeutic index, and concentrations above 3 nmol/L (2.3 ng/mL) are considered to be toxic. These relatively low concentrations require a sensitive measurement methodology which is commonly provided by immunochemistry. Digoxin analysis is often made in the presence of endogenous and exogenous interfering substances that can cross-react and potentially affect the accuracy of the results. The assays themselves can also be affected by noncross-reacting interfering substances whose effects are methodology-dependent.

9.2.1 Cross-Reacting Interfering Substances

Generally, interfering substances affecting digitalis-type immunoassays are grouped into cross-reacting and noncross-reacting categories. The majority of interfering substances are cross-reacting and exogenous in origin [3]. However, endogenous interference from digoxin-like immunoreactive factor (DLIF) has been known since the 1980s [4,5] and interference from bufadienolides has also been identified [6,7]. These compounds contain a steroid nucleus that permits some degree of binding with polyclonal antidigoxin antibodies. As with Fab fragments used as an antidote in digoxin poisoning (known as Digibind®), digoxin metabolites have also been shown to interfere with immunoassays by cross-reactivity [8]. Thus, cross-reacting interfering substances compete for binding to an analytical primary antibody, while noncross-reacting interfering substances bind to the ligand being measured and prevent its binding to the primary antibody in use [3].

9.2.2 Noncross-Reacting Interfering Substances

Immunoassays rely on various approaches to detect antibody-antigen interactions. For example, in radioimmunoassays, the change in the binding of ^{125}I-digoxin as a tracer is monitored by a gamma counter. In enzyme immunoassays, the generation of the product from the substrate can be monitored by colorimetric, fluorescent, or chemiluminescent methods. Almost all of these detection techniques can be affected by the variations in the matrix of the sample that is brought about by the presence of both endogenous molecules such as bilirubin, triglycerides, or excessive protein concentration. It is therefore, important to consider sample integrity and matrix as a source of discrepancy in digoxin results. In older immunoassay systems, the serum sample is pretreated with sulfosalicylic acid, which has been shown to alter the structure of digoxin and reduce its affinity for the primary antibody [9].

9.3 HPLC-IMMUNOASSAY (HPLC-IA) COMBINATION METHODOLOGY

In recent decades, HPLC has been used in clinical laboratories to provide a valuable means by which several drugs and their metabolites are measured. Some HPLC systems leave the molecules of interest intact, making them available for collection and further analysis. By taking advantage of this capability, we have developed a reference method for measurement of endogenous and exogenous digitalis-like compounds [10]. This technique involves the separation of the potentially immunoreactive components using chromatography, collecting the eluted fractions, and the processing and quantification of reacting substances in the fractions by immunoassay. In this section, we will briefly present the various components of this system.

9.3.1 System Components

There are several components in the system and these various components are discussed in the following sections.

9.3.1.1 Chromatographic Separation by High Performance Liquid Chromatography (HPLC)

Although many different options exist to separate digitalis-like immunoreactivity, a commonly used one uses a convex gradient acetonitrile/water mobile phase of 20% acetonitrile to 80% over 30 or 60 minutes (notated as 20:80:30 or 20:80:60). Alternative mobile phases, with a constant ratio of solvents (i.e., isocratic), are used for achieving greater separation of previously collected fractions [11]. The mobile phase pushes an injected sample through a 3–5 μm C18 capped column. The eluate passes through a UV (ultraviolet)-capable photo diode array (PDA) detector that detects the eluting compounds and permits determination of their λ_{max} that can be used for identification. In general, this mode of detection is limited for digitalis-like compounds, since they are often at very low concentrations and their UV detection is not possible. The outflow from the detector is routed to a fraction collector where fractions, by time or by peak detection, are collected for further analysis or purification (Figure 9.1). Frequently, 1 mL of a sample is extracted by solid phase extraction and injected into the HPLC. The mobile phase flow rate is kept at 1 mL/min resulting in 1 mL fractions. Following the collection and processing (drying down the mobile phase) of these fractions, they are reconstituted in 1 mL of drug-free matrix (e.g., phosphate-buffered saline) to be measured by immunoassay. Concentration measurements by immunoassay (see below) are therefore comparable to the original sample. There are times when the compound of interest is eluted over several minutes (i.e., milliliters of collected mobile phase). In these situations, each fraction is measured separately and the values added together to calculate the concentration of the compound in the sample (Figure 9.2). After separation and preparation of fractions, the discreet samples are analyzed by digoxin or digitoxin immunoassays. These can be done either by automated commercial methods such as microparticle enzyme immunoassay (MEIA), fluorescence polarization immunoassay (FPIA) or cloned enzyme donor immunoassay (CEDIA) or manual methods such as competitive-binding enzyme-linked immunosorbent assay (ELISA). Immunochemistry methods of detection are particularly important because they provide detailed cross-reactivity information for the primary antibody. Sample preparation is also important, as proteins and strong chromogens that act as potential interfering substances in the sample are partially or completely removed. This allows a more accurate determination of the concentration of the desired compound. Typical preparation involves sample clean-up using solid-phase extraction (SPE) columns containing a C18 resin. Various elution buffers can also be used to allow for differential elution of multiple compounds in the same sample.

9.3.1.2 Analysis of Collected Fractions by Immunoassay

There are many commercially available immunoassays for determination of concentrations of digoxin or digitoxin in serum or other biological matrix. Discrepant values are usually noted when correlation studies between two or more of these immunoassays are performed. On occasion, a measured digoxin or digitoxin value for a patient is not in agreement with the clinical condition of the patient. This occurs when a dosing regimen does not match the serum concentration of the drug. For example, a measurement of 10 ng/mL digoxin in a properly collected serum from a patient with no symptoms of digitalis poisoning calls into questions the validity of the immunoassay. The HPLC-IA reference method is very useful in either of the stated scenarios for resolution of the

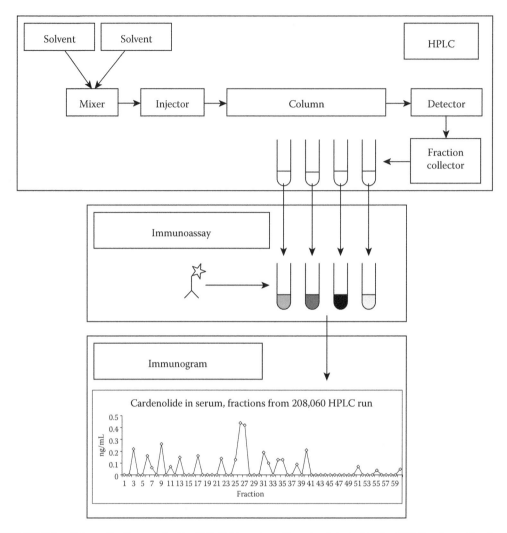

FIGURE 9.1   Schematic diagram for the HPLC-IA system. Samples injected in the HPLC column (top box) are separated using a gradient mobile phase with a flow of 1 mL/minute. The samples are fractionated by collecting the column eluate for discreet periods of time (1 minute, typically) using a fraction collector. Fractions are analyzed (middle box) by immunoassay and an immunogram (bottom box) is generated by plotting the sequential fraction number versus the measured concentration of the cardenolide in that fraction.

discrepancy. The power of this technology is the fact that the collected fractions can be reanalyzed by the same immunoassays which lead to the discrepant results. In this way, the actual concentration of the primary ligand (e.g., digoxin) is measured in addition to the immunoreactivity caused by the cross-reactants or the bias resulted from the presence of the interfering substances. The immunoassays often studied in discrepant digitalis cases have included the fluorescence polarization on the Roche FARA [12,13], chemiluminescence on the ACS:180 (currently known as Centaur), Abbott MEIA on either IMx or AxSYM [14,15], and the kinetic interaction of microparticles in solution (KIMS) on the Roche Integra [16]. ELISA detection of cardenolides has also proven to be a very useful and easy way to trace the immunoreactive compound elution from the HPLC system. The ELISA method requires an antibody specific for a cardenolide as well as the conjugated (typically to bovine serum albumin) and native cardenolide. Competitive assays such as ELISA are best suited to detecting cardenolides, since there are few available haptens for the molecule with a molecular

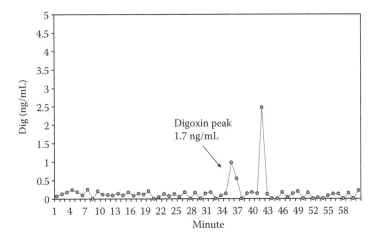

FIGURE 9.2 An immunogram generated using the HPLC-IA technique. A serum sample was extracted using a C18 extraction cartridge and eluted with 60% acetonitrile in water. The eluate was dried down, reconstituted in 1 mL mobile phase and shot using a 20:80:60 mobile phase at 1 mL/minute. One minute fractions were collected, dried down and reconstituted in the same matrix used for the immunoassay calibrators. A digoxin ELISA assay was used to measure digoxin in each fraction. The concentration in two fractions indicated the expected digoxin peak at approximately 37 minutes. The immunoreactivity measured in these two tubes was added to show the digoxin concentration for the peak. The peak at 41 minutes is an unidentified cross-reactant.

weight of 781 Daltons. The inherent cross-reactivity of polyclonal antibodies used in these assays presents a two-edged sword: cross-reactivity is a source of discrepant results as well as a means of identifying cross-reacting interfering substances. As an example, the endogenous form of digoxin (DLIF) also cross-reacts and interferes with quantitation of the plant-derived compounds [17–19]. Numerous studies have been performed on DLIF relying on its cross-reactivity with an antidigoxin antibody for detection and quantitation [9,20]. In fact, the HPLC-IA technique is currently the only accepted method for measuring DLIF and its related compounds [10,20,21].

9.4 RESOLUTION OF DISCREPANCIES IN DIGOXIN RESULTS BY HPLC-IA

Over the years, the HPLC-IA technique has been used to resolve discrepant digoxin results. In this section, we will present examples of applying this reference method to determine the source of digoxin like cross-reactivity in clinical samples.

9.4.1 RESOLUTION OF ANTIBODY-MEDIATED DIGOXIN DISCREPANCY

A rare convergence of a monoclonal gammopathy with digoxin therapy was discovered in an elderly female with a history of colon cancer in remission and newly diagnosed IgG-κ multiple myeloma (Figure 9.3). Three different immunoassays indicated her serum digoxin concentrations to be 3.73, 3.39, and 9.70 ng/mL digoxin equivalents. The patient had never been given Digibind® (antidigoxin Fab fragments) which is known to interfere with immunoassays. The patient was on a digoxin dosing regimen of 0.125 mg/day. HPLC fractionation of her serum sample and subsequent measurement by two different immunoassays showed 6.4 and 7.1 ng/mL of digoxin at the expected retention time (Figure 9.4). Subsequent spiking studies of the patient serum with ³H-digoxin demonstrated that a monoclonal antidigoxin antibody, a result of the multiple myeloma neoplasia, was interfering

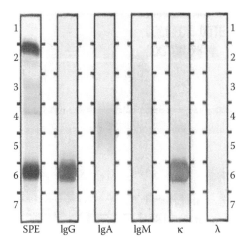

FIGURE 9.3 Urine immunofixation electrophoresis (IFE) results from a patient with multiple myeloma. The lower dark band in the SPE column and corresponding band in the IgG column indicate an IgG monoclonal gammopathy, κ type, (indicated by the lower band in the κ column) as a result of multiple myeloma. This antibody demonstrated specificity for digoxin and interfered with serum immunoassay digoxin measurement in the patient.

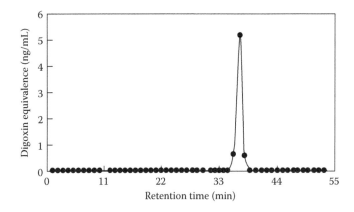

FIGURE 9.4 An immunogram showing the retention time and total concentration of digoxin in the patient sample. An HPLC mobile phase gradient of 20:80:60 was used and 1 minute fractions collected. The fractions were analyzed using an immunoassay, indicating a retention time of 37 minutes for digoxin and a total concentration of ~6 ng/mL.

in the various commercial digoxin immunoassays. The HPLC-IA technique was therefore, able to show the discrepancy source to be other than the cardenolides themselves. This investigation ultimately lead to the discovery of antidigoxin antibodies produced by the patient as an unusual and unexpected source of interference [22].

9.4.2 PRESENCE OF SEVERAL INTERFERING SUBSTANCES

The HPLC-IA method has been demonstrated to be very useful in cases where the apparent serum digoxin concentration measured is due to multiple sources as well as the principal ligand itself. In one particular case, a patient presented to an emergency room with symptoms of nausea, vomiting and dizziness yet without any apparent symptoms of cardiac toxicity. The patient's serum digoxin concentration was well above the toxic threshold and varied widely between six different immunoassays. HPLC separation and fractionation, followed by immunoassay, revealed that the patient had a therapeutically normal concentration of digoxin plus a larger concentration of a deglycosylated congener, digoxigenin bis-digitoxoside. DLIF was also detected which, along with digoxin bis-digitoxoside, was a source of cross-reactivity in the immunoassays. A third noncross-reacting substance interfering with the assay signal had compounded the seriousness of the matter. Therefore, the only means of teasing out the sources of cross-reactivity and interference was an initial separation by HPLC followed by measuring the cross-reactivities observed by the digoxin immunoassay [3].

9.4.3 OLEANDRIN POISONING BY CROSS-REACTIVITY AND SPECTRUM ANALYSIS

The PDA detector attached to the HPLC in the HPLC-IA method can play an important role in identifying unrecognized cardenolides. Cross-reactivity, while undesirable in most cases, can be used in identification, particularly when assay labeling is consulted for known cross-reacting compounds. These two HPLC-IA strategies were used to detect oleandrin poisoning in a 13-month-old

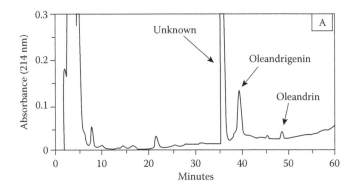

FIGURE 9.5 A 214 nm chromatogram from an HPLC separation of serum from a cardenolide poisoning case. A 20:80:60 HPLC gradient was used. The resulting peaks did not match the expected 37 minute digoxin retention time. Examination of the spectral profile of the later peaks indicated that they were related to oleandrin.

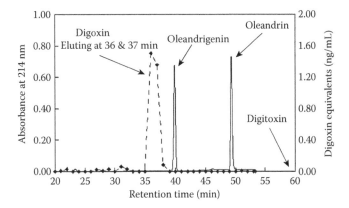

FIGURE 9.6 An overlay of a digoxin immunogram on an HPLC chromatogram comparing the retention time of digoxin and oleandrin. Digoxin was measured in discreet one minute fractions of an HPLC separation using an immunoassay, while oleandrin was detected using the photodiode array detector attached to the HPLC. The two separate peaks demonstrate different retention times, allowing the ability to separate and identify digoxin and oleandrin.

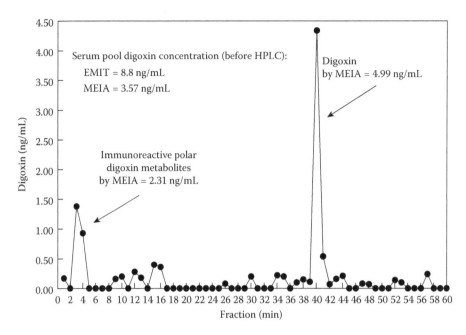

FIGURE 9.7 An immunogram generated from fractions collected from a 20:80:60 HPLC analysis of a discrepant sample. The sample was from a patient with several high initial measured serum digoxin concentrations. Subsequent HPLC-IA clarified the true digoxin concentration and identified the source of the difference between the initial and processed results. In this case, pharmacologically inactive digoxin polar metabolites were cross-reacting with the assay antibody to produce a falsely elevated measured concentration.

male with symptoms consistent with digoxin toxicity [23]. The patient's serum was tested by five different immunoassays, providing an apparent digoxin result ranging from 0.0 to 1.41 ng/mL. An HPLC chromatogram extracted at 214 nm showed three peaks (Figure 9.5) that did not correspond to digoxin retention times on the system. Determination of the λ_{max} narrowed down the possible compounds that would cause cardiotoxicity and cross-reactivity. Studies of the suspected compound (oleandrin) confirmed the phenomenon seen in the patient's digoxin measurements (Figure 9.6).

9.4.4 RESOLUTION OF DISCREPANT RESULTS DUE TO POLAR METABOLITES

Digoxin is eliminated as the parent compound as well as polar glucuronidated, sulfated and deglycosylated metabolites [24]. HPLC-IA was used to resolve discrepant serum digoxin concentrations in a patient who had measurements of 11.1 and 3.99 ng/mL by two different immunoassays. HPLC separation and fractionation revealed that inactive polar metabolites eluting shortly after injection in the HPLC column significantly contributed to the final serum concentration (Figure 9.7). The concentration of the active parent drug was lower, but still above the toxic threshold [25].

9.4.5 RESOLVING INTERFERENCE FROM AN HERBAL EPIMER OF DIGITOXIN

Uzarin is an epimer of digitoxin and has been found in the root of the uzara bush [26] and milk-weed [27]. It has a low affinity for the Na^+/K^+ ATPase pump, reducing its cardiotoxicity [28]. It is currently sold over-the-counter in Germany as an ethanol extracted antidiarrhea medication called Uzara®. Because of its structural similarities to digitoxin, uzarin has been detected in commercial digoxin [29] immunoassays by cross-reactivity with the antibodies used. A case study has been published where a patient taking Uzara® had an elevated serum digitoxin concentration [28]. Several of these studies used the HPLC-IA method to separate the immunoreactive components of the extract and characterize the degree of positive interference with digoxin immunoassays.

9.5 ADVANTAGES AND DISADVANTAGES OF HPLC-IMMUNOASSAY (HPLC-IA)

As demonstrated by the preceding case samples, the use of HPLC-IA to resolve a discrepant digoxin results is very versatile. This powerful approach allows for the simultaneous separation and collection of the pertinent fractions eluting from the column. Incorporation of immunoassays as a part of this technique allows for closure of the loop from an interfered-with immunoassay to an interference-free immunoassay resolution of the source of the discrepancy. Based on our experience, once the cross-reacting and noncross-reacting species have been separated, the eluting fractions (corresponding to that of digoxin) will yield increasingly more accurate digoxin results after reanalysis by the immunoassays. As stated in the above mentioned oleander case, the spectrum profile of a given peak monitored by PDA detector can also help with identification of the source of discrepancy. These peaks can be further analyzed by overlaying the PDA-generated chromatograms with the corresponding immunograms to compare retention times. The major disadvantages of this technique are the labor intensive steps of extraction, HPLC analysis, collection, and reanalysis of the fractions and the potential analysis of the PDA spectrum. Since this method is intended for resolution of discrepancies in clinical cases, its adaptation as a normal analytical process by a clinical laboratory is often not appropriate. However, implementation by a large referral lab may be of value for resolution of in-house or referred samples with discrepancies in digoxin results. It is of interest to note that a similar approach can be implemented for other drugs or substances for which there are multiple endogenous and exogenous sources of cross-reactivity and interference.

ACKNOWLEDGMENT

The authors would like to thank Rosemary Williams for her assistance in typographical and grammatical editing of this manuscript.

REFERENCES

1. Smith TW, Butler VP, Haber E. 1969. Determination of therapeutic and toxic digoxin concentrations by radio immunoassay. *N Engl J Med* 281:1212–1216.
2. Jortani SA, Valdes R, Jr. 1997. Digoxin and its related endogenous factors. *Crit Rev Clin Lab Sci* 34(3):225–274.
3. Jortani SA, Miller JJ, Valdes R, Jr. 1996. Resolving clinically discrepant digoxin results: A case study involving multiple interferences. *J Clin Lig Assay* 19:131–137.
4. Valdes R, Jr., Graves SW, Brown BA, Landt M. 1983. Endogenous substance in newborn infants causing false positive digoxin measurements. *J Pediatr* 102(6):947–950.
5. Valdes R, Jr. 1985. Endogenous digoxin-immunoactive factor in human subjects. *Fed Proc* 44(12):2800–2805.
6. Dasgupta A, Datta P. 1998. Rapid detection of cardioactive bufalin toxicity using fluorescence polarization immunoassay for digitoxin. *Ther Drug Monit* 20(1):104–108.
7. Dasgupta A, Biddle DA, Wells A, Datta P. 2000. Positive and negative interference of the Chinese medicine Chan Su in serum digoxin measurement. Elimination of interference by using a monoclonal chemiluminescent digoxin assay or monitoring free digoxin concentration. *Am J Clin Pathol* 114(2):174–179.
8. Valdes R, Jr., Miller JJ. 1995. Importance of using molar concentrations to express cross-reactivity in immunoassays. *Clin Chem* 41(2):332–333.

9. Qazzaz HM, Goudy S, Miller JJ, Valdes R, Jr. 1995. Treatment of human serum with sulfosalicylic acid structurally alters digoxin and endogenous digoxin-like immunoreactive factor. *Ther Drug Monit* 17(1):53–59.

10. Shaikh IM, Lau BW, Siegfried BA, Valdes R, Jr. 1991. Isolation of digoxin-like immunoreactive factors from mammalian adrenal cortex. *J Biol Chem* 266(21):13672–13678.

11. Qazzaz HM, El-Masri MA, Stolowich NJ, Valdes R, Jr. 1999. Two biologically active isomers of dihydroouabain isolated from a commercial preparation. *Biochim Biophys Acta* 1472(3):486–497.

12. Bonagura E, Law T, Rifai N. 1995. Assessment of the immunoreactivity of digoxin metabolites and the cross-reactivity with digoxin-like immunoreactive factors in the Roche-TDM ONLINE digoxin assay. *Ther Drug Monit* 17(5):532–537.

13. Brustolin D, Sirtoli M, Tarenghi G. 1992. An enzyme-labeled immunometric assay for quantitation of digoxin in serum or plasma. *Ther Drug Monit* 14(1):72–77.

14. Miller JJ, Straub RW, Jr., Valdes R, Jr. 1996. Analytical performance of a monoclonal digoxin assay with increased specificity on the ACS:180. *Ther Drug Monit* 18(1):65–72.

15. Dasgupta A, Risin SA, Reyes M, Actor JK. 2008. Rapid detection of oleander poisoning by Digoxin III, a new Digoxin assay: impact on serum Digoxin measurement. *Am J Clin Pathol* 129(4):548–553.

16. Domke I, Cremer P, Huchtemann M. 2000. Therapeutic drug monitoring on COBAS INTEGRA 400—evaluation results. *Clin Lab* 46(9–10):509–515.

17. Valdes R, Jr. 1992. Improving the specificity of digoxin immunoassays. *Wien Klin Wochenschr* Suppl 191:55–59.

18. Valdes R, Jr., Jortani SA. 2002. Unexpected suppression of immunoassay results by cross-reactivity: now a demonstrated cause for concern. *Clin Chem* 48(3):405–406.

19. Jortani SA, Valdes R, Jr. 1997. Digoxin and its related endogenous factors. *Crit Rev Clin Lab Sci* 34(3):225–274.

20. Qazzaz HM, Valdes R, Jr. 1996. Simultaneous isolation of endogenous digoxin-like immunoreactive factor, ouabain-like factor, and deglycosylated congeners from mammalian tissues. *Arch Biochem Biophys* 328(1):193–200.

21. Doris PA, Stocco DM. 1989. An endogenous digitalis-like factor derived from the adrenal gland: studies of adrenal tissue from various sources. *Endocrinology* 125(5):2573–2579.

22. Jortani SA, Harrison H, Johnson NA, Subudhi J Valdes Jr R. 2000. Monoclonal gammopathy associated with an anomalous digoxin measurement. *Clin Chem* 46:A38.

23. Gupta A, Joshi P, Jortani SA, Valdes R, Jr., Thorkelsson T, Verjee Z, Shemie S. 1997. A case of nondigitalis cardiac glycoside toxicity. *Ther Drug Monit* 19(6):711–714.

24. Gault MH, Longerich LL, Loo JC, Ko PT, Fine A, Vasdev SC, Dawe MA. 1984. Digoxin biotransformation. *Clin Pharmacol Ther* 35(1):74–82.

25. Keeling KL, Jortani SA, Staimer W, Valdes Jr R. 2004. Importance of evaluating the effects of polar metabolites on digoxin immunoassays. *Clin Chem* 50:A133.

26. Ghorbani M, Kaloga M, Frey HH, Mayer G, Eich E. 1997. Phytochemical reinvestigation of Xysmalobium undulatum roots (Uzara). *Planta Med* 63(4):343–346.

27. Abbott AJ, Holoubek CG, Martin RA. 1998. Inhibition of Na+ ,K+ -ATPase by the cardenolide 6'-O-(E-4-hydroxycinnamoyl) desglucouzarin. *Biochem Biophys Res Commun* 251(1):256–259.

28. Thurmann PA, Neff A, Fleisch J. 2004. Interference of Uzara glycosides in assays of digitalis glycosides. *Int J Clin Pharmacol Ther* 42(5):281–284.

29. Jortani SA, Helm RA, Johnson NJ, Valdes R, Jr. 1997. Interference of Uzara® (an anti-diarrheal medication) in digoxin assays. *Ther Drug Monit* 19(5):534.

10 Chromatographic Methods for Analysis of Cardioactive Drugs

Ronald W. McLawhon
University of California, San Diego, School of Medicine

CONTENTS

10.1   INTRODUCTION

Cardioactive drugs represent one of the most commonly prescribed groups of therapeutic agents to treat cardiac arrhythmias, congestive heart failure, and hypertension. In most instances, despite significant differences in chemical structure and properties and their therapeutic applications, many of these drugs exert their pharmacological effects by similar mechanism through controlling electrical conduction system and/or phases of the cardiac action potential [1,2]. Class I drugs, such as lidocaine and quinidine, block sodium influx in the first phase of the action potential, resulting in its prolongation. Class II agents include drugs like propranolol, which is a beta-adrenergic receptor antagonist that inhibits the chronotropic and sympathomimetic effects of epinephrine and norepinephrine on the heart, as well as the vasculature and circulatory system. Class III cardiotropic drugs, such as amiodarone, act to block repolarization by potassium currents and, thereby, prolong the refractory period and the overall action potential. Class IV drugs, characterized by verapamil and nifedipine, are calcium channel blockers that decrease conduction through the atrioventricular (A-V) node and shorten the plateau of the cardiac action potential.

Currently, routine therapeutic monitoring of cardioactive drugs in human serum or plasma is performed for those agents that with a very narrow therapeutic index, serious risks and complications of toxicity, and to ensure patient compliance and adjust dosages for optimal therapeutic benefit [3,4]. Many cardioactive agents that have been commonly used in medical practice for several decades are easily monitored in most clinical laboratories due to the development and widespread use of commercially developed homogeneous and heterogeneous immunoassays that are available in both automated and semiautomated formats [4,5]. Drugs such as digoxin, procainamide, disopyramide, quinidine and lidocaine are generally measured using these various immunoassay methods, which includes enzyme multiplied immunoassays, cloned donor enzyme immunoassays, fluorescence polarization immunoassay, chemiluminescence and electro-chemiluminescence immunoassays and immunoturbidimetry. In most cases, these techniques are rapid, inexpensive, easy to perform, reliable and infrequently have been found to have significant analytical limitations and interferences (except digoxin, which has been discussed in detail in Chapter 8). Thus, routine monitoring of these drugs in serum or plasma by immunoassay methods have been virtually supplanted by any chromatographic applications that may have developed over the years, and will not be discussed further in this chapter.

Over the last two decades, a host of next generation cardioactive drugs have been developed and introduced into the market, that are now widely prescribed as front line treatment for a range of cardiovascular disorders [2]. Many of these drugs are preferred because of their broad and diverse therapeutic benefits, while some offer wider therapeutic indices and lower risks for toxicity and more reliable absorption and bioavailability to achieve steady state concentrations without the need for regular monitoring. Some of the newer cardiotropic drugs Figure 10.1) including amiodarone, flecainide, tocainide, mexiletine and verapamil, in certain clinical situations, may require monitoring of serum or plasma levels to ensure better clinical outcome. Recommended therapeutic and toxic ranges of these cardiotropic agents are given in Table 10.1. At present, the only methods that are available for therapeutic drug monitoring of these drugs are chromatographic techniques—either gas liquid chromatography (GC) with various types of detectors as well as mass spectrometry (MS), high performance liquid chromatography (HPLC), or liquid chromatography/mass spectrometry (LC/MS). This chapter will focus on these cardiotropic agents and the methods currently employed in their analysis within clinical and reference laboratories.

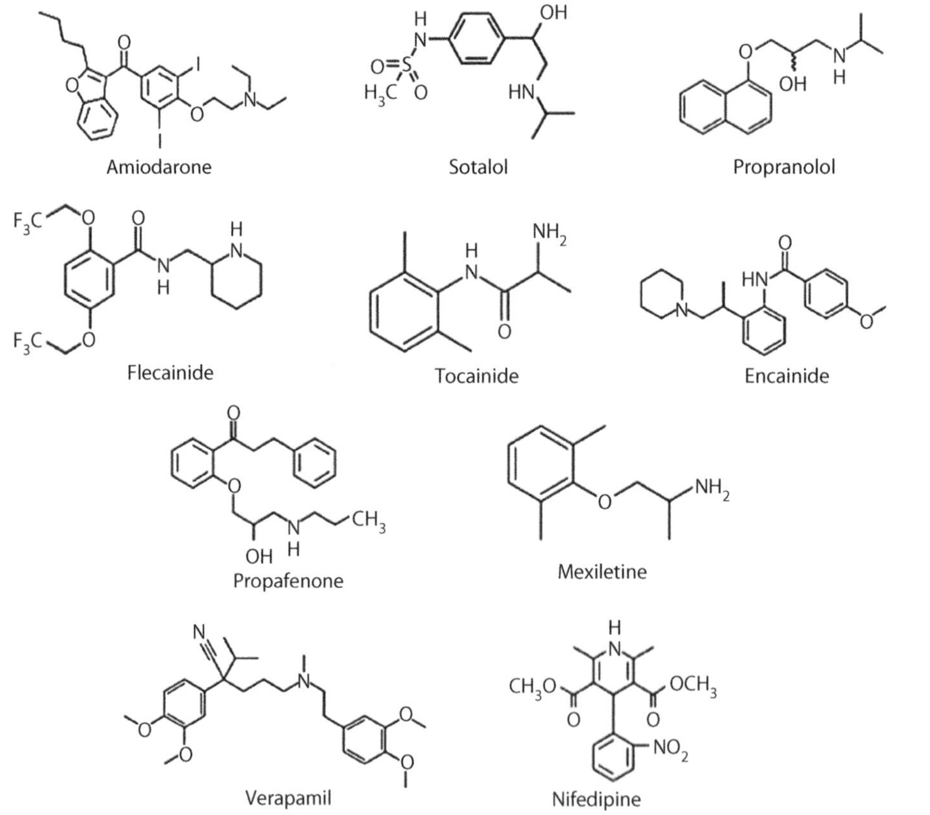

FIGURE 10.1 Chemical structures of commonly prescribed cardioactive drugs that are therapeutically monitored by chromatographic methods.

TABLE 10.1
Recommended Therapeutic of certain Cardiotropic Drugs

Drug	Specimen Requirement	Therapeutic Range	Toxic
Amiodarone	Serum or plasma	1.0–3.0 µg/ml	>3.0 µg/ml*
Flecainide	Serum or plasma	0.2–1.0 µg/ml	>1.5 µg/ml*
Mexiletine	Serum or plasma	1.0–2.0 µg/ml	1.5–3.0 µg/ml*
Nifedipine	Serum or plasma	25–100 ng/ml	>100 ng/ml
Propanolol	Serum or plasma	50–100 ng/ml	>1000 ng/ml^
Propafenone	Serum or plasma	0.5–2.0 µg/ml	>2.0 µg/ml*
Sotalol	Serum or plasma	1.0–4.0 µg/ml	>4.0 µg/ml*
Tocainide	Serum or plasma	5.0–12.0 µg/ml	
>15 µg/ml (peak)^			
Verapamil	Serum or plasma	50–200 ng/ml	>400 ng/ml (peak)^

* Recommended values based on reference ranges recommended by ARUP Laboratories (Salt Lake City, UT).
^ Recommended values based on reference ranges recommended by ARUP Laboratories (Salt Lake City, UT).

10.2 AMIODARONE

Amiodarone, a Class III antiarrhythmic agent, is most commonly used to treat supraventricular and life-threatening ventricular arrhythmias. It has been proven particularly useful for treatment of hemodynamically unstable ventricular tachycardia and recurrent fibrillation resistant to other therapy [1,2,8]. This drug is 95% protein bound, undergoes renal clearance and has a long, multi-phasic elimination (up to 53 days).

Unfortunately, despite its therapeutic benefits, amiodarone has numerous side effects and is often reserved as the treatment of last resort for severe, life-threatening arrhythmias [8,9]. Toxic side effects [8–11] are not concentration dependent but rather related to slow elimination, and include hypothyroidism (being a structural analog of thyroxine), interstitial pneumonitis and pulmonary fibrosis, keratopathy, and heart block or sinus bradycardia. These effects are generally noted at blood concentrations above 2.5 µg/mL. Amiodarone has also been observed to have numerous interactions with other drugs, including other cardioactive agents and potentiating the anticoagulant effects of warfarin.

While adverse effects of this drug can be severe, routine monitoring of serum or plasma concentrations of amiodarone and its potentially active metabolite, N-desethyl-amiodarone, are only rarely performed. Typical clinical indications for laboratory analysis are to monitor patient compliance and adequacy of blood concentrations (usually above 1.0 µg/mL), or when signs and symptoms of toxicity are manifested. The current methodology that is most widely employed is HPLC with ultraviolet (UV), fluorescence, or chemiluminescence detection, and using rapid and simple liquid extraction techniques [6,7,12,13]. Ou et al. described a liquid chromatographic technique for determination of amiodarone and its metabolite in human serum using HPLC and UV detection. The authors extracted amiodarone and its metabolite from 250 µl of human serum by adding 100 µl of 0.036 mol/L sodium dihydrogen phosphate buffer, 100 µl of internal standard (L8040, an analog of amiodarone) and then 200 µl of isopropyl ether. After vortex mixing and centrifugation, amiodarone, its metabolite and the internal standard were extracted into the organic extract and were analyzed by HPLC using a 5 µm spherical silica column (Waters Associates, Milford, MA). The elution of peaks was monitored at 254 nm wavelength. The mobile phase composition was methanol/17 mmol/L ammonium sulfate buffer (92:8 by vol). The assay was linear for serum concentration of amiodarone as well as its metabolite from 0.1 to 20.0 µg/mL [14]. In Figure 10.2a, chromatogram of representative patient sample analyzed by this protocol is shown [14]. In the method published by Juenke et al., the authors used 3 µm particle size CN column (cyano column: 100 mm×4.6 mm

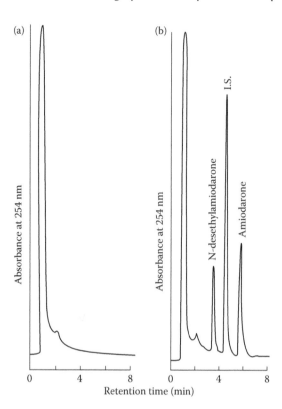

FIGURE 10.2   Chromatograms of representative patient's serum samples. (a) drug free serum, (b) sample from patient being treated with amiodarone. (From Ou CN, Rogneurud CL, Doung LT, and Frawley VL, *Clin Chem*, 36, 532–534, 1990. Copyright 1990 American Association for Clinical Chemistry. Reprinted with permission.)

internal diameter) and a mobile phase composition of acetonitrile/methanol/0.05 M ammonium acetate (40:56:3 by vol) [12]. The internal standard used was also L 8040 (Wyeth, Madison, NJ). Typical chromatograms demonstrating adequate separation and quantitation of both amiodarone and N-desethyl-amiodarone by HPLC are shown in Figure 10.3 (method and figures courtesy of Dr. G.A. McMillin, ARUP Laboratories, Salt Lake City, UT).

The limit of quantitation, linearity, imprecision and accuracy of various chromatographic assays described in the literature adequately cover the therapeutic range for appropriate patient monitoring and further allow for quantitation of both the parent compound and its metabolite. Imprecision has been reported to be <6% at therapeutic concentrations, with a broad analytical measuring range from 0.3 to 6.0 mg/L (0.3–6.0 μg/mL). While LC/MS methods (using electrospray ionization with an ion trap detector) have been developed [15], they offer little or no analytical performance advantages over well-established HPLC procedures for routine clinical monitoring and only offer marginal advantages for forensic applications where chemical identity needs to be confirmed.

10.3   SOTALOL AND PROPRANOLOL

Sotalol is a beta-adrenoreceptor blocker drug that also has class III antiarrhythmic properties and has been prescribed to patients with ventricular, atrial and supraventricular arrhythmias [2,3]. Because it inhibits the potassium ion channels in the heart, sotalol prolongs repolarization, and lengthens the QT interval and decreases automaticity. Sotalol is used to treat ventricular tachycardias, as well as specific indications for certain formulations in treating atrial fibrillation and atrial flutter. Several adverse effects, such as bradycardia, *torsades de pointes,* acute myocardial infarction, and cardiac heart failure [3,16], have been reported in patients with severe ventricular arrhythmia, and are most

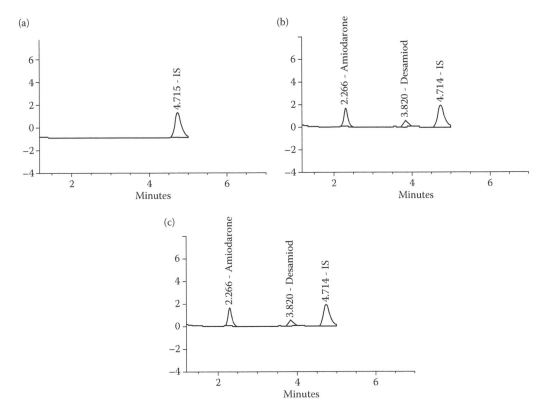

FIGURE 10.3 Amiodarone and desethylamiodarone as detected by HPLC-UV for a drug-free blank (a) internal standard, a calibrator containing 2.5 µg/ml amiodarone and 2.5 µg/ml desethylamiodarone, (b) and a typical patient with a amiodarone concentration of 1.5 µg/ml and desethylamiodarone concentration of 0.7 µg/ml in serum (c).

commonly the reason for therapeutic monitoring of drugs concentrations in serum and plasma. During the first week of treatment, adverse effects arise more frequently as a consequence of the prolongation of QT interval. Much like amiodarone, the current methodology that is most widely employed is HPLC with UV or fluorescence detection [7,17–19], following simple extraction. For example, in the method reported by Boutagy and Shenfield, plasma specimen was deproteinized with perchloric acid and sotalol was recovered into 4 M potassium hydrogen phosphate and analyzed by HPLC using a C-18 reverse phase column and a mobile phase composition of 6% acetonitrile in 0.08 M potassium dihydrogen phosphate buffer. Detection of peaks was achieved by fluorescence measurement with excitation wavelength at 235 nm and emission wavelength at 310 nm [18].

Chromatographic methods for analysis of sotalol in human serum or plasma have excellent limits of detection (<0.05 µg/mL) and imprecision in the range of 3–5%, with linear measurements that span well beyond (up to 10 µg/mL) the clinically relevant therapeutic range 1–4 µg/mL with toxic levels seen >4 µg/mL. These methods are also capable of resolving both R- and S-enantiomers of the drug. An example of a typical patient measurement is illustrated in Figure 10.4. Sotalol from patient's serum was analyzed by a 3 µm particle size CN column (cyano column: 100 mm×4.6 mm internal diameter). After adjusting pH of the sample with borate buffer and adding MJ-6564-1, the internal standard, sotalol along with the internal standard were extracted using an organic solvent mixture (chloroform/ isopropanol, 9:1 by vol). The internal standard was a sotalol analog available from Bristol Meyers and the mobile phase composition was acetonitrile/methanol/0.1 M ammonium acetate (72:18:5 by vol). Elution of peaks was monitored at 242 nm wavelength (method and figures courtesy of Dr. G.A. McMillin, ARUP Laboratories, Salt Lake City, UT).

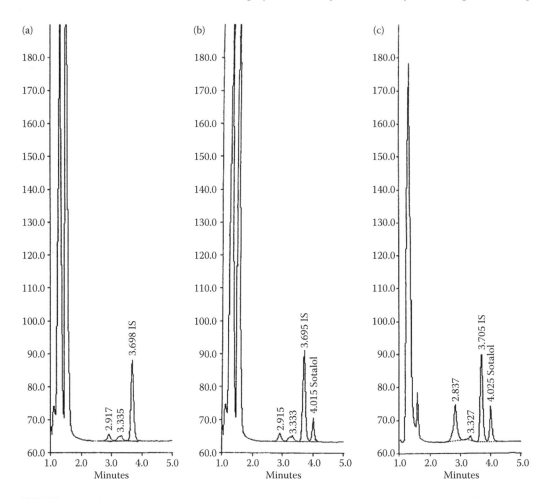

FIGURE 10.4   Sotalol as detected by HPLC-UV for a drug-free blank (a) internal standard, a calibrator containing 1.0 µg/ml of sotalol, (b) and a typical patient with a serum sotalol concentration of 1.4 µg/ml (c).

Propranolol is a nonselective beta-adrenergic antagonist that acts upon both beta-1 and beta-2 adrenergic receptors, and regulates both cardiac activity (Class II antiarrhythmic) and vascular smooth muscle. As such, it has wide clinical applications in treating atrial and ventricular arrhythmias, ischemic heart disease including myocardial infarction, and hypertension [1,2]. This drug is well absorbed, highly protein bound, and metabolized in the liver, but bioavailability is quite variable between individuals and with dosage. There is a dose dependent relationship of serum or plasma concentrations to slowing of heart rate, which can be monitored as equally effectively by clinical signs, and there is no demonstrated relationship between drug concentration and antihypertensive effects of this drug. Consequently, propranolol is rarely monitored in the laboratory except to assess patient compliance. Adverse reactions with high levels include nausea, vomiting, bradycardia, hypotension and congestive heart failure. Propranolol is easily measured using automated HPLC with fluorescence detection by well established methods [20], with concentrations measured to as low as 0.2 ng/mL and in excess of toxic limits of >1000 ng/mL.

10.4   FLECAINIDE

Flecainide is a sodium channel blocker and Class Ic antiarrhythmic agent with electrophysiologic properties that are similar to lidocaine, procainamide and quinidine [2,3]. It produces a dose dependent decrease intracardiac conduction and can suppress recurrence of ventricular tachycardia [21].

This drug is largely reserved for use in patients who failed to respond to other sodium channel blockers, due to severe cardiac toxicity as well as to excessive prolongation of PQ, QRS, and QT intervals on EKG. Reductions in heart rate, contractility, and conduction disturbances have been observed with flecainide in a dose and concentration dependent fashion. This drug is also contraindicated for use in patients with sick sinus syndrome and myocardial infarction. Death can occur from acute hypotension, respiratory failure and asystole [3,22,23]. Romain et al. also reported a fatal flecainide intoxication case where flecainide concentrations determined by GC coupled with electron capture detector (ECD) were 7.7 mg/kg in femoral blood, 0.26 mg/kg in bile, 18 mg/kg in liver and total amount of flecainide in gastric content as determined by GC/MS was 43 mg [24]. Given the toxicity and relatively narrow therapeutic window, routine therapeutic monitoring is important to assess toxicity and to optimize dosing in patients receiving this drug.

While a fluorescence polarization immunoassay had been developed nearly two decades ago for the analysis flecainide in serum or plasma, this assay is no longer commercially available [5] and was plagued with a number of problems including nonlinearity, limited specificity (recognizing primarily flecainide acetate), and differences in measured concentrations due to intraindividual variations in hepatic metabolism by CYP2D6 [4]. Currently, the most widely accepted and reliable method for analysis of flecainide in serum and plasma is HLPC with UV or fluorescence detection [6,7,25–27] after liquid-liquid extraction. Flecainide and its metabolites, *m-O*-dealkylated flecainide and the *m-O*-dealkylated lactam of flecainide can be reliably separated and measured with these techniques. For example, Doki et al. reported simultaneous determination of serum flecainide and its metabolites using C-18 reverse phase column and fluorescence detection after extracting flecainide and its metabolites from serum using ethyl acetate [26]. Figure 10.5 shows a typical sample chromatogram using a HPLC-UV method. Loxapine was used as the internal standard and HPLC analysis was carried out using a silica column (150 mm×4.6 mm internal diameter after extraction with methyl-tert-butyl ether and elution of peaks was monitored at 230 nm (method and figures courtesy of Dr. G.A. McMillin, ARUP Laboratories, Salt Lake City, UT). Breindahl reported a LC/MS method with electrospray ionization following solid phase extraction for analysis of flecainide [28] with analytical performance characteristics that are comparable to conventional HLPC techniques; while somewhat improved separation of parent compound, metabolites, and internal standards has been reported using smaller specimen volumes (0.25 mL of serum or plasma), it does not appear to represent a major improvement over the other existing chromatographic methods. The recommended therapeutic concentrations range for flecainide is from 0.2 to 1.0 μg/mL (with greatest benefit for suppression of premature ventricular contractions seen in this range), but adverse cardiotoxic effects such as bradycardia and conduction irregularities seen at levels above 1.5 μg/mL. Both HPLC and LC/MS methods perform acceptably and equivalently for clinical measurement within the clinically relevant concentration ranges. GC/MS techniques have also described, but have been utilized less frequently [23].

10.5 TOCAINIDE AND ENCAINIDE

Tocainide is another Class Ic antiarrhythmic agent that is structurally analogous and shares electrophysiological properties with lidocaine, but has the advantage of being administered orally and has a relatively long half-life in the circulation (13–16 hrs). This drug acts to reduce the amplitude and rate of depolarization of the cardiac action potential by decreasing the refractory period and has proven most useful in the treatment of life-threatening ventricular arrhythmias associated with prolonged QT intervals [2,3]. This drug is minimally protein bound and undergoes renal clearance without significant first pass metabolism. Therapeutic monitoring of serum and plasma levels of tocainide is performed to determine optimal dose and dose interval, and more importantly in patients who have congestive heart failure and severe renal dysfunction where clearance half-life of this drug is increased significantly. Toxicity occurs at concentrations greater than 15 μg/mL, and ranges from gastrointestinal and central nervous disturbances to cardiopulmonary depression (including arrest)

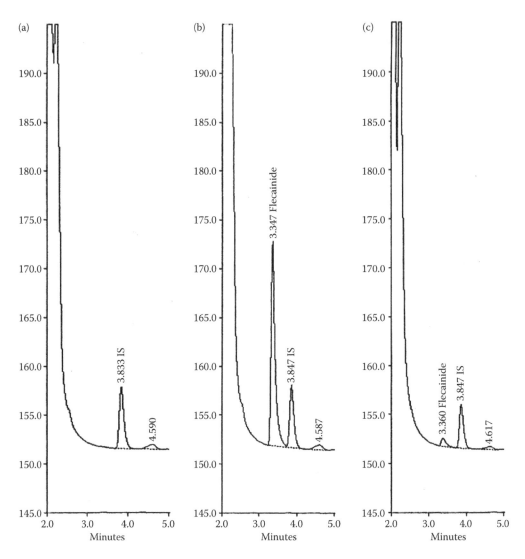

FIGURE 10.5 Flecainide as detected by HPLC-UV for a drug-free blank (a) internal standard, a calibrator containing 3.0 µg/ml of flecainide, (b) and a typical patient with a serum flecainide concentration of 0.2 µg/ml (c).

and the rare complications of leukopenia, agranulocytosis, and pulmonary fibrosis. Labor intensive GC (using flame ionization and ion capture detection) and HPLC methods following fluorescent derivatization have been described [6,7,29–31], although HPLC-UV methods using fast and simple extraction with *n*-butyl chloride or methylene chloride have been most widely adopted and provide analytical sensitivities down to 0.02–0.1 µg/mL. Due to the risks of bone marrow suppression, this drug is no longer commercially distributed in the United States, but remains available to physicians who had patients that were effectively managed on this medication prior to market withdrawal.

Encainide is a benzanilide derivative that has also been classified as a Class Ib antiarrhythmic agent. This drug is now strictly indicated for use in the suppression of documented life-threatening ventricular arrhythmias, including sustained ventricular tachycardia [32–34]. Encainide decreases excitability, conduction velocity, and automaticity as a result of slowed atrial, A-V nodal, His-Purkinje, and intraventricular conduction, as well as the rate of rise of the action potential without markedly affecting its duration. However, it should be noted that it is no longer accepted for treatment of less severe arrhythmias such as nonsustained ventricular tachycardias or frequent premature ventricular contractions, even if patients are symptomatic due to the risks of increased mortality associated with the development of proarrhythmia [2,3]. Like tocainide, encainide is no longer commercially available in the United States and its availability is limited to physicians who were prescribing and successfully managing patients of this drug prior to market withdrawal. Encainide and its two primary active metabolites, the O-demethyl (ODE) and 3-methoxy-O-demethyl (MODE) encainide, continues to be monitored therapeutically in academic and reference laboratory centers using HPLC methods with solid phase extraction using UV or fluorescence detection [35,36]. Typically, serum and plasma concentrations of these metabolites are expected to be higher than those of encainide and pharmacological effects correlate better with plasma metabolite concentrations than those of encainide itself [33,34]. In poor metabolizers, blood concentrations of active metabolites are low or undetectable and the effects of encainide therapy most closely correlated with concentrations of the parent drug. Excretion of encainide and its metabolites is impaired in individuals with renal disease, and dosages correspondingly should be decreased.

10.6   PROPAFENONE

Propafenone is another Class Ic antiarrhythmic drug that is structurally similar to flecainide and has beta-adrenergic receptor blocking and minor calcium channel antagonist activities [2]. This drug reduces the rate of rise in cardiac action potentials and, thereby, increases the threshold of excitability, depresses conduction velocity, and prolongs the refractory period. Propafenone currently is used for the treatment of supraventricular tachyarrhythmias, premature ventricular contractions, and ventricular tachycardia [37]. In contrast to some of the other Class I agents described above, propafenone undergoes significant first pass metabolism, with a half-life of approximately 6 hrs. Its clinical efficacy appears to be related to formation of 5-hydroxypropanfenone, a metabolite that is more pharmacologically active and has a half-life that is two-to-four times longer than the parent compound. Therapeutic monitoring of propafenone is useful to determine patient's compliance with this drug. However, therapeutic drug monitoring may also be useful when assessing adverse and toxic effects, such as hypersensitivity reactions, lupus-like syndrome, agranulocytosis, central nervous system (CNS) disturbances such as dizziness, lightheadedness, gastrointestinal upset, a metallic taste, and bronchospasm [2,3]. Therapeutic concentrations tend to be in the range of 0.5–2.0 µg/mL, with toxicity observed at levels greater than 2.0 µg/mL. Quantitation of both propafenone and the 5-hydroxypropanfenone can be simply and reliably performed by using a HPLC-UV method [6,7,38] following a liquid–liquid extraction with n-butyl chloride or methylene chloride. Chromatographic determination of propafenone concentration in human serum is shown Figure 10.6. Loxapine was use as the internal standard and a silica column was used for HPLC analysis using a mobile phase composition of methanol/0.1 M ammonium phosphate monobasic (pH: 2.25 (95:5 by vol). Elution of peaks was monitored at 254 nm (method and figures courtesy of Dr. McMillin GA, ARUP Laboratories, Salt Lake City, UT).

The chromatographic methods for analysis of propafenone show excellent within and between run imprecision, and remain linear over the clinically relevant ranges for both the parent compound (0.15–3.0 µg/ml) and the metabolite (0.075–1.5 µg/ml). No interference has been found from other commonly administered drugs, some of which may be quantitated simultaneously in some of these assays [6,7].

10.7   MEXILETINE

Mexiletine is another Class Ib antiarrhythmic drug that has electrophysiologic properties similar to lidocaine and is used to treat ventricular arrhythmias [2,4]. Compared to lidocaine, this drug has the advantage of a long half-life (7–14 hrs), with therapeutic concentrations in the range of 0.7–2.0 µg/mL. Mexiletine has a high degree of bioavailability, undergoes hepatic metabolism by the CYP2D6 cytochrome enzyme system, and is cleared from the circulation by the kidneys.

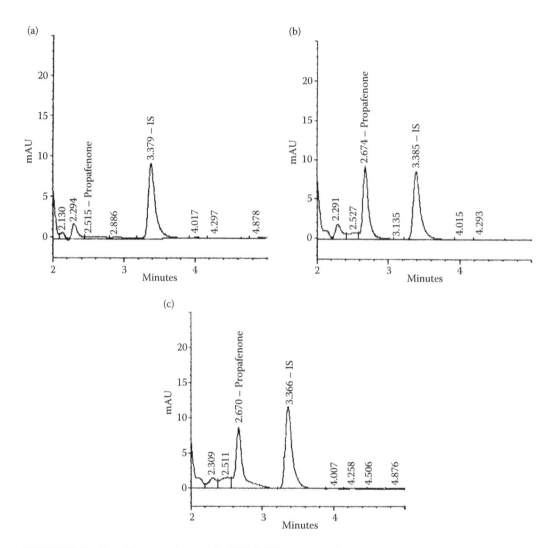

FIGURE 10.6 Propafenone as detected by HPLC-UV for a drug-free blank (a) internal standard, a calibrator containing 1.0 μg/ml of propafenone, (b) and a typical patient with a serum propafenone concentration of 0.8 μg/ml (c).

It is approximately 60% protein bound, with a large volume of distribution indicating that it is also highly tissue bound. Drug concentration is primarily monitored to assess optimal therapeutic levels as well as toxicity. This becomes particularly important in the clinical settings of myocardial infarction and uremia, where the half life of mexiletine will increase significantly with decreased renal clearance. Mexiletine toxicity is usually observed at blood concentrations above 2 μg/mL. The signs and symptoms of mexiletine toxicity include dizziness, tremor, ataxia, confusion, diplopia, dysarthria, hypotension, and hypotension.

Several chromatographic methods have been developed to measure mexiletine in serum and plasma. GC and GC/MS procedures have been widely employed [39–41] to assay mexiletine, including sensitive and precise applications that require derivatization (with 2,2,2-trochloroethyl chloroformate and perfluorooctanoyl chloride) prior to analysis; Figure 10.7 is a representative of a GC method (with nitrogen-phosphorus detector) used for the quantitative determination of mexiletine in human serum without derivatization. The internal standard used was N-propyl amphetamine. After

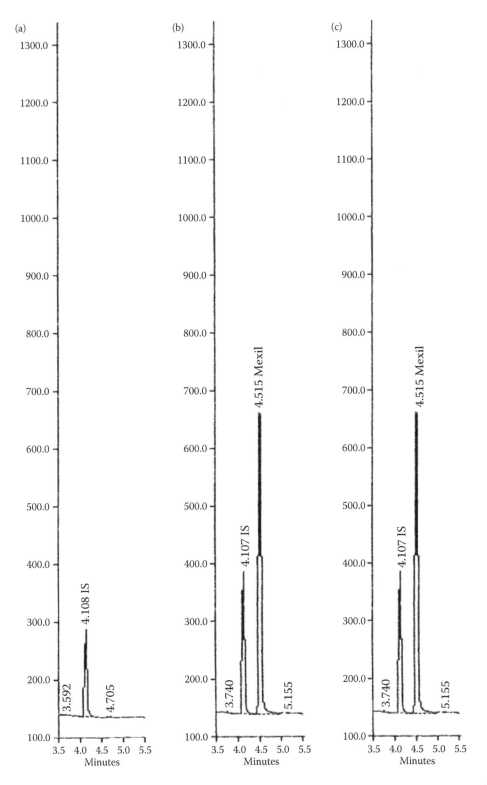

FIGURE 10.7 Mexiletine as detected by GC for a drug-free blank (a) internal standard, a calibrator containing 2.5 µg/ml of mexiletine, (b) and a typical patient containing 2.9 µg/ml in serum (c).

adding borate buffer and internal standard into the specimen, mexiletine along with the internal standard were extracted using ethyl acetate and analyzed by GC with flame ionization detector (method and figures courtesy of Dr. McMillin GA, ARUP Laboratories, Salt Lake City, UT).

HPLC methods using UV and fluorescence detection have also been described [7,42], for analysis of mexiletine using both liquid-liquid and solid phase extraction techniques. Several of these HPLC methods allow for simultaneous analyses of other class I antiarrhythmic drugs, such as lidocaine, procainamide, flecainide, tocainide and propafenone, and may offer added convenience to some laboratories [7]. However, both gas and liquid chromatography appear to be equally acceptable for therapeutic monitoring as they offer excellent within and between day imprecision (CV 2–5%), and adequately span the therapeutic and toxic ranges that are clinically relevant with mexiletine.

10.8 VERAPAMIL AND NIFEDIPINE

Verapamil is a voltage-dependent calcium channel blocker that is used extensively in the treatment of a wide range of cardiovascular disorders [2,4]. As a Class IV antiarrhythmic drug, these agents decrease impulse conduction through the AV node and has proven particularly effective in protecting the ventricles from supraventricular tachyarrhythmias (atrial arrhythmia, atrial flutter, and paroxysmal supraventricular tachycardia). Due to its additional vasodilatory actions on vascular smooth muscle, it is also used for treatment of stable and unstable angina pectoris, preservation of ischemic myocardium, hypertension, congestive heart failure, migraine headaches, and Raynaud's phenomenon.

Verapamil is metabolized by N-demethylation to its active metabolite, norverapamil, which is usually found in similar concentration to verapamil once steady state levels are reached in the circulation. This drug undergoes first pass metabolism in the liver and cleared from the circulation by the kidneys; with severe hepatic dysfunction, decreased clearance and increased bioavailability, volume of distribution, and half-life may be observed. Blood concentrations of verapamil (ranging from 50 to 250 ng/mL) appear to correlate well with cardiac response, and are most frequently monitored to ensure optimal dosing and levels are achieved to assess the potential toxic side effects. Frequent side effects of verapamil headaches, facial flushing, dizziness, swelling, increased urination, fatigue, nausea, ecchymosis, lightheadedness, and constipation; the most serious toxic complication is sinus bradycardia and heart block, particularly 3:2 Wenckebach-type atrioventricular block, at blood levels in excess of 450 ng/mL [4].

Both verapamil and its norverapamil can be reliably measured [7,43,44] in serum or plasma using GC and HPLC-UV techniques following simple liquid-liquid extraction. The imprecision with these methods are <5–7% and can detect parent drug and metabolite levels down to 5 ng/mL. More recently, an LC/MS method has been described [45] that allows for simultaneous determination of enantiomers of both verapamil and norverapamil using chiral column and a mobile phase composition of 85% aqueous ammonium acetate at pH 7.4 plus 15% acetonitrile. The electrospray tandem mass spectrometer was operated in selected reaction monitoring mode using deuterated internal standards. This rapid method allows for more sensitive limits of detection down to 0.1 ng/mL and 0.12 ng/mL for verapamil and its norverapamil, respectively.

Nifedipine is a dihydropyridine calcium channel blocker and primary uses are in the treatment of angina (particularly unstable angina) and hypertension [2]. A large number of other uses have also been found for this agent, such as Raynaud's phenomenon, premature labor, painful spasms of the esophagus in cancer, and a subset of patients with pulmonary arterial hypertension. Side effects of nifedipine are generally mild and reversible. Most side effects are expected consequences of the dilation of the arteries. The most common side effects of nifedipine include headache, dizziness, flushing, and edema (swelling) of the lower extremities. Less common side effects include dizziness, nausea and constipation. Therapeutic concentrations range between 25 and 100 ng/ml, with toxicity seen at levels above 100 ng/mL.

Both nifedipine and its metabolite dehydronifedipine can be measured by GC and HPLC methods, using either liquid-liquid or solid phase extraction with UV and fluorescence detection methods [46–48]. Analytical limits of detection are generally reported between 1–5 ng/mL, with upper limits of linearity of up to 300–500 ng/mL with HPLC methods; fluorescence detection offers a slight advantage improving sensitivity and enhanced precision particularly at lower concentration levels. LC/MS methods, using flow injection and electrospray ionization, have also been developed [49,50] that demonstrate acceptable accuracy, precision and sensitivity; these LC/MS further improves limits of quantitation (0.5 ng/mL), and appear to allows for improved resolution of parent and metabolites and may have additional value in assessing herbal drug interactions.

10.9 DETERMINATION OF MULTIPLE CARDIOTROPIC DRUGS IN A SINGLE ASSAY

There are several chromatographic methods reported in the literature that are capable of analyzing multiple cardiotropic drugs using one protocol. One advantage of these methods is that multiple sample preparation and chromatographic runs are not required for TDM purpose in patients receiving multiple drugs. For example, Bhamra et al. described a HPLC method for the measurement of mexiletine and flecainide in blood plasma or serum [51]. In another report the authors measured 12 antiarrhythmic drugs; amiodarone, aprindine, disopyramide, flecainide, lidocaine, lorcainide, mexiletine, procainamide, propafenone, sotalol, tocainide, and verapamil using HPLC after solid phase extraction of these drugs from plasma. As most antiarrhythmic drugs are basic in nature, good absorption on the extraction columns were obtained by alkalinization except for aprindine (at neutral pH) and amiodarone (pH 3.5). After washing with water, compounds were eluted with methanol except for amiodarone which as eluted with a mixture of acetonitrile and acetate buffer at pH 5 (80:20 by vol). The chromatographic separation was achieved using a hexyl column (5 μm particle size; 150 mm×4.6 mm internal diameter) and the mobile phase was consisted of mixtures of acetonitrile or methanol with phosphate or acetate buffer at different pH values [52]. More recently, Kristoffersen et al. described simultaneous determination of 6-beta blockers (atenolol, sotalol, metoprolol, bisoprolol, propranolol and carvedilol), 3-calcium channel antagonists (diltiazem, amlodipine, and verapamil), four angiotensin II-antagonists (losartan, irbesartan, valsartan, and telmisartan) and one antiarrhythmic drug (flecainide) in post mortem whole blood by automated solid phase extraction and liquid chromatography couple with MS. The authors used gradient elution with a mobile phase composition of 90% A (10 mM ammonium formate, pH adjusted to 3.1 using formic acid) and 10% B (acetonitrile) run over 10 min to 10% A and 90% B and this composition was maintained for additional 3 min. The detection of peaks and quantitation was achieved by electrospray ionization MS [53].

10.10 CONCLUSIONS

Therapeutic monitoring of many commonly prescribed cardioactive drugs has been facilitated by the development of rapid and easy to use immunoassay procedures. However, many other cardiotropic agents are currently used today that have broader therapeutic application and margins of safety. While these drug concentrations in human serum or plasma are generally not routinely monitored, there are certainly clinical situations (patient noncompliance, suboptimal clinical response, underlying renal or hepatic disease that alters clearance, bioavailability, or metabolism, and signs and symptoms of toxicity) where laboratory analysis may be warranted and will prove to be beneficial for patient management and safety. In general, HPLC methods have been developed for the quantitation of most commonly prescribed cardioactive drugs, and show acceptable analytical and clinical performance in most instances. GC, GC/MS, and, more recently, LC/MS applications have also been used, and perform roughly equivalently to the more commonly adopted HPLC techniques. While the latter LC/MS methods require more upfront equipment investment and operational support, they may yield lower specimen requirements, faster throughput, and enhanced sensitivity desired in many laboratories.

ACKNOWLEDGMENTS

Special thanks to Dr. Gwendolyn A. McMillin and Ms. JoEtta Juenke of ARUP Laboratories in Salt Lake City, UT, for generously providing sample chromatograms and sharing methodologies used within their laboratory.

REFERENCES

1. Roden DM. 2005. Antiarrhythmic drugs. In: *Goodman and Gilman's The Pharmacological Basis of Therapeutics*, 11th Edition (Brunton L, Lazo J, Parker K, eds). McGraw-Hill Professional, New York 899–932.
2. Darbar R, and Roden DM. 2006. The future of antiarrhythmic drugs. *Curr Opin Cardiol* 21:361–367.
3. Burton ME, Shaw LM, Schentag JJ, and Evans WE (eds). 2006. *Applied Pharmacokinetics and Pharmacodynamics, Principles of Therapeutic Drug Monitoring*, 4th Edition. Lippincott Williams & Wilkins, Baltimore, MD, 440–462.
4. Moyer TP. 2005. Therapeutic drug monitoring. In: *Tietz Textbook of Clinical Chemistry*. 4th Edition (Burtis CA, Ashwood ER, eds). WB Saunders Company, Philadelphia, PA, 1237–1285.
5. Dasgupta A, and Datta P. 2007. analytical techniques for measuring concentrations of therapeutic drugs in biological fluids. In: *Handbook of Drug Monitoring Methods* (Dasgupta A, ed.). Humana Press Inc., Totowa, NJ, 67–86.
6. Scott RE, Johnson P, and Moyer TP. 1988. Simultaneous analysis of five new class I anti-arrhythmic drugs. *Clin Chem* 34: 1251.
7. Verbesselt R, Tjandramaga TB, and de Schepper PJ. 1991. High performance liquid chromatographic determination of 12 antiarrhythmic drugs in plasma using solid phase extraction. *Ther Drug Monit* 13:157–165.
8. Siddoway LA. 2003. Amiodarone: guidelines for use and monitoring. *Am Family Physician* 68:2189–2196.
9. Heger JJ, Prystowsky EN, and Zipes DN. 1983. Relationships between amiodarone dosage, drug concentrations, and adverse side effects. *Am Hear J* 106:931–935.
10. Latini R, Tognoni G, and Kates RE. 1984. Clinical pharmacokinetics of amiodarone. *Clin Pharmacokinet* 9:136–156.
11. Riva E, Gerna M, and Latini R. 1982. Pharmacokinetics of amiodarone in man. *J Cardiovasc Pharmacol* 4:264–269.
12. Juenke JM, Brown PI, McMillin GA, and Urry FM. 2004. A rapid procedure for the monitoring of amiodarone and N-desethylamiodarone by HPLC-UV detection. *J Anal Toxicol* 28:63–66.
13. Pérez-Ruiz T, Martínez-Lozano C, and García-Martínez MD. 2008. Simultaneous determination of amiodarone and its metabolite desethylamiodarone by high-performance liquid chromatography with chemiluminescent detection. *Anal Chim Acta* 623:823–895.
14. Ou CN, Rogneurud CL, Doung LT, and Frawley VL. 1990. Liquid chromatographic determination of amiodarone and N-desmethylamiodarone in serum. *Clin Chem* 36:532–534.
15. Kollroser M, and Scober K. 2002. Determination of amiodarone and desethylamiodarone in human plasma by high-performance liquid chromatography–electrospray ionization tandem mass spectrometry with an ion trap detector. *J Chromatogr B Biomed Sci Appl* 766:219–226.
16. Waldo A, Camm A, deRuyter H, Friedman P, MacNeil D, Pauls J, Pitt B, Pratt C, Schwartz P, and Veltri E. 1996. Effect of d-sotalol on mortality in patients with left ventricular dysfunction after recent and remote myocardial infarction. *Lancet* 348:7–12.
17. Kárkkäinen S. 1984. High-performance liquid chromatographic determination of sotalol in biological fluids. *J Chromatogr* 336:313–319.
18. Boutagy J, and Shenfield, GM. 1991. Simplified procedure for the determination of sotalol in plasma by high-performance liquid chromatography. *J Chromatogr* 565:523–528.
19. Lefebvre MA, Girault J, Saux MC, and Fourtillan JB. 1980. Fluorimetric high-performance liquid chromatographic determination of sotalol in biological fluids. *J Pharmaceut Sci* 69:1216–1217.

20. Jatlow P, Bush W, and Hochster H. 1979. Improved liquid chromatographic determination of propranolol in plasma, with fluorescent detection. *Clin Chem* 25:777–779.

21. Gill J, Mehta D, Ward D and Camm A. 1992. Efficacy of flecainide, sotalol, and verapamil in the treatment of right ventricular tachycardia in patients without overt cardiac abnormality. *Br Heart J* 68 (4):392–397.

22. Echt D, Liebson P, Mitchell L, Peters R, Obias-Manno D, Barker A, Arensberg D, Baker A, Friedman L, and Greene H. 1991. Mortality and morbidity in patients receiving encainide, flecainide, or placebo. The Cardiac Arrhythmia Suppression Trial. *N Engl J Med* 324:781–788.

23. Winkelmann B, and Leinberger H. 1987. Life-threatening flecainide toxicity. A pharmacodynamic approach. *Ann Intern Med* 106:807–14.

24. Romain N, Giroud C, Michaud K, Augsburger M, et al. 1999. Fatal flecainide intoxication. *Forensic Sci Int* 106:115–123.

25. Fischer C, and Buhl K. 1992. Gas chromatography/mass spectrometry validation of high performance liquid chromatography analysis of flecainide enantiomers in serum. *Ther Drug Monit* 14:433–435.

26. Doki K, Homma M, Kuga K, Watanabe S, Yamaguchi I, and Kohda Y. 2004. Simultaneous determination of serum flecainide and its metabolites by using high performance liquid chromatography. *J Pharmaceut and Biomed Anal* 35:1307–1312.

27. Alessi-Severini S, Jamali F, Pasutto FM, Coutts RT, and Gulamhusein S. 2006. High-performance liquid chromatographic determination of the enantiomers of flecainide in human plasma and urine *J Pharmaceut Sci* 79:257–260.

28. Breindahl T. 2000. Therapeutic drug monitoring of flecainide in serum using high-performance liquid chromatography and electrospray mass spectrometry. *J Chromatogr B Biomed Sci Appl* 746:249–254.

29. Reece PA, and Stanley PE. 1980. High Performance liquid chromatography assay for tocainide in human plasma: comparison with gas-liquid chromatography. *J Chromatogr* 183:109–114.

30. vasBinder E, and Annesley T. 1991. Liquid chromatographic analysis of mexiletine in serum with alternate application to tocainide, procainamide and N-acetylprocainamide. *Biomed Chromatogr* 5:19–22.

31. Conings L, and Verbeke N. 1985. High performance liquid chromatographic analysis of tocainide in human plasma. *Pharmaceut Res* 2:311–313.

32. Brogden RN, and Todd PA. 1987. Encainide. A review of its pharmacological properties and therapeutic efficacy. *Drugs* 34:519–538.

33. Roden DM, and Woosley RL. 1988. Clinical pharmacokinetics of encainide. *Clin Pharmacokinet* 14:141–147.

34. Dresel PE. 1984. Effect of encainide and its two major metabolites on cardiac conduction. *J Pharmacol Exp Ther* 228:180–185.

35. Bartek MJ, Mayol RF, Boarman MP, Gammans RE, and Gallo DG. Analysis of encainide and metabolites in plasma and urine by high-performance liquid chromatography. *Ther Drug Monit* 10:446–452.

36. Dasgupta A, Rosenzweig IB, Turgeon J, and Raisys VA. 1990. Encainide and metabolites analysis in serum or plasma using a reversed-phase high performance liquid chromatographic technique. *J Chromatogr* 526:260–265.

37. Antman EM, Beamer AD, Cantillon C, et al. 1988. Long term oral propafenone therapy for suppression of refractory symptomatic atrial fibrillation and flutter. *J Am Coll Cardiol* 12:1005–1011.

38. Hoyer GL. 1988. A HPLC method for the quantitation of propafenone and 5-hydroxy propafenone. *Chromatographia* 25:1034–1038.

39. Minnigh MB, Alvin JD, and Zemaitis MA. 1994. Determination of plasma mexiletine levels with gas chromatography-mass spectrometry and selected ion monitoring. *J Chromatogr B Biomed Sci Appl* 662:118–122.

40. Dasgupta A, Appenzeller P, and Moore J. 1998. Gas chromatography-electron ionization mass spectrometric analysis of serum mexiletine concentration after derivatization with 2,2,2-trochloroethyl chloroformate: a novel derivative. *Ther Drug Monit* 20:313–318.

41. Dasgupta A, and Yousef O. 1998. Gas chromatographic-mass spectrometric determination of serum mexiletine concentration after derivatization with perfluorooctanoyl chloride, a new derivative. *J Chromatogr B Biomed Sci Appl* 705:282–288.

42. Mastropaolo W, Holmes DR, Osborn MJ, et al. 1984. Improved liquid chromatographic determination of mexiletine, an antiarrhythmic drug in plasma. *Clin Chem* 30:319–322.

43. Todd GD, Bourne DWA, and McAllister GA. 1980. Measurement of verapamil concentrations in plasma by gas chromatography and high performance liquid chromatography. *Ther Drug Monit* 2:411–416.

44. Harapat SR, and Kates RE. 1980. High performance liquid chromatographic analysis of verapamil: II. Simultaneous quantitation of verapamil and its active metabolite norverapamil. *J Chromatogr* 181:484–489.

45. Hedeland M, Fredriksson E, Lennernäs H, and Bondesson U. 2004. Simultaneous quantitation of the enantiomers of verapamil and N-demethylated metabolites in human plasma using liquid chromatography-tandem mass spectrometry. *J Chromatogr B Biomed Sci Appl* 804:303–311.

46. Mascher H, and Vergin H. 1988. HPLC-determination of nifedipine in plasma on normal phase. *Chromatographia* 25:919–922.

47. Zendelovska D, Simeska S, Sibinovska O, et al. 2006. Development of an HPLC method for the determination of nifedipine in human plasma by solid-phase extraction. *J Chromatogr B Biomed Sci Appl* 839:85–88.

48. Jankowski A, and Lamparczyk H. 1994. Evaluation of chromatographic methods for the determination of nifedipine in human serum. *J Chromatogr A* 668:469–473.

49. Dankers J, van den Elshout J, Ahr G, Brendel E, and van der Heiden C. 1998. Analytical determination of nifedipine in human plasma by flow-injection tandem mass spectrometry. *J Chromatogr B Biomed Sci Appl* 710:115–120.

50. Wang XD, Li JL, Lu Y, Chen X, Huang M, Chowbay B, and Zhou SFJ. 2007. Rapid and simultaneous determination of nifedipine and dehydronifedipine in human plasma by liquid chromatography-tandem mass spectrometry: application to a clinical herb-drug interaction study. *J Chromatogr B Biomed Sci Appl* 852:534–544.

51. Bhamra RK, Flanagan RJ, and Holt DW. 1984. High performance liquid chromatographic method for the measurement of mexiletine and flecainide in blood plasma or serum. *J Chromatogr* 307:439–444.

52. Verbesselt R, Tjandramaga TB, and De Schepper PJ. 1991. J+High performance liquid chromatographic determination of 12 antiarrhythmic drugs in plasma using solid phase column extraction. *Ther Drug Monit* 13:157–165.

53. Kristoffersen L, Oiestad EL, Opdal MS, Krogh M et al. 2007. Simultaneous determination of 6-beta blockers, 3-calcium channel antagonists, 4 angiotensin II-antagonists and 1 antiarrhythmic drug in post mortem whole blood by automated solid phase extraction and liquid chromatography mass spectrometry. Method development and robustness testing by experimental design. *J Chromatogr B Analyt Technol Biomed Life Sci* 850:147–160.

11 Immunoassays for Tricyclic Antidepressants: Unsuitable for Therapeutic Drug Monitoring?

Matthew D. Krasowski
University of Iowa Hospitals and Clinics

Mohamed G. Siam
University of Pittsburgh Medical Center Presbyterian-Shadyside
and Zagazig University

Sean Ekins
Collaborations in Chemistry

CONTENTS

11.1   INTRODUCTION

Tricyclic antidepressants (TCAs) are a class of drugs first discovered in the 1950s that have traditionally been used for the treatment of major depression [1] (see Figure 11.1 for examples of their chemical structures). TCAs were the dominant antidepressants in the United States for several decades extending into the late 1980s. Other important therapeutic uses of TCAs include treatment of chronic pain (especially amitriptyline), enuresis (imipramine), and obsessive-compulsive disorder (clomipramine) [1,2]. However, therapeutic use of TCAs for treatment of major depression has decreased significantly with the introduction of other newer classes of antidepressants such as selective serotonin reuptake inhibitors (SSRIs) and serotonin-norepinephrine reuptake inhibitors (SNRIs) [1].

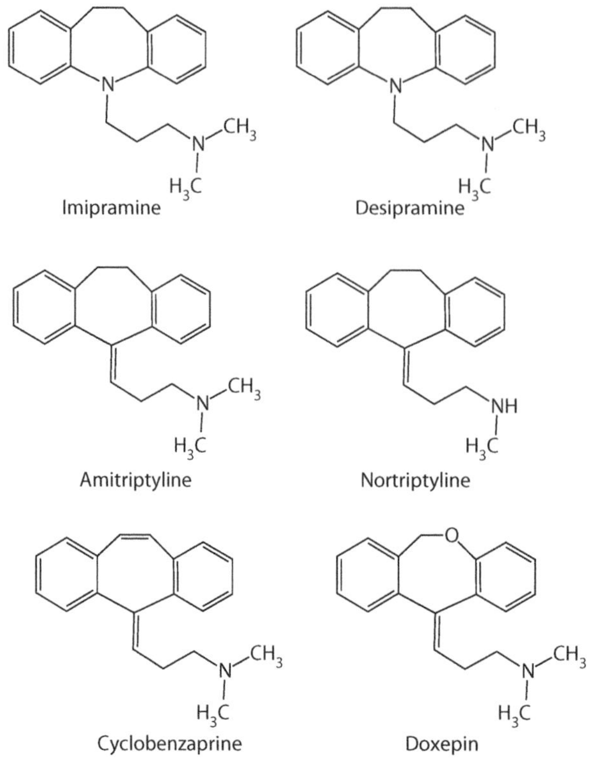

FIGURE 11.1 Structures of clinically used tricyclic antidepressants and the related tricyclic drug cycloben-zaprine (which differs from amitriptyline by one double bond).

11.2 THERAPEUTIC USES AND TOXICITY OF TRICYCLIC ANTIDEPRESSANTS (TCAs)

While the mechanism of action of TCAs for treatment of major depression is incompletely under-stood, much of the therapeutic action is attributed to inhibition of norepinephrine and serotonin transporters ("reuptake inhibition") [3]. This action serves to increase the amount of serotonin and norepinephrine in the synapses of neurons that release these neurotransmitters. Some of the TCAs also affect other molecular targets at clinically relevant concentrations. Other actions of TCAs include inhibition of muscarinic acetylcholine receptors ("anticholinergic effect") and α-adrenergic receptors ("antiadrenergic effect").

While the therapeutic effectiveness of TCAs in treating major depression is well-established, the occurrence of unpleasant side effects due to anticholinergic (e.g., dry mouth, sedation, blurred vision, or light sensitivity from mydriasis, urinary retention) or antiadrenergic (e.g., orthostatic hypotension) effects limits patient acceptance. In TCA overdose, particularly with amitriptyline, the anticholinergic symptoms can resemble severe atropine poisoning with dilated pupils, flushed skin, hyperthermia, tachycardia, and cardiac arrhythmias. Most of the newer antidepressants such as SSRIs and SNRIs are much safer in overdose situation than the TCAs and generally are better toler-ated than TCAs [1]. Overdose of several weeks supply of TCAs can lead to life-threatening toxicity, with cardiac arrhythmias being especially difficult to manage clinically. Even as prescriptions of TCAs have declined in the United States, fatalities due to TCA overdose, as tracked by the Drug

Abuse Warning Network (http://dawninfo.samhsa.gov/; DAWN), continue to be reported [4]. TCAs therefore, represent a class of compounds that are of interest for laboratory detection.

11.3   THERAPEUTIC DRUG MONITORING OF TRICYCLIC ANTIDEPRESSANTS (TCAs)

Therapeutic drug monitoring (TDM) of TCAs has two main possible advantages [5–7]. Firstly, for some TCAs, most notably nortriptyline, therapeutic serum concentrations have been well-defined empirically. Secondly, possible benefits of TDM are that TCA serum concentration may be affected by genetic variation of enzymes that metabolize TCAs (e.g., cytochrome P450s, CYPs) or by concomitant medications, herbal products, or foods that alter TCA metabolism, or by interference with transporter-mediated efflux. For example, amitriptyline is metabolized to nortriptyline by CYP2C9, an enzyme expressed in the liver that shows significant variation in expression due to genetic polymorphisms. It is widely known that CYP2C9 poor metabolizers convert amitriptyline slowly, potentially leading to excessively high amitriptyline concentrations and the associated adverse consequences [8,9]. Nortriptyline is converted to 10-hydroxynortriptyline by CYP2D6, an enzyme that also shows significant genetic variation. Like CYP2C9, CYP2D6 poor metabolizers of nortriptyline exist and are prone to toxic side effects when administered standard doses of nortriptyline [8,9].

The gene encoding CYP2D6 can be duplicated or even multiplied, leading to more than two functional copies of the gene and high CYP2D6 activity relative to the average population. These CYP2D6 ultra-rapid metabolizers have been observed to metabolize nortriptyline much more rapidly than the average population. In the most extreme case reported, a subject was found to have 13 functional copies of the gene for CYP2D6 and a very short half-life of nortriptyline [10]. Overall, TDM of TCAs like those described above can help guide dosing to maintain effective yet safe serum concentrations.

However, TDM of TCAs is complicated by multiple factors. First, clinically used TCAs often have multiple metabolites, some of which may also have significant antidepressant activity [5,6]. For example, amitriptyline is converted to nortriptyline and imipramine is converted to desipramine. Immunoassay measurement of total TCA concentrations in serum does not determine how much parent drug versus metabolite(s) is present. Second, some TCAs do not have well-defined concentration-efficacy relationships and therefore clinically useful therapeutic ranges are not available at present. Third, as will be discussed in detail below, measurement of TCA serum concentrations by immunoassay is prone to significant interference from structurally related compounds to TCAs. Concentrations of individual TCAs and their metabolites in serum/plasma can be more specifically determined by a variety of chromatographic techniques including gas chromatography and high-performance liquid chromatography, either alone or in combination with mass spectrometry.

Immunoassays for TCAs were first developed as toxicology screening tools starting with radioimmunoassays in the 1970s and 1980s [11–21]. Homogenous immunoassays for TCAs in serum were later developed [22–28], and multiple commercial assays are still on the market in the United States. Homogeneous immunoassay techniques for measuring TCA serum concentrations include the fluorescence polarization immunoassay (FPIA, Abbott Diagnostics) and enzyme-multiplied immunoassay techniques (EMIT, Dade–Behring—now Siemens Diagnostics; Microgenics). Immunoassays for TCAs have been widely applied in qualitative screening for the presence of TCAs in common "drug of abuse" and "toxicology" panels [4,29]. In these applications, the assays are often used to generate a qualitative result, e.g., presence or absence of total TCAs and metabolites that produce a reaction result equivalent or greater than that produced by desipramine at a concentration of 1000 ng/mL. Qualitative assays for TCAs have also been developed for urine [30]. One commercial example of this is the Biosite Triage system.

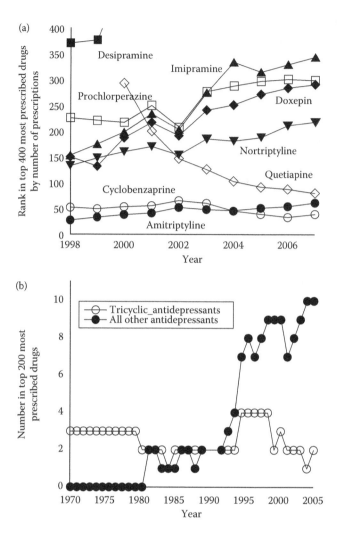

FIGURE 11.2 Trends in prescription frequency of tricyclic antidepressants (TCAs), drugs that cross-react with serum tricyclic immunoassays, and other (nontricyclic) antidepressants in the United States. (a) Rank of five TCAs, cyclobenzaprine, and quetiapine in terms of number of prescriptions written in the United States for 1998–2007. Prescriptions of TCAs have steadily declined over the last ten years, with desipramine no longer ranked in the top 400 most prescribed medications. Two compounds shown to cross-react with serum TCA immunoassays, cyclobenzaprine and quetiapine, are prescribed much more frequently than all TCAs except amitriptyline. (b) Number of different TCAs in the top 200 most prescribed medications in the United States in the time period from 1970 to 2007. Currently only one TCA (amitriptyline) ranks in the top 200 most prescribed drugs, while 10 non-tricyclic antidepressants are in the top 200 most prescribed medications for 2007. See text for references for which most prescribed data were derived.

11.4   TRENDS IN PRESCRIPTIONS FOR TRICYCLIC ANTIDEPRESSANTS (TCAs)

In the United States from 1970 through 2005 [31–66], between two to four TCAs have been among the top 200 most prescribed medications in the United States (Figure 11.2). The last 10 years, however, have seen marked steady declines in prescriptions for TCAs. The exception to this trend is amitriptyline, which continues to be among the top 60 most prescribed medications (Figure 11.2a), likely due in large part to its effectiveness as an adjunct medication in treating chronic pain [2].

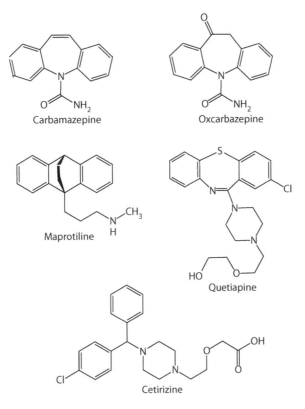

FIGURE 11.3   Structures of drugs shown to cross-react with serum tricyclic antidepressant immunoassays.

In contrast to TCAs, prescriptions of newer (nontricyclic) antidepressants have been increasing steadily, with ten of these medications now among the top 200 most prescribed drugs in the United States (Figure 11.2b).

11.5   COMPOUNDS WITH STRUCTURAL SIMILARITY TO TRICYCLIC ANTIDEPRESSANTS (TCAs)

TCAs share structural similarity with a number of other medications, notably other drugs that have three or four predominantly aromatic ring structures. Cyclobenzaprine is used as a skeletal muscle relaxant but is very closely related to TCAs, differing by only one double bond from amitriptyline (Figure 11.1). It is not well understood how such a subtle molecular change results in a markedly different clinical profile from amitriptyline and other TCAs [67].

Phenothiazine antipsychotics (e.g., chlorpromazine, fluphenazine, prochlorperazine, thioridazine), carbamazepine, and oxcarbazepine are examples of three-ringed molecules that also share structural similarity to TCAs (Figure 11.3). Phenothiazines were the dominant antipsychotics until the mid-1980s when "atypical" antipsychotics started to gain clinical popularity [68]. Currently, only a single phenothiazine (promethazine, often used to treat nausea and vomiting) is in the top 200 most prescribed medication in the United States [44]. Carbamazepine and oxcarbazepine are both widely used drugs to treat epilepsy [69]. Additionally, the class of tetracyclic (four-ringed) antidepressants include amoxapine, maprotiline, mianserin, and mirtazapine [1]. Some of these molecules demonstrate significant cross-reactivity with TCA immunoassays (Table 11.1).

TABLE 11.1

Immunoassay Cross-Reactivity and Molecular similarity of Tricyclic Antidepressants and Structurally Related Compounds

Drug or Metabolite	Class	Cross-reactivity in TCA Immunoassays[a]	MDL similarity to Desipramine[b]	Rank in Top Prescriptions 2007[c]
Amitriptyline	TCA	Strong	0.600	62
Clomipramine	TCA	Strong	0.750	Not ranked
Desipramine	TCA	Strong	1.000	Not ranked
Doxepin	TCA	Strong	0.529	292
Imipramine	TCA	Strong	0.837	345
Nortriptyline	TCA	Strong	0.628	219
Trimipramine	TCA	Strong	0.750	Not ranked
Cyclobenzaprine	TCA-like	Strong	0.565	40
Amoxapine	Tetracyclic antidepressant	None	0.508	Not ranked
Maprotiline	Tetracyclic antidepressant	Strong	0.659	Not ranked
Mianserin	Tetracyclic antidepressant	Strong	0.696	Not ranked
Mirtazapine	Tetracyclic antidepressant	None	0.653	147
Carbamazepine	Anticonvulsant	Weak	0.460	293
Carbamazepine epoxide	Anticonvulsant metabolite	Weak	0.397	Not applicable
Oxcarbazepine	Anticonvulsant	Weak	0.418	270
Prochlorperazine	Phenothiazine antipsychotic	Strong	0.630	303
Quetiapine	Atypical antipsychotic	Weak	0.485	81
Cetirizine	Antihistamine	Weak	0.429	20
Hydroxyzine	Antihistamine	Weak	0.467	98

[a] Based on review of package inserts for tricyclic antidepressant screening immunoassays from Abbott Diagnostics, Microgenics, and Siemens (formerly Dade–Behring) and by literature review (see text). Strong reactivity is when reactivity equivalent to 1000 ng/mL target compound (either desipramine or imipramine) is achieved by less than 10,000 ng/mL of the cross-reactive compound. Weak reactivity is when reactivity equivalent to 1000 ng/mL target compound is only seen at concentrations greater than 10,000 ng/mL but less than 100,000 ng/mL.

[b] Tanimoto coefficient (between 0.000 and 1.000) in comparison between compound and desipramine. Comparison of desipramine to itself by definition yields a coefficient of 1.000 (maximally similar).

[c] Rank in top prescriptions based on data in *Red Book, Montvale, NJ:* Thompson Healthcare, 2008.

11.6   CROSS-REACTIVITY OF IMMUNOASSAYS FOR TRICYCLIC ANTIDEPRESSANTS (TCAs) WITH OTHER DRUGS

Immunoassays for TCAs in serum have generally used antibodies that were raised with imipramine or desipramine as the hapten [22,26,29]. Such immunoassays typically show significant cross-reactivity with a variety of TCAs and their metabolites. However, these assays also cross-react with other structurally similar molecules. As mentioned above, cyclobenzaprine, while not generally classified as a TCA, differs only slightly from amitriptyline and cross-reacts well with marketed immunoassays [70] (Table 11.1). There are also multiple reports of positive TCA screening tests in patients with high plasma concentrations of carbamazepine and/or carbamazepine 10, 11-epoxide, as may occur during intentional or inadvertent overdose [71–75]. More recently, cross-reactivity of TCA assays with oxcarbazepine, an anticonvulsant very similar to carbamazepine has also been documented [75]. Phenothiazines, which were the dominant antipsychotics several decades ago, can also cross-react with TCA immunoassays [76–78]. This interference is likely to decline in observed frequency due to the steadily decreasing clinical use of phenothiazines [44].

The widely prescribed antihistamines cetirizine and hydroxyzine have also been shown to cross-react with TCA immunoassays at high plasma concentrations [79]. Cetirizine and hydroxyzine share less obvious structural similarity to TCAs than phenothiazine, carbamazepine, or oxcarbazepine (Figure 11.3). Lastly, several reports have shown cross-reactivity of TCA immunoassays with quetiapine, a relatively new atypical antipsychotic that contains a tricyclic ring feature in its chemical structure (Figure 11.3) [80–82]. Prescriptions for quetiapine in the United States have increased steadily for the past five years to the point that quetiapine is prescribed nearly as often as amitriptyline [44]. There are also reports of intentional abuse of quetiapine [83–85], sometimes in combination with illicit drugs such as cocaine [86]. This means that patients having high concentrations of quetiapine in their serum will likely be seen in increasing numbers in emergency departments or drug abuse clinics where TCA immunoassays may be performed as part of toxicology or drugs of abuse screening panels.

11.7　COMPUTATIONAL METHODS TO RATIONALIZE TRICYCLIC ANTIDEPRESSANT (TCA) IMMUNOASSAY CROSS-REACTIVITY

In order to help rationalize cross-reactivity of TCA immunoassays with drugs other than TCAs, we have utilized molecular descriptor-based chemoinformatics approaches that can rank how similar compounds are to the target compound of the immunoassays (e.g., either desipramine or imipramine). Molecular similarity analyses determine the similarity between molecules independent of any in vitro or other data [87–89]. Variables that can be included in similarity calculations are extensive and include those related to molecular structure, electrostatic potential, electron density, and basic physicochemical properties. For example, at the level of structure, two molecules may be similar if they possess the same functional group(s) or a common substructure. The key piece of a similarity searching system is the method used to measure structural similarity [90–93]. The most common approaches use two-dimensional fragment bit strings compared using the Tanimoto coefficient. The Tanimoto coefficient ranges from 0 to 1, with 0 being maximally dissimilar and 1 being maximally similar. Other similarity coefficients have been tested but the Tanimoto method is the most widely used and accepted and generally provides reliable results. To date, such similarity analysis methods have been used widely in the pharmaceutical industry to screen for drug-like molecules [87,88,94,95] and counter-screen for compounds associated with false positives in high-throughput assays [96].

We have found one particular similarity measure (MDL public keys) to be particularly useful in defining similarity of molecules to the target compound of an immunoassay. For example, in comparison to desipramine, other TCAs (not surprisingly) rank high in similarity (Tanimoto coefficient ~0.600 and above; Table 11.1). Phenothiazines such as prochlorperazine and thioridazine also rank high (Tanimoto coefficient ~0.6), correlating with their documented ability to cross-react with TCA immunoassays at therapeutic concentrations [76–78]. Other compounds that can cross-react with TCA immunoassays including carbamazepine, oxcarbazepine, cetirizine, hydroxyzine, and quetiapine have lower similarity (Tanimoto coefficient ~0.400–0.450) to desipramine than TCAs or phenothiazines but higher similarity than other prescribed or over-the-counter medications such as ibuprofen (Tanimoto coefficient 0.129, Figure 11.4; Table 11.1). Carbamazepine, oxcarbazepine, cetirizine, hydroxyzine, and quetiapine generally cross-react only at high serum concentrations seen during overdose, suggesting that interactions with these compounds with the assay antibodies are not optimal due to structural and chemical differences from the target TCA antigen (i.e., either desipramine or imipramine). Our analysis of ~800 other drugs and drug metabolites show that the majority of drugs marketed in the United States (prescription or over-the-counter) have low similarity to desipramine or imipramine (Tanimoto coefficient less than 0.350; for example, see ibuprofen in Figure 11.4) and would be unlikely to cause positive reactions even at very high concentrations.

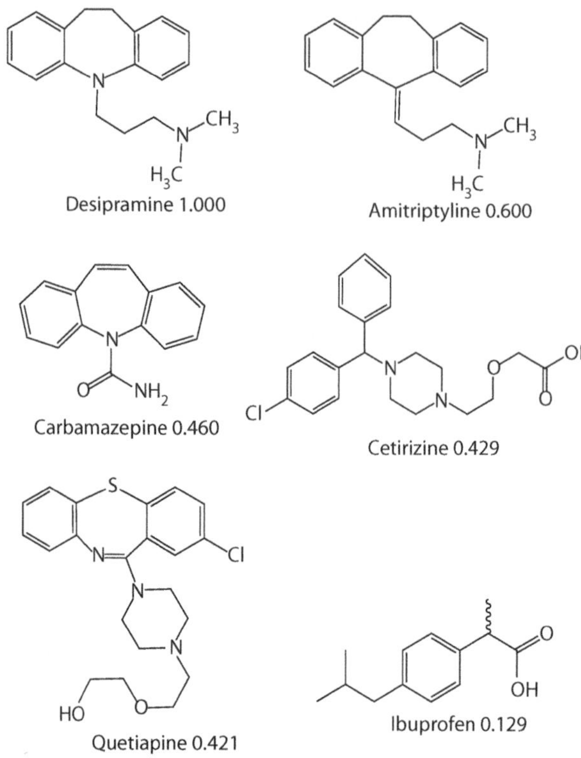

FIGURE 11.4 Similarity of five compounds to the target compound desipramine (target of some tricyclic antidepressants screening assays) calculated by MDL public keys using the Tanimoto similarity measure. Of the five compounds, amitriptyline is most similar (Tanimoto measure = 0.600) while ibuprofen is the least similar (Tanimoto measures = 0.146). Carbamazepine, cetirizine, and quetiapine have higher similarity to desipramine relative to most prescription drugs on the market in the United States but lower similarity to desipramine than TCAs such as amitriptyline.

We hope to use these chemoinformatics approaches to identify previously undocumented cross-reactive compounds for immunoassays for TCA and other compounds. The use of *in silico* approaches may be particularly useful for drug metabolites that might otherwise never be studied due to lack of available reference standards to test.

11.8 CONCLUSIONS

Immunoassays used to detect total TCAs in serum are typically used for qualitative screening in toxicology or drug of abuse testing panels. The broad specificity of these immunoassays allows for detection of multiple TCAs and metabolites, but also results in significant cross-reactivity with other medications that may be structurally similar but belong to different therapeutic classes. It is our opinion therefore that the apparent lack of specificity of TCA immunoassays currently limits their application to TDM. Consequently, more specific assays such as gas chromatography or high-performance liquid chromatography (discussed in Chapter 11) are preferred for TDM of TCA. Our findings using molecular similarity analysis approaches to predict immunoassay cross-reactivity are broadly applicable to other immunoassays and are currently ongoing.

REFERENCES

1. Rang, H.P., M.M. Dale, J.M. Ritter, and P.K. Moore. 2003. Drugs used in affective disorders. In *Pharmacology*. Edinburgh, UK: Churchill Livingstone, 535–549.
2. Jann, M.W., and J.H. Slade. 2007. Antidepressant agents for the treatment of chronic pain and depression. *Pharmacotherapy* 27 (11):1571–1587.
3. Frazer, A. 1997. Pharmacology of antidepressants. *J Clin Psychopharmacol* 17 (Suppl 1):2S–18S.
4. Wu, A.H.B., C. McKay, L.A. Broussard, R.S. Hoffman, T.C. Kwong, T.P. Moyer, E.M. Otten, S.L. Welch, and P. Wax. 2003. National Academy of Clinical Biochemistry laboratory medicine practice guidelines: recommendations for the use of laboratory tests to support poisoned patients who present to the emergency department. *Clin Chem* 49 (3):357–379.
5. Linder, M.W., and P.E. Keck. 1998. Standards of laboratory practice: antidepressant drug monitoring. National Academy of Clinical Biochemistry. *Clin Chem* 44 (5):1073–1084.
6. Preskorn, S.H., R.C. Dorey, and G.S. Jerkovich. 1988. Therapeutic drug monitoring of tricyclic antidepressants. *Clin Chem* 34 (5):822–828.
7. Van Brunt, N. 1983. The clinical utility of tricyclic antidepressant blood levels: a review of the literature. *Ther Drug Monit* 5 (1):1–10.
8. Kirchheiner, J., K. Brøsen, M.L. Dahl, L.F. Gram, S. Kasper, I. Roots, F. Sjöqvist, E. Spina, and J. Brockmöller. 2001. CYP2D6 and CYP2C19 genotype-based dose recommendations for antidepressants: a first step towards subpopulation-specific dosages. *Acta Psychiatr Scand* 104 (3):173–192.
9. Steimer, W., B. Müller, S. Leucht, and W. Kissling. 2001. Pharmacogenetics: a new diagnostic tool in the management of antidepressive drug therapy. *Clin Chim Acta* 308 (1–2):33–41.
10. Dalén, P., M.L. Dahl, M.L. Bernal Ruiz, J. Nordin, and L. Bertilsson. 1998. 10-Hydroxylation of nortriptyline in white persons with 0, 1, 2, 3, and 13 functional CYP2D6 genes. *Clin Pharmacol Ther* 63 (4):444–452.
11. Brunswick, D.J. 1979. Radioimmunoassay of tricyclic antidepressants. *Psychopharmacol Bull* 15 (1):56.
12. Brunswick, D.J., B. Needelman, and J. Mendels. 1979. Specific radioimmunoassay of amitriptyline and nortriptyline. *Br J Clin Pharmacol* 7 (4):343–348.
13. Hubbard, J.W., K.K. Midha, J.K. Cooper, and C. Charette. 1978. Radioimmunoassay for psychotropic drugs II: synthesis and properties of haptens for tricyclics antidepressants. *J Pharm Sci* 67 (11):1571–1578.
14. Lucek, R., and R. Dixon. 1977. Specific radioimmunoassay for amitriptyline and nortriptyline in plasma. *Res Commun Chem Pathol Pharmacol* 18 (1):125–136.
15. Maguire, K.P., G.D. Burrows, T.R. Norman, and B.A. Scoggins. 1978. A radioimmunoassay for nortriptyline (and other tricyclic antidepressants) in plasma. *Clin Chem* 24 (4):549–554.
16. Mason, P.A., K.M. Rowan, B. Law, A.C. Moffat, E.A. Kilner, and L.A. King. 1984. Development and evaluation of a radioimmunoassay for the analysis of body fluids to determine the presence of tricyclic antidepressant drugs. *Analyst* 109 (9):1213–1215.
17. Mould, G.P., G. Stout, G.W. Aherne, and V. Marks. 1978. Radioimmunoassay of amitriptyline and nortriptyline in body fluids. *Ann Clin Biochem* 15 (4):221–225.
18. Read, G.F., and D. Riad-Fahmy. 1978. Determination of tricyclic antidepressant, clomipramine (Anafranil), in plasma by a specific radioimmunoassay procedure. *Clin Chem* 24 (1):36–40.
19. Robinson, K., and R.N. Smith. 1985. Radioimmunoassay of tricyclic antidepressants and some phenothiazine drugs in forensic toxicology. *J Immunoassay* 6 (1–2):11–22.
20. Virtanen, R. 1980. Radioimmunoassay for tricyclic antidepressants. *Scand J Clin Lab Invest* 40 (2):191–197.
21. Virtanen, R., J.S. Salonen, M. Scheinin, E. Iisalo, and V. Mattila. 1980. Radioimmunoassay for doxepin and desmethyldoxepin. *Acta Pharmacol Toxicol (Copenh)* 47 (4):274–278.
22. Adamczyk, M., J. Fishpaugh, C. Harrington, D. Johnson, and A. Vanderbilt. 1993. Immunoassay reagents for psychoactive drugs. II. The method for the development of antibodies specific to imipramine and desipramine. *J Immunol Methods* 163 (2):187–197.
23. Cheret, P., and P. Brossier. 1986. Metalloimmunoassay of tricyclic antidepressant drugs: production and characterization of antiserum. *Res Commun Chem Pathol Pharmacol* 54 (2):237–253.
24. Dorey, R.C., S.H. Preskorn, and P.K. Widener. 1988. Results compared for tricyclic antidepressants as assayed by liquid chromatography and enzyme immunoassay. *Clin Chem* 34 (11):2348–2351.

25. Ernst, R., L. Williams, M. Dalbey, C. Collins, and S. Pankey. 1987. Homogeneous enzyme immunoassay (EMIT) protocol for monitoring tricyclic antidepressants on the COBAS-BIO centrifugal analyzer. *Ther Drug Monit* 9 (1):85–90.

26. Pankey, S., C. Collins, A. Jaklitsch, A. Izutsu, M. Hu, M. Pirio, and P. Singh. 1986. Quantitative homogeneous enzyme immunoassays for amitriptyline, nortriptyline, imipramine, and desipramine. *Clin Chem* 32 (5):768–772.

27. Poklis, A., D. Soghoian, C.R. Crooks, and J.J. Saady. 1990. Evaluation of the Abbott ADx total serum tricyclic immunoassay. *J Toxicol Clin Toxicol* 28 (2):235–248.

28. Rao, M.L., U. Staberock, P. Baumann, C. Hiemke, A. Deister, C. Cuendet, M. Amey, S. Härtter, and M. Kraemer. 1994. Monitoring tricyclic antidepressant concentrations in serum by fluorescence polarization immunoassay compared with gas chromatography and HPLC. *Clin Chem* 40 (6):929–933.

29. Schroeder, T.J., J.J. Tasset, E.J. Otten, and J.R. Hedges. 1986. Evaluation of Syva EMIT toxicology serum tricyclic antidepressant assay. *J Anal Toxicol* 10 (6):221–224.

30. Poklis, A., L.E. Edinboro, J.S. Lee, and C.R. Crooks. 1997. Evaluation of a colloidal metal immunoassay device for the detection of tricyclic antidepressants in urine. *J Toxicol Clin Toxicol* 35 (1):77–82.

31. *Red Book*. 1995. Montvale, NJ: Medical Economics Company, Inc.

32. *Red Book*. 1996. Montvale, NJ: Medical Economics Company, Inc.

33. *Red Book*. 1997. Montvale, NJ: Medical Economics Company, Inc.

34. *Red Book*. 1998. Montvale, NJ: Medical Economics Company, Inc.

35. *Red Book*. 1999. Montvale, NJ: Medical Economics Company, Inc.

36. *Red Book*. 2000. Montvale, NJ: Medical Economics Company, Inc.

37. *Red Book*. 2001. Montvale, NJ: Medical Economics Company, Inc.

38. *Red Book*. 2002. Montvale, NJ: Thompson Medical Economics, Inc.

39. *Red Book*. 2003. Montvale, NJ: Thompson PDR.

40. *Red Book*. 2004. Montvale, NJ: Thompson PDR.

41. *Red Book*. 2005. Montvale, NJ: Thomson PDR.

42. *Red Book*. 2006. Montvale, NJ: Thompson PDR.

43. *Red Book*. 2007. Montvale, NJ: Thompson PDR.

44. *Red Book*. 2008. Montvale, NJ: Thomson Healthcare.

45. Anonymous. 1971. Top 200 drugs in 1970. *Pharm Times* 37 (4):29–33.

46. Anonymous. 1972. Top 200 drugs in 1971. *Pharm Times* 38 (4):31–35.

47. Anonymous. 1974. Top 200 drugs...new generic Rxs continue to rise in 1973, accounting for 10.6% of new prescriptions. *Pharm Times* 40 (4):35–41.

48. Anonymous. 1975. Top 200 drugs...1973 vs. 1974: 4.3% decline refills spawns 0.9% dip in overall Rx volume. *Pharm Times* 41 (4):39–46.

49. Anonymous. 1976. Top 200 drugs...1974 vs. 1975: generics rise by 3.2% despite 1% dip in total Rx volume. *Pharm Times* 42 (4):37–44.

50. Anonymous. 1979. The top 200 drugs. *Pharm Times* 45 (4):29–37.

51. Anonymous. 1982. The top 200 prescription drugs of 1981. *Am Drug* 185 (2):20,24–25.

52. Anonymous. 1983. The top 200 prescription drugs of 1982. *Am Drug* 187 (2):13,16,19.

53. Anonymous. 1984. The top 200 prescription drugs of 1983. *Am Drug* 189 (2):42,47–48,50.

54. Anonymous. 1984. 1983 National Prescription Audit: top 200 drugs products account for 61.8% of all Rxs. *Pharm Times* 50 (4):27–35.

55. Anonymous. 1985. The top 200 prescription drugs of 1984. *Am Drug* 191 (2):30,32,36,40.

56. Anonymous. 1986. The top 200 prescription drugs of 1985. *Am Drug* 193 (2):18,21,27,30.

57. Anonymous. 1986. The top 200 drugs of 1985. *Pharm Times* 52 (4):25–33.

58. Anonymous. 1987. The top 200 Rx drugs of 1986. *Am Drug* 195 (2):19,23,26,28,32.

59. Anonymous. 1989. The top 200 Rx drugs of 1988. *Am Drug* 199 (2):38,40,45–46,48,51–52.

60. Anonymous. 1989. Top 200 drugs of 1989. *Am Drug* 201 (2):26,28,30,32,34,36,38–39.

61. Anonymous. 1991. The top Rx drugs of 1990. *Am Drug* 203 (2):56,58,60,62,65–66,68.

62. Anonymous. 1996. Top 200 drugs. *Am Drug* 215 (2):18–20,23–24,26.

63. Anonymous. 1997. Top 200 drugs 1996. *Pharm Times* 62 (4):27,29–30,32–34,36.

64. Simonsen, L.L. 1988. Top 200 drugs of 1987. *Pharm Times* 54 (4):38–46.

65. Simonsen, L.L. 1989. Top 200 drugs of 1988. *Pharm Times* 55 (4):40–48.

66. Simonsen, L.L. 1995. Top 200 drugs. *Pharm Times* 61 (4):17–20.

67. Lofland, J.H., D. Szarlej, T. Buttaro, S. Shermock, and S. Jalalil. 2001. Cyclobenzaprine hydrochloride is a commonly prescribed centrally acting muscle relaxant, which is structurally similar to tricyclic antidepressants (TCAs), and differs from amitriptyline by only one double bond. *Clin J Pain* 17 (1):103–104.

68. Rang, H.P., M.M. Dale, J.M. Ritter, and P.K. Moore. 2003. Antipsychotic drugs. In *Pharmacology*. Edinburgh, UK: Churchill Livingstone, 525–534.
69. Rang, H.P., M.M. Dale, J.M. Ritter, and P.K. Moore. 2003. Antiepileptic drugs. In *Pharmacology*. Edinburgh, UK: Churchill Livingstone, 550–561.
70. Van Hoey, N.M. 2005. Effect of cyclobenzaprine on tricyclic antidepressant assays. *Ann Pharmacother* 39 (7–8):1314–1317.
71. Chattergood, D.S., Z. Verjee, M. Anderson, D. Johnson, M.A. McGuigan, G. Koren, and S. Ito. 1998. Carbamazepine interference with an immune assay for tricyclic antidepressants in plasma. *J Toxicol Clin Toxicol* 36 (1–2):109–113.
72. Dasgupta, A., C. McNeese, and A. Wells. 2004. Interference of carbamazepine and carbamazepine 10,11-epoxide in the fluorescence polarization immunoassay for tricyclic antidepressants: estimation of the true tricyclic antidepressant concentration in the presence of carbamazepine using a mathematical model. *Am J Clin Pathol* 121 (3):418–425.
73. Flieschman, A., and V.W. Chiang. 2001. Carbamazepine overdose recognized by a tricyclic antidepressant assay. *Pediatrics* 107 (1):176–177.
74. Matos, M.E., M.M. Burns, and M.W. Shannon. 2000. False-positive tricyclic antidepressant drug screen results leading to the diagnosis of carbamazepine intoxication. *Pediatrics* 105 (5):E66.
75. Saidinejad, M., T. Law, and M.B. Ewald. 2007. Interference by carbamazepine and oxcarbazepine with serum- and urine-screening assays for tricyclic antidepressants. *Pediatrics* 120 (3):e504–e509.
76. Maynard, G.L., and P. Soni. 1996. Thioridazine interferences with imipramine metabolism and measurement. *Ther Drug Monit* 18 (6):729–731.
77. Nebinger, P., and M. Koel. 1990. Specificity data of the tricyclic antidepressants assay by fluorescent polarization immunoassay. *J Anal Toxicol* 14 (4):219–221.
78. Ryder, K.W., and M.R. Glick. 1986. The effect of thioridazine on the Automatic Clinical Analyzer serum tricyclic anti-depressant screen. *Am J Clin Pathol* 86 (2):248–249.
79. Dasgupta, A., A. Wells, and P. Datta. 2007. False-positive serum tricyclic antidepressant concentrations using fluorescence polarization immunoassay due to the presence of hydroxyzine and cetirizine. *Ther Drug Monit* 29 (1):134–139.
80. Caravati, E.M., J.M. Juenke, B.I. Crouch, and K.T. Anderson. 2005. Quetiapine cross-reactivity with plasma tricyclic antidepressant immunoassays. *Ann Pharmacother* 39 (9):1446–1449.
81. Henrickson, R.G., and A.P. Morocco. 2003. Quetiapine cross-reactivity among three tricyclic antidepressant immunoassays. *J Toxicol Clin Toxicol* 41 (2):105–108.
82. Sloan, K.L., V.M. Haver, and A.J. Saxon. 2000. Quetiapine and false-positive urine drug testing for tricyclic antidepressants. *Am J Psychiatr* 157 (1):148–149.
83. Hussain, M.Z., W. Waheed, and S. Hussain. 2005. Intravenous quetiapine abuse. *Am J Psychiatr* 162 (9):1755–1756.
84. Pararrigopoulos, T., D. Karaiskos, and J. Liappas. 2008. Quetiapine: another drug with potential for misuse? A case report. *J Clin Psychiatr* 69 (1):162–163.
85. Reeves, R.R., and J.C. Brister. 2007. Additional evidence of the abuse potential of quetiapine. *South Med J* 100 (8):834–836.
86. Waters, B.M., and K.G. Joshi. 2007. Intravenous quetiapine-cocaine use ("Q-ball"). *Am J Psychiatr* 164 (1):173–174.
87. Bender, A., and R.C. Glen. 2004. Molecular similarity: a key technique in molecular informatics. *Org Biomol Chem* 2 (2):3204–3218.
88. Ekins, S., J. Mestres, and B. Testa. 2007. *In silico* pharmacology for drug discovery: applications to targets and beyond. *Br J Pharmacol* 152 (1):21–37.
89. Hall, L.H. 2004. A structure-information approach to the prediction of biological activities and properties. *Chem Biodivers* 1 (1):183–201.
90. Gillet, V.J., P. Willett, and J. Bradshaw. 1998. Identification of biological activity using substructural analysis and genetic algorithms. *J Chem Inf Comput Sci* 38 (2):165–179.
91. Hert, J., P. Willett, D.J. Wilton, P. Acklin, K. Azzaoui, E. Jacoby, and A. Schuffenhauer. 2004. Comparison of fingerprint-based methods for virtual screening using multiple bioactive reference structures. *J Chem Inf Comput Sci* 44 (3):1177–1185.
92. Hert, J., P. Willett, D.J. Wilton, P. Acklin, K. Azzaoui, E. Jacoby, and A. Schuffenhauer. 2004. Comparison of topological descriptors for similarity-based virtual screening using multiple bioactive reference structures. *Org Biomol Chem* 2 (22):3256–3266.
93. Willett, P. 2003. Similarity-based approaches to virtual screening. *Biochem Soc Trans* 31 (3):603–606.

94. Fischer, P.M. 2008. Computational chemistry approaches to drug discovery in signal transduction. *Biotechnol J* 3 (4):452–470.

95. Reddy, A.S., S.P. Pati, P.P. Kumar, H.N. Pradeep, and G.N. Sastry. 2007. Virtual screening in drug discovery–a computational perspective. *Curr Protein Pept Sci* 8 (4):329–351.

96. Feng, B.Y., A. Simeonov, A. Jadhav, K. Babaoglu, J. Inglese, B.K. Shoichet, and C.P. Austin. 2007. A high-throughput screen for aggregation-based inhibition in a large compound library. *J Med Chem* 50 (10):2385–2390.

12 Chromatographic Techniques for the Analysis of Antidepressants

Uttam Garg
Children's Mercy Hospitals and Clinics

CONTENTS

12.1   INTRODUCTION

Depression is a common and widespread psychiatric disorder. It is estimated that 10–20% of adults in the United States experience depression in their lifetime and 3% of the population is depressed at any given time. Depression negatively impacts on individuals, families, economy, productivity and society in general. Patients with depression are at a greater risk of suicide and development of many other serious illnesses such as cardiovascular disease and myocardial infarction. Over the decades a number of antidepressant drugs have been developed and used clinically. Tricyclic antidepressants (TCAs) and monoamine oxidase inhibitors (MAOI) were one of the earliest developed medications and are generally referred as the first generation antidepressants. Though still in widespread use this class of antidepressant has a number of side effects resulting in a poor safety profile therefore, therapeutic drug monitoring (TDM) of these antidepressants is required. More recently developed antidepressants include selective serotonin reuptake inhibitors (SSRIs), tetracyclic antidepressants and other atypical noncyclic compounds. These newer antidepressants have an improved margin of safety but some of these drugs may still need monitoring due to side effects and other reasons such as compliance issues and drug–drug interactions. Immunoassays are available for monitoring of TCAs but lack specificity. For the most part, immunoassays are not available for newer antidepressants. Chromatographic methods are an essential part for TDM of antidepressants.

12.2   PHARMACOLOGY OF TRICYCLIC ANTIDEPRESSANTS (TCAs)

As the name indicates, TCAs have a three-ring structure. Commonly used TCAs include amitriptyline, clomipramine, desipramine, doxepin, imipramine, nortriptyline, protriptyline and trimipramine. TCAs are almost completely absorbed through the intestinal tract and reach peak plasma concentration within 2–12 h. However, due to first-pass hepatic metabolism, their bioavailability ranges from approximately 40 to 80%. TCAs are highly lipophilic and thus have a very high volume of distribution. These drugs are metabolized by two major pathways: demethylation and hydroxylation. Loss of one methyl group (demethylation) from the tertiary amine part of TCAs leads to the formation of active secondary amines. For example demethylation of amitriptyline and imipramine leads to formation of active metabolites nortriptyline and desipramine, respectively. The second pathway of TCAs metabolism is ring hydroxylation and conjugation to form glucuronides. These metabolites are then excreted in the urine. Some pharmacokinetic properties of TCAs and other antidepressants are shown in Table 12.1, and the structures of common TCAs are shown in Figure 12.1.

The exact mechanism of action of TCAs has not been completely elucidated. It is postulated that at least in part the mechanism of action includes inhibition of reuptake of norepinephrine and serotonin, thus increasing concentrations of neurotransmitters in the synapses. Although, the affect on neurotransmitters uptake is rapid, the clinical effect of TCAs may not seen for weeks. This suggests that the mechanism by which TCAs exert their antidepressant effect is more complicated. Furthermore, many other drugs such as amphetamines and cocaine which inhibit neurotransmitter uptake are not antidepressants. In fact concurrent use of nervous system stimulants and antidepressants is contraindicated. Other clinical uses of TCAs include the treatment of enuresis, chronic pain, obsessive-compulsive disorder (OCD), attention-deficit hyperactivity disorder, migraine prophylaxis and school phobia [1,2].

TCAs also have significant side effects. The adverse effects are generally mediated through inhibition of cholinergic, histaminic, and α_1-adreneric receptors. The anticholinergic effects of TCAs produce dry mouth, urinary retention and constipation due to decreased gastrointestinal motility, and dry eyes, dry nose, decreased sweating, and hyperthermia. Cardiac effects include inhibition of the fast sodium channels in the His–Purkinje system, and the atrial and ventricular myocardium. These effects are similar to class 1A antiarrhythmic drugs such as quinidine. The conduction abnormalities are seen in EKG as widening of the QRS, PR, and QT intervals. These conduction abnormalities along with TCAs inhibitory effect on peripheral α_1-adrenergic receptor may lead to severe hypotension. TCAs should be avoided in the patients with preexisting cardiac conduction problems due to risk of development of atrioventricular heart block. The CNS effects due to inhibition of antihistaminic, anticholinergic and GABA-A receptors include mental status changes including obtundation and delirium, and seizures.

12.3 INDICATIONS FOR THERAPEUTIC DRUG MONITORING (TDM) OF TRICYCLIC ANTIDEPRESSANTS (TCAs)

Although TDM of TCAs is frequently used, some investigators question its value. Studies have shown that certain changes such as prolonged QRS on EKG correlate better with cardiovascular and neurological toxicity as compared to the blood levels of TCAs [3]. Also plasma levels of TCAs may not correlate very well with clinical outcome and toxicity. This is particularly true in overdose situations. Despite these arguments, the measurement of TCAs levels is unequivocally useful in many clinical scenarios such as when there is a question about patient compliance, monitoring drug-drug interactions, establishing individual target concentration based on the patient's clinical response and metabolic differences due to age, gender and race. The other factors that justify TDM for TCAs include variation in bioavailability between different brands, change in patient's lifestyle such as weight loss/gain, smoking and exercise [4–9].

The case for TDM of TCAs is evident from a number of studies. Metabolism of TCAs varies significantly with age. Preskorn et al. [4] examined steady state concentrations of imipramine and its metabolite desipramine in hospitalized children and found that the interindividual variability for these drugs were 12 and 72 fold respectively, thus making a strong case for TDM of TCAs. The metabolism of TCAs varies significantly among different races and ethnic groups. Due to slower metabolism, African-Americans and Japanese have higher concentrations of TCAs as compared to

TABLE 12.1
Pharmacokinetic Properties of TCAs, SSRIs, and other Non-TCAs

Drug (Active Metabolite)	Class	Average Half-life (Hours)	Vd (L/kg)	Oral Bioavailability	Average Protein Binding	Therapeutic Range (ng/mL)	Toxic Level (ng/mL)
Amitriptyline (Nortriptyline)	TCA	21	15	50	95	120–250[b]	>500[b]
Amoxapine (8-hydroxyamoxapine)	Monoamines reuptake inhibitor	10	1	90	90	200–400[b]	>600[b]
Bupropion (Hydroxybupropion[a])	Dopamine reuptake inhibitor	15	45	90	85	25–100	>400
Citalopram (Norcitalopram[a])	SSRI	30	14	80	50	40–100	>250
Desipramine (NA)	TCA	20	42	40	80	75–300	>500
Doxepin (Nordoxepin)	TCA	17	20	27	90	150–250[b]	>500[b]
Fluoxetine (Norfluoxetine)	SSRI	60	50	100	94	300–1000[b]	>2000[b]
Fluvoxamine (NA)	SSRI	23	25	95	77	20–400	Not known
Imipramine (Desipramine)	TCA	12	18	40	90	150–250[b]	>500[b]
Maprotiline (NA)	Tetracyclic	33	24	100	88	150–300	>1000
Mirtazapine (Normirtazapine)	Tetracyclic	30	12	90	85	4–40	Not known
Nortriptyline (NA)	TCA	30	18	50	92	50–150	>500
Paroxetine (NA)	SSRI	22	15	90	95	20–200	>800
Protriptyline (NA)	TCA	80	13	75	95	70–250	>500
Sertraline (Norsertraline[a])	SSRI	28	20	90	98	30–200	>500
Trazodone (NA)	SSRI	9	1	80	90	800–1600	>5000
Trimipramine (NA)	TCA	27	32	50	90	100–250	>500
Venlafaxine (O-desmethyl venlafaxine)	SSRI	5	7	90	27	250–500[b]	>1000[b]

Notes: Vd, volume of distribution; NA, no significantly active metabolite.

[a] Significantly less active than parent drug.

[b] Total concentration of parent and active metabolite.

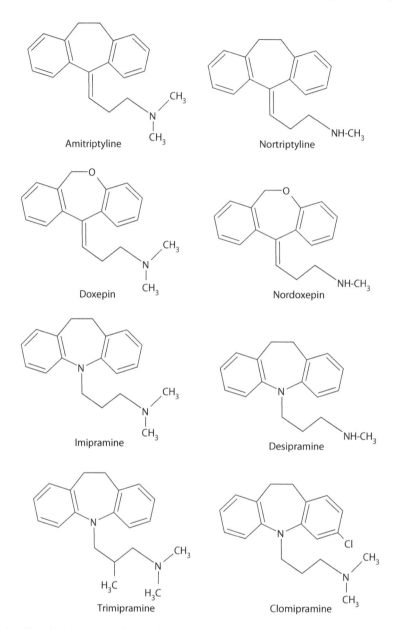

FIGURE 12.1 Chemical structure of some TCA.

Caucasians. Asians and Hispanics respond to lower doses of TCAs due to hypersensitivity recep-tors [5]. Another acquired factor which has been shown to significantly affect TCAs metabolism is alcoholism. A study showed that the metabolism for imipramine and desipramine in detoxified alcoholic men were 1.5–2.0 times higher as compared to healthy controls. The findings suggest that recently detoxified alcoholics may require higher doses and frequent monitoring of TCAs [6]. Mullar et al. [7] compared TCAs doses based on clinical judgment and serum levels. The authors found that treating depression based on TDM of TCAs was superior to clinical judgment.

TCAs are highly metabolized by the cytochrome P450 enzyme system, CYP2D6 being the major contributor. Drugs that inhibit cytochrome P450 lead to increased blood concentrations of TCAs, causing drug toxicity. CYP2D6 inhibitors include amiodarone, bupropion, celecoxib, chlorpromazine, cimetidine, citalopram, doxorubicin, haloperidol, methylphenidate, quinidine, ranitidine, ritonavir, terbinafine, ticlopidine, and histamine H1 receptor antagonists [8,9]. On the other hand drugs such as carbamazepine, phenobarbital, phenytoin and rifampin which induce CYP2D6, lead to increased metabolism of TCAs, thus reducing serum concentration.

Both tertiary and secondary amine forms of TCAs are prescribed to patients. Tertiary amines TCAs are metabolized to secondary amines and these compounds retain significant pharmacological activity. Therefore, when a patient is on tertiary TCAs, the secondary amine metabolites should also be measured. The secondary amines TCAs are further metabolized to hydroxy metabolites which have shorter half-lives. Though hydroxy metabolites have significant antidepressant activity, they are not monitored routinely. However, monitoring of these metabolites may be warranted in specific situations such as renal impairment where these metabolites may accumulate to significant concentrations.

12.4   ANALYSIS OF TRICYCLIC ANTIDEPRESSANTS (TCAs)

TCAs are very lipophilic in nature. Therefore, it is important to avoid serum or plasma gel separator tubes when collecting blood samples for analysis of TCAs [10]. TCAs are stable for one week in serum or plasma at room temperature, up to four weeks at 4°C and over one year at –20°C [8].

The concentrations of TCAs in serum or plasma can be determined by using immunoassays or chromatographic methods. Immunoassays for TCAs are available as point of care testing devices and for application on chemistry analyzers. Immunoassays are rapid and can provide useful information quickly, especially in the case of suspected overdose. However, immunoassays are prone to interferences and lack specificity. Many drugs including carbamazepine, quetiapine, phenothiazine, diphenhydramine, cyproheptadine, and cyclobenzaprine are known to interfere with TCAs immunoassays. Table 12.2 lists the drugs which commonly interfere with such immunoassays [11]. Therefore, results of immunoassays should be interpreted with caution along with patient's clinical and medication history.

Due to interferences in immunoassays, chromatographic methods are preferred for measurement of TCAs. Chromatographic methods include thin layer chromatography (TLC), gas chromatography (GC) and high performance liquid chromatography (HPLC). TLC is generally used for urine samples and is useful in ruling-in or ruling-out ingestion in overdose situations, and can reliably identify a number of TCAs. One commonly used TLC system is called Toxi-Lab (Varian Inc., Palo Alto, CA). TLC is fairly a simple technique but does not provide any quantitative information. Gas and liquid chromatographic techniques are commonly used in TDM of TCAs. In addition to parent TCAs, the metabolites are also generally monitored. The metabolites of parent tertiary amines, the secondary amines, are pharmacologically active and contribute to overall therapeutic and toxic effects. Furthermore, the monitoring of metabolites can give additional information on time of ingestion, drug metabolism, and drug–drug interactions.

GC equipped with capillary column and coupled with flame ionization detector, nitrogen phosphorus detector or mass spectrometer is commonly used for screening and quantification of TCAs [12–15]. The capillary columns are typically, 10–30 meters, fused silica columns, bonded nonpolar to intermediate polarity methyl silicone liquid phases (0–50% phenyl). The TCAs are generally extracted from serum or plasma using liquid–liquid extraction which involves alkalization of the sample followed by extraction with organic solvents. The organic extract is then concentrated and injected into the GC. Sometimes additional steps are taken to further purify the TCAs to reduce interferences. After alkaline organic solvent extraction, TCAs may be back extracted in acidic aqueous medium such as dilute hydrochloric acid. Acidic aqueous phase is then taken and alkalinized and TCAs are re-extracted with organic solvent(s). The organic extracts are then concentrated and injected into the gas chromatograph. In recent years a number of solid-phase extraction methods have also been reported. The solid-phase extraction methods provide cleaner preparation and better recovery [16–18]. With GC, most of the TCAs particularly tertiary amines can be separated without derivatization. However, TCAs metabolites, secondary amines and hydroxy compounds may need

TABLE 12.2
Drugs that Cause False Positive Results in Various Immunoassays

Drug	Comment/Reference(s)
Carbamazepine	Unresponsive patient with history of seizures and tic disorder tested falsely positive for TCAs. No evidence of TCAs toxicity by EKG [40].
Carbamazepine	False positives TCAs due to carbamazepine were confirmed by HPLC/GC-MS [41,42].
Iminostilbene (Carbamazepine metabolite)	Three false positive cases reported on Triage panel [43].
Quetiapine	34-year-old patient tested positive due to quetiapine. Quetiapine cross reactivity of 4.3% with TCAs was found in Diagnostic Reagents Inc. (now Microgenics) [44].
Quetiapine	Urine samples were spiked with various concentrations of quetiapine. Syva and Microgenics immunoassays tested positive at 100 and 10 μg/mL. Triage immunoassay was negative at up to 1000 μg/mL [45].
Quetiapine	False positive on Abbott Laboratories FPIA [46].
Quetiapine	Spiked plasma samples were used. Abbott's TDx, Syva and STAD-ACA immunoassays showed cross reactivity in a concentration dependent manner [47].
Phenothiazines	A patient on thioridazine and flurazepam tested false positive for TCAs due to thioridazine. Even therapeutic concentrations of thioridazine cause false positives [48]. Other studies with false positive immunoassays are published [49,50].
Diphenhydramine	21-year-old female ingested 2 g of diphenhydramine. It interfered in EMIT assay. Unlike other compounds which are tricyclics and have close structure to TCAs, diphenhydramine is an ethanolamine [51].
Cyproheptadine	A 14-year-old girl who ingested ~120 mg cyproheptadine tested positive for TCAs by EMIT [52].
Cyproheptadine	Pediatric case of false positive TCAs. Most likely false positive was due to cyproheptadine metabolite rather than the parent compound [53].
Cyclobenzaprine	Interferences in many different types of immunoassays [54–56].
Hydroxyzine and cetirizine	Interference in fluorescence polarization immunoassay [57]. Structurally unrelated to TCAs.

derivatization to increase sensitivity as well as to improve peak shape. The derivatives include trifluoroacetyl, heptafluorobutyryl, 4-carbethoxyhexafluorobutyryl chloride, fluoracyl, and silane. In one study, the stability of the 4-carbethoxyhexafluorobutyryl chloride derivatives of secondary amines of TCAs was found to be superior to that of trifluoroacetyl derivatives [19].

The common detectors used in GC for detection of TCAs are nitrogen phosphorus detector and mass spectrometer [17]. Although nitrogen phosphorus detector may have higher sensitivity than mass spectrometer, it lacks specificity and may impose problems in identification of closely eluting peaks. Mass spectrometers are preferred detectors due to their specificity and higher confidence in identification of closely eluting peaks. The analysis is performed using either electron impact mode or chemical ionization mode. Currently, electron impact mode is perhaps used more commonly than chemical ionization mode. However, mass spectrometers with chemical ionization mode are gaining popularity due to their higher sensitivity and selectivity. The mass spectrometers are operated either in full spectrum acquisition mode or selected ion monitoring mode. The former mode is generally used for identification and the latter for the quantification as it provides higher sensitivity. Gas chromatography-tandem mass spectrometry (GC-MS-MS) methods are now also available and provide better sensitivity and selectivity than GC-MS instruments. Relative retention times of some antidepressants using GC-MS is shown in Table 12.3. The instrument and the operating conditions are given in Table 12.4. Figure 12.2 shows the GC-MS chromatogram of several antidepressants, and Figures 12.3 and 12.4 show the electron impact ionization mass spectra of TCAs amitriptyline and doxepin, respectively.

TABLE 12.3
Relative Retention Times (RRTs) of some Antidepressants

Antidepressant	RRT
Bupropion	0.4570
Fluoxetine	0.6930
Fluvoxamine	0.7194
Venlafaxine	0.8605
Amitriptyline	0.9319
Nortriptyline	0.9398
Trimipramine	0.9471
Imipramine	0.9473
Doxepin	0.9492
Mirtazepine	0.9538
Desipramine	0.9548
Nordoxepin	0.9548
Protriptyline	0.9581
Maprotiline	1.0086
Sertraline	1.0238
Citalopram	1.0409
Clomipramine	1.0483
Paroxetine	1.1211
Amoxapine	1.1462
Trazodone	1.7387

Note: RRTs are based on promazine as an internal standard and retention time of ~9.25 minutes.

HPLC is another frequently used technique for TDM of TCAs [20–22]. In fact based on a recent College of American Pathologist (CAP) survey, HPLC with UV (ultraviolet) detection is the most common method for quantification of TCAs. Although, unlike GC-MS, HPLC-UV does not provide structural information and thus lacks selectivity, it overcomes many problems posed by polar secondary amines and hydroxyl metabolites on GC analysis. The columns used for HPLC separation of various TCAs include C18, C8, phenyl, and CN columns. These columns can effectively separate parent TCAs and the metabolites. Typical mobile phases contain phosphate or acetate buffers in organic solvents such as acetonitrile and methanol. Example of a typical TCAs chromatogram using HPLC with UV detector is shown in Figure 12.5.

A number of methods for the analysis of TCAs using HPLC have been published. A method for simultaneous determination of benzodiazepine and TCAs have also been published [23]. Like GC, HPLC may not separate all the TCAs of interest and may lack sensitivity for some TCAs. These problems can be overcome by using HPLC-MS or HPLC-MS-MS. A sensitive and specific HPLC-MS-MS method involving atmospheric pressure chemical ionization tandem mass-spectrometry (HPLC-APCI-MS-MS) has been described for the identification and quantitation of seven TCAs i.e., amitriptyline, nortriptyline, doxepin, dosulepin, dibenzepin, opipramol and melitracen. These method uses direct injection and on line sample deproteinization [24]. A HPLC-MS-MS method for the determination of TCAs and non-TCAs including amitriptyline, clomipramine, trimipramine, imipramine, doxepin, mianserin, maprotiline, dosulepine, amoxapine and their active metabolites desipramine, nortriptyline, desmethylclomipramine, and nordoxepin, along with MAOI toloxatone and moclobemide has been published [25].

TABLE 12.4
GC-MS Instrument and Conditions used to Obtain
Data shown in Table 12.3

Instrument	Agilent 5890 GC/5972 MS
GC column	DB-1, 15 m × 0.25 mm × 0.25 μm
Initial oven temperature	90°C
Initial time	1.0 min.
Ramp 1	32°C/min
Temperature 2	170°C
Hold time	2.0 min.
Ramp 2	20°C/min
Final temperature	270°C
Hold time	9.50 min.
Injector temperature	250°C
Detector temperature	280°C
Purge time on	1 min
Column pressure	5 psi

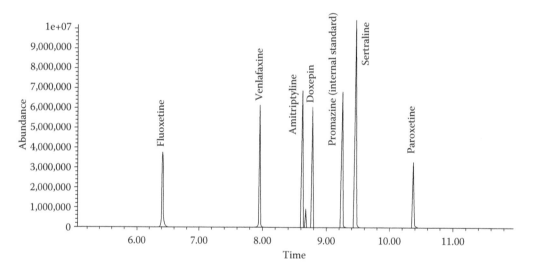

FIGURE 12.2   Example of GC-MS total ion chromatogram of several antidepressants (pure standards were analyzed without derivatization). GC-MS instrumentation and conditions' details are given in Table 12.4.

12.5 NEWER, SECOND, AND THIRD GENERATION, NON-TRICYCLIC ANTIDEPRESSANTS (TCAs)

With the better understanding of depression and mechanism of action of antidepressants action over the recent years many non-TCAs have been developed. Sometimes these antidepressants are referred to as second and third generation antidepressants. Unlike TCAs, they lack adrenergic, antihistaminic, and anticholinergic effects and thus have fewer side effects when compared to TCAs. These antidepressants include amoxapine and maprotiline which inhibit reuptake of monoamines, trazodone that inhibits serotonin reuptake, bupropion which inhibits reuptake of norepinephrine and dopamine, and venlafaxine as well as mirtazapine that inhibit uptake of both norepinephrine

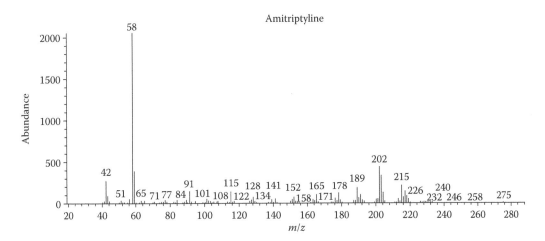

FIGURE 12.3   GC-MS electron impact mass spectrum of amitriptyline. In general mass spectra are normalized to the base ion peak with counts of 10,000. To show low abundant ions, the mass spectrum has been zoomed to the base ion peak counts of ~2000.

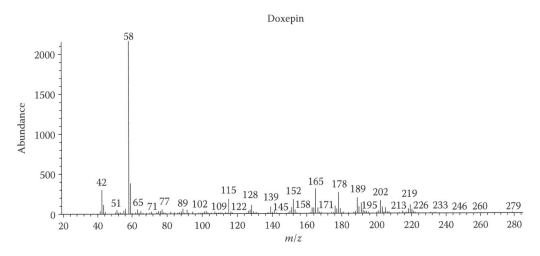

FIGURE 12.4   GC-MS electron impact mass spectrum of doxepin. In general mass spectra are normalized to the base ion peak with counts of 10,000. To show low abundant ions, the mass spectrum has been zoomed to the base ion peak counts of ~2000.

and serotonin. In addition, in this newer category of drugs there are SSRIs which include citalopram, escitalopram, fluoxetine, fluvoxamine, paroxetine, and sertraline. Currently SSRIs are the most commonly used antidepressants in the United States [1,26].

Some pharmacokinetic properties of these non-TCAs are summarized in Table 12.1. Structures of some of these newer antidepressants are shown in Figure 12.6. Fluoxetine was the first SSRI approved by the Federal Drug Administration (FDA) for treatment of depression. It contains the propylamine side chain as found in most TCAs. In addition to its use as antidepressant, fluoxetine is also used in the treatment of bulimia and obsessive compulsive disorder. The dose for the treatment of bulimia and obsessive compulsive disorder is generally two to three times higher than as antidepressant. Fluoxetine has a half-life of 2–4 days and is metabolized to an active metabolite norfluoxetine, which has a half-life of 7–9 days. Due to the long half-lives of the parent drug and its active metabolite, fluoxetine is now available in a special form for once a week dosing. Also due to the long

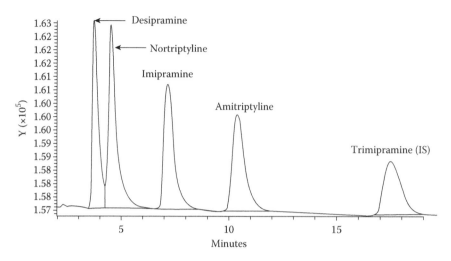

FIGURE 12.5 Example of TCAs chromatogram generated using reverse phase C18-10 cm column and HPLC-UV detector (254 nm). A sample spiked with different TCAs were alkalinized with NaOH and extracted with hexanes: isoamyl alcohol (99:1). TCAs were back extracted with 0.01 N HCl and injected into HPLC. The mobile phase was phosphate buffer (pH 6.7) containing acetonitrile and diethylamine.

half life, at least five weeks should be allowed before start of therapy with MAOI [27]. Citalopram is another widely used SSRI. In addition to its use as an antidepressant, it is used in the treatment of dementia, smoking cessation, ethanol abuse, OCD in children and diabetic neuropathy [1,27]. Escitalopram is the active isomer of racemic citalopram and is more selective SSRI as compared to citalopram. Fluvoxamine, another SSRI, is FDA-approved only for the treatment of OCD in children ≥8 years of age and adults [1]. Its investigational uses include the treatment of major depression, panic disorder and anxiety disorders in children [27]. Like other SSRIs, fluvoxamine is generally a safe drug. Common symptoms of mild to moderate toxicity are drowsiness, tremor, diarrhea, vomiting, abdominal pain, dizziness, mydriasis, and sinus tachycardia. At higher doses, seizures, sedation, hypokalemia, hypotension and sinus bradycardia may occur. TDM of fluvoxamine is important because its concentration varies significantly with age and sex. Steady-state plasma concentrations in children are two to three times higher than adults, and female children have significantly higher area under the curve for drug metabolism than males.

Paroxetine and sertraline are two other FDA approved SSRIs. In addition to their role in the treatment of depression, they are used in the treatment of many other disorders. Paroxetine was first approved by FDA for the treatment of social phobia and generalized anxiety disorder. Later the drug was approved for the treatment of post-traumatic stress disorder, panic disorder with or without agoraphobia and OCD in adults [1]. It is also used in the treatment of eating disorders, impulse control disorders, self-injurious behavior and premenstrual disorders [27]. Another SSRI, paroxetine has the highest rate of discontinuation syndrome because of its short half-life and lack of active metabolites. Symptoms of paroxetine discontinuation syndrome are generally mild such as nausea, dizziness, bad dreams, paresthesia, and a flu-like illness. If severe symptoms develop, restarting of paroxetine may be needed [28]. Paroxetine is extensively metabolized in the liver through oxidation and methylation, and further formation of glucuronide and sulfate conjugates which are eliminated in the urine. Sertraline is used in the treatment of major depression, OCD, panic disorder, post-traumatic stress disorder, premenstrual dysphoric disorder, and social anxiety disorder [29]. When administered orally, it is completely absorbed and is highly protein bound. The drug is metabolized by the liver through CYP2C19 and CYP2D6 enzyme systems. One of the major metabolite nor-sertraline is pharmacologically active. It has a half-life of about three days which is approximately three times longer than sertraline. Therefore, a two-week washout period is recommended before

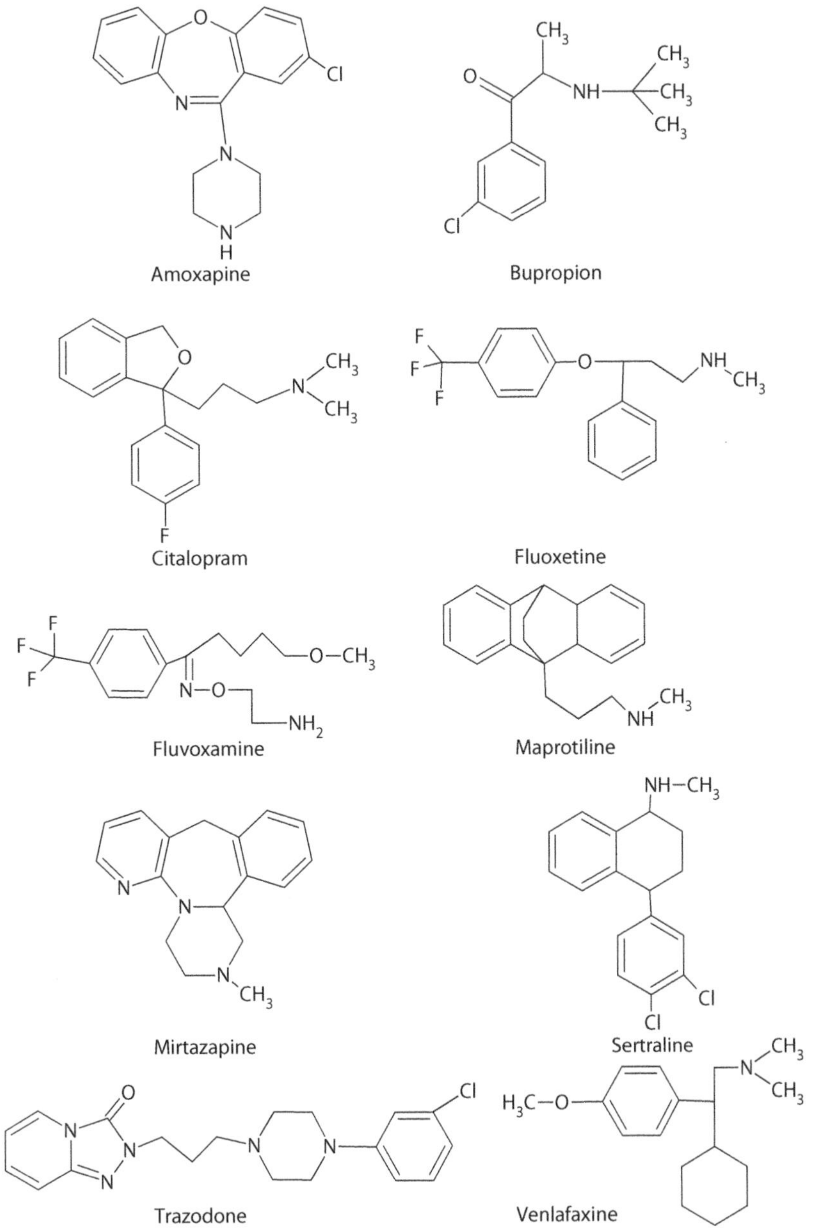

FIGURE 12.6 Chemical structure of some SSRIs and other non-TCAs.

initiation of therapy with MAOI. The common side effects of sertraline include nausea, dry mouth, fatigue and decreased libido. It is associated with more cases of diarrhea as compared to fluoxetine but has fewer cases of anxiety and insomnia [1].

Major mechanism of action of SSRIs is to inhibit serotonin reuptake. In addition, SSRIs also interact directly with various serotonin receptors (5-HT$_{1A}$, 5-HT$_2$, and 5-HT$_3$) to cause pharmacological response. In addition to their use as antidepressants, SSRIs are also used in the treatment of OCD, panic disorder, bulimia, and many other conditions [30]. Coadministration of any SSRI with a MAOI is highly contraindicated due to the potential for serotonin syndrome due to accumulation of very high levels of serotonin in the brain. Serotonin syndrome is characterized by agitation, hyperthermia, tachycardia, and neuromuscular disturbance including rigidity. Many drugs including MAOI, tramadol, sibutramine, meperidine, sumatriptan, lithium, St John's wort, gingko biloba, and atypical antipsychotic agents interact with SSRIs and can lead to serotonin syndrome [31]. The boxed warning for SSRIs includes the risk of suicidal thinking and behavior in children and adolescents with major and other depressive disorders.

12.6   ANALYSIS OF NON-TRICYCLIC ANTIDEPRESSANTS (TCAs)

Unlike TCAs, there are no immunoassays for the monitoring of non-TCAs. In addition, there is no reliable spot method for these antidepressants. Gas and liquid chromatographic methods are commonly used for the determination of SSRIs and other non-TCAs [32–35]. Like TCAs, GC methods for analysis of non-TCAs are equipped with capillary column and mass spectrometer. The drugs are extracted using liquid–liquid or solid phase extraction. To increase drug concentrations or purity, sometimes multiple extractions or back extractions are used. The extract is concentrated and injected into the GC with or without derivatization. Mass spectrometer is operated in full spectrum acquisition mode or selected ion monitoring mode. The former is preferred for identification and the latter for quantification. Wille et al. [33] reported solid phase extraction procedure for the analysis of 13 new generation antidepressants venlafaxine, fluoxetine, viloxazine, fluvoxamine, mianserin, mirtazapine, melitracen, reboxetine, citalopram, maprotiline, sertraline, paroxetine, and trazodone along with their eight metabolites O-desmethylvenlafaxine, norfluoxetine, desmethylmianserine, desmethylmirtazapine, desmethylcitalopram, didesmethylcitalopram, desmethylsertraline, and m-chlorophenylpiperazine. The extract is suitable for both GC and HPLC analysis. Relative retention times of some antidepressants are shown in Table 12.3. The instrument and the operating conditions, generated to produce data in Table 12.3, are given in Table 12.4. Figure 12.2 shows the GC-MS chromatogram of several antidepressants, and Figures 12.7 through 12.10 show the electron impact ionization mass spectra of fluoxetine, venlafaxaine, sertraline, and paroxetine, respectively.

Many non-TCA such as trazodone and nefazodone are heat labile and are not suitable for determination with GC. Furthermore, many antidepressants require derivatization before analysis by GC. HPLC is a method of choice for these antidepressants and is also the most commonly used method. Number of HPLC methods for the determination of SSRIs and other non-TCA has been described. A method for the simultaneous determination of the citalopram, fluoxetine, paroxetine

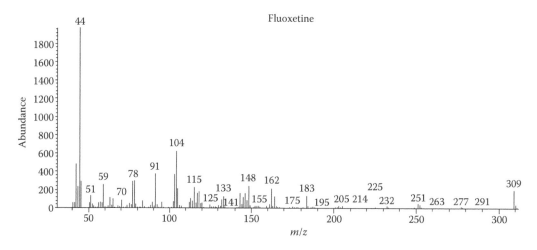

FIGURE 12.7   GC-MS electron impact mass spectrum of fluoxetine. In general mass spectra are normalized to the base ion peak with counts of 10,000. To show low abundant ions, the mass spectrum has been zoomed to the base ion peak counts of ~2000.

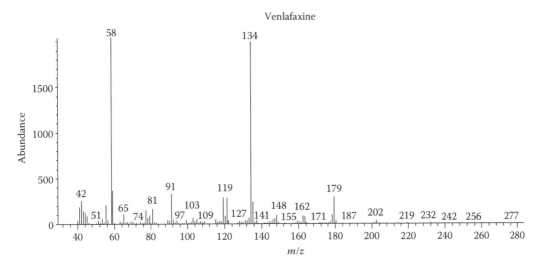

FIGURE 12.8   GC-MS electron impact mass spectrum of venlafaxaine. In general mass spectra are normalized to the base ion peak with counts of 10,000. To show low abundant ions, the mass spectrum has been zoomed to the base ion peak counts of ~2000.

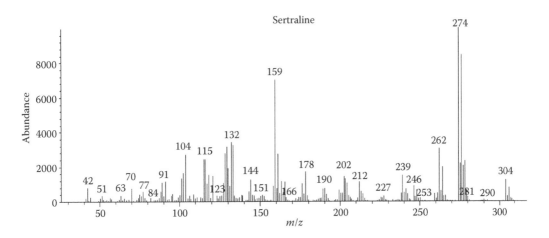

FIGURE 12.9   GC-MS electron impact mass spectrum of sertraline.

and their metabolites in whole blood and plasma has been published. The method used a solid-phase extraction and reverse-phase HPLC equipped with fluorescence and ultraviolet detection [36]. Another HPLC method for the determination of 10 frequently prescribed TCA and non-TCA: imipramine, amitriptyline, clomipramine, fluoxetine, sertraline, paroxetine, citalopram, mirtazapine, moclobemide, and duloxetine has also been described [37]. Due to their increased sensitivity and selectivity, recently HPLC tandem mass spectrometry methods have been developed [38,39]. Sauvage et al. [38] reported turbulent-flow liquid chromatography coupled to tandem-mass spectrometry method for determination of 13 antidepressants—amoxapine, amitriptyline, citalopram, clomipramine, dothiepin, doxepin, fluoxetine, imipramine, maprotiline, mianserin, paroxetine, sertraline, trimipramine and their metabolites- nortriptyline, monodesmethylcitalopram, desmethylclomipramine, desipramine, norfluoxetine, desmethylmianserin, and N-desmethylsertraline. Castaing et al. [39] described a liquid chromatography-tandem mass spectrometry method for the determination of SSRIs including fluoxetine, paroxetine, sertraline,

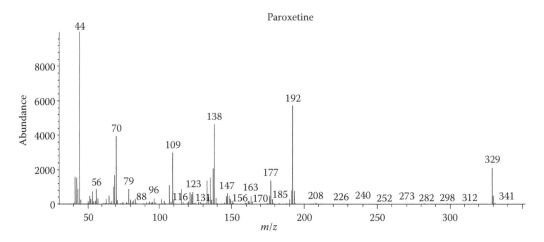

FIGURE 12.10   GC-MS electron impact mass spectrum of paroxetine.

fluvoxamine, and citalopram; serotonin noradrenaline reuptake inhibitors milnacipran and venla-faxine; a noradrenergic and specific serotoninergic antidepressant mirtazapine, and five of their active metabolites norfluoxetine, desmethylcitalopram, didesmethylcitalopram, desmethylvenla-faxine, and desmethylmirtazapine.

12.7   CONCLUSIONS

In conclusion, depression is a major medical problem and the number of patients with depression is increasing as well as the number of prescriptions. The major classes of antidepressants are TCAs, SSRIs, and other non-TCAs non-SSRI drugs. Of all these antidepressants, TCAs have higher mor-bidity and mortality. Although toxicity of TCAs may correlate well with clinical findings of specific changes in EKG, the role of TDM of TCAs remains unequivocal. The monitoring of TCAs can be done by immunoassays or chromatographic methods. Although immunoassays are rapid and conve-nient methods for monitoring TCAs, they lack specificity due to interference by a number of drugs and may lead to misdiagnosis and mistreatment. Chromatographic methods, although not routinely available, are preferred methods for TDM of TCAs. The newer generations of antidepressants such as SSRIs and tetracyclic antidepressants are safer as compared to TCAs. Despite their safety, there are number of circumstances when their monitoring is warranted. Due to lack of immunoassays, non-TCAs are generally monitoring through chromatographic methods.

REFERENCES

1. Ables AZ, Baughman OL, 3rd. 2003. Antidepressants: update on new agents and indications. *Am Fam Physician* 67:547–54.
2. Sindrup SH, Otto M, Finnerup NB, Jensen TS. 2005. Antidepressants in the treatment of neuropathic pain. *Basic Clin Pharmacol Toxicol* 96:399–409.
3. Liebelt EL, Ulrich A, Francis PD, Woolf A. 1997. Serial electrocardiogram changes in acute tricyclic antidepressant overdoses. *Crit Care Med* 25:1721–26.
4. Preskorn SH, Bupp SJ, Weller EB, Weller RA. 1989. Plasma levels of imipramine and metabolites in 68 hospitalized children. *J Am Acad Child Adolesc Psychiatry* 28:373–75.
5. Ziegler VE, Biggs JT. 1977. Tricyclic plasma levels. Effect of age, race, sex, and smoking. *JAMA* 238:2167–69.
6. Ciraulo DA, Barnhill JG, Jaffe JH. 1988. Clinical pharmacokinetics of imipramine and desipramine in alcoholics and normal volunteers. *Clin Pharmacol Ther* 43:509–18.

7. Muller MJ, Dragicevic A, Fric M, Gaertner I, Grasmader K, Hartter S, et al. 2003. Therapeutic drug monitoring of tricyclic antidepressants: how does it work under clinical conditions? *Pharmacopsychiatry* 36:98–104.

8. Linder MW, Keck PE, Jr. 1998. Standards of laboratory practice: antidepressant drug monitoring. National Academy of Clinical Biochemistry. *Clin Chem* 44:1073–84.

9. Wilkinson GR. 2005. Drug metabolism and variability among patients in drug response. *N Engl J Med* 352:2211–21.

10. Dasgupta A, Yared MA, Wells A. 2000. Time-dependent absorption of therapeutic drugs by the gel of the Greiner Vacuette blood collection tube. *Ther Drug Monit* 22:427–31.

11. Garg U. 2008. Pitfalls in measuring antidepressant drugs. In: Dasgupta A, ed. *Handbook of drug monitoring methods: Therapeutics and drugs of abuse.* Totowa, NJ: Humana Press, 133–63.

12. Van Brunt N. 1983. Application of new technology for the measurement of tricyclic antidepressants using capillary gas chromatography with a fused silica DB5 column and nitrogen phosphorus detection. *Ther Drug Monit* 5:11–37.

13. Bredesen JE, Ellingsen OF, Karlsen J. 1981. Rapid isothermal gas-liquid chromatographic determination of tricyclic antidepressants in serum with use of a nitrogen-selective detector. *J Chromatogr* 204:361–67.

14. Dorrity F, Jr., Linnoila M, Habig RL. 1977. Therapeutic monitoring of tricyclic antidepressants in plasma by gas chromatography. *Clin Chem* 23:1326–28.

15. Martinez MA, Sanchez de la Torre C, Almarza E. 2004. A comparative solid-phase extraction study for the simultaneous determination of fluvoxamine, mianserin, doxepin, citalopram, paroxetine, and etoperidone in whole blood by capillary gas-liquid chromatography with nitrogen-phosphorus detection. *J Anal Toxicol* 28:174–80.

16. Lee XP, Hasegawa C, Kumazawa T, Shinmen N, Shoji Y, Seno H, et al. 2008. Determination of tricyclic antidepressants in human plasma using pipette tip solid-phase extraction and gas chromatography-mass spectrometry. *J Sep Sci* 31:2265–71.

17. de la Torre R, Ortuno J, Pascual JA, Gonzalez S, Ballesta J. 1998. Quantitative determination of tricyclic antidepressants and their metabolites in plasma by solid-phase extraction (Bond-Elut TCA) and separation by capillary gas chromatography with nitrogen-phosphorous detection. *Ther Drug Monit* 20:340–46.

18. Lee XP, Kumazawa T, Sato K, Suzuki O. 1997. Detection of tricyclic antidepressants in whole blood by headspace solid-phase microextraction and capillary gas chromatography. *J Chromatogr Sci* 35:302–8.

19. Way BA, Stickle D, Mitchell ME, Koenig JW, Turk J. 1998. Isotope dilution gas chromatographic-mass spectrometric measurement of tricyclic antidepressant drugs. Utility of the 4-carbethoxyhexafluorobutyryl derivatives of secondary amines. *J Anal Toxicol* 22:374–82.

20. Theurillat R, Thormann W. 1998. Monitoring of tricyclic antidepressants in human serum and plasma by HPLC: characterization of a simple, laboratory developed method via external quality assessment. *J Pharm Biomed Anal* 18:751–60.

21. Queiroz RH, Lanchote VL, Bonato PS, de Carvalho D. 1995. Simultaneous HPLC analysis of tricyclic antidepressants and metabolites in plasma samples. *Pharm Acta Helv* 70:181–86.

22. Dorey RC, Preskorn SH, Widener PK. 1988. Results compared for tricyclic antidepressants as assayed by liquid chromatography and enzyme immunoassay. *Clin Chem* 34:2348–51.

23. Uddin MN, Samanidou VF, Papadoyannis IN. 2008. Development and validation of an HPLC method for the determination of benzodiazepines and tricyclic antidepressants in biological fluids after sequential SPE. *J Sep Sci* 31:2358–70.

24. Kollroser M, Schober C. 2002. Simultaneous determination of seven tricyclic antidepressant drugs in human plasma by direct-injection HPLC-APCI-MS-MS with an ion trap detector. *Ther Drug Monit* 24:537–44.

25. Titier K, Castaing N, Le-Deodic M, Le-Bars D, Moore N, Molimard M. 2007. Quantification of tricyclic antidepressants and monoamine oxidase inhibitors by high-performance liquid chromatography-tandem mass spectrometry in whole blood. *J Anal Toxicol* 31:200–7.

26. Pacher P, Kecskemeti V. 2004. Trends in the development of new antidepressants. Is there a light at the end of the tunnel? *Curr Med Chem* 11:925–43.

27. Lacy CF, Armstrong LL, Goldman MP, Lance LL. 2004. *Lexi-Comp's Drug Information Handbook.* Hudson, OH: Lexi-Comp, 595–98.

28. Tonks A. 2002. Withdrawal from paroxetine can be severe, warns FDA. *BMJ* 324:260.

29. Brady K, Pearlstein T, Asnis GM, Baker D, Rothbaum B, Sikes CR, et al. 2000. Efficacy and safety of sertraline treatment of posttraumatic stress disorder: a randomized controlled trial. *JAMA* 283:1837–44.

30. Schatzberg AF. 2000. New indications for antidepressants. *J Clin Psychiatry* 61 Suppl 11:9–17.

31. Garg U. 2007. Therapeutic drug monitoring of antidepressants. In: Dasgupta A, ed. *Therapeutic drug monitoring data*. Washington, DC: AACC Press, 107–128.

32. Wille SM, Van Hee P, Neels HM, Van Peteghem CH, Lambert WE. 2007. Comparison of electron and chemical ionization modes by validation of a quantitative gas chromatographic-mass spectrometric assay of new generation antidepressants and their active metabolites in plasma. *J Chromatogr A* 1176:236–45.

33. Wille SM, Maudens KE, Van Peteghem CH, Lambert WE. 2005. Development of a solid phase extraction for 13 'new' generation antidepressants and their active metabolites for gas chromatographic-mass spectrometric analysis. *J Chromatogr A* 1098:19–29.

34. Bickeboeller-Friedrich J, Maurer HH. 2001. Screening for detection of new antidepressants, neuroleptics, hypnotics, and their metabolites in urine by GC-MS developed using rat liver microsomes. *Ther Drug Monit* 23:61–70.

35. Namera A, Watanabe T, Yashiki M, Iwasaki Y, Kojima T. 1998. Simple analysis of tetracyclic antidepressants in blood using headspace-solid-phase microextraction and GC-MS. *J Anal Toxicol* 22:396–400.

36. Kristoffersen L, Bugge A, Lundanes E, Slordal L. 1999. Simultaneous determination of citalopram, fluoxetine, paroxetine and their metabolites in plasma and whole blood by high-performance liquid chromatography with ultraviolet and fluorescence detection. *J Chromatogr B Biomed Sci Appl* 734:229–46.

37. Malfara WR, Bertucci C, Costa Queiroz ME, Dreossi Carvalho SA, Pires Bianchi Mde L, Cesarino EJ, et al. 2007. Reliable HPLC method for therapeutic drug monitoring of frequently prescribed tricyclic and nontricyclic antidepressants. *J Pharm Biomed Anal* 44:955–62.

38. Sauvage FL, Gaulier JM, Lachatre G, Marquet P. 2006. A fully automated turbulent-flow liquid chromatography-tandem mass spectrometry technique for monitoring antidepressants in human serum. *Ther Drug Monit* 28:123–30.

39. Castaing N, Titier K, Receveur-Daurel M, Le-Deodic M, Le-bars D, Moore N, et al. 2007. Quantification of eight new antidepressants and five of their active metabolites in whole blood by high-performance liquid chromatography-tandem mass spectrometry. *J Anal Toxicol* 31:334–41.

40. Fleischman A, Chiang VW. 2001. Carbamazepine overdose recognized by a tricyclic antidepressant assay. *Pediatrics* 107:176–7.

41. Chattergoon DS, Verjee Z, Anderson M, Johnson D, McGuigan MA, Koren G, et al. 1998. Carbamazepine interference with an immune assay for tricyclic antidepressants in plasma. *J Toxicol Clin Toxicol* 36:109–13.

42. Saidinejad M, Law T, Ewald MB. 2007. Interference by carbamazepine and oxcarbazepine with serum- and urine-screening assays for tricyclic antidepressants. *Pediatrics* 120:e504–9.

43. Tomaszewski C, Runge J, Gibbs M, Colucciello S, Price M. 2005. Evaluation of a rapid bedside toxicology screen in patients suspected of drug toxicity. *J Emerg Med* 28:389–94.

44. Sloan KL, Haver VM, Saxon AJ. 2000. Quetiapine and false-positive urine drug testing for tricyclic antidepressants. *Am J Psychiatry* 157:148–49.

45. Hendrickson RG, Morocco AP. 2003. Quetiapine cross-reactivity among three tricyclic antidepressant immunoassays. *J Toxicol Clin Toxicol* 41:105–8.

46. Schussler JM, Juenke JM, Schussler I. 2003. Quetiapine and falsely elevated nortriptyline level. *Am J Psychiatry* 160:589.

47. Caravati EM, Juenke JM, Crouch BI, Anderson KT. 2005. Quetiapine cross-reactivity with plasma tricyclic antidepressant immunoassays. *Ann Pharmacother* 39:1446–49.

48. Ryder KW, Glick MR. 1986. The effect of thioridazine on the Automatic Clinical Analyzer serum tricyclic anti-depressant screen. *Am J Clin Pathol* 86:248–49.

49. Maynard GL, Soni P. 1996. Thioridazine interferences with imipramine metabolism and measurement. *Ther Drug Monit* 18:729–31.

50. Benitez J, Dahlqvist R, Gustafsson LL, Magnusson A, Sjoqvist F. 1986. Clinical pharmacological evaluation of an assay kit for intoxications with tricyclic antidepressants. *Ther Drug Monit* 8:102–5.

51. Sorisky A, Watson DC. 1986. Positive diphenhydramine interference in the EMIT-st assay for tricyclic antidepressants in serum. *Clin Chem* 32:715.

52. Wians FH, Jr., Norton JT, Wirebaugh SR. 1993. False-positive serum tricyclic antidepressant screen with cyproheptadine. *Clin Chem* 39:1355–56.

53. Yuan CM, Spandorfer PR, Miller SL, Henretig FM, Shaw LM. 2003. Evaluation of tricyclic antidepressant false positivity in a pediatric case of cyproheptadine (periactin) overdose. *Ther Drug Monit* 25:299–304.

54. Wong EC, Koenig J, Turk J. 1995. Potential interference of cyclobenzaprine and norcyclobenzaprine with HPLC measurement of amitriptyline and nortriptyline: resolution by GC-MS analysis. *J Anal Toxicol* 19:218–24.
55. Van Hoey NM. 2005. Effect of cyclobenzaprine on tricyclic antidepressant assays. *Ann Pharmacother* 39:1314–17.
56. Melanson SE, Lewandrowski EL, Griggs DA, Flood JG. 2007. Interpreting tricyclic antidepressant measurements in urine in an emergency department setting: comparison of two qualitative point-of-care urine tricyclic antidepressant drug immunoassays with quantitative serum chromatographic analysis. *J Anal Toxicol* 31:270–75.
57. Dasgupta A, Wells A, Datta P. 2007. False-positive serum tricyclic antidepressant concentrations using fluorescence polarization immunoassay due to the presence of hydroxyzine and cetirizine. *Ther Drug Monit* 29:134–39.

13 Pharmacokinetics and Therapeutic Drug Monitoring of Immunosuppressants

Kathleen A. Kelly and Anthony W. Butch
University of California at Los Angeles

CONTENTS

13.1 INTRODUCTION

It has now been more than 50 years since the first successful kidney transplant was performed between monozygotic twins [1]. At that time, the field of immunology was in its infancy and transplants between nonidentical twins ended in organ failure as a result of acute graft rejection. It was not until the introduction of azathioprine (a nucleotide analog less toxic than 6-mercaptopurine) in the early 1960s that chemical immunosuppression and prolonged kidney allograft survival became possible [2]. Azathioprine by itself was not potent enough to prevent acute graft rejection. However, the combination of azathioprine and corticosteroids was shown to provide effective chemical immunosuppression, with 1-year kidney allograft survival rates ranging from 40 to 50% [3]. This combination of chemical immunosuppression continued to be the cornerstone of transplant programs for the next 20 or so years until cyclosporine A (CsA) entered the transplantation arena in the late 1970s [4].

In the late 1980s, other immune cell modulators such as tacrolimus and sirolimus were discovered and added to the arsenal of chemical immunosuppressive agents [5,6]. Mycophenolic acid (MPA) (as the prodrug mycophenolate mofetil) became available in the mid 1990s based on reports from multicenter clinical trials demonstrating that it could further reduce the incidence of renal graft rejection when used in combination with CsA and steroids [7–9].

The number of solid organ transplants performed in the United States continues to increase each year (Table 13.1) [10]. There has been a 13% increase in kidney, a 18% increase in liver, a 2% increase in heart, and an overall increase of 13% over the last 5 years, when comparing organ transplants performed in 2006 with 2002 [10]. Sadly, the limiting factor in the number of transplanted organs is the availability of donor organs. There were more than 94,000 patients on the United States organ transplant waiting list at the end of 2006 [11]. The overall increase in transplanted organs from 2005 to 2006 was due to a 5% increase in the number of organs recovered from deceased donors.

The discovery that CsA had immunosuppressive activity that specifically targeted T lymphocytes was a major breakthrough in organ transplantation because it dramatically reduced acute graft rejection and improved long-term graft and patient survival [12,13]. The identification of other immunosuppressive drugs that modulate immune responses by additional molecular pathways enabled treatment options to evolve and has permitted combination therapies to be individualized based on patient requirements. Classes of immunosuppressive drugs, along with generic and brand

TABLE 13.1
Solid Organ Transplants in the United States

Organ Transplanted	Year				
	2002	2003	2004	2005	2006
Kidney	14,527	14,856	15,671	16,076	16,646
Liver	5061	5364	5780	6000	6136
Heart	2112	2026	1961	2062	2147
All organs[a]	24,552	25,083	26,539	27,530	28,291

[a] Includes pancreas, kidney-pancreas, intestine, lung, and heart-lung transplants.

TABLE 13.2

Immunosuppressive Drugs used in Solid Organ Transplantation

Drug Class	Generic Name	Brand Names
Corticosteroids	Prednisone	Orasone, Deltasone
	Methylprednisolone	Solu-Medrol, A-methaPred, Medrol
	Dexamethasone	Decadron
Antimetabolites	Azathioprine	Imuran
	Cyclophosphamide	Cytoxan, Neosar
	Mycophenolate mofetil	CellCept
	Mycophenolate sodium	Myfortic
Calcineurin inhibitors	Cyclosporine A	Sandimmune, Neoral, many generic
	Tacrolimus (FK-506)	forms of Cyclosporine A
		Prograf
mTOR inhibitors	Sirolimus (Rapamycin)	Rapamune
	Everolimus[a] (RAD0001)	Certican

[a] Everolimus is currently in phase III clinical trials in the United States and has not been approved by the FDA for use an immunosuppressive agent.

names currently approved by the United States Food and Drug Administration (FDA) for use in solid organ transplantation are listed in Table 13.2.

13.2 RATIONAL FOR MONITORING OF IMMUNOSUPPRESSANTS

A prerequisite for optimizing and individualizing immunosuppressive therapy is a reliable and precise method for monitoring drug concentrations. However, not all immunosuppressive drugs require routine monitoring of blood concentrations. For instance, corticosteroids are dosed based on empirical guidelines and are not routinely monitored. Although methods have been developed to measure blood concentrations of azathioprine [14–16], this antiproliferative agent is seldom monitored by transplant centers. Blood concentrations of CsA, tacrolimus, sirolimus, and MPA, are routinely monitored at transplant centers for the following reasons: [1] there is a clear relationship between drug concentration and clinical response; [2] these drugs have a narrow therapeutic index; [3] the drug levels exhibit a high degree of inter- and intrapatient variability; [4] the pharmacological response can be difficult to distinguish from unwanted side effects; [5] there is a risk of poor or noncompliance because the drugs are administered for the lifetime of the graft or patient; and [6] there are significant drug-drug interactions.

The potential for drug interactions is not limited to nonimmunosuppressive agents, but can also occur among the various classes of immunosuppressive drugs. For instance, CsA inhibits transport of a MPA metabolite from the liver into bile resulting in lower MPA concentrations when the two drugs are used together for immunosuppressive therapy [17,18]. The combination of CsA and sirolimus or tacrolimus and sirolimus results in increased blood concentrations of sirolimus [17,19]. The majority of kidney, liver and heart transplant patients receive tacrolimus and MPA, followed by CsA and MPA for immunosuppression, prior to hospital discharge [20]. Tacrolimus and sirolimus or CsA and sirolimus are less commonly used, and sirolimus and mycophenolate mofetil are the least common drugs used after discharge. All these drug regiments typically include corticosteroids [20]. This illustrates the widespread use of combination immunosuppression and the importance of therapeutic drug monitoring, given the potential for various drug interactions.

This chapter will focus primarily on FDA-approved immunosuppressive drugs routinely monitored by clinical laboratories supporting solid organ transplant programs. These include CsA, tacrolimus, sirolimus, and MPA. Everolimus will only be discussed briefly because it is not FDA-approved and is awaiting additional phase III clinical trials. Interestingly, everolimus, is approved in Europe and about 60 other countries as an immunosuppressive drug in organ transplantation. Other drugs that are not commonly monitored, such as corticosteroids, azathioprine and cyclophosphamide, will not be discussed further. Clinical pharmacokinetics, unwanted adverse effects and various drug interactions will be provided for each of the chemical immunosuppressive agents. A comprehensive review of analytical methods will also be provided, along with detailed information regarding limitations and potential sources of error associated with each of the testing methodologies.

13.3 CALCINEURIN INHIBITORS

The chemical structures of CsA and tacrolimus, calcineurin inhibitors commonly used in organ transplantation, are shown in Figure 13.1. The calcineurin inhibitors block the activation and proliferation of CD4+ and CD8+ T lymphocytes by inhibiting IL-2 production [21,22]. Under normal circumstances, binding of major histocompatibility complex-peptide complexes to T cell receptors result in the formation of an activated form of the calcium/calmodulin-dependent serine/threonine phosphatase calcineurin. This leads to de-phosphorylation of the nuclear factor of activated T cells (NF-AT) (among others) and nuclear translocation of NF-AT. Once in the nucleus, NF-AT binds genes encoding proinflammatory cytokines such as IL-2, resulting in up-regulated gene transcription and proliferation of CD4+ and CD8+ T lymphocytes [23]. CsA and tacrolimus freely cross lymphocyte membranes and form complexes with specific cytoplasmic binding proteins called immunophilins. CsA binds to the immunophilin, cyclophilin and tacrolimus binds to the immunophilin FK506-binding protein-12 [24,25]. The drug-immunophilin complexes inhibit calcineurin activity, which prevents nuclear translocation of NF-AT. The end result is down-regulated cytokine gene transcription that prevents the activation of CD4+ and CD8+ lymphocytes [26–28].

13.3.1 CYCLOSPORINE A (CsA)

CsA is a small cyclic polypeptide (molecular weight of 1204) that was originally isolated from fungal cultures of *Tolypocladium inflatum Gams* in 1970 [29]. It is currently approved in the United States as an immunosuppressive drug to prolong organ and patient survival in kidney, liver, heart, and bone marrow transplants. CsA is available for both oral and intravenous administration

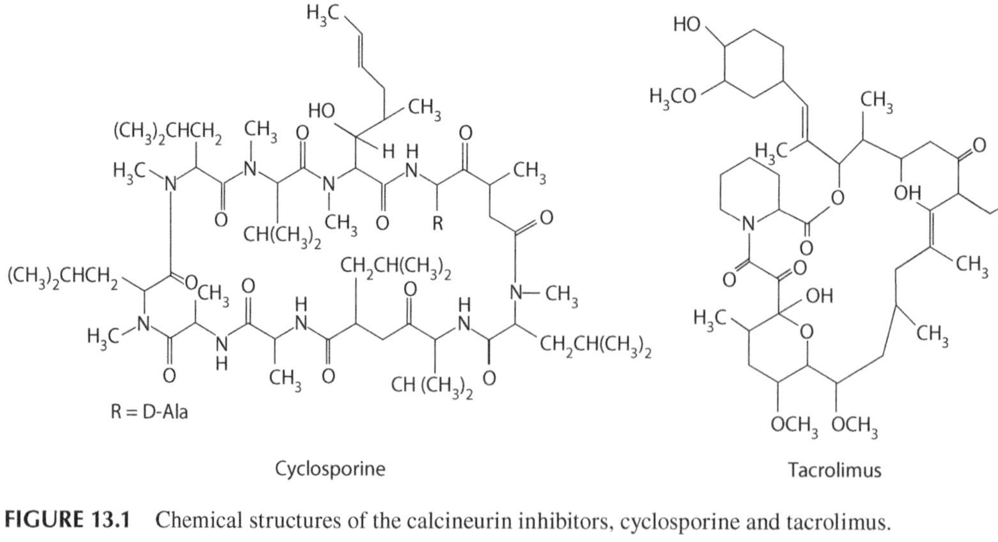

Cyclosporine   Tacrolimus

FIGURE 13.1   Chemical structures of the calcineurin inhibitors, cyclosporine and tacrolimus.

(Sandimmune). A microemulsion formulation of CsA, called Neoral, exhibiting more reproducible absorption characteristics is also available for oral administration [30]. In addition, several generic microemulsion formulations are now available and are often referred to as CsA modified [31,32].

13.3.1.1 Pharmacokinetics

Oral absorption of Sandimmune is low (5–30%) and highly variable, ranging from 4% to 89% in renal and liver transplant patients [33,34]. Absorption of the microemulsion formulation is more consistent, averaging ~40% [35]. Peak blood concentrations typically occur between 1–3 hours and 2–6 hours following oral administration of Neoral and Sandimmune, respectively [33,36,37]. Absorption can be delayed for several hours in a subgroup of patients. Because CsA is lipophilic, it crosses most biologic membranes and has a wide tissue distribution [38]. CsA is highly bound to plasma proteins (>90% to lipoproteins), with the majority of CsA located within erythrocytes. The distribution of CsA between plasma and erythrocytes is temperature-dependent and varies with changes in hematocrit [39]. Because of the potential for artifactual redistribution of CsA during specimen processing due to ambient temperature fluctuations, EDTA-anticoagulated whole blood should be used to measure CsA concentrations [40–42].

CsA is extensively metabolized by cytochrome P450 enzymes (CYP3A isoenzymes) located in the small intestine and liver [43]. There is also a cellular transporter of immunosuppressive drugs, called P-glycoprotein that influences metabolism by regulating CsA bioavailability. P-glycoprotein pumps some of the CsA out of enterocytes back into the lumen of the gut [44,45]. This efflux pump probably contributes to the poor absorption rates observed after oral administration of CsA. CYP3A isoenzymes and P-glycoprotein genetic polymorphisms can also influence the oral bioavailability of CsA and are probably involved in the delayed absorption that has been noted in some patients [44]. CsA is oxidized or N-demethylated to more than 30 metabolites [46,47]. Most of the metabolites do not possess immunosuppressive activity and are not clinically significant [48]. However, there is growing evidence indicating that a few of the inactive metabolites may contribute to CsA toxicity [48]. Two of the hydroxylated metabolites, AM1 and AM9 exhibit 10–20% of the immunosuppressive activity of the parent compound [49,50] and can account for as much as 33% of the whole blood CsA concentration [51]. The major route of CsA elimination is biliary excretion into the feces. As expected, dosage adjustments are necessary in patients with hepatic dysfunction. Only a small fraction (6%) of CsA and metabolites appear in the urine [36], making dosage adjustments unnecessary in patients with renal insufficiency.

13.3.1.2 Adverse Effects

Serious side effects related to CsA treatment are concentration-dependent and include nephrotoxicity, neurotoxicity, hepatotoxicity, hirsutism, hypertrichosis, gingival hypertrophy, glucose intolerance, hypertension, hyperlipidemia, hypomagnesemia, hyperuricemia, and hypokalemia. In general, over suppression leads to an increased risk for viral infections and lymphoproliferative disease, especially in children [52].

13.3.1.3 Drug-interactions

Numerous drugs influence the absorption and metabolism of CsA. Any drug that inhibits the cytochrome P450 system or the P-glycoprotein efflux pump increases blood CsA concentrations due to decreased metabolism and increased absorption. Drugs having the opposite effect (P450 and/or P-glycoprotein inducers) produce decreased CsA concentrations. Drugs causing increased CsA blood concentrations include calcium channel blockers, several antifungal agents, and the antibiotic erythromycin. Several anticonvulsants and antibiotics, including antituberculosis agents reduce blood CsA concentrations. In addition, there are many other drugs that synergize with CsA and potentiate nephrotoxicity. There are several excellent reviews that discuss specific drug interactions with CsA [53,54]. Not all of the interactions are caused by pharmaceuticals since various foods and herbal remedies can influence CsA concentrations. For instance, grapefruit juice increases CsA blood concentrations by increasing absorption whereas St John's Wort decreases CsA concentrations by increasing metabolism [55].

13.3.1.4 Preanalytic Variables

Whole blood anticoagulated with EDTA is the recommended sample type based on numerous consensus documents [40–42]. EDTA whole blood is stable at least 11 days at room temperature or higher temperatures (37°C) [56]. For long-term storage, whole blood samples should be placed at –20°C and are stable at least 3 years [57]. As previously mentioned, CsA should only be measured in whole blood samples. Plasma is not acceptable because partitioning of CsA between plasma and erythrocytes is a temperature and time-dependent process that can be altered during in vitro specimen processing [41]. In addition, plasma CsA concentrations are two-fold lower than whole blood concentrations and results in poor analytical precision at low plasma CsA concentrations.

The timing of specimen collection has always been right before administration of the next dose (i.e., trough levels) [40,41]. For standardization purposes, the timing should be within one-hour before the next dose [42]. The introduction of Neoral in 1995, a microemulsion CsA formulation with more predictable absorption kinetics has resulted in higher peak concentrations and increased drug exposure, based on area under the concentration time curves [58]. The highest and most variable CsA concentrations typically occur within the first four hours after Neoral dosing [59]. However, similar trough concentrations are observed for both the conventional and microemulsion CsA formulations, demonstrating that trough concentrations are not predictive of total drug exposure [60–62]. Increased exposure to CsA using Neoral results in decreased rejection rates with slightly higher serum creatinine concentrations, compared with conventional CsA therapy [58,63,64]. Thus, a better predictor of immunosuppressive efficacy was needed when administering Neoral. Pharmacokinetic and pharmacodynamic studies demonstrated that maximal inhibition of calcineurin and IL-2 production is correlated with the highest CsA concentrations 1–2 hours after dosing [59,65], indicating that drug levels shortly after dosing may be a better predictor of total drug exposure and clinical outcome [66]. Because multiple time points after dosing are not practical in a clinical setting, different time points were examined and CsA concentrations 2 hours after dosing (called C2 monitoring) was shown to correlate best with total drug exposure and improved clinical outcomes [67–70]. These finding have resulted in C2 monitoring of CsA becoming standard practice at many transplant centers. However the clinical benefits of C2 monitoring has recently been challenged by meta-analysis of ten randomized clinical trials comparing trough CsA levels with C2 monitoring in renal, hepatic and cardiac transplant recipients [71]. This study found that C2 monitoring did not result in a significant improvement in long-term organ survival suggesting that single point monitoring (either trough or C2 monitoring) may not be appropriate for all transplant recipients due to delayed or inadequate absorption of CsA [71].

C2 monitoring creates various nursing and phlebotomy challenges because blood samples have to be drawn very close to the two-hour time point after dosing, ideally 10 minutes on either side of the 2-hour mark [72]. At the authors' institution, C2 testing is performed on 18% of all whole blood samples (annual volume ~11,400) received in the laboratory for CsA testing. To avoid confusion and prevent testing delays due to the need for sample dilution of C2 specimens, our laboratory has created a separate test for C2 monitoring and reports all CsA C2 results in µg/mL to avoid misinterpreting C2 results as tough levels. We still report CsA trough results in ng/mL.

13.3.1.5 Methods of Analysis

Monitoring of CsA is critical for optimizing immunosuppression and organ survival while minimizing unwanted toxic side effects. Improvements in immunosuppressive regiments, along with demands for narrower and tighter control of CsA blood levels have placed greater demand on clinical laboratories to provide timely and reliable drug concentrations. There are many methods currently available to measure CsA. Factors that need to be considered when selecting a CsA assay include metabolite cross-reactivity, cost of instrumentation and reagents, ease of operation, level of technical expertise required to perform testing, test volume, expected turn-around times, and the familiarity of the transplant physicians with various assays. For example, turnaround times can be a critical issue in an outpatient setting when it is desirable to have CsA test results available when patients are being seen by their physicians. Depending on the institution, this may require 2–4 hour turnaround times for anywhere from ten to 50 specimens that have been drawn a few hours before the scheduled clinic visit.

CsA can be measured by radioimmunoassay (RIA), semiautomated and automated nonisotopic immunoassays, and high performance liquid chromatography (HPLC) with ultra-violet detector (HPLC-UV) or mass spectrometric detection systems (HPLC-MS). There are five different nonisotopic CsA assays manufactured by three companies that are used by the majority of laboratories in the United States (Table 13.3). None of the individual RIAs, including the Cyclo-Trac SP assay from Diasorin (Stillwater, MN), are used by more than ten laboratories. RIAs are not popular because of the manual format and/or need to handle radioisotopes. The Abbott polyclonal fluorescence polarization immunoassay (FPIA; Abbott Park, IL) is also not used by many laboratories because of extensive metabolite cross-reactivity. Interestingly, the Abbott monoclonal FPIA is used by >60% of all laboratories. This is somewhat surprising because the Abbott monoclonal FPIA has considerable cross-reactivity with CsA metabolites and recommendations by numerous consensus panels specify that the analytical method should be specific for parent compound [40–42]. HPLC methods to measure CsA are specific for parent compound and are considered the comparative method or "gold standard" for CsA quantitation. However, HPLC methods are used by only 10% of all laboratories and are primarily restricted to larger transplant centers. The lack of widespread acceptance of HPLC methods to measure CsA may reflect high initial equipment costs for MS detection systems and the need for specialized training. HPLC systems with UV detection are considerably less expensive and easier to operate, but can suffer from a wide variety of chemical interferences depending on the specific protocol utilized. There are several excellent protocols to measure CsA using HPLC-MS and HPLC-MS/MS systems [73,74]. In addition, simultaneous measurement of two or more immunosuppressive drugs in individual samples can be performed by HPLC-MS because sample requirements are the same for many of the immunosuppressants (CsA, tacrolimus, sirolimus, everolimus) [75].

All of the immunoassays, with the exception of the Dimension antibody conjugated magnetic immunoassay (ACMIA; Siemens Healthcare Diagnostics Inc., Deerfield, IL) are semiautomated

TABLE 13.3
Currently used Methods to Measure Whole Blood Concentrations of CsA

Method	Assay	Manufacturer	Labs using Assay (%)[a]
RIA immunoassay	Cyclo-Trac SP	DiaSorin	≤1
Semiautomated	Polyclonal FPIA	Abbott	1
	Monoclonal FPIA	Abbott	62
	CEDIA PLUS	Microgenics	9
	Syva EMIT 2000	Siemens	6
Automated	Dimension ACMIA	Siemens	11
HPLC-UV			2
HPLC-MS			8

Notes: RIA, radioimmunoassay; FPIA, fluorescence polarization immunoassay; CEDIA, cloned enzyme donor immunoassay; EMIT, enzyme-multiplied immunoassay technique; ACMIA, antibody conjugated magnetic immunoassay; HPLC-UV, high performance liquid chromatography with ultraviolet detection; HPLC-MS, high performance liquid chromatography with mass spectrometry detection.

[a] Percentages are based on the College of American Pathologists Immunosuppressive Drug Monitoring First survey of 2008.

because they require a whole blood pretreatment step. This typically involves preparing a whole blood hemolysate by adding an extraction reagent such as methanol to an aliquot of whole blood. The hemolysate is then centrifuged and the separated supernatant is either analyzed by the FPIA or Syva enzyme-multiplied immunoassay (EMIT) (Siemens). The cloned enzyme donor immunoassay (CEDIA) PLUS (Microgenics Corp., Fremont, CA) pretreatment step is simpler and does not require centrifugation after adding the extraction reagent. The Dimension ACMIA (Siemens) does not require any sample pretreatment allowing whole blood samples to be placed directly on the instrument. Instruments that currently have applications for the various CsA immunoassays are provided in Table 13.4. In addition, Siemens has developed a CsA assay with a simplified pretreatment step using direct chemiluminescence technology for use on the ADVIA Centaur [76]. Abbott has also developed a chemiluminescent microparticle immunoassay (CMIA) for measuring CsA on the Architect family of instruments [77].

13.3.1.6 Metabolite Cross-Reactivity

The Abbott polyclonal antibody-based FPIA is nonspecific and has extensive cross-reactivity with CsA metabolites. Its use has been declining over the years as immunoassays with less metabolite cross-reactivity have been developed. CsA results using the Abbott polyclonal FPIA are approximately four-times higher than those obtained by HPLC methods [78]. Because of the magnitude of metabolite cross-reactivity and the poor correlation with clinical outcomes and toxicity, the use of this polyclonal assay should be discouraged. Cross-reactivity of the monoclonal immunoassays with CsA metabolites is shown in Table 13.5. The Dimension ACMIA has the least overall metabolite cross-reactivity whereas the monoclonal FPIA and CEDIA PLUS are reported to have the highest overall metabolite cross-reactivity. AM1 and AM9 are typically present in the highest concentrations after transplantation [51] and cross-reacts the least in the Dimension ACMIA and Syva EMIT, but the most in the monoclonal FPIA (Table 13.5). The magnitude of metabolite cross-reactivity contributes to the degree of CsA overestimation when comparing immunoassays with HPLC. Mean CsA concentrations have been found to be approximately 12%, 13%, 17%, 22%, and 40% higher than HPLC when measured by the Dimension ACMIA, Syva EMIT, CEDIA PLUS, FPIA on the TDx, and FPIA on the AxSYM, respectively [79–83]. Thus, it is important to consider metabolite cross-reactivity and the degree of CsA overestimation when selecting the "right" CsA immunoassay to support a solid organ transplant program.

TABLE 13.4
Instrument Applications for CsA Immunoassays

Immunoassay	Instrument Application	Manufacturer
Monoclonal FPIA	TDx, AxSYM	Abbott Laboratories
CEDIA PLUS	MGC240	Microgenics Corp.
	SYNCHRON LX, UniCel Dx	Beckman Coulter
	Hitachi 902, 911, 912, 917, Modular P	Roche Diagnostics
	AU 400, 640, 2700, 5400	Olympus America
	Aeroset	Abbott Laboratories
Syva EMIT 2000	COBAS Mira[a], INTEGRA 400, 800	Roche Diagnostics
	Dimension RxL Max, Xpand, Xpand Plus, V-Twin, Viva, Viva-E	Siemens Healthcare
Dimension ACMIA	Dimension ExL, RxL Max, Xpand,	Siemens Healthcare
	Xpand Plus, Vista 1500, V-twin, Viva, Viva-E	
RIA	Cyclo-Trac SP	Diasorin

Notes: FPIA, fluorescence polarization immunoassay; CEDIA, cloned enzyme donor immunoassay; EMIT, enzyme-multiplied immunoassay technique; ACMIA, antibody conjugated magnetic immunoassay; RIA, radioimmunoassay.

[a] This instrument is no longer manufactured or supported by the company.

TABLE 13.5
CsA Metabolite Cross-Reactivity of Immunoassays

	% CsA Metabolite Cross-Reactivity[a]			
Immunoassay	AM1	AM4n	AM9	AM19
Monoclonal FPIA	6–12	≤6	14–27	≤4
CEDIA PLUS	8	30	18	2
Syva EMIT 2000	≤5	8–13	≤4	0
Dimension ACMIA	0	4	0	0

Notes: FPIA, fluorescence polarization immunoassay; CEDIA, cloned enzyme donor immunoassay; EMIT, enzyme-multiplied immunoassay technique; ACMIA, antibody conjugated magnetic immunoassay.

[a] Each metabolite was evaluated at 1000 µg/L except AMI, which was tested at 500 µg/L in the CEDIA PLUS assay. Data are derived from References 79–83.

13.3.1.7 Analytical Considerations

Consensus conference recommendations for CsA immunoassays are that the slope of the line should be 1.0 ± 0.1, with a y-intercept and $S_{y/x} \leq 15$ µg/L, when compared with HPLC [41]. None of the current immunoassays satisfy all three requirements [78–83]. For instance, the Dimension ACMIA satisfies the slope and intercept requirements but exceeds the $S_{y/x}$ limit, while the CEDIA PLUS and Syva EMIT satisfies only one requirement. The FPIA fails to satisfy any of the requirements. Between-day precision recommendations require a CV of $\leq 10\%$ at a CsA concentration of 50 µg/L and a CV of $\leq 5\%$ at 300 µg/L [41,42]. Most of the immunoassays satisfy the precision recommendation at 300 µg/L, but it is important that each laboratory determine between-day precision studies at CsA concentrations of 50 µg/L. This is particularly important since recent immunosuppressive drug regiments are designed to reduce CsA trough concentrations in order to minimize toxicity. Another potential problem is bias due to incorrect assay calibration. Results from the September 2008 International Proficiency Testing Scheme reveal that the FPIA (TDx) and CEDIA PLUS overestimate CsA concentrations by 2–7%, whereas the Syva EMIT and Dimension ACMIA underestimate CsA by 3–11% at a target concentration of 150 µg/L [84]. Lastly, for assays involving a manual extraction step, poor technique can significantly contribute to the overall imprecision of the assay. Careful attention to detail and good technique can minimize variations at this important preanalytical step. This holds true for all whole blood immunosuppressive drug assays requiring a manual extraction step (tacrolimus, sirolimus, everolimus).

13.3.1.8 C2 Monitoring and Specimen Dilution

Therapeutic ranges for CsA are often organ-specific and can vary widely between transplant centers. They also differ based on various immunosuppressive drug combinations, the time after transplant, and during periods of toxicity and organ rejection. Trough whole blood CsA levels following kidney transplants are typically between 125 and 350 µg/L shortly after transplant and are tapered down to <150 µg/L during maintenance therapy. Recommended levels after liver and heart transplants are 120–325 µg/L shortly after transplant and <150 µg/L during maintenance therapy. These target ranges were determined by HPLC and will vary considerably when measured by immunoassay, depending on metabolite cross-reactivity.

For C2 monitoring, target concentrations vary between 600 and 1700 µg/L depending on the type of graft and the time after transplantation [66]. C2 concentrations often exceed the analytical range of most immunoassays since typical calibration curves are designed to measure trough CsA levels. The FPIA and Syva EMIT have analytical ranges up to 1500 and 500 µg/L, respectively. The CEDIA PLUS and Dimension ACMIA have separate calibration curves for C2 monitoring, with an analytical range from 450–2000 to 350–2000 µg/L, respectively. However, 28% of labs using the

CEDIA PLUS reported using only the low-range calibration curve and would have to dilute samples above 450 μg/L [85]. Sample dilution can also lead to major inaccuracies in test results and dilution protocols need to be carefully validated before implementation [85,86]. This is because CsA metabolites may not dilute in a linear fashion and there may be differences in the amount of time needed for diluted samples to re-equilibrate, depending on the immunoassay and dilution protocol. Proficiency testing programs have demonstrated that laboratories produce widely varying results when challenged with samples with CsA concentrations outside the analytical range of immunoassays. For instance, at a CsA concentration of 2000 μg/L, 125 laboratories reported CsA values ranging from 1082 to 3862 μg/L [86]. These findings indicate that laboratories need to develop carefully validated dilution protocols. A validated dilution protocol for the monoclonal FPIA on the TDx has been described [87].

Another concern with C2 monitoring is metabolite concentrations and the need for therapeutic ranges that are assay-specific. This is clearly necessary when measuring trough CsA concentrations. A recent study monitoring C2 concentrations in kidney and liver transplant patients obtained similar CsA concentrations when C2 samples were measured by the FPIA, CEDIA PLUS, and Syva EMIT [88]. In contrast, there were widely different CsA concentrations when the paired trough samples were measured by the same immunoassays. These data indicate that for C2 monitoring, assay-specific therapeutic ranges may not be necessary.

13.3.2   TACROLIMUS

Tacrolimus (also known as FK-506) is a macrolide antibiotic with a molecular weight of 822 (Figure 13.1) that was originally isolated from the fungus *Streptomyces tsukubaensis* [5]. In the United States, tacrolimus (brand name Prograf) was approved for use in liver and kidney transplantation in 1994 and 1997, respectively. Tacrolimus is ~100 times more potent than CsA and is associated with a decrease in acute and chronic rejection, and better long-term graft survival [89]. At the authors' institution, ~four times more tacrolimus tests are performed compared with CsA.

13.3.2.1   Pharmacokinetics

Tacrolimus is available for both oral and intravenous administration. Similar to CsA, oral absorption of tacrolimus from the gut is poor and highly variable, averaging 25% [90]. Peak blood concentrations occur within 1.5–4 hours. Tacrolimus is primarily bound to albumin, α_1-acid glycoprotein and lipoproteins in the plasma. However, the majority of tacrolimus is found within erythrocytes [91]. Tacrolimus is metabolized by cytochrome P450 isoenzymes (CYP3A) located in the small intestine and liver. Similar to CsA, the bioavailability of tacrolimus is influenced by CYP3A and the mutidrug efflux pump (P-glycoprotein) located in intestinal enterocytes. Biotransformation of tacrolimus occurs by demethylation, hydroxylation and oxidative reactions [92]. At least nine metabolites have been identified based on in vitro studies [93], and all, with the exception of 31-*O*-demethyl tacrolimus (M-II) have very little immunosuppressive activity. M-II has been shown in vitro to have the same immunosuppressive activity as parent compound [94]. Metabolites represent 10–20% of whole blood tacrolimus concentrations [95]. Tacrolimus is eliminated primarily by biliary excretion into the feces. Patients with hepatic dysfunction require dosage adjustments. Very little tacrolimus is found in urine and blood concentrations are not altered in renal dysfunction.

13.3.2.2   Adverse Effects

Tacrolimus shares many dose-dependent side effects with CsA [96]. These include nephrotoxicity, neurotoxicity, hepatotoxicity, hypertension and glucose intolerance. Nephrotoxicity with tacrolimus may be less of a problem than with CsA, especially in renal transplantation [97]. Diabetogenesis is approximately three times more common with tacrolimus than CsA [98]. Hyperkalemia, hyperuricemia, hyperlipidemia, hirsutism, and gingival hypertrophy are also observed following tacrolimus use, but less commonly than with CsA [99]. Alopecia is also associated with tacrolimus use [94].

13.3.2.3 Drug-Interactions

Because tacrolimus is metabolized mainly by the cytochrome P450 system, the majority of drug-interactions described for CsA also apply to tacrolimus [90]. St John's Wort also decreases blood tacrolimus concentrations.

13.3.2.4 Preanalytic Variables

For quantitation of tacrolimus, EDTA anticoagulated whole blood is the specimen of choice for the same reasons provided for CsA. Whole blood samples are stable for one week when shipped by mail without coolant [100,101], 1–2 weeks at room temperature [101,102], 2 weeks at refrigerator temperatures [102], and almost 1 year at –70°C [102]. Trough blood tacrolimus concentrations are almost exclusively used for routine monitoring and are believed to be a good indicator of total drug exposure [103]. However, recent experience with CsA has challenged this notion, and alternative draw times 1–6 hours after dosing have been proposed [104]. While some investigators have found a poor correlation between trough tacrolimus concentrations and total drug exposure, others have found good correlation [105,106]. Overall, the findings suggest that trough tacrolimus concentrations are predictive of total drug exposure and that measuring tacrolimus at specified times after dosing may not result in dramatic improvements. Until this issue is fully resolved, trough levels will continue to be used for reasons of convenience and reproducibility.

13.3.2.5 Methods of Analysis

Monitoring of tacrolimus is an integral part of any organ transplant program because of variable dose-to-blood concentrations and the narrow therapeutic index. Tacrolimus can be measured by enzyme-linked immunosorbent assay (ELISA), semiautomated and automated immunoassay, and HPLC-MS (Table 13.6). The ELISA and semiautomated immunoassays require a manual whole blood pretreatment step. The Dimension ACMIA does not require a pretreatment step allowing whole blood samples to be directly placed on the instrument. Sample extraction can be semiautomated using modern HPLC-MS systems [107]. The ELISA takes about 4 hours to complete, requires numerous manual steps, and is used by <10 clinical laboratories in the United States. The Abbott microparticle enzyme immunoassay (MEIA) II on the IMx instrument is currently used by more than 70% of the laboratories participating in the immunosuppressive proficiency testing program (Table 13.6). The MEIA II has a reported detection limit of 2 μg/L and replaced an earlier version (MEIA I) with a detection limit of 5 μg/L. A fully automated

---

TABLE 13.6

Analytical Methods to Measure whole Blood Concentrations of Tacrolimus

Method	Assay	Manufacturer	Labs using Method (%)[a]
ELISA	Pro-Trac II	DiaSorin	<1
Immunoassay			2
Semiautomated	MEIA II	Abbott	73
	Syva EMIT	Siemens	2
	CEDIA	Microgenics	<1
Automated	Dimension ACMIA	Siemens	13
HPLC-MS			11

Notes: ELISA, enzyme-linked immunosorbent assay; MEIA, microparticle enzyme immunoassay; EMIT, enzyme-multiplied immunoassay technique; CEDIA, cloned enzyme donor immunoassay; ACMIA, antibody conjugated magnetic immunoassay; HPLC-MS, high performance liquid chromatography with mass spectrometry detection.

[a] Percentages are based on the College of American Pathologists Immunosuppressive Drugs Monitoring First Survey of 2008.

TABLE 13.7
Instrument Applications for Tacrolimus Immunoassays

Immunoassay	Instrument Application	Manufacturer
ELISA	Pro-Trac II	Diasorin
CMIA	Architect i1000$_{SR}$/i2000$_{SR}$	Abbott Laboratories
MEIA	IMx	Abbott Laboratories
CEDIA PLUS	Hitachi 911, 912, 917, Modular P	Roche Diagnostics
Dimension ACMIA	Dimension ExL, RxL Max,	Dade Behring

Notes: ELISA, enzyme-linked immunosorbent assay; CMIA, chemiluminescent microparticle immunoassay; MEIA, microparticle enzyme immunoassay; CEDIA, cloned enzyme donor immunoassay; ACMIA, antibody conjugated magnetic immunoassay.

Dimension ACMIA has been available since 2006 and is the second most popular immunoassay after the MEIA II method. The Syva EMIT for tacrolimus has recently received FDA approval and is used by only 2% of laboratories. The Microgenics CEDIA for tacrolimus is also not widely used, despite being available on several Roche instruments. Instrument applications for tacrolimus immunoassays are shown in Table 13.7.

HPLC-MS methods are used by the majority of laboratories not using the MEIA II or Dimension ACMIA. Tacrolimus cannot be measured by HPLC-UV because the molecule does not possess a chromophore. It is noteworthy that HPLC-MS is the only method that is specific for parent drug and meets the recommendations set forth in Consensus documents [42]. There are numerous protocols to quantitate tacrolimus by HPLC-MS or HPLC-MS/MS with detection limits <0.5 ng/mL [107,108]. A major advantage of HPLC-MS over immunoassays is the ability to simultaneously measure other immunosuppressant drugs in the same whole blood sample, such as CsA, sirolimus and everolimus [109].

13.3.2.6   Metabolite Cross-Reactivity

All of the immunoassays have significant cross-reactivity with tacrolimus metabolites. The ELISA, MEIA II and EMIT cross-react with M-II (31-*O*-demethyl), M-III (15-*O*-demethyl) and M-V (15,13-di-*O*-demethyl) metabolites of tacrolimus [110]. The CEDIA has significant cross-reactivity with M-I (13-*O*-demethyl), but does not cross react with M-II or M-III. Cross-reactivity of the CEDIA with M-V has not been examined [111]. The ACMIA is expected to have metabolite cross-reactivity similar to the EMIT since both assays use the same monoclonal antibody. The extent of positive bias due to metabolite cross-reactivity is dependent on the transplant group studied. Metabolite cross-reactivity in patients with good liver function is typically not a problem because metabolite concentrations are relatively low compared to parent drug [112]. However, metabolites tend to accumulate during reduced liver function and immediately after liver transplant, resulting in significant assay interference and falsely high blood tacrolimus concentrations [113]. Overall, the MEIA II produces tacrolimus results that are 15–20% higher, the EMIT produces results 17% higher, and the CEDIA produces results 19% higher than those obtained by HPLC-MS, in kidney and liver transplant patients [110,111,114–116]. Calibration error may also contribute to some of the overall positive bias.

13.3.2.7   Analytical Considerations

The recommended therapeutic range for whole blood tacrolimus concentrations after kidney and liver allograft transplants is 5–20 µg/L when measured by HPLC-MS [117]. When tacrolimus is used with other immunosuppressive agents such as sirolimus, the desired target concentration for tacrolimus can be considerably reduced to <5 µg/L. In view of this, it is important for each laboratory to determine performance characteristics of their tacrolimus assay at concentrations <5 µg/L and make transplant services aware of the lower limit of detection and the imprecision (%CV) at this

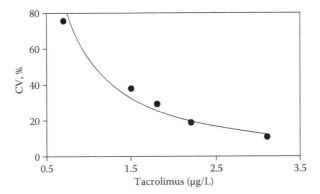

FIGURE 13.2   Functional sensitivity of the Abbott tacrolimus MEIA II on the IMx instrument. Whole blood patient pools at varying tacrolimus concentrations were analyzed in duplicate on ten separate days. The coefficient of variation (CV) is the standard deviation of the mean tacrolimus concentration divided by the mean. The value is multiplied by 100 and is expressed as a percentage (%).

concentration. The functional sensitivity (between-day CV $<20\%$) of the MEIA II and CEDIA are reported to be around 2 µg/L [110,115,118,119], whereas the detection limit of the EMIT is around 3 µg/L [114]. At our institution we examined functional sensitivity of the MEIA II tacrolimus assay by measuring whole blood pools at various concentrations in duplicate during a 10-day period. As shown in Figure 13.2, a 20% CV was observed at a tacrolimus concentration of ~2 µg/L. In addition, we found that the MEIA II produced tacrolimus concentrations ranging from 0.8 to 1.7 µg/L when testing samples from patients not receiving tacrolimus (n=8). Homma et al., also found false positive results when measuring tacrolimus in whole blood samples from patients not receiving tacrolimus using the MEIA II [120]. Based on our data, we use a cutoff of 2 µg/L for tacrolimus, and report lower values as <2 µg/L. The Abbott CMIA for tacrolimus has recently been approved for use in the United States and preliminary studies have demonstrated improved precision at low tacrolimus concentrations, with a CV of 20% at a concentration of 0.8 µg/L [121].

The MEIA II has been shown to produce falsely elevated tacrolimus concentrations when the hematocrit is $<25\%$ [122,123]. The EMIT for tacrolimus is not affected by changes in hematocrit values [123]. Hematocrit bias in the MEIA II could result in therapeutic tacrolimus blood concentrations in under-immunosuppressed patients due to low hematocrit values. This would potentially be most problematic shortly after transplant when hematocrit values are typically at their lowest concentrations. This tacrolimus bias could also make it difficult to appropriately dose patients with widely fluctuating hematocrit values.

The reliability of the MEIA II at low whole blood tacrolimus concentrations has recently been questioned. At tacrolimus concentrations <9 µg/L, the MEIA II exhibited greater between-day imprecision and a weaker correlation with results obtained by HPLC-MS/MS [124]. Recovery experiments also demonstrated that the degree of over-estimation of tacrolimus using the MEIA II was more pronounced at lower drug concentrations [124] Poor precision at low tacrolimus concentrations was also noted in the College of American Pathologists longitudinal immunosuppressive drug study. The study found that the major source of imprecision was within-lab variation over time and it was postulated that the variation might be due to changes in assay standardization or reagent lot-to-lot changes [125]. Taken together, these performance variables are important to consider when selecting a whole blood tacrolimus immunoassay.

13.4   MAMMALIAN TARGET OF RAPAMYCIN (mTOR) INHIBITORS

The chemical structures of the mTOR inhibitors, sirolimus and everolimus are shown in Figure 13.3. Both are macrocyclic lactones. Sirolimus (also known as rapamycin) is a lipophilic molecule

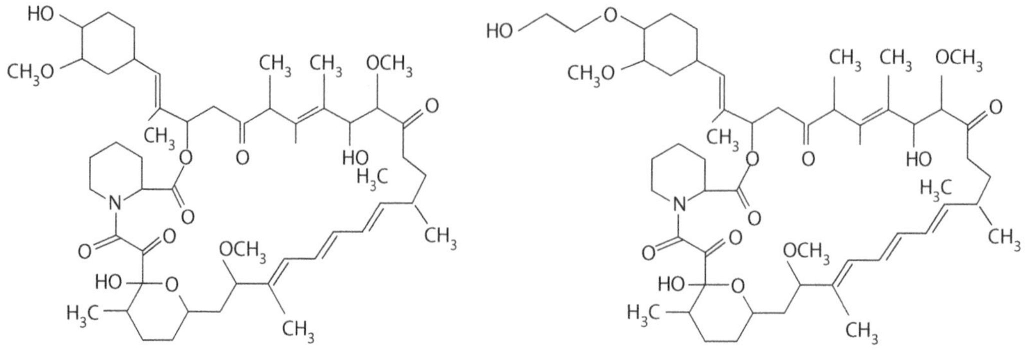

FIGURE 13.3   Chemical structures of the mammalian target of rapamycin (mTOR) inhibitors, sirolimus and everolimus.

(molecular weight of 914) derived from *Streptomyces hygroscopicus*. This actinomycete fermentation product was identified in the early 1970s and was approved by the FDA in 1999 for use with CsA to reduce the incidence of acute rejection in renal transplantation [126]. Everolimus is a chemically modified version that is more hydrophilic than sirolimus, and has improved pharmacokinetic characteristics and improved bioavailability [127]. Everolimus is still in phase III trials and is only available for investigational use in the United States.

Sirolimus and everolimus readily cross the lymphocyte plasma membrane and bind to the intracellular immunophilin, FK506 binding protein-12 [128]. In contrast to tacrolimus, sirolimus-immunophilin and everolimus-immunophilin complexes do not inhibit calcineurin activity. Instead, the complexes are highly specific inhibitors of the mammalian target of rapamycin (mTOR), a cell cycle serine/threonine kinase involved in the protein kinase B signaling pathway. This results in suppressed cytokine-induced T lymphocyte proliferation, with a block in progression from the G1 to S phase of the cell cycle [129]. The mTOR inhibitors synergize with calcineurin inhibitors to produce a profound immunosuppressive effect on T lymphocytes.

13.4.1   SIROLIMUS

13.4.1.1   Pharmacokinetics

Sirolimus is available for both oral and intravenous administration. The long half-life of ~60 hours allows once a day dosing [130]. Sirolimus is rapidly absorbed from the gastrointestinal tract and peak blood concentrations occur two hours after an oral dose [131]. Oral bioavailability is low, ranging from 5 to 15% [132] and is considerably reduced (~five-fold) when administered within four hours or concomitantly with CsA [133]. There is considerable interpatient variability in total drug exposure that can vary by as much as 50% [133]. Sirolimus is primarily found within erythrocytes (96%), with approximately 3% and 1% partitioning into the plasma and lymphocytes/granulocytes, respectively [134]. Almost all of the plasma sirolimus is bound to proteins, with lipoproteins being the major binding protein. Similar to the calcineurin inhibitors, sirolimus is metabolized in the intestine and liver by cytochrome P450 enzymes (CYP3A) [135]. The multidrug efflux pump P-glycoprotein in the gastrointestinal tract also controls metabolism by regulating bioavailability. Sirolimus is hydroxylated and demethylated to more than seven metabolites with the hydroxyl forms being the most abundant [136]. Metabolites represent approximately 55% of whole blood sirolimus levels [136]. The biologic activity of metabolites has not been fully investigated because the metabolites are difficult to isolate. However, preliminary studies indicate that the immunosuppressive activity of metabolites is <30% of that observed for the parent compound [137]. Sirolimus is eliminated primarily by biliary and fecal pathways, with small quantities appearing in urine [135]. As with the calcineurin inhibitors, dosage adjustments are needed in patients with hepatic dysfunction.

13.4.1.2 Adverse Effects

The incidence of adverse effects is dose related and includes metabolic, hematological, and dermatological effects [138]. Metabolic side effects include hypercholesterolemia, hyper- and hypokalemia, hypophosphatemia, hyperlipidema, and increased liver function tests. Anemia can be problematic, with decreases in leukocyte, erythrocytes, and platelet counts being common. Skin rashes, acne and mouth ulcers are also observed in patients being switched to mTOR inhibitors. As with other immunosuppressive drugs, there is an increased risk of infection and an association with lymphoma development. Interstitial pneumonitis can also occur with sirolimus therapy [139].

13.4.1.3 Drug-Interactions

CYP3A inhibitors such as antifungal agents (itraconazole, ketoconazole), clarithromycin, erythromycin, and verapamil increase blood levels of sirolimus. CYP3A inducers such as carbamazepine, phenobarbital, phenytoin, and rapamycin may decrease sirolimus blood levels. Grapefruit juice can increase sirolimus by decreasing drug clearance. St John's Wort can decrease sirolimus levels. As previously noted, the concomitant use of CsA can result in increased sirolimus concentrations [140]. Although tacrolimus and sirolimus compete for sites on the same binding protein, the two drugs do not appear to have significant drug–drug interactions in clinical practice [106].

13.4.1.4 Preanalytic Variables

EDTA anticoagulated whole blood is the recommended specimen matrix [132]. This is because almost all of the sirolimus (~95%) is concentrated in erythrocytes and plasma levels are too low for most analytical methods [134]. Whole blood samples are stable for 10 days at ambient temperature [141], at least 1 week at 30–34°C [141,142], 30 days at 4°C [143] and at least two months at –40°C [143]. Whole blood samples can withstand three freeze-thaw cycles without altering sirolimus concentrations [141,142]. In contrast to the calcineurin inhibitors, there is good correlation between predose sirolimus concentrations and total drug exposure based on area under the curve measurements [106,144]. This also holds true when sirolimus is used in combination with CsA or tacrolimus [106,144]. Thus, whole blood 24-hour trough specimens are recommended when monitoring sirolimus [132].

13.4.1.5 Methods of Analysis

Therapeutic monitoring of sirolimus is critical because the administered dose is a poor predictor of total drug exposure due to individual patient variables. Because of the long drug half-life, daily monitoring of sirolimus is typically not necessary. Weekly monitoring may be needed shortly after transplantation, followed by monthly monitoring. Target concentrations for sirolimus range between 4 and 12 µg/L when used in combination with a calcineurin inhibitor [145]. Similar to tacrolimus, these relatively low whole blood concentrations can be a challenge analytically for some of the currently available assay methods. As combination immunosuppressant therapies continue to evolve, target concentrations for sirolimus may become even lower, further challenging the analytical performance of some of the currently utilized immunoassays.

Sirolimus can be measured by immunoassay and by HPLC with UV or MS detection. According to the College of American Pathologist proficiency testing program (first survey of 2008) more than 190 laboratories currently perform sirolimus testing. Approximately 70% of the labs measure whole blood sirolimus by the Abbott MEIA using the IMx, which became commercially available in 2004. The original Abbott MEIA kit was never available for routine monitoring of sirolimus and was used only in support of early clinical studies (investigational use only) until the assay was discontinued in 2001. Abbott has recently launched a CMIA for use on their ARCHITECT family of analyzers [146] that is currently used by a few laboratories in the United States. A CEDIA for sirolimus (Microgenics) is also available for use on several Roche automated analyzers (Hitachi 911, 912, 917, and modular P), but is not widely used. Siemens has developed an ACMIA for sirolimus testing on the Dimension RxL Max and ExL that is currently pending FDA approval.

The majority of labs not using the Abbott MEIA use HPLC-MS (~26% of all labs) to measure sirolimus. The major advantage of HPLC-MS is increased sensitivity and specificity, despite the need for highly skilled personnel. A few labs measure sirolimus by HPLC-UV, although this method requires elaborate sample cleanup procedures and long chromatographic run times [147–149]. This results in higher labor costs, making HPLC-UV methods unsuitable for laboratories supporting large transplant programs. A rapid liquid chromatography-MS/MS method with turbulent flow technology has recently been introduced with markedly reduced run times of < 20 minutes, compared with 2 hour run times for traditional HPLC-MS methods [150].

13.4.1.6 Metabolite Cross-Reactivity

The currently available immunoassays have significant cross-reactivity with sirolimus metabolites. The MEIA method has 58 and 63% cross-reactivity with 41-O-demethyl-sirolimus and 7-O-demethyl-sirolimus, respectively [150]. The CEDIA has 44% cross-reactivity with 11-hydroxy-sirolimus and 73% cross-reactivity with 41-O- and 32-O-demethyl-sirolimus [151]. This degree of metabolite cross-reactivity results in significant assay bias. The MEIA produces whole-blood sirolimus concentrations that are 9–49% higher than those obtained by HPLC-UV and HPLC-MS, depending on the study and transplant group studied [151,153–157]. One study found that the CEDIA method produces whole blood sirolimus levels with a mean positive bias of 20.4%, compared with HPLC-MS [158]. However, immunoassay metabolite cross-reactivity may be less of an issue from a clinical standpoint since the distribution of metabolites in whole blood are similar among patients and are relatively stable over long periods of time [159].

13.4.1.7 Analytical Considerations

The therapeutic window for sirolimus appears to be between 5 and 15 μg/L when used in combination with CsA and between 12 and 20 μg/L when used alone [130]. Sirolimus levels slightly below the currently used therapeutic range can be a challenge for some of the HPLC-UV methods, with functional sensitivities (based on between-day CV's of < 20%) of 2–3 μg/L [148,149]. This can also be a problem when using an immunoassay. The MEIA method has a functional sensitivity that varies among laboratories, with values ranging from 1.3 to 3.0 μg/L [151,153–157]. Technical variations at the manual extraction step most likely contribute to the differences in functional sensitivity that were observed among laboratories evaluating the MEIA. One study found that the CEDIA has a functional sensitivity of 3.0 μg/L [158]. HPLC-MS methods have excellent sensitivity, with functional sensitivities <1 μg/L [160,161]. It is important that laboratories experimentally determine their own lower limit of detection based on long-term between day imprecision data (using whole blood samples), and not rely on package insert information or published data.

The sirolimus MEIA is prone to error that is dependent on hematocrit levels. There is an inverse relationship between hematocrit and measured sirolimus levels. At a sirolimus concentration of 5 μg/L results can be 20% higher for hematocrits of <35% and as much as 20% lower for hematocrits >45% [151,162]. When the hematocrit is between 35 and 45%, MEIA bias is <10% at sirolimus concentrations ranging from 5 to 22 μg/L. Incomplete extraction of sirolimus from erythrocyte binding proteins is the most probable mechanism leading to the hematocrit interference. The CEDIA does not appear to be affected by variations in hematocrit between 20 and 60% [152], however, there are no independently published studies supporting the manufacturer's claim.

13.4.2 Everolimus

Everolimus (also known as SZD RAD) is a structural analog of sirolimus with an additional hydroxyethyl group (Figure 13.3). Everolimus is currently in phase III clinical trials in the United States and has not received FDA approval for use as an immunosuppressive agent.

13.4.2.1 Pharmacokinetics

Everolimus has improved bioavailability [163,164] and a shorter elimination half-life (~24 hours) than sirolimus [165]. Everolimus also has less intrapatient drug variability than sirolimus [144,166]. Concomitant use of CsA results in increased everolimus blood concentrations due to inhibition of everolimus metabolism [167]. Similar to sirolimus, everolimus is metabolized in the intestine and liver by cytochrome P450 enzymes. At least 20 metabolites have been identified [168], with mono-hydroxyl, di-hydroxyl, demethylated and an open ring form being major metabolites [169]. Metabolites are in relatively low concentrations when monitoring trough blood levels [169].

13.4.2.2 Methods of Analysis

Immunoassays to measure everolimus are currently not available in the United States and most likely will lag behind FDA approval of the drug. Seradyn has developed a FPIA (Innofluor Certican Assay System) to measure whole blood everolimus outside the United States on Abbott TDx instrumentation [170]. The FPIA method has a functional sensitivity of 2 μg/L [170], which is just below the therapeutic trough blood concentration lower limit of 3 μg/L [171]. When compared with HPLC-MS, the FPIA has a positive mean bias of 24.4% in renal transplant recipients [172]. The positive bias is due to differences in calibrator assigned values and antibody cross-reactivity with everolimus metabolites [172]. Metabolite cross-reactivity ranges from 5 to 72% [168]. HPLC-UV and HPLC-MS methods are also available to measure everolimus [173,174].

13.5 MYCOPHENOLIC ACID (MPA)

MPA is a fermentation product of *Penicillium* species that originally was shown to have antibacterial, antifungal and immunosuppressive potential in animal studies [175]. To improve the bioavailability of MPA, mycophenolate mofetil (brand name CellCept), the 2-morpholinoethyl ester of MPA was developed for oral and intravenous administration [176]. Mycophenolate mofetil received FDA approval for use as an immunosuppressive agent to prevent organ rejection in 1995. The sodium salt of MPA, mycophenolate sodium (brand name Myfortic), has recently become available for oral administration as delayed-release tablets. MPA has primarily replaced azathioprine in organ transplantation. The chemical structure of the active compound MPA, and the two parent compounds are shown in Figure 13.4.

MPA is a potent noncompetitive inhibitor of inosine monophosphate dehydrogenase (IMPDH) enzymatic activity [177]. IMPDH is the rate-limiting enzyme in the production of guanosine nucleotides, which are required for DNA synthesis and cellular proliferation. Guanosine nucleotides are synthesized in most cell types by the IMPDH pathway and a separate salvage pathway. However, the salvage pathway is not found in lymphocytes and MPA blockage of the IMPDH pathway selectively inhibits lymphocyte proliferation [178,179]. There are two isoforms of IMPDH and MPA selectively inhibits the type II isoform, which is predominantly expressed by activated but not resting lymphocytes [180].

13.5.1 PHARMACOKINETICS

Mycophenolate mofetil and mycophenolate sodium are rapidly and completely absorbed, and quickly de-esterified in the blood and tissues to MPA, the active form of the drug. The half-life of mycophenolate mofetil during intravenous administration is <2 minutes [181]. Following an oral dose of mycophenolate mofetil, MPA reaches a maximum concentration within one hour [182]. Almost all the drug (>99%) can be found in the plasma compartment [183]. For this reason, serum or plasma is used for MPA quantitation.

MPA has an elimination half-life of 18 hours and is glucuronidated in the liver to the primary inactive metabolite, 7-*O*-glucuronide mycophenolic acid (MPAG) [184]. Small quantities of the

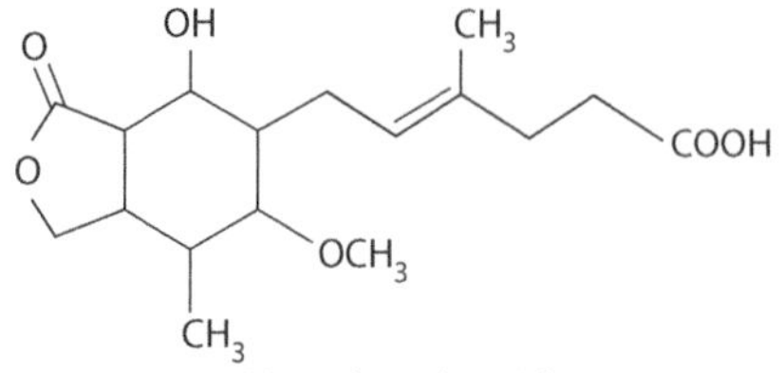

Mycophenolic acid

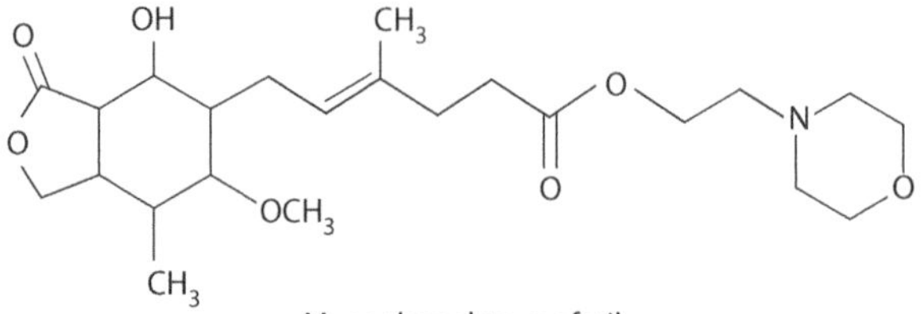

Mycophenolate mofetil

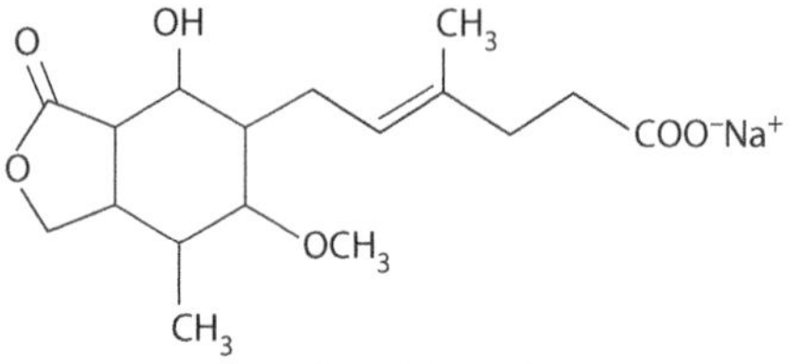

Mycophenolate sodium

FIGURE 13.4 Chemical structures of the active compound mycophenolic acid, and the two prodrugs, mycophenolate mofetil and mycophenolate sodium.

inactive metabolite 7-*O*-glucoside are also produced in the liver [182,185]. Another metabolite produced in small quantities is acyl glucuronide, an active metabolite that may contribute to the adverse gastrointestinal effects of MPA [186]. MPAG exhibits significant enterohepatic recirculation with a second MPA plasma peak occurring 4–12 hours after drug administration. The kidneys primarily clear MPAG and concentrations rapidly accumulate in patients with severe renal impairment (glomerular filtration rates <25 mL/min) [187]. MPA is extensively bound in the circulation to albumin and typical concentrations of free (unbound) MPA range from 1.25 to 2.5% of the total concentration [183]. Free MPA concentrations are increased in hypoalbuminemia, hyperbilirubinemia and uremia [188]. It has been shown that the immunosuppressive effects of MPA are related to free and not total MPA concentrations [183]. In chronic renal failure the free MPA concentration can dramatically rise and the patient can be over immunosuppressed even though the total MPA concentration is within the therapeutic range [188,189].

13.5.2 Adverse Effects

Adverse effects from mycophenolate mofetil and mycophenolate sodium are similar. The most common dose limiting unwanted side effects are diarrhea, nausea, vomiting, and abdominal pain [190]. Marrow suppression and anemia can also occur [96]. An increased risk of cytomegalovirus, candida and herpes simplex infections has also been reported [96,191].

13.5.3 Drug-Interactions

Coadministration of CsA results in significantly lower trough concentrations of MPA [192], most likely as a result of diminished enterohepatic recirculation of MPAG and MPA [193]. The antibiotics mycostatin, tobramycin, and cefuroxime also decrease MPA bioavailability by a similar mechanism [194]. Tacrolimus may increase the bioavailability of MPA by inhibiting MPAG formation [195], however, additional studies are needed to confirm this potential drug interaction. Steroids such as dexamethasone lower MPA concentrations by augmenting the activity of the enzyme responsible for MPA metabolism. Several nonsteroidal inflammatory drugs such as niflumic acid, diflunisal, flufenamic acid, mefenamic acid and salicylic acid increase MPA concentrations by inhibiting MPA glucuronidation [196]. Antacids (aluminum and magnesium hydroxide) lower total MPA exposure by reducing drug absorption in the gastrointestinal tract. Other drugs such as calcium polycarbophil and iron ion preparations also result in decreased MPA concentrations by the same mechanism [197]. Lastly, salicylic acid and furosemide increase the free fraction of MPA by altering albumin binding.

13.5.4 PREANALYTIC VARIABLES

Plasma or serum can be used to measure MPA and free MPA blood concentrations [189]. However, plasma from EDTA anticoagulated whole blood is the recommended specimen of choice since the same sample can be used to measure whole blood CsA, tacrolimus and sirolimus [198]. MPA and MPAG are stable in whole blood and plasma samples at room temperature for at least 4 hours [199]. Plasma samples are stable at 4°C for four days and at least 11 months when stored at –20°C [198]. Free MPA is stable for at least six months when stored at –20°C [200]. Thawing and refreezing of plasma samples can be performed up to four times without significant loss of MPA [201]. When monitoring MPA during intravenous infusion of mycophenolate mofetil, whole blood samples should be immediately placed in ice and the plasma separated within 30 minutes [202,203]. This is because mycophenolate mofetil is very unstable and rapidly undergoes temperature-dependent degradation to MPA in whole blood samples placed at room temperature [202].

Trough concentrations of MPA are routinely used for drug monitoring and are generally believed to be a relatively good indicator of total drug exposure [204]. This is somewhat surprising since numerous studies have shown that area under the curve (0–12 hours) measurements are more predictive of total drug exposure and acute graft rejection than trough concentrations [205–207]. In addition, MPA trough concentrations can vary considerably depending upon time after transplantation [207]. Nevertheless, the superiority of area under the curve measurements is probably overshadowed by practical considerations such as additional testing costs and difficulties associated with the collection of multiply timed samples.

13.5.5 METHODS OF ANALYSIS

When MPA was originally approved for use (as mycophenolate mofetil) therapeutic drug monitoring was considered unnecessary. However, recent studies have found wide variations in total drug exposure (as high as 10-fold) following a fixed dose, suggesting that individualized dosing may be of considerable benefit [208,209]. A roundtable meeting recently recommended therapeutic drug monitoring based on the interpatient variability and the significant drug interactions associated with combination immunosuppressive therapy [210]. At the present time fewer than 40 laboratories in the United States currently measure MPA (first CAP proficiency survey of 2008). Roughly 40% the labs measure MPA by HPLC and another 30% use HPLC-MS methods. Roche has recently developed an automated enzyme receptor assay to measure total MPA and free MPA using the COBAS INTEGRA system (Indianapolis, IN) that is used by only a handful of laboratories [211,212]. Numerous HPLC methods with UV, fluorimetric and MS detection systems have been described to measure MPA in plasma samples [200,201,213–215]. The HPLC methods primarily differ in sample extraction, analytical column, run-time, and lower limit of detection. Free MPA can be measured by HPLC methods after separation of protein-bound MPA by ultrafiltration [187,216]. However, free MPA is typically more difficult to measure and does not appear to be superior to total MPA in predicting clinical outcomes in most transplant patients [217].

A few companies are currently developing product applications for various automated instruments that test either serum and/or plasma samples. For instance, Siemens has developed an ACMIA to measure MPA on the Dimension that is pending FDA approval [218]. Microgenics is developing a CEDIA to measure MPA on Hitachi, Olympus, and Microgenics (MGC 240) instruments [219]. A Syva EMIT 2000 MPA immunoassay has been developed that is widely used outside the United States. The assay can be performed on the Dimension, Roche COBAS and Hitachi instruments. The antibody used in the EMIT assay cross-reacts with acyl glucoronide [220] and produces MPA values that are approximately 10–30% higher than those obtained by HPLC [221–224]. The bias can be considerably higher in patients with impaired renal function due to accumulation of acyl glucoronide [221,225]. The positive bias due to acyl glucoronide cross-reactivity may turn out to be advantageous since this metabolite has in vitro anti-IMPDH activity [208,226].

13.5.6   ANALYTICAL CONSIDERATIONS

The generally accepted therapeutic range for trough MPA plasma concentrations is 1.0–3.5 mg/L [198,227,228]. This range of values can be easily measured by currently available analytical methods with good precision. Concentrations of free MPA are typically 2% of the total MPA level and can be analytically challenging for some of the HPLC-UV methods [229]. In these situations the functional sensitivity of the free MPA assay needs to be carefully validated.

HPLC is the reference method for measuring MPA that other methods are validated against. This is because HPLC is highly specific for parent compound and is free from coadministered drug interferences [202,213–215]. As more immunoassays to measure MPA become available, metabolite cross-reactivity and assay bias will have to be taken into account when interpreting MPA concentrations.

13.6   CONCLUSIONS

Advances in immunosuppressive therapy are largely responsible for the success and improved outcomes following allogeneic organ transplantation. Today, very few allografts are lost from immune-mediated acute rejection and there are remarkable improvements in patient and graft survival. A major goal of immunosuppressive drug therapy is to optimize therapeutic effectiveness while minimizing unwanted adverse effects. Toward this end, therapeutic drug monitoring plays a central role in order to achieve optimal drug therapy requiring individualized dosing. Therapeutic monitoring of CsA, tacrolimus and sirolimus is now considered an integral part of organ transplant programs and several arguments have been made for monitoring MPA.

Although HPLC with UV or MS detection is considered the reference method for monitoring immunosuppressive drugs, the majority of laboratories still use automated immunoassays to measure CsA, tacrolimus, and sirolimus. An exception is MPA, which is primarily measured by HPLC because immunoassays have only recently become commercially available. Immunoassays have gained widespread use because they can be either semi- or fully automated, have low start-up costs, and do not require specialized testing personnel. The major drawback of immunoassays is metabolite cross-reactivity, which results in varying degrees of positive and negative bias. In addition, immunoassay cross-reactivity is not always predictable and can be highly variable depending on the type of organ transplanted and the time after transplant. This makes drug levels difficult to interpret in the context of therapeutic ranges, which have been established using other analytical methods such as HPLC. Advantages of HPLC include excellent specificity since the methods can distinguish between drug metabolites and the parent compound. Drawbacks of HPLC include extensive sample cleanup, long analytical run times and the need for specialized training. These limitations can be partially overcome by using HPLC with MS detection, which requires less sample cleanup and has shorter run times. Unfortunately, HPLC-MS systems are considerably more expensive and require highly specialized testing personnel. Although newer HPLC-MS systems with automated sample preparation are easier to operate, automated immunoassays will continue to be used by the majority of laboratories except those that support very large organ transplant programs.

REFERENCES

1. Merrill JP, Murray JE, Harrison JH, Guild WR. 1956. Successful homotransplantation of the human kidney between identical twins. *JAMA* 160:277–82.
2. Murray JE, Merrill JP, Harrison JH, Wilson RE, Dammin GJ. 1963, Prolonged survival of human-kidney homographs by immunosuppressive drug therapy. *N Engl J Med* 268:1315–23.
3. Starzl TE, Marchioro TL, Waddell WR. 1963. The reversal of rejection in human renal homografts with subsequent development of homograft tolerance. *Surg Gynecol Obstet* 117:385–95.
4. Calne RY, White DJ, Thiru S, Evans DB, McMaster P, Dunn DC, Craddock GN, Pentlow BD, Rolles K. 1978. Cyclosporin A in patients receiving renal allografts from cadaver donors. *Lancet* 2:1323–27.
5. Goto T, Kino T, Hatanaka H, Nishiyama M, Okuhara M, Kohsaka M, Aoki H, Imanaka H. 1987. Discovery of FK-506, a novel immunosuppressant isolated from *Streptomyces tsukubaensis*. *Transplant Proc* 19:4–8.
6. Singh K, Sun S, Vezina C. 1979. Rapamycin (AY-22,989), a new antifungal antibiotic. IV. Mechanism of action. *J Antibiot (Tokyo)* 32:630–45.
7. Sollinger HW. 1995. Mycophenolate mofetil for the prevention of acute rejection in primary cadaveric renal allograft recipients. U.S. Renal Transplant Mycophenolate Mofetil Study Group. *Transplantation* 60:225–32.
8. The Tricontinental Mycophenolate Mofetil Renal Transplantation Study Group. 1996. A blind, random-ized clinical trial of mycophenolate mofetil for the prevention of acute rejection in cadaveric renal trans-plantation. *Transplantation* 61:1029–37.
9. European Mycophenolate Mofetil Cooperative Study Group. 1995. Placebo-controlled study of myco-phenolate mofetil combined with cyclosporin and corticosteroids for prevention of acute rejection. *Lancet* 345:1321–25.
10. Scientific Registry of Transplant Recipients. Trends in organ organ donation and transplantation in the United States, 1997–2007. Table I-1. http://www.ustransplant.org/annual_reports/current/Chapter_I_AR_CD.htm?cp=2 (Accessed November 2008).
11. Scientific Registry of Transplant Recipients. Trends in organ organ donation and transplantation in the United States, 1997–2007. Table I-3. http://www.ustransplant.org/annual_reports/current/Chapter_I_AR_CD.htm?cp=2 (Accessed November 2008).
12. Lindholm A, Albrechtsen D, Tufveson G, Karlberg I, Persson NH, Groth CG. 1992. A randomized trial of cyclosporine and prednisolone versus cyclosporine, azathioprine, and prednisolone in primary cadaveric renal transplantation. *Transplantation* 54:624–31.
13. Anon. 1983. Cyclosporin in cadaveric renal transplantation: one-year follow-up of a multicentre trial. *Lancet* 2:986–89.
14. Bruunshuus I, Schmiegelow K. 1989. Analysis of 6-mercaptopurine, 6-thioguanine nucleotides and 6-thiuric acid in biological fluids by high-performance liquid chromatography. *Scand J Clin Invest* 49:779–84.
15. Kreuzenkamp-Jansen CW, De Abreu RA, Bokkerink JPM, Trijbels JMF. 1995. Determination of extra-cellular and intracellular thiopurines and methylthiopurines with HPLC. *J Chromatogr* 672:53–61.
16. Rabel SR, Stobaugh JF, Trueworthy R. 1995. Determination of intracellular levels of 6-mercaptopurine metabolites in erythrocytes utilizing capillary electrophoresis with laser-induced fluorescence detection. *Anal Biochem* 224:315–22.
17. Filler G, Lepage N, Delisle B, Mai I. 2001. Effect of cyclosporine on mycophenolic acid area under the concentration-curve in pediatric kidney transplant recipients. *Ther Drug Monit* 23:514–19.
18. van Gelder T, Klupp J, Barten MJ, Christians U, Morris RE. 2001. Comparison of the effects of tacroli-mus and cyclosporine on the pharmacokinetics of mycophenolic acid. *Ther Drug Monit* 23:119–28.
19. Undre NA. 2003. Pharmacokinetics of tacrolimus-based combination therapies. *Nephrol Dial Transplant* 18(Suppl 1):i12–i15.
20. Scientific Registry of Transplant Recipients. Trends in organ donation and transplantation in the United States, 1997–2007. Table III-2. http://www.ustransplant.org/annual_reports/archives/2005/Chapter_III_AR_CD.htm?cp=4 (Accessed November 2008)
21. Shibasaki F, Hallin U, Uchino H. 2002. Calcineurin as a multifunctional regulator. *J Biochem (Tokyo)* 131:1–15.

22. Siekierka JJ, Hung SH, Poe M, Lin CS, Sigal NH. 1989. A cytosolic binding protein for the immunosuppressant FK506 has peptidylprolyl isomerase activity but is distinct from cyclophilin. *Nature* 341:755–57.
23. Schreiber SL, Crabtree GR. 1992. The mechanism of action of cyclosporin A and FK-506. *Immunol Today* 13:136–42.
24. Flanagan WM, Corthesy B, Bram RJ, Crabtree GR. 1991. Nuclear association of a T-cell transcription factor blocked by FK506 and cyclosporin A. *Nature* 352:803–7.
25. Clipstone NA, Crabtree GR. 1992. Identification of calcineurin as a key signaling enzyme in T-lymphocyte activation. *Nature* 357:695–97.
26. Schreiber SL. 1991. Chemistry and biology of immunophilins and their immunosuppressive ligands. *Science* 251:283–87.
27. Gummert JF, Ikonen T, Morris RE. 1999. Newer immunosuppressive drugs: a review. *J Am Soc Nephrol* 10:1366–80.
28. Jorgensen KA, Koefoed-Nielsen PB, Karamperis N. 2003. Calcineurin phosphatase activity and immunosuppression. A review on the role of calcineurin phosphatase activity and the immunosuppressive effect of cyclosporin A and tacrolimus. *Scand J Immunol* 57:93–98.
29. Borel JF, Feurer C, Gubler HU, Stahelin H. 1976. Biological effects on cyclosporine A: a new antilymphocytic agent. *Agents and Actions* 6:468–75.
30. Vonderscher J, Meinzer A. 1994. Rationale for the development of Sandimmune Neoral. *Transplant Proc* 26:2925–27.
31. Bartucci MR. 1999. Issues in cyclosporine drug substitution: implications for patient management. *J Transpl Coord* 9:137–42.
32. Alloway RR. 1999. Generic immunosuppressant use in solid organ transplantation. *Transplant Proc* 31(Suppl 3A):2S–5S.
33. Kovarik JM, Mueller EA, van Bree JB, Fluckinger SS, Lange H, Schmidt B, Boesken WH, Lison AE, Kutz K. 1994. Cyclosporine pharmacokinetics and variability from a microemulsion formulation-a multicenter investigation in kidney transplant patients. *Transplantation* 58:658–63.
34. Ptachcinski RJ, Venkataramanan R, Burckart GJ. 1986. Clinical pharmacokinetics of cyclosporin. *Clin Pharmacokinet* 11:107–32.
35. Hoppu K, Jalanko H, Laine J, Holmberg C. 1996. Comparison of conventional oral cyclosporine and cyclosporine microemulsion formulation in children with a liver transplant. *Transplantation* 62:66–71.
36. Faulds D, Goa KL, Benfield P. 1993. Cyclosporin. A review of its pharmacodynamic and pharmacotherapeutic properties, and therapeutic use in immunoregulatory disorders. *Drugs* 45:953–1040.
37. Noble S, Markham A. 1995. Cyclosporin. A review of the pharmacokinetic properties, clinical efficacy and tolerability of a microemulsion-based formulation (Neoral). *Drugs* 50:924–41.
38. Fahr A. 1993. Cyclosporin clinical pharmacokinetics. *Clin Pharmacokinet* 24:472–95.
39. Wenk M, Follath F, Abisch E. 1983. Temperature dependency of apparent cyclosporine A concentrations in plasma. *Clin Chem* 29:1865.
40. Kahan BD, Shaw LM, Holt D, Grevel J, Johnston A. 1990. Consensus document: Hawk's meeting on therapeutic drug monitoring of cyclosporine. *Clin Chem* 36:1510–16.
41. Shaw LM, Yatscoff RW, Bowers LD, Freeman DJ, Jeffery JR, Keown PA, McGilveray IJ, Rosano TG, Wong PY. 1990. Canadian consensus meeting on cyclosporine monitoring: Report of the consensus panel. *Clin Chem* 36:1841–46.
42. Ollerich M, Armstrong VW, Kahan B, Shaw L, Holt DW, Yatscoff R, Lindholm A, Halloran P, Gallicano K, Wonigeit K, Schutz E, Schran H, Annesley T. 1995. Lake Louise consensus conference on cyclosporin monitoring in organ transplantation: report of the consensus panel. *Ther Drug Monit* 17:642–54.
43. Zhang YC, Benet L. 2001. The gut as a barrier to drug absorption. *Clin Pharmacokinet* 40:159–68.
44. Wu CY, Benet LZ, Hebert MF, Gupta SK, Rowland M, Gomez DY, Wacher VJ. 1995. Differentiation of absorption and first-pass gut and hepatic metabolism in humans: studies with cyclosporine. *Clin Pharmacol Ther* 58:492–97.
45. Lown KS, Mayo RR, Leichtman AB, Hsiao HL, Turgeon DK, Schmiedlin-Ren P, Brown MB, Guo W, Rossi SJ, Benet LZ, Watkins PB. 1997. Role of intestinal P-glycoprotein (mdr1) in interpatient variation in the oral bioavailability of cyclosporine. *Clin Pharmacol Ther* 62:248–60.
46. Wallemacq PE, Lhoest G, Dumont P. 1989. Isolation, purification and structure elucidation of cyclosporine A metabolites in rabbit and man. *Biomed Mass Spectrom* 18:48–56.
47. Chrintians U, Sewing KF. 1993. Cyclosporin metabolism in transplant patients. *Pharmacol Ther* 57:291–345.

48. Yatscoff RW, Rosano TG, Bowers LD. 1991. The clinical significance of cyclosporine metabolites. *Clin Biochem* 24:23–35.
49. Radeke HH, Christians U, Sewing KF, Resch K. 1992. The synergistic immunosuppressive potential of cyclosporin metabolite combinations. *Int J Immunopharmacol* 14:595–604.
50. Rosano TG, Brooks CA, Dybas MT, Cramer SM, Stevens C, Freed BM. 1990. Selection of an optimal assay method for monitoring cyclosporine therapy. *Transplant Proc* 22:1125–28.
51. Ryffel B, Foxwell BM, Mihatsch MJ, Donatsch P, Maurer G. 1988. Biologic significance of cyclosporine metabolites. *Transplant Proc* 20(suppl 2):575–84.
52. Smets F, Sokal EM. 2002. Lymphoproliferation in children after liver transplantation. *J Pediatr Gastroenterol Nutr* 34:499–505.
53. Scott JP, Higenbottam TW. 1988. Adverse reactions and interactions of cyclosporin. *Med Toxicol* 3:107–27.
54. Yee GC, McGuire TR. 1990. Pharmacokinetic drug interactions with cyclosporin. *Clin Pharmacol* 19:319–32 and 400–15.
55. Durr D, Stieger B, Kullak-Ublick GA, Rentsch KM, Steinert HC, Meier PJ, Fattinger K. 2000. St. John's Wort induces intestinal P-glycoprotein/MDR1 and intestinal and hepatic CYP3A4. *Clin Pharmacol Ther* 68:598–604.
56. Smith MC, Sephel GC. 1990. Long-term in vitro stability of cyclosporine in whole-blood samples. *Clin Chem* 36:1991–92.
57. Schran HF, Rosano TG, Hasse AE, Pell MA. 1987. Determination of cyclosporine concentrations with monoclonal antibodies. *Clin Chem* 33:2225–29.
58. Keown P, Landsberg D, Hollaran P, Shoker A, Rush D, Jeffery J et al. 1996. A randomized, prospective multicenter pharmacoepidemiologic study of cyclosporine microemulsion in stable renal graft recipients. Report of the Canadian Neoral Renal Transplantation Study Group. *Transplantation* 27:1744–52.
59. Halloran PF, Helms LM, Noujaim J. 1999. The temporal profile of calcineurin inhibition by cyclosporine in vivo. *Transplantation* 15:1356–61.
60. Lindholm A, Kahan BD. 1993. Influence of cyclosporine pharmacokinetics, trough concentrations, and AUC monitoring on outcome after kidney transplantation. *Clin Pharmacol Ther* 54:205–18.
61. Lindholm A. 1991. Review: factors influencing the pharmacokinetics of cyclosporine in man. *Ther Drug Monit* 13:465–77.
62. Grevel J, Welsh MS, Kahan B. 1989. Cyclosporine monitoring in renal transplantation: area under the curve monitoring is superior to trough-level monitoring. *Ther Drug Monit* 11:246–48.
63. Belitsky P, Levy GA, Johnston A. 2000. Neoral absorption profiling: an evolution in effectiveness. *Transplant Proc* 32(suppl 3A):S45–S52.
64. Keown P, Niese D. 1998. Cyclosporine microemulsion increases drug exposure and reduces acute rejection without incremental toxicity in de novo renal transplantation. International Sandimmune Neoral Study Group. *Kidney Int* 54:938–44.
65. Stein CM, Murray JJ, Wood AJ. 1999. Inhibition of stimulated interleukin-2 production in whole blood: a practical measure of cyclosporine effect. *Clin Chem* 45:1477–84.
66. Oellerick M, Armstrong VW. 2002. Two-hour cyclosporine concentration determination: an appropriate tool to monitor neoral therapy? *Ther Drug Monit* 24:40–46.
67. Mahalati K, Belitsky P, Sketris I, West K, Panek R. 1999. Neoral monitoring by simplified sparse sampling area under the concentration-time curve. *Transplantation* 68:55–62.
68. Grant D, Kneteman N, Tchervenkow J, Roy A, Murphy G, Tan A, Hendricks L, Guilbault N, Levy G. 1999. Peak cyclosporine levels (Cmax) correlate with freedom from liver graft rejection: results of a prospective, randomized comparison of neoral and sandimmune for liver transplantation (NOF-8). *Transplantation* 67:1133–37.
69. Cantarovick M, Barkun JS, Tchervenkov JI, Besner JG, Aspeslet L, Metrakos P. 1998. Comparison of Neoral dose monitoring with cyclosporine through levels versus 2-hour postdose levels in stable liver transplant patients. *Transplantation* 66:1621–27.
70. Cantarovick M, Elstein E, de Varennes B, Barkun JS. 1999. Clinical benefit of Neoral dose monitoring with cyclosporine 2-hour post-dose levels compared with trough levels in stable heart transplant patients. *Transplantation* 68:1839–42.
71. Knight SR, Morris PJ. 2007. The clinical benefits of cyclosporine C2-level monitoring: a systemic review. *Transplantation* 83:1525–35.
72. Wallemacq PE. 2004. Therapeutic monitoring of immunosuppressant drugs. Where are we? *Clin Chem Lab Med* 42:1204–11.

73. Whitman DA, Abbott V, Fregien K, Bowers LD. 1993. Recent advances in high-performance liquid chromatography/mass spectrometry and high-performance liquid chromatography/tandem mass spectrometry: detection of cyclosporine and metabolites in kidney and liver tissue. *Ther Drug Monit* 15:552–56.

74. Zhou L, Tan D, Theng J, Lim L, Liu YP, Lam KW. 2001. Optimized analytical method for cyclosporine A by high-performance liquid chromatography-electrospray ionization mass spectrometry. *J Chromatogr B Biomed Sci Appl* 754:201–7.

75. Taylor PJ. 2004. Therapeutic drug monitoring of immunosuppressant drugs by high-performance liquid chromatography-mass spectrometry. *Ther Drug Monit* 26:215–19.

76. Belensky A, Lazzaro P, Shuaib A, Natrajan A, Costello J, Barbarakis M. 1996. Bayer ADVIA Centaur® cyclosporine assay: an analytical evaluation. *Clin Chem* 52(suppl):A60 (abstract).

77. Maine GT, Wallemacq P, Ait-Youcet H, Berg K, Schmidt E, Young J et al. 2008. Analytical multi-site evaluation of the Abbott ARCHITECT cyclosporine assay. *Clin Chem* 54(suppl):A13 (abstract).

78. Tredger JM, Roberts N, Sherwood R, Higgins G, Keating J. 2000. Comparison of five cyclosporin immunoassays with HPLC. *Clin Chem Lab Med* 38:1205–7.

79. Steimer W. 1999. Performance and specificity of monoclonal immunoassays for cyclosporine monitoring: how specific is specific? *Clin Chem* 45:371–81.

80. Schutz E, Svinarov D, Shipkova M, Niedmann PD, Armstrong VW, Wieland E, Oellerich M. 1998. Cyclosporin whole blood immunoassays (AxSYM, CEDIA, and Emit): a critical overview of performance characteristics and comparison with HPLC. *Clin Chem* 44:2158–64.

81. Hamwi A, Veitl M, Manner G, Ruzicka K, Schweiger C, Szekeres T. 1999. Evaluation of four automated methods for determination of whole blood cyclosporine concentrations. *Am J Clin Pathol* 112:358–65.

82. Terrell AR, Daly TM, Hock KG, Kilgore DC, Wei TQ, Hernandez S, Weibe D. 2002. Evaluation of a no-pretreatment cyclosporin A assay on the Dade Behring Dimension RxL clinical analyzer. *Clin Chem* 48:1059–65.

83. Butch AW, Fukuchi AM. 2004. Analytical performance of the CEDIA® cyclosporine PLUS whole blood immunoassay. *J Anal Toxicol* 28:204–10.

84. Analytical Services International. Ciclosporin International Proficiency Testing Scheme. http://www.bioanalytics.co.uk/pt/dates_and_results/Cic295.pdf (Accessed November 2008).

85. Morris RG, Holt DW, Armstrong VW, Griesmacher A, Napoli KL, Shaw LM. 2004. Analytical aspects of cyclosporine monitoring, on behalf of the IFCC/IATDMCT joint working group. *Ther Drug Monit* 26:227–30.

86. Holt DW, Johnston A, Kahan BD, Morris RG, Oellerich M, Shaw LM. 2000. New approaches to cyclosporine monitoring raise further concerns about analytical techniques. *Clin Chem* 46:872–74.

87. Juenke JM, Brown PI, Urry FM, McMillin GA. 2004. Specimen dilution for C2 monitoring with the Abbott TDxFLx cyclosporine monoclonal whole blood assay. *Clin Chem* 50:1430–3.

88. Johnston A, Chusney G, Schutz E, Oellerich M, Lee TD, Holt DW. 2003. Monitoring cyclosporin in blood: between-assay differences at trough and 2 hours post-dose (C2). *Ther Drug Monit* 25:167–73.

89. First MR. 2004. Tacrolimus based immunosuppression. *J Nephrol* 17:25–31.

90. Venkataramanan R, Swaminathan A, Prasad T, Jain A, Zuckerman S, Warty V, McMichael J. 1995. Clinical pharmacokinetics of tacrolimus. *Clin Pharmacokinet* 29:404–30.

91. Zahir H, Nand RA, Brown KF, Tattam BN, McLachlan AJ. 2001. Validation of methods to study the distribution and protein binding of tacrolimus in human blood. *J Pharmacol Toxicol Methods* 46:27–35.

92. Iwasaki K, Shiraga T, Nagase K, Tozuka Z, Noda K, Sakuma S, Fujitsu T. 1993. Isolation, identification, and biological activities of oxidative metabolites of FK506, a potent immunosuppressive macrolide lactone. *Drug Metab Dispos* 21:971–77.

93. Kelly P, Kahan BD. 2002. Review: metabolism of immunosuppressant drugs. *Curr Drug Metab* 3:275–87.

94. Tamura K, Fujimura T, Iwasaki K, Sakuma S, Fujitsu T, Nakamura K. et al. 1994. Interaction of tacrolimus (FK506) and its metabolites with FKBP and calcineurin. *Biochem Biophys Res Commun* 202:437–43.

95. Beysens J, Wigner RMH, Beuman GH, van der Heyden J, Kootstra G, van As H. 1991. FK 506: Monitoring in plasma or in whole blood? *Transplant Proc* 23:2745–47.

96. Taylor AL, Watson CJE, Bradley JA. 2005. Immunosuppressive agents in solid organ transplantation: mechanisms of action and therapeutic efficacy. *Crit Rev Oncol/Hematol* 56:23–46.

97. Artz MA, Boots JM, Ligtenberg G, Roodnat JI, Christiaans MH, Vos PF, Moons P et al. 2004. Conversion from cyclosporine to tacrolimus improves quality-of-life indices, renal graft function and cardiovascular risk profile. *Am J Transplant* 4:937–45.

98. Mentzer Jr RM, Jahania MS, Lasley RD.1998. Tacrolimus as a rescue immunosuppressant after heart and lung transplantation. The U.S. Multicenter FK506 Study Group. *Transplantation* 65:109–13.

99. Laskow DA, Neylan JF, Shapiro RS, Pirsch JD, Vergne-Marini PJ, Tomlanovich SJ. 1998. The role of tacrolimus in adult kidney transplantation: a review. *Clin Tranplant* 12:489–503.

100. Annesley TM, Hunter BC, Fidler DR, Giacherio DA. 1995. Stability of tacrolimus (FK 506) and cyclosporine G in whole blood. *Ther Drug Monit* 17:361–5.

101. Alak AM, Lizak P. 1996. Stability of FK506 in blood samples. *Ther Drug Monit* 18:209–11.

102. Freeman DJ, Stawecki M, Howson B. 1995. Stability of FK 506 in whole blood samples. *Ther Drug Monit* 17:266–67.

103. Holt DW. 2002. Therapeutic drug monitoring of immunosuppressive drugs in kidney transplantation. *Curr Opin Nephrol Hypertens* 11:657–63.

104. Staatz CE, Tett SE. 2004. Clinical pharmacokinetics and pharmacodynamics of tacrolimus in solid organ transplant. *Clin Pharmacokinet* 43:623–53.

105. Wong KM, Shek CC, Chau KF, Li CS. 2000. Abbreviated tacrolimus area-under-the-curve monitoring for renal transplant recipients. *Am J Kidney Dis* 35:660–66.

106. McAlister VC, Mahalati K, Peltekian KM, Fraser A, MacDonald AS. 2002. A clinical pharmacokinetic study of tacrolimus and sirolimus combination immunosuppression comparing simultaneous to separated administration. *Ther Drug Monit* 24:346–50.

107. Lensmeyer GL, Poquette MA. 2001. Therapeutic monitoring of tacrolimus concentrations in blood: semi-automated extraction and liquid chromatography-electrospray ionization mass spectrometry. *Ther Drug Monit* 23:239–49.

108. Keevil BG, McCann SJ, Cooper DP, Morris MR. 2002. Evaluation of a rapid micro-scale assay for tacrolimus by liquid chromatography-tandem mass spectrometry. *Ann Clin Biochem* 39:487–92.

109. Deters M, Kirchner G, Rewsch K, Kaever V. 2002. Simultaneous quantification of sirolimus, everolimus, tacrolimus and cyclosporine by liquid chromatography-mass spectrometry (LM-MS). *Clin Chem Lab Med* 40:285–92.

110. Iwasaki K, Shiraga T, Matsuda H, Nagase K, Tokuma Y, Hata T et al. 1995. Fujioka M. Further metabolism of FK506 (tacrolimus). Identification and biological activities of the metabolites oxidized at multiple sites of FK506. *Drug Metab Dispos* 23:28–34.

111. *CEDIA® Tacrolimus Assay* (package insert). Microgenics Corporation, Fremont, CA, 2005.

112. Staatz CE, Taylor PJ, Tett SE. 2002. Comparison of an ELISA and an LC/MS/MS method for measuring tacrolimus concentrations and making dosage decisions in transplant recipients. *Ther Drug Monit* 24:607–15.

113. Gonschior AK, Christians U, Winkler M, Linck A, Baumann J, Sewing KF. 1996. Tacrolimus (FK506) metabolite patterns in blood from liver and kidney transplant patients. *Clin Chem* 42:1426–32.

114. LeGatt DF, Shalapay CE, Cheng SB. 2004. The EMIT 2000 tacrolimus assay: an application protocol for the Beckman Synchron LX20 PRO analyzer. *Clin Biochem* 37:1022–30.

115. Oellerich M, Armstrong VW, Schutz E, Shaw LM. 1998. Therapeutic drug monitoring of cyclosporine and tacrolimus. *Clin Biochem* 31:309–16.

116. Cogill JL, Taylor PJ, Westley IS, Morris RG, Lynch SV, Johnson AG. 1998.Evaluation of the tacrolimus II microparticle enzyme immunoassay (MEIA II) in liver and renal transplant recipients. *Clin Chem* 44:1942–46.

117. Busuttil RW, Klintmalm GB, Lake JR, Miller CM, Porayko M. 1996. General guidelines for the use of tacrolimus in adult liver transplant patients. *Transplantation* 61:845–47.

118. Schambeck CM, Bedel A, Keller F. 1998. Limit of quantification (functional sensitivity) of the new IMx tacrolimus II microparticle enzyme immunoassay. *Clin Chem* 44:2217.

119. *Tacrolimus II (package insert)*. Abbott Laboratories, Diagnostics Division, Abbott Park, IL, 2003.

120. Homma M, Tomita T, Yuzawa K, Takada Y, Kohda Y. 2002. False positive blood tacrolimus concentration in microparticle enzyme immunoassay. *Biol Pharm Bull* 25:1119–20.

121. Kahn SE, Vazquez P, Meyer P, Dickson D, Schmidt E, Castellani W, et al. 2008. Analytical multi-site evaluation of the Abbott ARCHITECT tacrolimus assay. *Clin Chem* 54(suppl):A19 (abstract).

122. Kuzuya T, Ogura Y, Motegi Y, Moriyama N, Nabeshima T. 2002. Interference of hematocrit in the tacrolimus II microparticle enzyme immunoassay. *Ther Drug Monit* 24:507–11.

123. Akbas SH, Ozdem S, Caglar S, Tuncer M, Gurkan A, Yucetin L. et al. 2005. Effects of some hematological parameters on whole blood tacrolimus concentration measured by two immunoassay-based analytical methods. *Clin Biochem* 38:552–57.

124. Ghoshal AK, Soldin SJ. 2002. IMx tacrolimus II assay: is it reliable at low blood concentrations? A comparison with tandem MS/MS. *Clin Biochem* 35:389–92.

125. Steele BW, Wang E, Soldin SJ, Klee G, Elin RJ, Witte DL. 2003. A longitudinal replicate study of immunosuppressive drugs. A College of American Pathologists Study. *Arch Pathol Lab Med* 127:283–88.

126. Miller JL. 1999. Sirolimus approved with renal transplant indication. *Am J Health Syst Pharm* 56:2177–78.
127. Sedrani R, Cottens S, Kallen J, Schuler W. 1998. Chemical modification of rapamycin: the discovery of SZD RAD. *Transplant Proc* 30:2192–94
128. Abraham RT, Wiederrecht GJ.1996. Immunopharmacology of rapamycin. *Ann Rev Immunol* 14:483–510.
129. Kimball PM, Derman RK, Van Buren CT, Lewis RM, Katz S, Kahan BD. 1993. Cyclosporine and rapamycin affect protein kinase C induction of intracellular activation signal, activator of DNA replication. *Transplantation* 55:1128–32.
130. Mahalati K, Kahan BD. 2001. Clinical pharmacokinetics of sirolimus. *Clin Pharmacokinet* 40:573–85.
131. Zimmerman JJ, Kahan BD. 1997. Pharmacokinetics of sirolimus in stable renal transplant patients after multiple oral dose administration. *J Clin Pharmacol* 37:405–15.
132. Yatscoff RW, Boeckx R, Holt DW, Kahan BD, LeGatt DF, Sehgal S et al. 1995. Consensus guidelines for therapeutic drug monitoring of rapamycin: report of the consensus panel. *Ther Drug Monit* 17:676–80.
133. Cattaneo D, Merlini S, Pellegrino M, Carrara F, Zenoni S, Murgia S, Baldelli S et al. 2004. Therapeutic drug monitoring of sirolimus: effect of concomitant immunosuppressive therapy and optimization of drug dosing. *Am J Transplant* 4:1345–51.
134. Yatscoff R, LeGatt D, Keenan R, Chackowsky P.1993. Blood distribution of rapamycin. *Transplantation* 56:1202–6.
135. Sattler M, Guengerich FP, Yun CH, Christians U, Sewing KF. 1992. Cytochrome P-450 3A enzymes are responsible for biotransformation of FK506 and rapamycin in man and rat. *Drug Metab Dispos* 20:753–61.
136. Gallant-Haidner HL, Trepanier DJ, Freitag DG, Yatscoff RW. 2000. Pharmacokinetics and metabolism of sirolimus. *Ther Drug Monit* 22:31–35.
137. Leung LY, Zimmeman J, Lim HK. 1997. Metabolic disposition of [14C]-rapamycin (sirolimus) in healthy male subjects after a single oral dose. *Proceedings of the International Society for the Study of Xenobiotics* 12:26 (abstract).
138. Montalbano M, Neff GW, Yamashiki N, Meyer D, Bettiol M, Slapak-Green G et al. 2004. A retrospective review of liver transplant patients treated with sirolimus from a single center: an analysis of sirolimus related complications. *Transplantation* 78:264–68.
139. Haydar AA, Denton M, West A, Rees J, Goldsmith DJ. 2004. Sirolimus-induced pneumonitis: three cases and a review of the literature. *Am J Transplant* 4:137–39.
140. Kaplan B, Meier-Kriesche HU, Napoli KL, Kahan BD. 1998. The effects of relative timing of sirolimus and cyclosporine microemulsion formulation coadministration on the pharmacokinetics of each agent. *Clin Pharmacol Ther* 63:48–53.
141. Jones K, Saadat-Lajevardi S, Lee T, Horwatt R, Hicks D, Johnston A, Holt DW. 2000. An immunoassay for the measurement of sirolimus. *Clin Therapeutics* 22(suppl):B49–B61.
142. Salm P, Tresillian MJ, Taylor PJ, Pillans PI. 2000. Stability of sirolimus (rapamycin) in whole blood. *Ther Drug Monit* 22:423–26.
143. Yatscoff RW, Faraci C, Bolingbroke P. 1992. Measurement of rapamycin in whole blood using reverse-phase high-performance liquid chromatography. *Ther Drug Monit* 14:138–41.
144. Kahan BD, Napoli KL, Kelly PA, Podbielski J, Hussein I, Urbauer DL. 2000. Therapeutic drug monitoring of sirolimus: correlations with efficacy and toxicity. *Clin Transplant* 14:97–109.
145. Holt DW, Denny K, Lee TD, Johnston A. 2003. Therapeutic monitoring of sirolimus: its contribution to optimal prescription. *Transplant Proc* 35(suppl 3):157S–161S.
146. Kahn SE, Vazquez D, Meyer P, Dickson D, Kenney D, Edwards M, et al. 2008. Analytical evaluation of the Abbott ARCHTECT sirolimus assay. *Clin Chem* 54(suppl):A14 (abstract).
147. Napoli KL, Kahan BD. 1996. Routine clinical monitoring of sirolimus (rapamycin) whole-blood concentrations by HPLC with ultraviolet detection. *Clin Chem* 42:1943–48.
148. Napoli KL. 2000. A practical guide to the analysis of sirolimus using high-performance liquid chromatography with ultraviolet detection. *Clin Ther* 22(suppl):B14–B24.
149. Maleki S, Graves S, Becker S, Horwatt R, Hicks D, Stroshane RM, Kincaid H. 2000. Therapeutic monitoring of sirolimus in human whole-blood samples by high-performance liquid chromatography. *Clin Ther* 22(suppl):B25–B37.
150. Wang S, Miller A. 2008. A rapid liquid chromatography-tandem mass spectrometry analysis of whole blood sirolimus using turbulent flow technology for online extraction. *Clin Chem Lab Med* 46:1631–34.

151. Wilson D, Johnston F, Holt D, Moreton M, Engelmayer J, Gaulier J-M et al. 2006. Multi-center evaluation of analytical performance of the microparticle enzyme immunoassay for sirolimus. *Clin Biochem* 39:378–86.

152. *CEDIA® Sirolimus Assay (package insert).* Microgenics Corporation, Fremont, CA, 2004.

153. Vicente FB, Smith FA, Peng Y, Wang S. 2006. Evaluation of an immunoassay of whole blood sirolimus in pediatric transplant patients in comparison with high-performance liquid chromatography/tandem mass spectrometry. *Clin Chem Lab Med* 44:497–99.

154. Holt DW, Laamanen MK, Johnston A. 2005. A microparticle enzyme immunoassay to measure sirolimus. *Transplant Proc* 37:182–84.

155. Zochowska D, Bartlomiejczyk I, Kaminska A, Senatorski G, Paczek L.2006. High-performance liquid chromatography versus immunoassay for the measurement of sirolimus: comparison of two methods. *Transplant Proc* 38:78–80.

156. Fillee C, Mourad M, Squifflet JP, Malaise J, Lerut J, Reding R et al. 2005. Evaluation of a new immunoassay to measure sirolimus blood concentrations compared to a tandem mass-spectrometric chromatographic analysis. *Transplant Proc* 37:2890–91.

157. Morris RG, Salm P, Taylor PJ, Wicks FA, Theodossi A. 2006. Comparison of the reintroduced MEIA® assay with HPLC-MS/MS for the determination of whole-blood sirolimus from transplant recipients. *Ther Drug Monit* 28:164–68.

158. Westley IS, Morris RG, Taylor PJ, Salm P, James MJ. 2005. CEDIA® sirolimus assay compared with HPLC-MS/MS and HPLC-UV in transplant recipient specimens. *Ther Drug Monit* 27:309–14.

159. Holt DW, McKeown DA, Lee TD, Hicks D, Cal P, Johnston A. 2004. The relative proportions of sirolimus metabolites in blood using HPLC with mass-spectrometric detection. *Transplant Proc* 36:3223–25.

160. Christians U, Jacobsen W, Serkova N, Benet LZ, Vidal C, Sewing KF. Et al. 2000. Automated, fast and sensitive quantification of drugs in blood by liquid chromatography-mass spectrometry with on-line extraction: immunosuppressants. *J Chromatogr B Biomed Sci Appl* 748:41–53.

161. Holt DW, Lee T, Jones K, Johnston A. 2000. Validation of an assay for routine monitoring of sirolimus using HPLC with mass spectrometric detection. *Clin Chem* 46:1179–83.

162. Salm P, Taylor PJ, Pillans PI. 2000. The quantitation of sirolimus by high-performance liquid chromatography-tandem mass spectrometry and microparticle enzyme immunoassay in renal transplant recipients. *Clin Ther* 22(suppl):B71–B85.

163. Kirchner GI, Meier-Wiedenbach I, Manns MP. 2004. Clinical pharmacokinetics of everolimus. *Clin Pharmacokinet* 43:83–95.

164. Hoyer PF, Ettenger R, Kovarik JM, Webb NJ, Lemire J, Mentser M et al. 2003. Everolimus Pediatric Study Group. Everolimus in pediatric de nova renal transplant patients. *Transplantation* 75:2082–85.

165. Kahan BD, Kaplan B, Lorber MI, Winkler M, Cambon N, Boger RS. 2001. RAD in de novo renal transplantation: comparison of three doses on the incidence and severity of acute rejection. *Transplantation* 71:1400–6.

166. Kovarik JM, Kahan BD, Kaplan B, Lorber M, Winkler M, Rouilly M et al. 2001. Everolimus Phase 2 Study Group. Longitudinal assessment of everolimus in de novo renal transplant recipients over the first post-transplant year: pharmacokinetics, exposure-response relationships, and influence on cyclosporine. *Clin Pharmacol Ther* 69:48–56.

167. Kahan BD, Podbielski J, Napoli KL, Katz SM, Meir-Kriesche HU, Van Buren CT. 1998. Immunosuppressive effects and safety of a sirolimus/cyclosporine combination regimen for renal transplantation. *Transplantation* 66:1040–46.

168. Nashan B. 2002. Review of the proliferation inhibitor everolimus. *Expert Opin Investig Drug* 11:1842–50.

169. Kirchner GI, Winkler M, Mueller L, Vidal C, Jacobsen W, Franzke A. 2000. Pharmacokinetics of SDZ RAD and cyclosporin including their metabolites in seven kidney graft patients after the first dose of SDZ RAD. *Br J Clin Pharmacol* 50:449–54.

170. *Innofluor® Certican® Assay System (package insert).* Seradyn Inc, Indianapolis, IN, 2003.

171. Lehmkuhl H, Ross H, Eisen H, Valantine H. 2005. Everolimus (Certican) in heart transplantation: optimizing renal function through minimizing cyclosporine exposure. *Transplant Proc* 37:4145–49.

172. Salm P, Warnholtz C, Boyd J, Arabshahi L, Marbach P, Taylor PJ. 2006. Evaluation of a fluorescent polarization immunoassay for whole blood everolimus determination using samples from renal transplant recipients. *Clin Biochem* 39:732–38.

173. Baldelli S, Murgia S, Merlini S, Zenoni S, Perico N, Remuzzi G, Cattaneo D. 2005. High-performance liquid chromatography with ultraviolet detection for therapeutic drug monitoring of everolimus. *J Chromatogr B* 816:99–105.

174. Salm P, Taylor PJ, Lynch SV, Pillans PI. 2002. Quantification and stability of everolimus (SDZ RAD) in human blood by high-performance liquid chromatography-electrospray tandem mass spectrometry. *J Chromatogr B Anal Technol Biomed Life Sci* 772:283–90.

175. Quinn CM, Bugeja VC, Gallagher JA, Whittaker PA. 1990. The effect of mycophenolic acid on the cell cycle of *Candida abicans*. *Mycopathologia* 111:165–68.

176. Lee WA, Gu L, Miksztal AR, Chu N, Leung K, Nelson PH. 1990. Bioavailability improvement of mycophenolic acid through amino ester derivatization. *Pharm Res* 7:161–66.

177. Franklin TJ, Cook JM. 1969. The inhibition of nucleic acid synthesis by mycophenolic acid. *Biochem J* 113:515–24.

178. Wu JC. 1994. Mycophenolate mofetil: molecular mechanisms of action. *Perspect Drug Discov Design* 2:185–204.

179. Eugui EM, Allison A. 1993. Immunosuppressive activity of mycophenolate mofetil. *Ann NY Acad Sci* 685:309–29.

180. Allison AC, Eugui EM. 1996. Purine metabolism and immunosuppressive effects of mycophenolate mofetil (MMF). *Clin Transplant* 10:77–84.

181. Bullingham R, Monroe S, Nicholls A, Hale M. 1996. Pharmacokinetics and bioavailability of mycophenolate mofetil in healthy subjects after single-dose oral and intravenous administration. *J Clin Pharmacol* 36:315–24.

182. Bullingham RE, Nicholls AJ, Kamm BR. 1998. Clinical pharmacokinetics of mycophenolate mofetil. *Clin Pharmacokinet* 34:429–55.

183. Nowak I, Shaw LM. 1995. Mycophenolic acid binding to human serum albumin: characterization and relation to pharmacodynamics. *Clin Chem* 41:1011–17.

184. Korecka M, Nikolic D, van Breemen RB, Shaw LM. 1999. Inhibition of inosine monophosphate dehydrogenase by mycophenolic acid glucuronide is attributable to the presence of trace quantities of mycophenolic acid. *Clin Chem* 45:1047–50.

185. Shipkova M, Armstrong VW, Wieland E, Niedmann PD, Schutz E, Brenner-Weiss G et al. 1999. Identification of glucoside and carboxyl-linked glucuronide conjugates of mycophenolic acid in plasma of transplant recipients treated with mycophenolate mofetil. *Br J Pharmacol* 126:1075–82.

186. Wieland E, Shipkova M, Schellhaas U, Schutz E, Niedmann PD, Armstrong VW, Oellerich M. 2000. Induction of cytokine release by acyl glucuronide of mycophenolic acid: a link to side effects? *Clin Biochem* 33:107–13.

187. Shaw LM, Korecka M, van Breeman R, Nowak I, Brayman KL. 1998. Analysis, pharmacokinetics and therapeutic drug monitoring of mycophenolic acid. *Clin Biochem* 31:323–28.

188. Kaplan B, Meier-Kriesche HU, Friedman G, Mulgaonkar S, Gruber S, Korecka M et al. 1999. The effect of renal insufficiency on mycophenolic acid protein binding. *J Clin Pharmacol* 39:715–20.

189. Holt DW. 2002. Monitoring mycophenolic acid. *Ann Clin Biochem* 39:173–83.

190. Mourad M, Malaise J, Chaib Eddour D, De Meyer M, Konig J, Schepers R, Squifflet JP, Wallemacq P. 2001. Pharmacokinetic basis for the efficient and safe use of low-dose mycophenolate mofetil in combination with tacrolimus in kidney transplantation. *Clin Chem* 47:1241–48.

191. Sollinger HW. 2004. Mycophenolates in transplantation. *Clin Transplant* 18:485–92.

192. Vidal E, Cantarell C, Capdevila L, Monforte V, Roman A, Pou L. 2000. Mycophenolate mofetil pharmacokinetics in transplant patients receiving cyclosporine or tacrolimus in combination therapy. *Pharmacol Toxicol* 87:182–84.

193. Shipkova M, Armstrong VW, Kuypers D, Perner F, Fabrizi V, Holzer H, Wieland E, Oellerich M. 2001. MMF Creeping Creatinine Study Group. *Ther Drug Monit* 23:717–21.

194. Schmidt LE, Rasmussen A, Norrelykke MR, Poulsen HE, Hansen BA. 2001. The effect of selective bowel decontamination on the pharmacokinetics of mycophenolate mofetil in liver transplant recipients. *Liver Transplant* 7:739–42.

195. Undre NA, van Hooff J, Christiaans M, Vanrenterghem Y, Donck J, Heeman U et al. 1998. Pharmacokinetics of FK 506 and mycophenolic acid after the administration of a FK 506-based regimen in combination with mycophenolate mofetil in kidney transplantation. *Transplant Proc* 30:1299–302.

196. Vietri M, Pietrabissa A, Mosca F, Pacifici GM. 2000. Mycophenolic acid glucuronidation and its inhibition by non-steroidal anti-inflammatory drugs in human liver and kidney. *Eur J Clin Pharmacol* 56:659–64.

197. Kato R, Ooi K, Ikura-Mori M, Tsuchishita Y, Hashimoto H, Yoshimura H et al. 2002. Impairment of mycophenolate mofetil absorption by calcium polycarbophil. *J Clin Pharmacol* 42:1275–80.

198. Shaw LM, Holt DW, Oellerich M, Meiser B, van Gelder T. 2001. Current issues in therapeutic drug monitoring of mycophenolic acid: report of a roundtable discussion. *Ther Drug Monit* 23:305–15.

199. Tsina I, Chu F, Hama K, Kaloostian M, Tam YL, Tarnowski T, Wong B. 1996. Manual and automated (robotic) high-performance liquid chromatography methods for the determination of mycophenolic acid and its glucuronide conjugate in human plasma. *J Chromatogr B* 675:119–29.

200. Streit F, Shipkova M, Armstrong VW, Oellerich M. 2004. Validation of a rapid and sensitive liquid chromatography-tandem mass spectrometry method for free and total mycophenolic acid. *Clin Chem* 50:152–59.

201. Saunders DA. 1997. Simple method for the quantitation of mycophenolic acid in human plasma. *J Chromatogr B Biomed Sci Appl* 704:379–82.

202. Tsina I, Kaloostian M, Lee R, Tarnowski T, Wong B.1996. High-performance liquid chromatographic method for the determination of mycophenolate mofetil in human plasma. *J Chromatogr B* 681:347–53.

203. Shipkova M, Armstrong VW, Kiehl MG, Niedmann PD, Schutz E, Oellerich M, Wieland E. 2001. Quantification of mycophenolic acid in plasma samples collected during and immediately after intravenous administration of mycophenolate mofetil. *Clin Chem* 47:1485–88.

204. Mahalati K, Kahan BD. 2005. Pharmacological surrogates of allograft outcome. *Ann Transplant* 5:14–23.

205. Filler G, Mai I. 2000. Limited sampling strategy for mycophenolic acid area under the curve. *Ther Drug Monit* 22:169–73.

206. Pawinski T, Hale M, Korecka M, Fitzsimmons WE, Shaw LM. 2002. Limited sampling strategy for the estimation of mycophenolic acid area under the curve in adult renal transplant patients with concomitant tacrolimus. *Clin Chem* 48:1497–504.

207. Le Guellec C, Buchler M, Giraudeau B, Le Meur Y, Gakoue JE, Lebranchu Y, Marquet P, Paintaud G. 2002. Simultaneous estimation of cyclosporin and mycophenolic acid areas under the curve in stable renal transplant patients using a limited sampling strategy. *Eur J Clin Pharmacol* 57:805–11.

208. van Gleder T, Shaw LM. 2005. The rationale for and limitations of therapeutic drug monitoring for mycophenolate mofetil in transplantation. *Transplantation* 80(suppl 2):S244–253.

209. Brunet M, Cirera I, Martorell J, Vidal E, Millan O, Jimenez O, Rojo I, Londono MC, Rimola A. 2006. Sequential determination of pharmacokinetics and pharmacodynamics of mycophenolic acid in liver transplant patients treated with mycophenolate mofetil. *Transplantation* 81:541–46.

210. van Gelder T, Meur YL, Shaw LM, Oellerich M, DeNofrio D, Holt C et al. 2006. Therapeutic drug monitoring of mycophenolate mofetil in transplantation. *Ther Drug Monit* 28:145–54.

211. Domke I, Engelmayer J, Langmann T, Liebisch G, Streit F, Luthe H, Dorn A, Schmitz G, Oellerich M. 2005. Measurement of total and free mycophenolic acid with new enzyme receptor methods on COBAS INTEGRA Systems. *Clin Chem* 51(suppl):A148 (abstract).

212. Bunch DR, Wang S. 2008. Therapeutic drug monitoring of plasma and serum mycophenolic acid by Roche Integra 400 in comparison with a high performance liquid chromatography method. *Clin Chem* 54(suppl):A10 (abstract).

213. Teshima D, Kitagawa N, Otsubo K, Makino K, Itoh Y, Oishi R. 2002. Simple determination of mycophenolic acid in human serum by column-switching high-performance liquid chromatography. *J Chromatogr B Analyt Technol Biomed Life Sci* 780:21–6.

214. Sparidans RW, Hoetelmans RM, Beijnen JH. 2001. Liquid chromatographic assay for simultaneous determination of abacavir and mycophenolic acid in human plasma using dual spectrophotometric detection. *J Chromatogr B Biomed Sci Appl* 750:155–61.

215. Renner UD, Thiede C, Bornhauser M, Ehninger G, Thiede HM. 2001. Determination of mycophenolic acid and mycophenolate mofetil by high-performance liquid chromatography using postcolumn derivatization. *Anal Chem* 73:41–46.

216. Jain A, Venkataramanan R, Hamad IS, Zuckerman S, Zhang S, Lever J, Warty VS, Fung JJ. 2001. Pharmacokinetics of mycophenolic acid after mycophenolate mofetil administration in liver transplant patients treated with tacrolimus. *J Clin Pharmacol* 41:268–76.

217. Weber LT, Shipkova M, Armstrong VW, Wagner N, Schutz E, Mehls O et al. 2002. The pharmacokinetic-pharmacodynamic relationship for total and free mycophenolic acid in pediatric renal transplant recipients: a report of the German Study Group on Mycophenolate Mofetil Therapy. *J Am Soc Nephrol* 13:759–68.

218. Gross SP, Driscoll JA, McClafferty TA, Edwards RL, Chun A. 2006. Performance of the mycophenolic acid method on the Dade Behring Dimension® Clinical Chemistry System. *Clin Chem* 52(suppl):A63 (abstract).

219. Luo W, Nimmagadda S, Ruzicka R, Tsai A, Loor R. 2006. Development of application protocols for CEDIA® mycophenolic acid assay on the Hitachi 911, Olympus AU640, and MGC 240 Clinical Chemistry Analyzers. *Clin Chem* 52(suppl):A67 (abstract).

220. Shipkova M, Schutz E, Armstrong VW, Niedmann PD, Weiland E, Oellerich M. 1999. Overestimation of mycophenolic acid by EMIT correlates with MPA metabolite. *Transplant Proc* 31:1135–37.
221. Weber LT, Shipkova M, Armstrong VW, Wagner N, Schutz E, Mehls O, Zimmerhackl LB, Oellerich M, Tonshoff B. 2002. Comparison of the EMIT immunoassay with HPLC for therapeutic drug monitoring of mycophenolic acid in pediatric renal-transplant recipients on mycophenolate mofetil therapy. *Clin Chem* 48:517–25.
222. Beal JL, Jones CE, Taylor PJ, Tett SE. 1998. Evaluation of an immunoassay (EMIT) for mycophenolic acid in plasma from renal transplant recipients compared with a high-performance liquid chromatography assay. *Ther Drug Monit* 20:685–90.
223. Schutz E, Shipkova M, Armstrong VW, Niedmann PD, Weber L, Tonshoff B et al. 1998. Therapeutic drug monitoring of mycophenolic acid: comparison of HPLC and immunoassay reveals new MPA metabolites. *Transplant Proc* 30:1185–87.
224. Westley IS, Sallustio BC, Morris RG. 2005. Validation of a high-performance liquid chromatography method for the measurement of mycophenolic acid and its glucuronide metabolites in plasma. *Clin Biochem* 38:824–29.
225. Premaud A, Rousseau A, Le Meur Y, Lachatre G, Marquet P. 2004. Comparison of liquid chromatography-tandem mass spectrometry with a commercial enzyme-multiplied immunoassay for the determination of plasma MPA in renal transplant recipients and consequences for therapeutic drug monitoring. *Ther Drug Monit* 26:609–19.
226. Schutz E, Shipkova M, Armstrong VW, Wieland E, Oellerich M. 1999. Identification of a pharmacologically active metabolite of mycophenolic acid in plasma of transplant recipients treated with mycophenolate mofetil. *Clin Chem* 45:419–22.
227. Oellerich M, Shipkova M, Schutz E, Wieland E, Weber L, Tonshoff B, Armstrong VW. 2000. Pharmacokinetic and metabolic investigations of mycophenolic acid in pediatric patients after renal transplantation: implications for therapeutic drug monitoring. German Study Group on Mycophenolate Mofetil Therapy in Pediatric Renal Transplant Recipients. *Ther Drug Monit* 22:20–26.
228. Shaw LM, Korecka M, Aradhye S, Grossman R, Bayer L, Innes C. et al. 2000. Mycophenolic acid area under the curve values in African American and Caucasian renal transplant patients are comparable. *J Clin Pharmacol* 40:624–33.
229. Mandla R, Line PD, Midtvedt K, Bergan S. 2003. Automated determination of free mycophenolic acid and its glucuronide in plasma from renal allograft recipients. *Ther Drug Monit* 25:407–14.

14 Analysis of Immunosuppressants by Liquid Chromatography or Liquid Chromatography with Mass Spectrometry

Kimberly Napoli Eaton (Retired)
University of Texas Medical School at Houston

CONTENTS

14.1 INTRODUCTION

The revolution in organ transplantation began in the early 1980s with the discovery of a powerful, yet selective, immunosuppressive agent, cyclosporine. Later, tacrolimus, sirolimus, mycophenolic acid and everolimus were introduced and all continue to be used widely with great success in reducing the risk for organ rejection. These agents (see Figure 14.1 for structures) or their analogues are also being used to alleviate symptoms of auto-immune disease, to treat cancer, to reduce scar tissue formation around drug-eluting stents, and a variety of other applications. However, success with cyclosporine, and the other innovator agents that followed, has been achieved with a common belief in the benefits of therapeutic drug monitoring (TDM). These agents, except possibly mycophenolic acid, are critical dose drugs; that is, they exhibit narrow therapeutic ranges that overlap subtherapeutic and toxic indices. Moreover, individualized tailoring of drug regimen and dosage is required because of their wide intra- and interindividual pharmacokinetic variabilities that are due, in part, to type of transplant, time after transplant, race, concomitant drugs, and other factors. Thus, estimation of drug level is either required or recommended for each of these agents and TDM is critical to achieve optimal clinical outcome. Numerous task forces, expert panels and consensus panels have been convened to review issues related to TDM of these immunosuppressive agents and to make recommendations for guidance to industry and to practitioners with regard to specimen of choice, timing of sample collection and specifications for analytical methods and other factors [1–13]. The United States Food and Drug Administration (FDA) has also developed guidance documents intended for use by industry and FDA staff regarding the safety and effectiveness of cyclosporine, sirolimus and tacrolimus assays [14,15].

14.2 TECHNOLOGIES APPLIED TO QUANTITATION OF IMMUNOSUPPRESSANT DRUGS

With the advent of clinical application of cyclosporine in the early 1980s, transplant physicians, faced with learning how to administer this powerful new drug demanded that clinical laboratories provide TDM services to assist in patient management. As early as 1981 a chromatographic method for analysis of cyclosporine was published [16]. At the time RIA (radioimmunoassay) for cyclosporine was also commercially available and was also widely used due to faster turnaround of results compared to the chromatographic technique.

Today four major immunosuppressive drugs are administered commonly, usually in combination but sometimes alone (cyclosporine, tacrolimus, sirolimus and mycophenolic acid), and a fifth outside of the United States (everolimus) for which TDM is required or recommended. Since the release of the original RIA for cyclosporine, many immunoassays are commercially available using over ten different technologies and various analyzers. These technologies are identified in brief below using information primarily from package inserts or manufacturers' websites. Some products have limited availability. Additional specifications of particular assays that use these technologies are listed in Table 14.1a–e [17–80].

- Antibody Conjugate Magnetic Immunoassay (ACMIA, heterogeneous) products available commercially from Siemens (formerly Dade Behring) are CSA Flex® (Cyclosporine), CSA-E Flex® reagent cartridges (Cyclosporine Extended Range) and TAC-R Flex® reagent cartridges (Tacrolimus) for use on Siemens Dimension® systems. The ACMIA principle relies on on-line mixing and ultrasonic lysing of whole blood (no pretreatment) followed by exposure to β-galactosidase-antibody conjugate, removal of free conjugate using analyte-coated magnetic particles and detection via a spectrometric β-galactosidase reaction.
- Cloned Enzyme Donor Immunoassay (CEDIA) products are available commercially from Microgenics (now part of ThermoFisher) as CEDIA® Cyclosporine Plus Assay (also

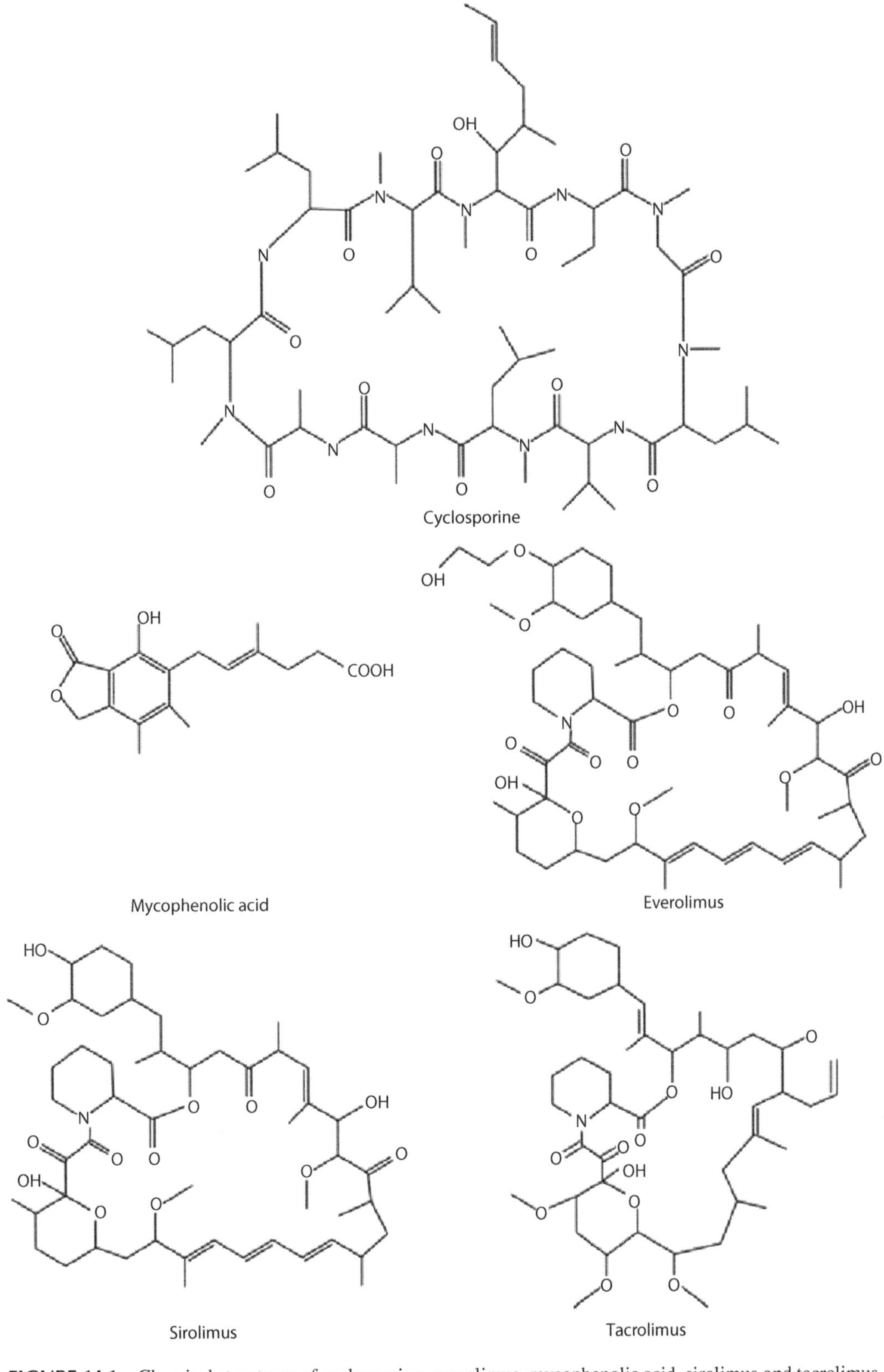

FIGURE 14.1   Chemical structures of cyclosporine, everolimus, mycophenolic acid, sirolimus and tacrolimus.

TABLE 14.1A

Cyclosporine Product Performance Specifications

Techno-logy	Product	Refer-ences	Functional Sensitivity Concen-tration[a]	Reportable Range Concen-tration	Samples	Concen-tration	n	Within	Total or Between
						Imprecision			
ACMIA	Cyclosporine Flex®	17, 18	25	to 500	Blood pool, Low	134	40	6.6%	5.8%
					Blood pool, Med	223	40	4.6%	5.9%
					Blood pool, High	360	40	4.8%	4.8%
ACMIA	Cyclosporine Extended Range Flex®	19	350	350 to 2000	Blood pool, Low	368	80	3.3%	5.2%
					Blood pool, Med	1123	80	2.7%	5.1%
					Blood pool, High	1750	80	2.7%	6.0%
CEDIA®	Cyclosporine Plus	20	40	25 to 450	Blood pool, Low	54	63	8.8%	12.2%
					Blood pool, Med	ND	ND	ND	ND
					Blood pool, High	435	63	1.6%	4.5%
CEDIA®	Cyclosporine Plus High Range	20	450	450 to 2000	Blood pool, Low	472	63	4.8%	7.5%
					Blood pool, High	1695	63	2.3%	5.2%
CMIA	Cyclosporine	21	21	30 to 1500	Blood panel, Low	89	80	12.1%	12.8%
					Blood panel, Med	261	80	9.1%	10.0%
					Blood panel, High	950	80	7.3%	7.7%
EMIT	EMIT® 2000 Cyclosporine Assay	22-26	25	to 500	"Control," Low	56	10	4.2%	8.1%
					"Control," Med	148	10	2.7%	4.2%
					"Control," High	340	10	2.9%	5.4%
EMIT	EMIT® 2000 CSAE Cyclosporine Specific Assay	27	<350	350 to 2000	Blood pool, Low	~400	80	3.3 to 4.8%	5.9 to 8.7%
					Blood pool, Med	~900	80		
					Blood pool, High	~1400	80		

Method Comparison

Reference	Samples	Concentration Range	n	Regression Slope (95% CI)	r	Metabolite Cross-reactivity (Concentration)
HPLC-UV	Kidney	25 to 550	273	1.03 (1.00-1.10)	0.92	AM4n, 5%; AM1, AM9, AM19, AM1c9, AM4n9,
HPLC-UV	Liver	25 to 550	201	1.18 (1.16-1.21)	0.96	0 to 2% (1000)
HPLC-UV	Heart	25 to 550	111	1.10 (1.04-1.15)	0.89	
LC-MS	Kidney	350 to 1600	60	1.09	0.97	AM1, AM4n, AM9, AM19, AM1c9, 2 to 5% (500)
LC-MS	Liver	350 to 1600	40	1.11	0.97	
LC-MS	Heart	350 to 1600	35	1.00	0.98	
LC-MS	Kidney troughs	26 to 379	122	1.09	0.94	AM9, 20%; AM4n, 16%; AM1, AM19, AM1c,
LC-MS	Liver troughs	41 to 386	80	1.18	0.91	AM4c9, <5% (1000)
LC-MS	Heart/lung troughs	31 to 383	109	0.93	0.94	
LC-MS	Kidney within 8 hrs	486 to 1882	47	1.02	0.97	Same as above
LC-MS	Liver within 8 hrs	529 to 1417	46	0.98	0.96	
LC-MS	Kidney, liver, heart	31 to 1457	227	1.20 (1.17-1.23)	0.99	AM1, AM4n, AM9, AM1c, AM19, ±1% (1000)
HPLC-UV	Kidney	~25 to 500	100	1.30	ND[b]	AM9, 7%; AM1, AM4n, AM19, AM1c9,
HPLC-UV	Liver	~25 to 500	96	1.24	ND	"insignificant" (1000)
LC-MS	Kidney	350 to 2000	60	1.12	0.95	AM1, AM4n, AM9, AM19, AM1c, AM4c9, <6% (1000)
LC-MS	Liver	350 to 2000	39	0.99	0.96	
LC-MS	Heart	350 to 2000	33	1.05	0.98	

(Continued)

TABLE 14.1A (Continued)

Technology	Product	References	Functional Sensitivity Concentration[a]	Reportable Range Concentration	Samples	Concentration	n	Within	Total or Between
							Imprecision		
EMIT	Cyclosporine	28, 29	22	to 500	Test procedure control, Low	74	30	4.4%	6.8
					Test procedure control, Med	208	30	3.6%	4.1
					Test procedure control, High	358	30	4.1%	5.7
FPIA	Cyclosporine Monoclonal Whole Blood	30	25	25 to 1500	Supplemented blood, Low	148	320	2.2%	3.4%
					Supplemented blood, Med	404	320	2.0%	2.5%
					Supplemented blood, High	783	320	2.4%	3.1%
FPIA	Cyclosporine and Metabolites Whole Blood	31	65	65 to 2000	Test procedure control, Low	361	150	4.6%	6.1%
					Test procedure control. Med	1226	149	3.2%	3.9%
					Test procedure control, High	1746	149	2.8%	4.6%
FPIA	Cyclosporine	32	23	to 800	Test procedure control, Low	71	640	7.6%	8.5%
					Test procedure control, Med	304	640	4.9%	5.9%
					Test procedure control, High	592	640	6.2%	6.7%
RIA	CYCLO-Trac SP	33, 34	15	25 to 1000	ND	50 to 1000	ND	3.4 to 10.0%	6.4 to 10.0%
HPLC-UV	"Home brew"	16, 35–37	10 to 25	to 3000	Supplemented blood	200 to 600	6, 18	~3–7%	~4–8%

			Method Comparison			

Reference	Samples	Concentration Range	n	Regression Slope (95% CI)	r	Metabolite Cross-reactivity (Concentration)
other EMIT	Kidney, liver, heart	43 to 485	262	0.94 (0.92–0.96)	0.96	AM9, 13%; AM4n, 5%; AM19, 3%; AM1, NDA[c] (500 or 667)
HPLC-UV	Kidney	ND	325	1.14	0.96	AM9, 19%; AM1, 7%; AM4n, AM1c, AM19, <5% (250 or 500)
HPLC-UV	Liver	ND	457	1.02	0.88	
HPLC-UV	Heart	ND	388	1.17	0.91	
HPLC-UV	Kidney, heart	ND	234	3.19	0.71	AM1, 96%; AM4n, 62%; AM1c, 60%; AM9, 19%; AM19, 9% (250)
HPLC-UV	Kidney	~50 to 1000	327	1.04 (1.00–1.08)	0.94	AM9, 11%; AM1, 7%; AM4n, AM1c, AM19, <5% (250 or 500)
HPLC-UV	Liver	~50 to 1000	228	1.16 (1.10–1.23)	0.93	
HPLC-UV	Heart	~50 to 1000	192	1.08 (1.02–1.14)	0.90	
HPLC-UV	Kidney	~0 to 700	134	1.01	ND	ND
HPLC-UV	Liver	~0 to 1200	51	1.00	ND	
HPLC-UV	Heart	~50 to 1100	84	0.93	ND	
ND	ND	ND	ND	ND	ND	ND

(Continued)

TABLE 14.1A   (Continued)

Techno-logy	Product	Refer-ences	Functional Sensitivity Concen-tration[a]	Reportable Range Concen-tration	Imprecision				
					Samples	Concen-tration	n	Within	Total or Bet-ween
LC-MS	"Home brew"	38–43	<1.0 to 10	usually to 2000, up to 5000	Supplemented blood	25	30	2.4%	3.8%
					Supplemented blood	125	30	2.1%	3.3%
					Supplemented blood	500	30	2.2%	3.3%
					Supplemented blood	1250	30	2.5%	2.8%

TABLE 14.1B
Mycophenolic Acid Product Performance Specifications

Techno-logy	Product	Refer-ences	Functional Sensitivity Concen-tration[a]	Reportable Range Concen-tration	Imprecision				
					Samples	Concen-tration	n	Within	Total or Bet-ween
CEDIA®	Mycophenolic Acid	44	0.3	0.3 to 10	Plasma pool, Low	1.0	126	5.6%	7.7%
					Plasma pool, Med	2.4	126	2.8%	4.0%
					Plasma pool, High	6.0	126	1.5%	2.3%
EMIT	EMIT® 2000 Myco-phenolic Acid (MPA) Assay	45–47	0.1	0.1 to 15	Test procedure control, Low	1.0	80	3.4 to 4.0%	5.0 to 6.0%
					Test procedure control, Med	7.5	80	2.4 to 3.6%	3.1 to 4.5%
					Test procedure control, High	12.0	80	3.8 to 4.9%	4.3 to 6.5%
ENZYM-ATIC	Total Myco-phenolic Acid	48	0.4	0.4 to 15	Plasma pool, Med	1.6	63	0.8%	2.2%
					Plasma pool, High	6.4	63	0.7%	1.8%
HPLC-UV	"Home brew"	49, 50	0.2 to 0.25	to 20	Supplemented plasma, Low	0.5	10	12.5%	7.6%
					Supplemented plasma, Med	7.5	10	3.0%	4.1%
					Supplemented plasma, High	30	10	6.2%	6.1%

Method Comparison

Reference	Samples	Concentration Range	n	Regression Slope (95% CI)	r	Metabolite Cross-reactivity (Concentration)
HPLC-UV	"Random"	38 to 1960	60	1.02	1.00	ND
other LC-MS	Supplemented blood, patient pools	1 to 1200	21	Mean bias = 2.8%	ND	ND

Method Comparison

Reference	Samples	Concentration Range	n	Regression Slope (95% CI)	r	Metabolite Cross-reactivity (Concentration)
LC-MS	Kidney, plasma	ND[b]	111	1.14 (1.08 to 1.19)	0.96	AcMPAG, 192% (10); MPAG, NDA[c] (1000)
LC-MS	Heart, plasma	ND	65	0.98 (0.88 to 1.07)	0.93	
LC-MS	Kidney, serum	ND	54	1.09 (0.99 to 1.20)	0.94	
LC-MS	Heart, serum	ND	41	1.07 (0.95 to 1.19)	0.94	
HPLC-UV	Kidney receiving tacrolimus	~0 to 40	89	1.07	0.99	AcMPAG, up to 185%; MPAG, NDA (1000)
HPLC-UV	Kidney receiving cyclosporine	~0 to 60	40	1.12	0.99	
HPLC-UV	Various	ND	155	1.04	0.99	
HPLC-UV	Kidney, plasma	0.5 to 13.6	89	1.06 (1.04 to 1.08)	1.00	AcMPAG, 6% (10); MPAG, NDA (1000)
HPLC-UV	Heart, plasma	0.6 to 14.2	70	1.09 (1.05 to 1.13)	0.99	
EMIT	Kidney	ND	120	1.03	0.92	ND

(Continued)

TABLE 14.1B   (Continued)

Techno-logy	Product	Refer-ences	Functional Sensitivity Concen-tration[a]	Reportable Range Concen-tration	Imprecision				
					Samples	Concen-tration	n	Within	Total or Bet-ween
LC-MS	"Home brew"	51–53	0.05 to 0.1	to 50	Supplemented serum, Low	0.2	15	8.5%	7.0%
					Supplemented serum, Med	1.0	15	5.5%	6.8%
					Supplemented serum, High	25	15	4.2%	5.5%

TABLE 14.1C
Sirolimus Product Performance Specifications

Techno-logy	Product	Refer-ences	Functional Sensitivity Concen-tration[a]	Reportable Range Concen-tration	Imprecision				
					Samples	Concen-tration	n	Within	Total or Bet-ween
CEDIA®	Sirolimus Assay	54	5.0	5.0 to 30	Blood pool 1	6.1	30	8.4%	9.7%
					Blood pool 2	7.0	30	9.6%	9.0%
					Blood pool 3	8.8	30	8.5%	9.5%
CMIA	Sirolimus	55	0.7	2.0 to 30	Blood panel, Low	5.0	80	3.1%	4.9%
					Blood panel, Med	11.2	80	4.0%	4.9%
					Blood pool, High	21.9	80	2.3%	3.7%
MEIA	Sirolimus	56	1.8	2.5 to 30	Test procedure control, Low	5.04	80	8.1%	10.1%
					Test procedure control, Med	10.4	80	4.1%	6.8%
					Test procedure control, High	20	80	5.7%	7.1%
HPLC-UV	"Home brew"	57, 58	1.0 to 2.5	usually to 50, up to 75	Supplemented blood, Low	7.5	20	8.5%	6.9%
					Supplemented blood, Med	22.5	20	1.8%	2.5%
					Supplemented blood, High	58	20	1.6%	2.9%
LC-MS	"Home brew"	38, 40, 59–62	0.25 to 1.0	usually to 50, up to 100	Blood pool, Low	1.8	16	ND	8.2%
					Blood pool, Med	13.1	16	ND	5.3%
					Blood pool, High	21.2	16	ND	4.9%

Method Comparison

Reference	Samples	Concentration Range	n	Regression Slope (95% CI)	r	Metabolite Cross-reactivity (Concentration)
HPLC-UV	Kidney	ND	46	0.97	1.00	ND
HPLC-UV	ND	0.2 to 24.0	106	0.98	0.98	
EMIT	Kidney	0.15 to 34.5	805	0.91	0.95	

Method Comparison

Reference	Samples	Concentration Range	n	Regression Slope (95% CI)	r	Metabolite Cross-reactivity (Concentration)
LC-MS	Kidney	4.0 to 30.0	165	1.19 (1.09 to 1.29)	0.864	41-O-demethyl SRL, 73%; 11-hydroxy SRL, 44%; numerous others, 7 to 22% (30)
LC-MS	Kidney	2.1 to 29.7	167	1.18 (1.11 to 1.27)	0.91	11-hydroxy SRL, 37%; 41-O-demethyl SRL, 20%; 41-O-demethyl-hydroxy SRL, 8% (10)
LC-MS	Kidney	2.9 to 23.6	215	1.23 (1.17–1.30)	0.93	7-O-demethyl SRL, 63% (3); 41-O-demethyl SRL, 58% (10); 11-hydroxy SRL, 37% (10); 41-O-demethyl hydroxy SRL, 6% (10)
LC-MS	Kidney	ND[b]	385	1.07	0.95	ND
LC-MS	Kidney	2.5 to 75	86	0.98	0.98	
HPLC-UV	ND	0 to 45	208	1.02	0.98	ND

TABLE 14.1D
Tacrolimus Product Performance Specifications

Technology	Product	References	Functional Sensitivity Concentration[a]	Reportable Range Concentration	Samples	Concentration	n	Within	Total or Between
									Imprecision
ACMIA	TAC-R Flex®	63	2.4	1.2 to 30	Blood pool, Low	3.4	40	5.6%	9.7%
					Blood pool, Med	11.5	40	2.5%	3.3%
					Blood pool, High	20.3	40	1.5%	2.1%
CEDIA®	Tacrolimus Assay	64, 65	2.0	2.0 to 30	Blood pool, Low	6.3	126	6.8%	7.8%
					Blood pool, Med	9.2	126	4.7%	6.1%
					Blood pool, High	15.2	126	3.1%	4.3%
CMIA	Tacrolimus	66	0.8	2.0 to 30	Blood panel, Low	4.8	80	4.4%	5.2%
					Blood panel, Med	10.1	80	2.4%	4.4%
					Blood panel, High	21.2	80	3.3%	4.4%
ELISA	PRO-Trac® II FK506	67	1.0	1.0 to 30	Supplemented blood, Low	3.9	10, 40	3.2%	7.9%
					Supplemented blood, Med	8.2	40	ND	6.8%
					Supplemented blood, High	16.5	10, 40	3.2%	7.8%
EMIT	Emit®2000 Tacrolimus Assay	68	2.8	2.0 to 30	Supplemented blood, Level 1	5.1	80	7.8%	16.4%
					Supplemented blood, Level 2	10.0	80	5.0%	10.3%
					Supplemented blood, Level 3	15.1	80	3.9%	8.4%
					Supplemented blood, Level 4	23.4	80	3.4%	6.8%
MEIA	Tacrolimus II	69	4.1	3.0 to 30	Test procedure control, Low	5.0	800	8.7%	12.0%
					Test procedure control, Med	10.9	800	5.3%	7.9%
					Test procedure control, High	21.4	800	4.1%	6.6%

			Method Comparison			
Reference	**Samples**	**Concentration Range**	**n**	**Regression Slope (95% CI)**	**r**	**Metabolite Cross-reactivity (Concentration)**
LC-MS	Kidney	1.3 to 20.3	103	1.16	0.88	12-O-demethyl TAC, 15%; 12-hydroxy TAC, 18%; 6
LC-MS	Liver		81	1.06	0.87	others, <3% (50)
MEIA	Kidney, liver		175	0.92	0.85	
LC-MS	Kidney	0 to 30	118	1.16	0.98	13-O-demethyl TAC, 38%; 3 others, <5% (20)
LC-MS	Liver		69	1.19	0.96	
MEIA	Liver		50	0.95	0.82	
LC-MS	Kidney, liver	2.1 to 14.8	125	1.07 (1.01 to 1.12)	0.92	31-O-demethyl TAC, 94%; 15-O-demethyl TAC, 45%;
MEIA	Kidney, liver	2.2 to 14.8	124	0.81 (0.75–0.88)	0.90	12-hydroxy TAC, 8%; 13-O-demethyl TAC, 6% (10)
LC-MS	ND[b]	1.0 to 25	95	0.95	0.83	31-O-demethyl TAC, 84%; 15,31-O-didemethyl TAC, 42%; 15-O-demethyl TAC, 36%; 4 others, NDA[c] (5)
LC-MS	Kidney, liver	ND	155	1.06	0.92	12-hydroxy TAC, 21%; 13-O-demethyl TAC, 10%; 6 others, <3% (100)
MEIA		ND	150	0.80	0.84	
LC-MS	ND	3.7 to 24.3	105	0.94 (0.91 to 0.97)	0.99	15-O-demethyl TAC, 67%; 15,31-O-didemethyl TAC, 62%; 31-O-demethyl TAC, 54%; 5 others, insignificant (10)

(Continued)

TABLE 14.1D   (Continued)

Techno-logy	Product	Refer-ences	Functional Sensitivity Concen-tration[a]	Reportable Range Concen-tration	Imprecision				
					Samples	Concen-tration	n	Within	Total or Bet-ween
HPLC-MS	"Home brew"	38, 40, 70–72	0.2 to 0.5	usually to 100	Blood pool, Low	2.7	15, 10	6.4%	5.2%
					Blood pool, Med	6.6	15, 10	5.1%	4.1%
					Blood pool, High	14.8	15, 10	3.5%	3.0%
HPLC-MS	MassTrak® Immunosup-pressants Kit (for tacrolimus)	73	0.5	to 30	Blood pool, Low	2.8	80	3.4%	4.7%
					Blood pool, Med	9.0	80	2.7%	3.4%
					Blood pool, High	20	80	1.9%	3.6%

TABLE 14.1E
Everolimus Product Performance Specifications

Techno-logy	Product	Refer-ences	Functional Sensitivity Concen-tration[a]	Reportable Range Concen-tration	Imprecision				
					Samples	Concen-tration	n	Within	Total or Bet-ween
FPIA	Innofluor® Certican® Assay	74, 75	2.0	2.0 to 40	Blood samples, Level 1	3.3	80	11.0%	19.0%
					Blood samples, Level 2	12.4	80	6.0%	9.0%
					Blood samples, Level 3	36.6	80	9.0%	11.0%
HPLC-UV	"Home brew"	76–78	1.0 to 2.5	to 100	Supplemented blood, Low	2.0	25	4.8%	12.1%
					Supplemented blood, Med	8.0	25	6.6%	7.0%
					Supplemented blood, High	30	25	4.2%	4.3%

Method Comparison

Reference	Samples	Concentration Range	n	Regression Slope (95% CI)	r	Metabolite Cross-reactivity (Concentration)
other LC-MS	Supplemented blood, patient pools	2.6 to 24.8	18	1.02	0.98	TAC metabolites, CSA or CSA metabolites, NDA (ND)
MEIA	Heart, lung	~3 to 30	99	0.92	0.93	
MEIA	ND	~3 to 30	156	0.91	0.98	
other LC-MS	Kidney	ND	51	1.08 (1.06–1.10)	1.00	12-hydroxy TAC, 13-O-demethyl TAC, 15-O-demethyl TAC, 31-O-demethyl TAC, 13,31-didemethyl TAC, NDA (ND)
other LC-MS	Liver	ND	58	1.10 (1.09–1.18)	1.00	

Method Comparison

Reference	Samples	Concentration Range	n	Regression Slope (95% CI)	r	Metabolite Cross-reactivity (Concentration)
LC-MS	Kidney	2.4 to 33.2	110	1.00 (0.90–1.09)	0.95	Sirolimus, 74% (10); phosphocholine RAD, 70%; 25-hydroxy RAD, 6%; 4 others, ≤3% (25)
LC-MS	Heart	2.1 to 20.6	111	1.03 (0.97–1.09)	0.96	
HPLC-UV	Heart	1.6 to 15	113	1.22	0.91	
ND[b]						ND

(*Continued*)

TABLE 14.1E (Continued)

					Imprecision				
Techno-logy	Product	Refer-ences	Functional Sensitivity Concen-tration[a]	Reportable Range Concen-tration	Samples	Concen-tration	n	Within	Total or Bet-ween
HPLC-MS	"Home brew"	79, 80	0.5 to 1.0	to 50	Supplemented blood, Low	1.3	10	10.6%	8.7%
					Supplemented blood, Med	12.5	10	3.3%	3.4%
					Supplemented blood, High	30	10	2.9%	6.1%

[a] Concentrations in ng/mL except Mycophenolic acid, ug/ml
[b] ND No data
[c] NDA No detectable amount

available are reagents for a High Range Assay), CEDIA® Mycophenolic Acid Assay, CEDIA® sirolimus assay and CEDIA® Tacrolimus Assay. Analyses can be performed on a variety of instrument systems including the Hitachi 911, 912, 917; Beckman Synchron, Olympus, and other automated analyzers. The principle of the CEDIA technology is to lyse whole blood, followed by exposure to enzyme donor (analyte-inactive β-galactosidase fragment conjugate) and antianalyte antibody, then bind remaining free enzyme donor to enzyme acceptor (second inactive β-galactosidase fragment) to produce active enzyme that catalyzes a spectrometric reaction. To achieve expected performance specifications, collection tubes must be at least 1/3 full, otherwise mycophenolic acid concentration will be overestimated, sirolimus will be underestimated and tacrolimus will be "impacted."
- Chemiluminescent Microparticle Immunoassay (CMIA) is a new product line from Abbott Diagnostics. Reagent kits are available for Sirolimus and Tacrolimus for analysis on the Abbott Diagnostics architect *i* system (Cyclosporine has just been released). The principle of CMIA technology is to lyse whole blood with subsequent exposure to antian-alyte coated paramagnetic particles, followed by addition of acridinium-labeled analyte conjugate then pretrigger and trigger solutions to initiate a chemiluminescent reaction.
- Enzyme-Linked Immunosorbent Assay (ELISA) technology has been utilized in a commercial reagent kit from Diasorin for tacrolimus (PRO-Trac II TAC). This procedure is no longer used clinically.
- Enzyme Multiplied Immunoassay Technique (EMIT, homogenous also HEIT [81]) reagents are available commercially from Siemens as the Dade Behring Syva® product line. EMIT® 2000 reagent kits are available for Cyclosporine Specific (and include extended range calibrators), Mycophenolic Acid and Tacrolimus on Viva E® or V-Twin® Drug Testing Systems. Roche Diagnostics offers an EMIT assay for cyclosporine while COBAS-based techniques for sirolimus and tacrolimus are under development. EMIT technology employs whole blood pretreatment followed by exposure to analyte-glucose-6-phosphate dehydrogenase conjugate and specific antibody, remaining free enzyme conjugate forms NADH (nicotinamide adenine dinucleotide) in a spectrometric reaction [81].

Method Comparison

Reference	Samples	Concentra-tion Range	n	Regression Slope (95% CI)	r	Metabolite Cross-reactivity (Concentration)
other LC-MS	ND	~2.5 to 20	100	0.97	0.98	ND
other LC-MS	Supplemented blood, patient pools	~1.0 to 30	71	0.97	0.99	

- Enzyme-Mediated Spectrometric Assay is an antibody-independent technology recently commercialized by Roche Diagnostics for mycophenolic acid (total MPA). This product is approved for use on COBAS INTEGRA systems. The principle of the test mimics inhibition by mycophenolic acid of the nicotinamide adenine dinucleotide (NAD)-dependent enzymatic reaction of inosine monophosphate dehydrogenase II (IMPDH) with inosine monophosphate (IMP), but utilizes a mutant enzyme. NADH product formation is proportional to absorbance at 340 nm.
- Fluorescence Polarization Immunoassay (FPIA) is a technology originally developed by Abbott Laboratories that is applied on the Abbott TDx® and TDx/FLx® analyzers (Cyclosporine and Metabolites, Cyclosporine Monoclonal, and Seradyn Incorporated's Innofluor® Certican® assay) and Abbott AxSYM/ AxSYM Plus analyzers. The principle of FPIA technology relies on specimen pretreatment. Then upon mixing, fluorescein-labeled analyte tracer and authentic analyte bind in competitive fashion to an analyte specific antibody. The extent of signal is proportional to the fluorescence polarization of the bound tracer.
- Microparticle Enzyme-Linked Immunoassay (MEIA) technology has been available for many years from Abbott Diagnostics for tacrolimus and, more recently, for sirolimus determination on the IMx® analyzer. The principle of MEIA requires sample pretreatment before exposure to analyte specific antibody-coated microparticle and analyte-alkaline phosphate conjugate, whereby unbound conjugate is removed from conjugate-antibody microparticle complexes bound irreversibly to a glass fiber matrix to which substrate is added that initiates a fluorescent reaction. It should be noted that hematocrit values outside of the 35–45% range (15–35%, 45–60%) result in up to a 23% difference from the expected sirolimus concentration.
- Radioimmunoassay RIA technology is, available commercially only as a cyclosporine reagent kit (CYCLO-Trac SP) from Diasorin.

In addition to these immunoassays, high performance liquid chromatography (HPLC) is also used for TDM of immunosuppressants. HPLC methods may be more accurate than immunoassays because of less chance of interference from metabolites or matrix.

- HPLC with Ultraviolet Detection (HPLC-UV) is another well developed technology with many published procedures. The only exception is a commercial kit (Mycophenolic Acid in Plasma/Serum) offered by Chromsystems Instruments and Chemicals for (total) mycophenolic acid. In principle, analyte is extracted from the biological matrix using an organic solvent, preferably in the presence of an internal standard. Further purification using solid phase extraction or other manipulation of the extract maybe required to ensure suitability prior to injection onto an HPLC system, whereupon reverse-phase chromatography selectively separates analyte from coextracted substances. Ultraviolet light at a wavelength selective for analyte and internal standard is used for detection of eluting compounds: concentration is proportional to the amount of light absorbed. However, tacrolimus cannot be quantified by HPLC-UV because it lacks a significant chromophore.

- Liquid Chromatography with Mass Spectrometric Detection (LC-MS) technology has been applied to TDM of all of the immunosuppressive drugs. Like HPLC-UV, the LC-MS knowledge base is limited to published "home brew" procedures, except for the recently released MassTrak™ Immunosuppressives Kit (tacrolimus) offered by Waters Corporation (other instrument manufacturers have products in development). In principle, analyte must be separated from the biological matrix before application onto a short LC column where water-soluble substances are washed away, then the compounds of interest are eluted (sometimes selectively) from the column using a methanol- or acetonitrile-based mobile phase. Per user-defined instrument specifications, column eluate is vaporized and compounds are ionized in the mass spectrometer source where specific ions are directed into the mass spectrometer. Because only ions with specific mass-to-charge ratios (e.g., analyte and internal standard) are permitted to pass though the quadrupoles to the photomultiplier for detection, this technology is highly selective. However, electrospray ionization that is commonly used for immunosuppressive drug analysis is prone to matrix-associated problems.

14.3   RECENT TRENDS IN METHOD UTILIZATION

Proficiency testing programs are a good source of information regarding utilization of technologies in clinical laboratories. The most widely used proficiency program in the United States for assessment of immunosuppressive drug testing is the College of American Pathologists (CAP) Immunosuppressives Survey. The most widely used international programs for assessment of immunosuppressive drug testing are the Ciclosporin, Tacrolimus, Sirolimus, Mycophenolic Acid and everolimus International Proficiency Testing Schemes (IPTS) from Analytical Services International Ltd. (London, England).

In the United States, accredited clinical laboratories are required to participate in the CAP program. As of early 2008 there were 471, 399, 188 and 26 laboratories assessing cyclosporine, tacrolimus, sirolimus and mycophenolic acid, respectively (Table 14.2). The position of LC-MS technology, for the most part, is increasing both in the United States and internationally. According to CAP data, since 2005 the percentage of United States laboratories using this technology has doubled for cyclosporine (up to 9% from 5%), tacrolimus (up to 11% from 6%) and mycophenolic acid (up to 46% from 21%). However, although the actual number of laboratories performing sirolimus analysis by LC-MS has increased by 46%, a large number of new laboratories enrolling in this survey have chosen to use MEIA technology. In effect the percentage using LC-MS for sirolimus testing has decreased (down to 28% from 85%). Internationally, the use of LC-MS technology has been much more widely adopted for cyclosporine, tacrolimus, sirolimus and mycophenolic acid (up to 13% from 2%, up to 23% from 15%, up to 51% from 38%, up to 18% from 12%, respectively).

TABLE 14.2
Recent Numbers of Laboratories Utilizing Methods

Analyte	Method (Manufacturer, Platform)	CAP[a]				IPTS[b]			
		2005[c]	2006	2007	2008	2005	2006	2007	2008
Cyclosporine	ACMIA (Siemens, Dimension)	24	26	45	55	79	96	106	113
	CEDIA (Microgenics)	25	37	44	44	60	66	71	77
	EMIT (Roche, COBAS Integra)	16	21	23	21	NC[d]	NC	NC	NC
	EMIT (Siemens, numerous)	NC	NC	NC	6	92	92	82	76
	FPIA (Abbott, AxSYM)	12	13	13	12	96	101	84	78
	FPIA (Abbott, TDx)	324	306	283	277	134	124	100	92
	FPIA, Drug+Metabolites (Abbott, TDx)	7	7	5	6	13	9	9	5
	RIA (Diasorin)	NC	NC	6	NC	23	19	15	12
	Others	NC	NC	NC	NC	10	14	9	19
	HPLC	9	10	8	9	40[e]	6	5	4
	HPLC-MS	22	29	33	41	0[e]	9	56	73
	TOTAL	**439**	**449**	**460**	**471**	**547**	**536**	**537**	**549**
	% HPLC and HPLC-MS	**7**	**9**	**9**	**11**	**7**	**3**	**11**	**14**
Mycophenolic acid	EMIT (Siemens, numerous)	NC	NC	NC	NC	79	61	62	63
	Others	NC	NC	NC	NC	NC	2	3	0
	HPLC	11	13	12	14	46	37	41	44
	HPLC-MS	3	10	9	12	13	13	18	23
	TOTAL	**14**	**23**	**21**	**26**	**138**	**113**	**124**	**130**
	% HPLC and HPLC-MS	**100**	**100**	**100**	**100**	**43**	**44**	**48**	**52**

(Continued)

TABLE 14.2 (Continued)

Analyte	Method (Manufacturer, Platform)	CAP[a]				IPTS[b]			
		2005[c]	2006	2007	2008	2005	2006	2007	2008
Sirolimus	CMIA (Abbott, Architect)	NC	NC	NC	8	NC	NC	NC	NC
	MEIA (Abbott, IMx)	NC	87	120	129	41	78	74	72
	HPLC	6	NC	NC	NC	51	35	26	15
	HPLC-MS	35	45	50	51	56	70	81	92
	TOTAL	**41**	**132**	**170**	**188**	**148**	**183**	**181**	**179**
	% HPLC and HPLC-MS	**100**	**34**	**29**	**27**	**72**	**57**	**59**	**60**
Tacrolimus	ACMIA (Siemens, Dimension)	NC	NC	10	58	NC	NC	35	66
	CMIA (Abbott, Architect)	NC	NC	NC	17	NC	NC	NC	16
	ELISA (Diasorin)	NC	NC	NC	NC	6	3	2	0
	EMIT (Siemens)	NC	NC	5	8	85	95	74	63
	MEIA (Abbott, IMx)	311	323	313	273	209	200	155	127
	Others	NC	NC	NC	NC	NC	4	9	11
	HPLC-MS	20	33	37	43	36	53	75	89
	TOTAL	**331**	**356**	**365**	**399**	**336**	**355**	**350**	**372**
	% HPLC-MS	**6**	**9**	**10**	**11**	**11**	**15**	**21**	**24**
Everolimus	FPIA (Seradyn, TDx)					6	40	50	59
	HPLC and HPLC-MS					19	22	35	54
	TOTAL					**25**	**62**	**85**	**113**
	% HPLC and HPLC-MS					**76**	**35**	**41**	**48**

a   College of American Pathologists.
b   International Proficiency Testing Scheme.
c   Data from the evaluation reports for the first distribution (A) of each year (CAP) or April of each year (IPTS).
d   Not charted by the program.
e   The data for HPLC and HPLC-MS are combined under HPLC.

14.3.1 Cyclosporine

In early 2008, CAP indicated eight technologies were in use in the United States for monitoring cyclosporine. The most widely used technology is FPIA on the Abbott Diagnostics TDx system. However, the popularity of this platform is decreasing (down to 58% from 74% in 2005) as utilization of ACMIA (up to 12% from 5% in 2005), CEDIA (up to 9% from 6% in 2005) and LC-MS (up to 9% from 5% in 2005) are increasing. Interestingly, although the number is small, a few remaining labs employ EMIT technology on the Roche COBAS INTEGRA platform, HPLC-UV or the old "Cyclosporine and Metabolites" FPIA for cyclosporine. Internationally FPIA is the most popular technology, although utilization is down from 2005 (31% from 42%). ACMIA is next (up to 21% from 14% in 2005), followed closely by CEDIA, EMIT and HPLC-MS at 13–14%. Interestingly 3% of laboratories continue to employ RIA.

14.3.2 Mycophenolic Acid

To date, the few laboratories participating in the CAP program who perform mycophenolic acid testing have utilized either HPLC-UV or LC-MS technology approximately equally. A commercial product is now available for mycophenolic acid testing in the United States (Total Mycophenolic Acid Assay by Roche Diagnostics). This nonantibody-mediated enzymatic reaction technique utilizes spectrometric detection. Testing for mycophenolic acid internationally is almost as popular as sirolimus testing (130 and 179 laboratories, respectively). Both LC-MS and HPLC-UV have been more widely applied than in the United States and EMIT technology that can be performed on common laboratory analyzers is available internationally.

14.3.3 Sirolimus

In 2005 only a handful of laboratories in the United States were participating in the CAP program for sirolimus and all of those labs were utilizing either LC-MS or HPLC-UV "home brew" methods. However, with the availability of an MEIA assay, the majority of participating labs (69%) currently use it. Internationally, LC-MS technology is widely used (51%) while a few labs (8%) still employ HPLC-UV technology. The other 40% are MEIA users with some laboratories apparently switching from HPLC-UV or adding MEIA as a new technology for sirolimus analysis since 2005.

14.3.4 Tacrolimus

In 2005 only two technologies were employed in the United States as reported by the CAP program (94% MEIA, 6% LC-MS). In 2008, tacrolimus analysis was distributed amongst four technologies. MEIA remains the most popular but use has decreased to 68% with ACMIA now commanding 15% and LC-MS 11% of users. The new CMIA technology (Abbott Diagnostics Architect system) likely will replace their older MEIA technology.

Internationally more technologies are available than in the United States and, while MEIA still commands 34% of utilization, approximately only 50% of the MEIA users in 2005 continue with this technology. Use of LC-MS has increased dramatically (up to 24% from 11% in 2005). ACMIA and CMIA have become available recently and will likely pull more users away from MEIA. An EMIT assay is used by approximately 17% of labs.

14.3.5 Everolimus

An immunoassay based on FPIA technology is available outside of the United States for analysis for everolimus and it is applied as commonly as are LC-MS and HPLC-UV technologies (59 and 54 sites, respectively). However, usage of both has grown in popularity since 2005 with 88 new laboratories participating in the Everolimus IPTS program.

## 14.4	BENEFITS/LIMITATIONS OF ANTIBODY-MEDIATED AND OTHER COMPETITIVE BINDING TECHNOLOGIES

Immunoassays and the new enzymatic assay for total mycophenolic acid are well suited for use in clinical laboratories. However, the benefits of the commercial immunoassays are in large part related to faster turnaround time (<1 hour). Some of the newer procedures require no sample pre-treatment. The stability of method calibration, which is usually in terms of weeks, is an important benefit that enhances between run reproducibility, permits quick turnaround time and saves costs because quality control materials may be analyzed less frequently. The limitations of immunoassay relate more to analytical performance. Accuracy of measurement is of primary importance, as recommended therapeutic ranges and panic concentration levels are based broadly on dosing regimen and physicians interpret drug level values following "universal" recommendations that are independent of a particular method of analysis. The inability of antibody to discriminate between parent compound and chemically and structurally similar drug metabolites is the most commonly cited limitation of immunoassay technology. Because the presence of such metabolites in clinical specimens varies with time, the performance of the unique antibodies, each with specific binding characteristics, contributes to inconsistent overestimation of drug concentration. Variability in the biological matrix also can compromise accuracy of measurement for specific clinical specimens. The most well documented matrix effect is that of hematocrit with the Abbott Diagnostics MEIA for tacrolimus [69,82–87]. In addition, standardization of assay material, lot to lot variation and other factors may influence accuracy of immunoassay methods.

A comparison for accuracy of performance according to technology is made clearly using results of IPTS samples that have been supplemented with drug compound by gravimetric methods, as these samples are free of the complicating factors of metabolite cross-reactivity and variable matrix influences. Table 14.3 presents data from the January through June 2008 distributions and highlights values with >15% deviation. The data provide convincing evidence that standardization is a serious limitation with some test procedures (chromatographic techniques included).

- EMIT, FPIA (monoclonal, TDx and AxSYM) and LC-MS technologies performed equally well with cyclosporine-supplemented samples averaging <5% difference from target concentrations between 40 and 1000 ng/mL. CEDIA did not perform accurately below 150 ng/mL and neither did HPLC-UV, nor did the old Cyclosporine and Metabolites FPIA below 100 ng/mL. Current RIA and ACMIA practices produced values that averaged approximately +16% and –14% of the expected cyclosporine target concentrations across the entire range of assessment, respectively.
- LC-MS and HPLC-UV procedures applied to sirolimus provided values that averaged approximately –6% across the 3–20 ng/mL target concentration range, whereas MEIA technology was far from accurate with values that ranged between –40 and –20% of the target concentrations (average –31.9%).
- MEIA and LC-MS procedures for tacrolimus assessed supplemented samples with equal accuracy, exhibiting an average 3–4% overestimation between 3 and 12 ng/mL. However, ACMIA technology gave a misleadingly superior –0.5% average difference from the target concentrations, exhibiting large inaccuracies for individual samples (–17.8 to +43.3%) that appeared to be independent of concentration. EMIT technology for tacrolimus was highly inaccurate below 9 ng/mL (+16 to +30% overestimation), providing more accurate values only in the 9 and 12 ng/mL range (+5.6 to +8.9%). A comparison for determination of tacrolimus between the Dade Behring Dimension and EMIT 2000 procedure on a COBAS Mira Plus using clinical specimens verified the current observations [88].
- FPIA technology underestimated everolimus concentrations by 19.6% across a 3 to 12 ng/mL range. This is less accurate than the combined HPLC-UV/LC-MS method group which averaged –10% of the target concentrations.

TABLE 14.3
Method Inaccuracy (Interlaboratory % Deviation from Target Concentration) from International Proficiency Testing Scheme Data

Drug	PT Sample/ Parameter	Target Concentration	LCMS	HPLC-UV	ACMIA	CEDIA	CMIA	EMIT	FPIA (AxSYM)	FPIA (TDx)	FPIA (TDx Mets)	MEIA	RIA
Cyclosporine	289B	40 ng/mL	5.0	**25.0**	-5.0	**27.5**		7.5	-5.0	10.0	**20.0**[b]		**22.5**
	286B	100	5.0	1.0	**-22.0**	-0.0		-4.0	-7.0	3.0	**15.0**		**12.0**
	287B	120	2.5	3.3	**-50.8**	**-20.0**		**-11.7**	-10.0	-4.2	5.8		3.3
	288B	150	6.7	0.7	**-12.0**	0.7		-2.0	0.0	6.0	**13.3**		**14.0**
	287C	200	5.5	**13.0**	**-14.0**	-2.0		-5.0	-3.0	3.0	6.0		**17.0**
	291C	200	2.5	5.5	-5.0	2.5		-4.0	0.5	3.0	8.5		**22.0**
	286A	250	6.0	-2.4	**-14.4**	7.2		-3.6	-3.6	0.8	2.8		**10.4**
	288C	300	5.7	1.0	-7.3	8.0		-2.0	-3.3	2.0	2.3		**15.3**
	289A	300	3.7	-0.7	**-11.7**	-1.3		-0.7	-2.7	0.7	1.7		**15.3**
	290A	300	2.3	1.3	**-10.3**	-2.0		-0.7	-1.7	1.3	6.0		**20.7**
	287A	400	2.0	6.0	**-31.3**	**-12.0**		-7.8	-5.8	-4.3	-6.8		**10.5**
	291A	400	4.3	-2.0	-2.0	3.8		-1.3	-2.5	3.3	-0.8		**20.8**
	286C	450	5.6	0.4	-4.0	5.1		-3.1	-4.4	0.4	-2.9		**20.4**
	290C	1000	1.8	-1.4	-4.4	**-12.0**		-0.5	-5.7	-3.3	5.9		**16.6**
	Mean		4.2	3.6	**-13.9**	1.0		-2.8	-3.9	1.6	5.5		**15.8**
	Min		1.8	-2.4	**-50.8**	**-20.0**		**-11.7**	-10.0	-4.3	-6.8		3.3
	Max		6.7	**25.0**	-2.0	**27.5**		-7.5	0.5	10.0	**20.0**[b]		**22.5**
Mycophenolic acid	44B	2 μg/mL	**-30.0**	**-30.0**				-15.0					
	45B	4	-2.5	-2.5				7.5					
	Mean		-16.3	-16.3				-3.8					
	Min		-30.0	-30.0				-15.0					
	Max		-2.5	-2.5				7.5					

(Continued)

TABLE 14.3 (Continued)

Drug	PT Sample[a]/Parameter	Target Concentration	LCMS	HPLC-UV	ACMIA	CEDIA	CMIA	EMIT	FPIA (AxSYM)	FPIA (TDx)	FPIA (TDx Mets)	MEIA	RIA
Sirolimus	114B	3 ng/mL	−10.0	3.3								−40.0	
	112C	4	5.0	2.5								−32.5	
	110C	5	−4.0	4.0								−22.0	
	114C	7	−14.3	−12.9								−37.1	
	113A	8	−10.0	−10.0								−38.8	
	109A	10	−8.0	−9.0								−32.0	
	110B	10	−10.0	−13.0								−33.0	
	111B	10	−10.0	−19.0								−36.0	
	113C	12	−10.0	−11.7								−30.8	
	109B	14	3.6	2.9								−22.1	
	111A	17	−4.7	−10.0								−28.8	
	112A	20	1.5	−4.0								−29.5	
	Mean		**−5.9**	**−6.4**								**−31.9**	
	Min		**−14.3**	**−19.0**								**−40.0**	
	Max		**5.0**	**4.0**								**−22.0**	
Tacrolimus	152A	3 ng/mL	3.3		43.3			30.0[b]				6.7[b]	
	154C	4	2.5		10.0		0.0	22.5				5.0	
	153C	5	2.0		−16.0			16.0				8.0	
	156C	6	8.3		6.7		5.0	16.7				8.3	
	157C	8	10.0		8.7		2.5	17.5				11.3	
	153B	9	1.1		−10.0			6.7				0.0	
	154A	9	1.1		−17.8		−1.1	8.9				−2.2	
	155A	9	1.1		−17.8		−2.2	5.6				−2.2	
	152C	10	2.0		−5.0			8.0				3.0	
	155B	12	2.5		−7.5		−0.8	5.8				1.7	
	Mean		**3.4**		**−0.5**		**0.6**	**13.8**				**3.9**	
	Min		**1.1**		**−17.8**		**−2.2**	**5.6**				**−2.2**	
	Max		**10.0**		**43.3**		**5.0**	**30.0**				**11.3**	

Everolimus	2 ng/mL		
40C		0.0	5.0[b]
43C	3	**–23.3**	**–30.0**
42A	4	–10.0	**–15.0**
40B	5	–2.0	**–20.0**
43A	6	**–25.0**	**–35.0**
42C	8	–7.5	**–17.5**
41A	9	–5.6	**–23.3**
40A	12	–6.7	**–20.8**
Mean		–10.0	–19.6
Min		–25.0	–35.0
Max		0.0	5.0

a Ordered by ascending target concentration.
b At or below functional sensitivity.
This table highlights values with >15%.

- Too few data were available within this time period to permit evaluation of mycophenolic acid measurement methods.

Imprecision and the related parameter, functional specificity, are limitations for some technologies (Table 14.1). For the clinical laboratory, applying a technology with poor precision results in data with low reliability; a condition which complicates drug level interpretation and may necessitate more frequent monitoring. For instance, many transplant centers now recommend minimal drug exposure via a specific synergistic (i.e., cyclosporine and sirolimus) or additive (i.e., cyclosporine and mycophenolic acid) combination of immunosuppressive agents to avoid long term toxicity. Therefore, reliable results are important for proper dosing of patients. For illustrating the ability of a given technology to produce the same result across laboratories, data from the IPTS is again useful, although dependence on "n" must be kept in mind. Table 14.4 presents interlaboratory imprecision data for supplemented samples that were distributed between January and June 2008. It becomes apparent that a technology may provide acceptable performance for one analyte but not another and that some technologies are inherently more precise than others, while some fail to meet reported specifications.

- When applied to cyclosporine, the most precise technologies were FPIA (TDx), HPLC-UV and LC-MS, averaging 6.4, 8.2 and 8.8%, respectively. Precision at low cyclosporine concentrations (40–120 ng/mL) was problematic for immunoassay (and LC-MS) but EMIT technology exhibited consistently high imprecision across the entire 40–1000 ng/mL target concentration range (average 10.8%, range 7.0–20.4%). Even at a concentration of 120 ng/mL, six of nine technologies displayed >10% imprecision and ACMIA performed unacceptably (19.1%).
- Significant imprecision problems were evident with all three of the technologies that are applied to sirolimus. The commercial MEIA provided increasingly poorer precision with decreasing concentration, although performance was acceptable (6.8–9.8%) above 10 ng/mL. LC-MS displayed a consistently high degree of imprecision (average 12.4%, range of 9.5–16.7%), illustrating the difficulty of achieving acceptable performance for this analyte (compare this to data for cyclosporine and tacrolimus by LC-MS). Precision using HPLC-UV was generally unacceptable (average 19.1%, range 12.1–28.2%) among 14 participants.
- Precision for the EMIT, ACMIA, and MEIA technologies applied to tacrolimus is poor especially across a 3 to 9 ng/mL target concentration range, with averages of 15.4, 13.4 and 12.2%, respectively. LC-MS technology was well-controlled, exhibiting an average 8.1% level of impression. The new CMIA technology (16 users) showed good precision (average 6%, range 3.1–8.0%).
- No technology for the determination of everolimus provided an acceptable degree of precision at any level across the 2–12 ng/mL target concentration range. The current FPIA procedure (second generation due to be released in 2009) provided no better than 20% imprecision (average 34.2%) and LC-MS and HPLC-UV technologies performed at >12% imprecision (average 14.9%).
- The limited data available for mycophenolic acid suggested that nonstandardized "home brew" LC-MS and HPLC-UV methods are less well controlled than the commercial EMIT technology.

14.5   BENEFITS/LIMITATIONS OF HPLC-UV AND LC-MS TECHNOLOGIES

Through a combination of the power of chromatographic and spectrometric principles HPLC-UV and LC-MS technologies take advantage of the chemical properties of the analyte and test

TABLE 14.4
Method Imprecision (% CV) from International Proficiency Testing Scheme Data

Drug	PT sample[a]/ Parameter	Target Concentration	LCMS	HPLC-UV	ACMIA	CEDIA	CMIA	EMIT	FPIA (AxSYM)	FPIA (TDx)	FPIA (TDx Mets)	MEIA	RIA
Cyclosporine	289B	40 ng/mL	12.3	ID[b]	21.5	17.9		20.4	22.2	16.1	109.9[c]		14.9
	286B	100	12.0	5.6	16.4	14.9		11.4	8.3	9.2	5.7		9.4
	287B	120	9.7	6.4	19.1	11.3		12.1	10.4	6.8	11.2		10.9
	288B	150	7.8	9.3	12.0	8.5		10.3	9.1	6.1	7.0		6.7
	287C	200	8.4	10.7	9.1	8.7		10.5	9.3	5.7	2.5		7.2
	291C	200	11.1	9.6	9.9	10.3		8.0	9.0	5.9	15.9		7.3
	286A	250	8.7	3.9	8.2	9.4		10.3	7.5	5.8	6.7		9.9
	288C	300	7.6	11.9	9.5	6.1		8.4	8.8	4.7	4.2		8.1
	289A	300	7.7	5.0	9.3	6.5		7.0	8.8	5.5	9.9		9.0
	290A	300	6.5	11.8	9.1	7.9		10.2	8.0	4.5	1.7		4.8
	287A	400	7.4	6.3	7.9	6.7		11.5	8.9	4.1	6.3		11.2
	291A	400	8.3	9.3	8.3	9.0		10.0	8.6	4.5	8.3		14.6
	286C	450	8.6	4.4	7.1	8.6		10.1	8.5	5.9	4.7		11.8
	290C	1000	6.8	12.4	13.0	12.9		11.6	10.0	5.4	8.1		13.2
	Mean		8.8	8.2	11.5	9.9		10.8	9.8	6.4	14.4		9.9
	Min		6.5	3.9	7.4	6.1		7.0	7.5	4.1	1.7		4.8
	Max		12.3	12.4	21.5	17.9		20.4	22.2	16.1	109.9		14.9
	n[d] (291C)		74	3	117	74		73	74	88	3		9
Mycophenolic acid	44B	2 µg/mL	14.7	16.4				7.8					
	45B	4	12.7	10.7				6.8					
	Mean		13.7	13.6				7.3					
	Min		12.7	10.7				6.8					
	Max		14.7	16.4				7.8					
	n (45B)		29	45				63					

(Continued)

TABLE 14.4 (Continued)

Drug	PT sample[a]/ Parameter	Target Concentration	LCMS	HPLC-UV	ACMIA	CEDIA	CMIA	EMIT	FPIA (AxSYM)	FPIA (TDx)	FPIA (TDx Mets)	MEIA	RIA
Sirolimus	114B	3 ng/mL	16.7	28.2								41.3	
	112C	4	13.7	23.9								16.1	
	110C	5	13.3	25.1								12.1	
	114C	7	11.2	15.3								14.8	
	113A	8	13.5	28.2								10.7	
	109A	10	9.5	17.7								8.8	
	110B	10	12.5	15.7								8.0	
	111B	10	11.3	12.6								7.5	
	113C	12	12.4	20.6								9.8	
	109B	14	11.7	16.4								7.4	
	111A	17	11.1	12.9								6.8	
	112A	20	12.0	12.1								8.3	
	Mean		**12.4**	19.1								**12.6**	
	Min		9.5	12.1								6.8	
	Max		**16.7**	28.2								**41.3**	
	n (114C)		93	14								71	
Tacrolimus	152A	3 ng/mL	**10.1**		**17.0**			23.2[c]				16.4[e]	
	154C	4	8.4		19.2		5.8	**18.9**				17.4	
	153C	5	8.9		18.9			18.9				15.9	
	156C	6	8.0		14.3		3.1	**16.3**				13.0	
	157C	8	7.5		12.7		7.0	12.8				11.3	
	153B	9	7.4		10.3			13.0				11.9	
	154A	9	7.6		12.1		8.0	**13.0**				10.6	
	155A	9	7.5		11.8		6.0	14.8				9.0	
	152C	10	8.8		8.7			10.1				8.0	
	155B	12	6.9		8.9		5.8	**12.5**				8.3	

Mean	8.1	13.4	6.0	15.4	12.2
Min	6.9	8.7	3.1	10.1	8.0
Max	10.1	19.2	8.0	23.2	17.4
n (155B)	90	66	16	63	126

Everolimus		2 ng/mL		
	40C		24.9	58.8[c]
	43C	3	12.4	53.5
	42A	4	15.0	33.2
	40B	5	14.2	32.8
	43A	6	12.8	31.0
	42C	8	12.6	20.3
	41A	9	14.6	21.5
	40A	12	12.7	22.6
	Mean		14.9	34.2
	Min		12.4	20.3
	Max		24.9	58.8
	n (42C)		53	64

[a] Ordered by ascending target concentration.
[b] Insufficient data.
[c] At or below functional sensitivity.
[d] Number of participating laboratories for specified PT sample.

procedures do not rely on time- and temperature-dependent formation of a biological reaction product or equilibrium in a competitive binding reaction of an immunoassay. LC-MS in particular offers the potential for superior precision, increased accuracy and lower functional sensitivity than test methods based on biological principles because the electronic components of a mass spectrometer can be focused narrowly on specific signals and have the speed to rapidly discriminate among numerous signals. HPLC-UV and LC-MS test procedure specifications are enhanced even more when an internal standard is used to control for variable in-process losses of the analyte.

Simultaneous determination of multiple analytes (including metabolites) from the same sample is possible, provided a compatible sample preparation procedure, chromatographic conditions and detection method can be developed. Although sample preparation is required, techniques are straightforward and have the potential to be automated. Chromatographic technology currently favors determination of immunosuppressive drugs by LC-MS. It overcomes the many limitations of HPLC-UV, namely requirement for larger sample volume, more intensive sample preparation, longer chromatographic run times with concomitantly higher solvent consumption and less functional sensitivity and specificity.

Probably the most difficult aspect of integration of LC-MS technology into the clinical laboratory is in the necessity to develop and fully validate analytical procedures in house. But neither development nor validation of any procedure can commence without drug or internal standard materials. There are now several suppliers of calibration standard and control materials (Table 14.5). It is also possible, if desired, to obtain some form of calibration or control materials from in vitro diagnostic device manufacturers. Ready availability of actual source material is critical for success, as these compounds are needed for method development and then quality control. The manufacturers of the innovator drugs are undoubtedly the preferred choice for obtaining high quality drug compound, and sometimes internal standard, but it may take long time to obtain necessary paper work and legal clearance for obtaining these compounds from the manufacturer. Fortunately, there are now several commercial suppliers of these compounds (Table 14.6), however, supply is limited at times and the degree of purity of available material must be proven to be acceptable for critical applications. Some of these suppliers also offer internal standard material; however, the more commonly used internal standards must be obtained through the drug manufacturer (hydroxy-propyl rapamycin, Novartis; carboxy butoxy ether of mycophenolic acid, Roche; desmethoxy-rapamycin, Wyeth). An arrangement between Novartis and the International Association of Therapeutic Drug Monitoring and Clinical Toxicology makes deuterated forms of everolimus and cyclosporine available to members through Bioanalytical Services International.

Preparation of calibrators and controls from fresh whole blood is preferable, but requires a ready and reliable source of analyte-free blood, analyte materials of proven quality and purity and adequate time, technical skill and facilities to permit proper preparation, testing and storage. Usually a protocol for collection of blood from healthy volunteers or use of residuals of nonanalyte-containing clinical specimens must be approved by the local institutional review board.

In house preparation of calibration and control materials may also be the least expensive route, but purchased materials provide a much more convenient solution, provided their performance mimics that of the clinical specimens at all stages of the analytical process.

The current difficulty for any laboratory to successfully meet all of the analytical criteria during routine service was illustrated with distribution of a set of whole blood samples supplemented with sirolimus to six clinical laboratories. Interlaboratory biases of −40 to +20% from the target concentrations were observed although intra-laboratory precision was excellent ($r=0.986$): this suggested less than optimal standardization, matrix effects, procedural differences, or storage problems [89]. However, LC-MS technology, or HPLC-UV for that matter, for many reasons is well-suited to clinical applications and there are no limitations to the integration of either of these technologies into the clinical laboratory.

TABLE 14.5
Suppliers of Products for Calibration and Control

Supplier	Product	Cyclosporine	Mycophenolic Acid	Sirolimus	Tacrolimus	Everolimus
Bio-Rad Laboratories	Lyphochek® Whole Blood Immunosuppressant Control (five levels)	✓		✓	✓	
	Lyphochek® Elevated Immunosuppressant Control (two levels)	✓				
Chromsystems	Immunosuppressants in Whole Blood Calibration Standard (one level)	✓		✓	✓	✓
	Immunosuppressants in Whole Blood Calibrator Set (six levels)	✓		✓	✓	✓
	Immunosuppressants Whole Blood Controls (four levels)	✓		✓	✓	✓
	Mycophenolic Acid Plasma calibration Standard (one level)		✓			
	Mycophenolic Acid Control Bilevel (two levels)		✓			
More Diagnostics	Extended Range (CSAE) Cyclosporine Control (three levels)	✓				
	Mycophenolic Acid (MPA) Liquid Control (four levels)		✓			
	Rap/Tac/CsA Immunosuppressant Control for Immunoassay Methods (three levels)	✓		✓	✓	
	Rap/Tac/CsA Immunosuppressant Control Multiassay Liquid (four levels)	✓		✓	✓	
	Tac/CsA Immunosuppressant Control Multiassay Liquid (four levels)	✓			✓	
Recipe	ClinCal® Plasma Calibrator for Mycophenolic Acid (one level)		✓			
	ClinChek® Plasma Control for Mycophenolic Acid (three levels)		✓			
	ClinCal® Thoroughbred Calibrator Set for Immunosuppressants (six levels)	✓		✓	✓	✓
	ClinChek® Thoroughbred Controls for Immunosuppressants (three levels)	✓		✓	✓	✓
	ClinChek® Thoroughbred Control for Cyclosporine (two levels)	✓				
UTAK Laboratories	Bi-level Cyclosporine A Whole Blood Control (two levels)	✓				
	Immunosuppressants Levels 1–3 Whole Blood Controls (three levels)	✓		✓	✓	✓
	MPA Levels 1, 2 and 3 Serum Controls		✓			

TABLE 14.6
Commercial Suppliers of Source Materials

Supplier	Cyclosporine	Mycophenolic Acid	Sirolimus (Rapamycin)	Tacrolimus (FK506)	Everolimus
A.G. Scientific	✓	✓	✓	✓	
Alexis Biochemicals	✓	✓	✓	✓	
BIOMOL Research Laboratories	✓	✓	✓	✓	
EMD Biosciences (CalBiochem)	✓	✓	✓		
Fermentek Biotechnology		✓	✓	✓	
GenWay	✓				
LC Laboratories	✓		✓	✓	✓
Sigma Aldrich	✓	✓	✓	✓	✓
Toronto Research Chemicals	✓	✓	✓	✓	✓
USP Pharmacopeia	✓	✓		✓	

The author does not recommend the quality of these products.

14.6 EVOLUTION OF HPLC-UV ANALYSIS

In the early 1980s cyclosporine became the first of the targeted immunosuppressants approved for clinical use and HPLC-UV methods were developed for TDM of cyclosporine. Tacrolimus, lacking a chromophore with sufficient absorption for UV detection at critical levels, could not be analyzed by HPLC-UV, but mycophenolic acid can be determined by HPLC-UV with relative ease. Today, HPLC-UV is applied primarily to mycophenolic acid testing, as LC-MS procedures have all but replaced HPLC-UV for cyclosporine and sirolimus.

14.6.1 Cyclosporine

Procedures for quantitative determination of cyclosporine using HPLC-UV were developed out of necessity, as the original radioimmunoassay available as a kit from the drug manufacturer Novartis (then Sandoz) was highly nonspecific due to significant cross-reactivity of cyclosporine metabolites with the polyclonal antibody. The decision to use whole blood as the matrix of choice circumvented the problem of temperature-dependent distribution of cyclosporine between the cellular and extra-cellular (plasma) compartments. However, extraction of the drug from whole blood was not straightforward because this hydrophobic drug was active at such low concentrations (ng/mL) that large sample volume (1–2 ml) was required in order to provide a sufficient amount of compound to detect. Additionally, because the peptide-based structure exhibited UV absorbance only at low wavelengths (190–215 nm), extensive sample clean up was necessary to achieve interference-free extracts [16,90]. One procedure took advantage of cyclosporine's high solubility in diethyl ether, and then acidified the extract to permit removal of neutral lipophilic components with a hexane or heptane wash, neutralization before re-extraction into diethyl ether prior to analysis using a suitable mobile phase. Adapting, combining or eliminating steps [35,36,91,92], or use of solid phase extraction [93] provided alternative, yet sometimes less than optimal solutions for sample preparation [94]. Under isocratic HPLC conditions Gaussian chromatographic peak shape and a reasonable retention time could be achieved using C_8- or C_{18}-based column material but only with elevated column temperature (70–80°C). An alternative to "home brew" procedures, a kit consisting of whole blood-based calibrators and quality control materials, an HPLC column and instructions was available for many years from Bio-Rad Laboratories (Irvine, CA) [95].

14.6.2 MYCOPHENOLIC ACID

Compared to the more complex HPLC-UV techniques required to determine cyclosporine, sirolimus and everolimus, HPLC-UV procedures for mycophenolic acid are relatively straightforward. However, availability of enzyme inhibition assay from Roche Diagnostics [96] may lead many laboratories to switch from HPLC-UV methods to this automated one for analysis of (total) mycophenolic acid. Laboratory personnel must consult with the treating physicians to decide if parent compound only or parent and metabolite(s) are desired or if measurement of free drug (and/or metabolites) would be useful because neither of these latter measurements is possible with current commercially available products.

Relatively interference-free measurement of mycophenolic acid is possible because sample cleanup begins with plasma (or serum) rather than whole blood [97] and therapeutic trough levels are in the μg/mL rather than ng/mL range. In addition, mycophenolic acid exhibits two relatively unique and one more commonly used ultraviolet absorbance maxima (216, 251 and 305 nm) from which detection wavelength can be selected [98]. Importantly, changing detection to 254 from 214 nm has been shown to reduce base line noise by 87% but peak height by only 15% [50].

Early publications presented relatively tedious sample cleanup procedures that utilized protein precipitation with perchloric acid or solid phase extraction followed by C_{18} reverse-phase chromatography for determination mycophenolic acid, the active metabolite of mycophenolate mofetil, and its major metabolite, the pharmacologically inactive phenolic glucuronide (MPAG) [99–101]. Since then, numerous procedures have been published for quantitation of MPA using HPLC-UV, each with a simpler sample cleanup procedure [49], different chromatographic technique [102,103] or use of a unique internal standard [104–107]. An example of a situation where the choice of internal standard was shown to adversely affect quantitation was when a common internal standard (carboxy butoxy ether derivative of mycophenolic acid) was used in determination of the phenol glucuronide metabolite. Greater than 20% bias was observed. However, no bias was observed when phenolphthalein glucuronic acid was used as the internal standard [108].

With regard to turnaround time, determination of mycophenolic acid alone allows for a "quick" isocratic chromatographic method (<10 minutes), whereas when both parent drug and metabolite(s) are measured simultaneously, a time-consuming isocratic or gradient mobile phase program must be applied which may require up to 30 min. One novel way to circumvent this problem is to use ß-glucuronidase on a portion of the sample to hydrolyze the glucuronide metabolites to mycophenolic acid and then calculate the difference between the two mycophenolic acid measurements in order to estimate the amount of metabolites [109]. Moreover, automation of sample preparation has replaced tedious solid phase extraction without sacrificing technologist's time [110].

Accurate measurement of low concentrations of the active component (ng/mL range), free mycophenolic acid, as well as the free phenol glucuronide is possible using HPLC-UV and may be requested by the clinicians to assess certain clinical conditions [111–113] although LC-MS technology with greater sensitivity is perhaps a more suitable choice. An additional ultrafiltration step is required in either case. Free mycophenolic acid is stable through at least one freeze-thaw cycle [114].

Measurement of the reactive acyl glucuronide metabolite (AcMPAG), with known immunosuppressive and toxic potentials [46], may require stabilization using acidification [115]. Procedures which include measurement of the acyl glucuronide tend to be more complex [46,50].

Both short term and long term stability of mycophenolic acid in storage has been reported [116].

Capillary electrophoresis technology has recently been applied to determination of mycophenolic acid and its metabolites from plasma [117,118]. The benefits of this technique are simplicity, limited reagent consumption (no organic solvent), indefinite column lifetime, good sensitivity and excellent precision.

14.6.3 SIROLIMUS

Although there is significant interest in measurement of sirolimus, there have been only a few procedures published for sirolimus by HPLC-UV because such techniques are difficult to develop and apply. Like cyclosporine, whole blood is the matrix of choice for TDM of sirolimus: in this case more than 95% of the drug is sequestered into red blood cells. Therapeutic trough levels of sirolimus in the low ng/mL range the necessitate of large sample volume. Furthermore the lone chromophore in sirolimus, a triene system, exhibits only a weak absorbance maximum at 277. Thus, compounds which contain aromatic compounds that exhibit strong UV absorbance at 280 nm (i.e., proteins) must be eliminated either during sample cleanup or through selective chromatography.

The first published procedure, although exhibiting a sensitivity of 1 ng/mL, was able to achieve only a modest 35% recovery from the sample cleanup procedure [119]. The second published procedure and its modifications for routine clinical application described a rigorous multi-step liquid-liquid extraction with methyl *tert*-butyl ether and 28-min chromatographic run that required removal of late eluting substances from the tandem C_{18} reversed phase columns with tetrahydrofuran after each sample [57,120,121]. Other investigators were able to simplify or shorten the sample extract preparation or chromatographic procedure somewhat, although multistep liquid-liquid extraction using organic (acetone, 1-cholobutane, hexane) or solid phase extraction sample cleanup and long chromatographic run times of up to 35 min were still necessary [58,122–126] for successful determination of sirolimus. The commonly used internal standard for HPLC-UV, desmethoxy rapamycin, is no longer commercially available and this will force users to switch to LC-MS technology eventually.

14.6.4 EVEROLIMUS

The first description of an HPLC-UV procedure for whole blood everolimus [76] was an adaptation of a procedure developed for sirolimus [58]. Few other published procedures describe quantitation of everolimus using HPLC-UV [77]. These procedures begin with steps similar to those commonly applied to sample preparation for HPLC-MS analysis; that is, protein precipitation using a strong organic solvent in the presence of zinc metal ions. However, to remove interfering lipophilic substances it was necessary to apply the resulting supernatant to solid phase extraction or basify the supernatant and extract into the same or another solvent and finally to wash with hexane or heptane. Chromatography accomplished on C_8 or C_{18}-based columns using elevated column temperature (55–60°C) in order to improved peak shape reduced run time to less than 15 minutes per sample. A technique has been published where everolimus and cyclosporine were determined simultaneously by switching the UV detector from 278 nm after appearance of everolimus and its internal standard to 214 nm until the end of the chromatographic run in order to detect cyclosporine and its internal standard at later retention times [127]. The chromatopathic analysis time was 36 min (Figure 14.2).

14.7 EVOLUTION OF LC-MS ANALYSIS

Continual improvement in quantitative procedures for determination of the immunosuppressive drugs by LC-MS has been documented over the last decade, primarily with tandem quadrupole systems using electrospray in the positive ionization mode. Interestingly, a few clinical centers have been successful with the more cost-efficient single quadrupole systems. Others have tried electrospray in the negative ionization mode, atmospheric pressure chemical ionization or ion trap systems. The capability of LC-MS technology to sort through the unintended interfering compounds in biological matrices and to selectively and sensitively detect compounds of interest is far greater than any other technology applied to quantification of immunosuppressive drugs.

The compounds of interest must be ionizable for detection using commonly employed mass spectrometric techniques such as electrospray ionization and atmospheric pressure chemical

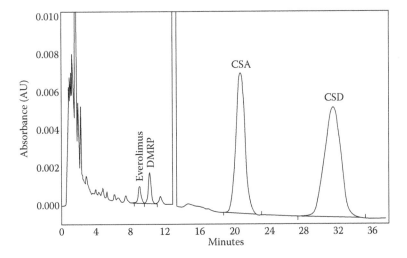

FIGURE 14.2   Chromatogram illustrating simultaneous analysis of whole blood supplemented with everolimus and cyclosporine, 20 and 700 ng/mL, respectively, by HPLC with detection at 278 nm (0–13 min) and 214 nm (13–38 min). Everolimus is baseline separated from its internal standard (desmethoxy-rapamycin, DMRP); retention times were 9.0 and 10.2 minutes, respectively. Cyclosporine and its internal standard (cyclosporin D, CsD) appear at retention times of 21.5 and 31.0 minutes, respectively. (Previously unpublished illustration kindly submitted to the author by D. Cattaneo).

ionization. The immunosuppressants (to differing degrees) fall into this category of compounds. Mobile phase additives such as acetic and formic acids facilitate ionization [128,129]. Conditions that promote labile ammoniated ions as compared to the more stable sodiated species, such as supplementation of the mobile phase with ammonium acetate or ammonium formate, as compared to the more stable sodiated species are preferred in many of the LC-MS procedures for determination of the immunosuppressive drugs. The environment in the ionization chamber of the mass spectrometer must be such that a consistent ratio of these species is maintained during ionization of both analyte and internal standard and from sample to sample. To achieve the most accurate measurements, the performance of the internal standard must parallel that of the analyte as closely as possible, including chromatographic retention time and ionization efficiency. Correction for aberrant ionization can be made only if the chemical nature of the internal standard is well-matched to the analyte.

Quantifier mass transitions are monitored by selection of only ions with specific mass-to-charge ratios (i.e., ammoniated adducts of the intact analyte and internal standard), followed by fragmentation of these precursor or parent ions into one or more product or daughter ions and then selective detection of only the most abundant product ions. For confirmation, employment of the ratio of the quantifier mass transition and qualifier mass transition response (fragmentation of the precursor ion to a second product ion) for each compound of interest is recommended [130,131] especially for TDM of immunosuppressants [132]. Unfortunately, this technique has been used in only a few of the LC-MS procedures for immunosuppressive drugs.

Matrix effects may profoundly affect the accuracy of quantitation using LC-MS. Matrix effects cause perturbations in ionization efficiency and result in ion suppression or enhancement. They are caused by the presence of unintended substances in the ionization chamber at the same time as the compound of interest. Matrix effects occur more often to polar compounds with electrospray (a liquid phase technique), but can also occur with atmospheric pressure chemical ionization (a gas phase technique). These effects are not resolved or detected as easily as in the case of interferences with HPLC-UV [133,134]. The source of substances that induce matrix effects may be the sample extract (actual extraction reagents or compounds present in the clinical specimen that were coextracted during sample preparation), other sample extracts (compounds from the previous sample(s) that were retained tightly on the HPLC column and that elute with subsequent samples), the HPLC column (breakdown and release of column material) or the mobile phase itself. Matrix effects can be minimized in a variety of ways: optimization of sample preparation, manipulation of chromatography, compensation through use of a suitable internal standard or, if possible, change to a different mass spectrometer interface.

Complex biological matrices contain high and variable levels of amines, amino acids, fatty acids, nucleotides, peptides, phospholipids, proteins, salts and triglycerides. In addition, clinical specimens contain drug metabolites [135–137]. The polymeric substances present in collection tubes, extraction tubes or plates may leach into the sample or extract [138]. The lower or higher ionization potentials and proton affinities of these substances in comparison to the compounds of interest may influence ionization efficiency.

Sample pretreatment to precipitate proteins can be executed effectively by several means that use different mechanisms [139].

- Organic solvents such as acetonitrile, methanol or ethanol lower the dielectric constant of proteins by displacing water molecules, but such solvents also increase the solubility of hydrophobic interfering compounds
- Acids such as trichloroacetic acid or phosphoric acid form insoluble salts with positively charged amino acid groups
- Salts such as aluminum chloride or ammonium sulfate reduce available water by becoming hydrated and thereby increase hydrophobic protein-protein interactions
- Metal ions such as zinc sulfate reduce protein stability by changing the isoelectric points and by displacing protons on proteins, thereby lowering the pH

Zinc sulfate with either acetonitrile or methanol is commonly used in LC-MS procedures for determination of immunosuppressive drugs. Zinc sulfate (10% in a 1:1 ratio with 0.5 N sodium hydroxide) in a 4:1 ratio with human plasma removes >99.9% of proteins, acetonitrile remove 92–95% while methanol removes 91–92% of proteins. However, sulfate causes severe ion suppression and may pollute the mass spectrometer interface [140]. Therefore, for each sample extract injected into the HPLC system, aqueous mobile phase must be flushed through the HPLC column and to waste through use of a diverter valve before the compounds of interest are eluted into the ionization chamber of the mass spectrometer. Ionization effects are worse with the organic solvents than acids used in protein precipitation but these can be reduced with the addition of ammonium formate or formic acid into the mobile phase.

Protein precipitation does not completely remove phospholipids (acetonitrile removes more phospholipids than methanol does) which may impact robustness and sensitivity of the assay [137]. Liquid-liquid extraction can produce clean extracts but recovery of the compounds of interest may be low or variable. Mixed-mode (reverse phase and ion-exchange) solid phase extraction produces the cleanest extracts but adds a multiple-step procedure to sample treatment. Of potential implication to determination of immunosuppressive agents are the glycerophosphocholine with mass-to-charge ratios between 496 and 807 (protonated ions): these values are within the range of that of ascomycin and the product ions of tacrolimus and sirolimus.

Retention of phospholipids on HPLC columns is independent of pH, so altering the mobile phase pH may be an effective means of moving the analyte and internal standard away from these interfering substances. Often a 100% organic solvent mobile phase is needed to elute these residual phospholipids. If they are not fully eluted from the HPLC column, these compounds can build up on the column until they reach a point when they will "bleed off" into subsequent analytical runs. As might be expected, their presence on the HPLC column can also reduce its effective lifetime.

The HPLC or solid-phase extraction column material itself (silica, Zirconia, polymer, bonded or unbonded hybrid) can leach out into the mobile phase or sample extract, respectively, depending on operating conditions (i.e., temperature, pH). Reversed phase material is generally not ionized with electrospray [134,136].

The choice of mobile phase organic solvent, usually acetonitrile or methanol, can also influence ionization efficiency [141]. An amazingly large ten-fold difference on the ionization response of desmethoxy-rapamycin by the brand and sometimes lot, but not grade, of methanol used in the mobile phase was recently reported [142]. Such changes had a direct impact on sensitivity but, in addition, some methanols altered the proportion of the ammoniated to sodiated adducts of sirolimus and the internal standard differentially, thus reducing the accuracy of the measurements. Certain brands of methanol also affected quantitation of the phenol glucuronide metabolite of mycophenolic acid because it was eluted from the HPLC column into the ionization chamber before its internal standard and at a lower methanol percentage. This situation caused the ionization efficiencies of the two compounds to differ. Unique effects on both single and tandem quadrupole mass spectrometer responses by brand and lot of methanol have also been noticed with the procedures used for determination of sirolimus, but not cyclosporine or tacrolimus, in the author's laboratory [unpublished observations]. Such problems might be minimized with use of a flow splitter or use of an alternative form of liquid chromatography that employs significantly lower flow rates, namely capillary or ultra-performance liquid chromatography.

Commercial calibration and control materials and proficiency testing samples, as well as materials or clinical specimens that have been frozen before analysis, also can be problematic with regard to differential instrument response to the compounds of interest. Measures must be taken during method development to ensure that the compounds of interest in all materials perform equally under the established conditions [143,144].

Matrix effects should be assessed using postcolumn infusion and postextraction spiking methods, although most of the published LC-MS procedures for the immunosuppressants report either one or the other or neither. Postcolumn infusion with a solution of the analyte and internal standard while analyte-free sample extracts are injected and monitored will provide information on the section(s) of the chromatographic run where ion suppression or enhancement is present but not a quantitative understanding of matrix effects on the compounds of interest [137]. Comparison of the instrument responses of neat solutions of analyte and internal standard compared to analyte-free sample extracts spiked with analyte and internal standard after extraction and to analyte-free sample matrix spiked with analyte and internal standard before extraction will provide measures of overall chromatographic system and detector performance, absolute and relative matrix effects and overall effect of matrix on recoveries and method performance, respectively [145].

Determination of mycophenolic acid is a special case, not only because the preferred biological matrix is plasma (or serum), but because its glucuronidated metabolites, especially the phenol with its relatively high concentration, can easily decompose into the parent compound in the ionization chamber of the mass spectrometer. Thus, the chromatographic program must be sufficient to separate the metabolites from the parent compound. A similar problem due to interference from metabolites has been observed with cyclosporin D, an internal standard commonly used in the determination of cyclosporine. This problem can be eliminated with choice of another internal standard or with alternative chromatographic conditions.

As the immunosuppressants are commonly administered in combination and requests for levels are often concurrent, the application of LC-MS can pay off in the ability to quantify numerous compounds simultaneously. However, in this case, matrix effects and related ion suppression/enhancement issues must be considered for all compounds. Equal applicability of a single analytical process to all analytes and internal standards must be considered and the capacity of the mass spectrometer to achieve the needed sensitivity while monitoring multiple mass transitions must be assured.

14.7.1 Cyclosporine

The earliest published procedures using LC-MS for quantitation of cyclosporine alone were hampered by long cycle times (14 minutes), in part due to the use of isocratic mobile phases. The orifice (or cone) voltage was either set quite high (100 V), to form preferentially protonated species that would produce sufficient quantities of specific low molecular weight fragment ions, or the collision energy was set low. In the latter case, the desire was to prevent collision-induced fragmentation of the protonated species which were the products of labile ammoniated ions [39,146]. Cyclosporine analogues were used as internal standards, however, caution was urged when it was shown that elution times shorter than 6 minutes caused interference with cyclosporin D (the interference was assumed to be caused by a metabolite that followed the same mass-to-charge (m/z) transition pattern) [147]. A few years later, a procedure that utilized deuterated cyclosporin as the internal standard was successful using an isocratic mobile phase with a 2-minute LC-MS cycle time, however a tedious multi-step solid phase extraction was required [42]. In the same year there were two important discoveries: (1) ions of the hydroxylated cyclosporine metabolites AM1, AM9 and AM19 were confirmed to suffer loss of water in-source under certain conditions to form species that were isobaric with cyclosporine or cyclosporin D [148] and (2) the superiority of deuterated cyclosporine (cyclosporine-d_{12}) to both cyclosporin D and ascomycin as an internal standard was also demonstrated [149] to be accounted for by absolute recovery, a fragmentation pattern that followed cyclosporine closely, and parallelism of ionization efficiency that was dependent on the percentage of the doubly-charged precursor ion. At that time, cyclosporine-d_{12} was not readily available although now it can be obtained by International Association of Therapeutic Drug Monitoring and Clinical Toxicology members through Analytical Services International at www. bioanalytics.co.uk.

14.7.2 Mycophenolic Acid

Analysis of mycophenolic acid by LC-MS presents a unique challenge in relation to those posed by the other major immunosuppressive agents. Dissociation of labile ions such as glucuronides and ethers can occur in the mass spectrometer source prior to the detection process. The phenol glucuronide metabolite, usually present in high concentration in specimens collected for mycophenolic acid determination, and the mycophenolic acid analogue (the carboxy butoxy ether of mycophenolic acid) used commonly as internal standard are two such compounds that can decompose to mycophenolic acid [150]. Thus, there is considerable risk for inaccurate measurements of mycophenolic acid unless proper cautions are exercised.

Determination of the concentration of total amount (protein bound plus free) of immunosuppressive drug has been standard procedure, in part, because available technologies were not sufficiently sensitive to accurately quantitate the very low quantities of free cyclosporine, sirolimus or tacrolimus. However, with therapeutic concentrations of mycophenolic acid in the μg/mL rather than ng/mL range, as for the other major immunosuppressants, accurate determination of free drug is feasible using HPLC-UV or LC-MS. Preparation of sample for free drug involves filtration of the sample. Importantly, free mycophenolic acid cannot be determined from samples that have been acidified in order to preserve the neutral pH-unstable acyl glucuronide metabolite because acidic conditions disrupt protein binding [151].

One of the first LC-MS procedures determined mycophenolic acid within 4 minutes using on-line sample cleanup followed by reverse-phase chromatography with a triphasic acetic acid-fortified mobile phase. Mass transitions of ammoniated ions were monitored for quantitation purposes, and with the protonated ion of mycophenolic acid were used as a qualifier the analytical specifications met all requirements for application to TDM [51]. Another procedure with a simple acetonitrile/ formic acid protein precipitation sample cleanup utilized a gradient chromatographic program at pH 3 to selectively elute the phenol glucuronide metabolite, mycophenolic acid and then indomethacin, the chosen internal standard, within a 6-minute run time. Unique among these methods, transitions of negative ions were monitored [52].

Shortly thereafter a procedure for simultaneous quantification of mycophenolic acid and its phenol glucuronide metabolite within 7 minutes was reported employing the same type of solid phase extraction cartridge, instrument system and mobile phase components as for cyclosporine, sirolimus and tacrolimus, but with a different chromatographic column. None of the phenol metabolite was hydrolyzed to mycophenolic acid under the acidic conditions employed and only a small fraction of the metabolite fragmented into mycophenolic acid in the mass spectrometer [153].

Inability to selectively detect the acyl glucuronide metabolite of mycophenolic acid by HPLC-UV in a significant percentage of samples prompted development of an LC-MS procedure for quantitation of mycophenolic acid and both of its phenol and acyl metabolites. The conditions set forth in a previously published procedure were closely followed [51], but with the necessary additions of dissolution of the acyl glucuronide metabolite in dimethyl sulfoxide as opposed to methanol, and additional stabilization of the compound through acidification of the plasma used in preparing calibrators and quality control materials. Even though both the phenol and acyl glucuronide metabolites follow the same positive ionization mass transition pattern, accurate measurement of all of the compounds of interest was permitted using chromatographic separation.

Recently a versatile procedure that can be applied to measurement of total or free mycophenolic acid as well as to its phenol and acyl glucuronide metabolites in both plasma and urine was developed and validated [153]. Careful specimen processing and storage procedures preceding sample treatment by solid phase extraction in the presence of an indomethacin internal standard ensured clean sample extracts. Baseline separation of components was provided by a linear gradient chromatography under acidic conditions between samples on a 100 mm reverse-phase column within 6 minutes. However an additional 3 minutes was required to recondition the column to starting conditions.

Although not observed directly in the procedures above, the choice of indomethacin as internal standard may have led to decreased precision or other variations in method performance. The chemical composition of indomethacin, but not mycophenolic acid or its metabolites, includes a chlorine atom. The presence of chlorine changes the charge distribution on the compound which may result among unacceptable differences in the ionization efficiencies of indomethacin and the analytes [154].

14.7.3 SIROLIMUS

An early LC-MS procedure for sirolimus alone borrowed a lengthy sample extraction procedure from an HPLC-UV method [58] and utilized an uncommon internal standard, namely nor-rapamycin (a dimethyl derivative) [59]. Using reverse-phase chromatography with an isocratic methanol mobile phase the compounds were eluted within 8 minutes; one positive ion mass transition was monitored for each compound. A more recent procedure utilized the same liquid-liquid sample preparation but employed a linear gradient on a reverse-phase column in this case an ion trap mass spectrometer was used to optimize fragmentation pattern of the more stable sodiated ions of sirolimus and the desmethoxy-rapamycin internal standard to multiple product ions [155]. Although the analytical specifications compared favorably to a similar procedure applied to a triple quadrupole analyzer, the 21-minute run time and separation of two isomeric forms of desmethoxy-rapamycin ultimately may limit the clinical application of this method.

A procedure that utilized a simple sample pretreatment with zinc sulfate and methanol supplemented with desmethoxy-rapamycin internal standard relied on on-line sample removal of hydrophilic substances followed by reverse-phase chromatography with an isocratic mobile phase. Detection of positive ion mass transitions was made within a 5-minute run time [60]. Using a similar sample extraction procedure, except with ascomycin as internal standard, the run time was reduced to 2.5 minutes by use of a simple on-line wash with a 50% methanolic mobile phase and step gradient to 100% to effect elution [62]. Although the analytical specifications compared favorably to other published procedures a drawback to this procedure was that the mean recovery was only 72 to 76%.

Recently postextraction addition experiments suggested variable suppression or enhancement of the desmethoxy-rapamycin internal standard ion in many patient samples that were analyzed for sirolimus using a modification of the previous procedure [62]. The authors contested that such effects on the internal standard could not be eliminated readily or completely in this desirable high-throughput method [156]. Therefore, the authors undertook an important comparison between desmethoxy-rapamycin and deuterated sirolimus. The authors used sirolimus-free clinical specimens which when supplemented with known amounts of sirolimus, demonstrated considerable differences in matrix effect, absolute recovery and process efficiency compared to when internal standard was included. The inter-sample imprecision was lower with the isotopically labeled internal standard than with desmethoxy-rapamycin (2.7–4.5% compared to 7.6–9.7%). These differences in imprecision amongst clinical specimens were masked when blood pools were used (3.7% vs 3.4%). Importantly, with desmethoxy-rapamycin, an unacceptable overestimation of sirolimus concentration of approximately 20% was observed using a cohort of 72 clinical patient samples and with external proficiency testing samples.

14.7.4 TACROLIMUS

The most reasonable early LC-MS procedures for tacrolimus alone required 500–1000 µL of sample to be subjected to protein precipitation and solid phase extraction prior to chromatography for 2 or 4 minutes [157,158]. Supplementation of the mobile phase with ammonium acetate and a relatively low orifice voltage setting promoted the presence of the ammonium ion adducts of tacrolimus and the ascomycin (FR900520), internal standard which were then fragmented in the collision cell into specific product ions. Superior specificity, sensitivity and a more rapid turnaround time than existing immunoassays suggested that LC-MS technology would be ideal for TDM of tacrolimus.

Subsequently, it was shown that a single quadrupole system in the positive electrospray ionization mode could be applied successfully for tacrolimus analysis [71]. A comprehensive semi-automated sample preparation using styrene-divinylbenzene solid phase extraction disk cartridges overcame the drawback of "dirty" extracts and ion suppression. Using reverse-phase chromatography on a relatively short C_{18} column (30 mm) with an isocratic 90% acetonitrile and water mobile phase, the analysis was complete within 1 minute. Electrospray ionization in the positive mode was used to establish the sodiated adducts of tacrolimus and the ascomycin internal standard for quantitation whereby, collision-induced fragments were used for qualification.

In that same year a tandem mass spectrometry procedure promoted a simple zinc sulfate and acetonitrile "protein crash" sample preparation in the presence of ascomycin. A methanolic mobile phase step gradient was applied to a short reverse-phase on-line sample cleanup column [72]. This technique, with the potential of an approximate 2.5-minute cycle time, became the basis for numerous other high-throughput applications [87]. This author also found that an adaptation of a previously published single quadrupole system [38] procedure was an acceptable alternative in the same laboratory to the more selective tandem mass spectrometric method and both provided superior analytical performance in comparison to micro-particle enzyme-linked immunoassay.

Recently a limitation of current LC-MS practice that involved a combination of differing instrument configurations, use of commercial calibration materials, and nonisotopically labeled internal standard was reported [144]. These investigators found that application of a previously published procedure for determination of sirolimus to tacrolimus [60] was successful in routine operation until a third tandem mass spectrometric system was recruited into service. While using calibration material from a one specific source but not another, and ascomycin as internal standard, the results of samples that were analyzed on the third system were significantly lower than those that were produced on the other two conforming instrument systems operating under similar conditions. It was concluded that a modulation of the ionization efficiency of tacrolimus, but not ascomycin, in this case by matrix constituents in the calibration material, would have been overcome (or masked) with use of an isotopically-labeled tacrolimus internal standard. These observations highlighted the importance of instrument-specific validation and use of best practices.

14.7.5   EVEROLIMUS

The concern over choice of internal standard continued with publication of an LC-MS procedure for everolimus alone. Using either ascomycin or hydroxyl-propyl rapamycin (SDZ RAD 223-756) as internal standard and a zinc sulfate and methanol pretreatment, the compounds of interest were eluted from a long C_{18} column (150 mm) via a step gradient over a 2.8-minute cycle time [79]. Using the positive electrospray mode, detection was made with one mass transition. Between-day precision was better when hydroxy-propyl rapamycin was used, as compared to ascomycin (0.6–7.0%, 3.0–10.1%). Moreover, the everolimus concentrations in 100 samples were nearly equivalent to those of an LC-MS method performed by a reference laboratory when hydroxyl-propyl rapamycin but not ascomycin was used (slope of regression=0.97, 0.73); the goodness of fit parameter (r^2) behaved in a similar manner (0.97, 0.86). Ascomycin clearly caused underestimation of everolimus concentrations. Meanwhile only a minimally acceptable limit of quantitation, 1.0 ng/mL, was achieved, due in part to the low ionization efficiency of everolimus [159]. A similar LC-MS procedure [80] soon followed where the limit of quantitation was 0.5 ng/mL. Underestimation of everolimus concentration when asco-mycin was used as internal standard in clinical and proficiency testing samples, as compared to desmethoxy-rapamycin, was also confirmed by another group [160].

Deuterated everolimus, perhaps the most appropriate suitable internal standard, is available from the International Association of Therapeutic Drug Monitoring and Clinical Toxicology members through Analytical Services International (www.bioanalytics.co.uk).

14.7.6   COMBINATION METHODS

Simultaneous determination of multiple immunosuppressive drugs, a major advantage of the application of LC-MS technology, was sought early on in the development of these techniques. One of the first procedures described quantification of cyclosporine, sirolimus, tacrolimus and SDZ-RAD (everolimus) using a single quadrupole system [38]. Sample pretreatment with zinc sulfate and methanol in the presence of three internal standards, cyclosporin D, ascomycin and 28, 40-diacetyl rapamycin, was followed by turbulent flow on-line sample cleanup on an ODS-1 HPLC column maintained at 65°C. The compounds were then back flushed onto a C_8 analytical column and eluted with a methanolic gradient over 9 minutes. The sodiated adducts were detected between 6.4 and 8.2 minutes. Sensitivity, accuracy and precision could be maintained for up to 500 injections on the extraction column and 2500 injections on the analytical column. Other procedures that used tandem mass spectrometry quickly appeared. Simultaneous determination of sirolimus and tacrolimus, with ascomycin as the common internal standard, was achieved using a zinc sulfate and acetonitrile protein precipitation, C_{18} reverse-phase chromatography with an isocratic mobile phase, and positive electrospray ionization facilitated detection. The run time was over 12 minutes [70].

Cyclosporine and everolimus, two drugs that are often administered concomitantly, were measured using deuterated cyclosporine and hydroxy-propyl rapamycin as internal standards [161]. Samples were treated with zinc sulfate and acetonitrile in the presence of ammonium hydroxide followed by solid phase extraction before reverse-phase chromatography under isocratic conditions (run time over 6 minutes). Interestingly, atmospheric pressure chemical ionization (APCI) in the negative mode was chosen for producing the protonated adduct of everolimus and APCI in the positive mode for cyclosporine. The limits of quantification were 0.37 and 7.0 ng/mL for everolimus and cyclosporine, respectively. This procedure was later followed by a more efficient method from the same laboratory [162]. The same internal standards were employed but the sample preparation was changed to a semi-automated liquid-liquid extraction using ammonium hydroxide and methyl *tert*-butyl ether. A 3.6-minute isocratic reverse-phase chromatography was followed by positive mode electrospray ionization of the ammoniated adducts.

All four major whole blood immunosuppressive agents were quantified successfully on a tandem quadrupole system. The positive electrospray ionization mode was used under conditions to promote ammoniated ions for all except cyclosporine for which a protonated species was used. Low molecular weight product ions were formed by increasing the orifice voltage and collision energy [61]. A simple protein precipitation with zinc sulfate and methanol in the presence of ascomycin and cyclosporin D internal standards served as sample pretreatment before application onto a reverse-phase HPLC column from which all compounds were eluted within 4 minutes by a methanolic step gradient.

Another group performed a similar sample pretreatment but took a different approach to chromatography of the four immunosuppressants [163]. In a method similar to that used previously [38] sample extracts were cleaned up with an on-line procedure using a 50% methanol wash of a "perfusion" column at high flow rate and then back flushed onto a phenyl hexyl column with elution of the compounds with a 97% methanol mobile phase. The cycle time was 2.5 minutes. Nevertheless, monitoring both quantifier and qualifier mass transitions for all compounds was insufficient to provide a high degree of precision.

Improvements to chromatographic efficiency and detector sensitivity were sought by consideration of a cyano HPLC column and negative ionization mode [164]. Following a simple protein precipitation sample pretreatment with acetonitrile, sample extracts were applied to either a reverse-phase (Atlantis™ C18) or cyano (YMC™ CN) HPLC column under identical conditions. The acetonitrile/water mobile phase was supplemented with either acetic or formic acid to promote formation of negative ions or positive ions, respectively. These authors considered use of reverse-phase column chromatography to be disadvantageous in that process efficiency can be compromised because gradient elution and time for re-equilibration (ten column volumes optimally) are required to elute the strongly retained immunosuppressive compounds. Moreover, unless a temperature in excess of 60°C is used, partial separation of the numerous conformations taken by these compounds in solution results in excessive band broadening. The high column temperatures on the other hand lead to shorter lifetime of silica-based columns. Cyano stationary phase chemistry was considered to be more advantageous because cyclosporine does not show radically different retention from the other immunosuppressant drugs; it is possible to completely resolve cyclosporine, sirolimus and tacrolimus within 3 minutes without gradient elution using approximately 50% acetonitrile at 50°C. Another advantage of a cyano column is that the individual conformers did not separate to the same extent as they did on C_{18} column. Therefore better peak shapes and higher efficiencies in analysis could be achieved. These authors also observed positive mode electrospray ionization to be less beneficial than the negative mode. Under their conditions (no ammonium acetate in the mobile phase), difficult to fragment sodiated adducts were promoted that produced multiple low intensity fragments rather than one diagnostic fragment. The mass transitions selected were cyclosporine (1225 > 1114), sirolimus (937 > 409), and tacrolimus (827 > 616). However with negative ionization mode electrospray, cyclosporine formed one strong structurally diagnostic fragment from the deprotonated precursor ion (m/z 1201 > 1089), whereas sirolimus and tacrolimus produced fewer fragments than with the positive mode (913 > 591; 803 > 561). This combined use of a cyano HPLC column and negative mode electrospray resulted in the distinct advantage of reducing the limits of detection by as much as 50-fold: cyclosporine from 5 to 0.1 ng/mL; sirolimus from 2 to 0.05 ng/mL; tacrolimus from 1 to 0.2 ng/mL [164].

Whereas column chemistry and mass spectrometric conditions were considered above, sample preparation methods were the focus of another group [40] because the highly proteinacous blood matrix reacts unfavorably with acetonitrile. It can cause precipitation as clumps which must be broken up through manual intervention to ensure complete recovery of the analyte(s). This was found to be especially true of commercial controls and proficiency testing samples that require reconstitution before use. Substitution with methanol was insufficient for full or consistent recovery [62]. With a slightly more complex sample treatment procedure in which blood cells were lysed with water prior to addition of zinc sulfate and methanol (containing cyclosporin D, desmethoxy-rapamycin and ascomycin internal standards), well-mixed extracts were held for 10 minutes before centrifugation. In this case, recoveries of cyclosporine, sirolimus and tacrolimus were 95–103%. Following this step with solid phase extraction provided for cleaner extracts that displayed minimal ion suppression, even with the difficult matrices of commercial calibrators and controls [143].

Single quadrupole mass spectrometric systems can also be used for determination of multiple immunosuppressive drugs: automated extraction economized on time in combination thoughtful consideration of instrument conditions that ensured reliable results [41].

A novel approach using atmospheric pressure chemical ionization in the negative mode was recently reported to avoid the problem of ion suppression often experienced with electrospray technique [165]. After a simple zinc sulfate/acetonitrile sample treatment and 1.5-minute binary step gradient across a short C_{18} column, the deprotonated species of cyclosporine, tacrolimus and their respective internal standards, cyclosporin D and ascomycin, were fragmented to one suitable product ion each. Little or no ion suppression was evidenced although there was some in-source fragmentation noted that did not adversely affect the performance of the method. However, the observed 25 and 1.0 ng/mL limits of quantitation for cyclosporine and tacrolimus, respectively, may not be sufficient for some clinical centers.

14.8   EXPERIENCE FROM THE AUTHOR'S LABORATORY

For analysis of immunosuppressants using LC-MS, we used a single quadrupole system configuration that was similar to a published method by Christians and his colleagues [38]. On-line sample cleanup was performed on a short extraction column at 65°C and then the compounds of interest were eluted with a stronger mobile phase onto an analytical column and into the mass spectrometer for detection of the sodiated adducts using electrospray in the positive ionization mode. The operation was facilitated by two six-port switching valves. The wash solution for the extraction column (40% methanol for cyclosporine and tacrolimus and 60% for sirolimus) was relatively strong in order to remove as many of the less tightly retained substances as possible. The isocratic elution mobile phase was even stronger, 83% methanol for sirolimus and tacrolimus, 86% for cyclosporine. The run time was 3.5 minutes plus a 45-second injection cycle. Both columns were washed overnight with 98% methanol to remove any lipophilic substances that had accumulated during the day's work. The lifetime of the extraction column was usually about three weeks and the analytical column was three months. The mass spectrometer source was kept clean by diverting eluent flow from entering the mass spectrometer, except during data acquisition. The cone required changing about once every three months.

Later a tandem quadrupole system was available in the laboratory and methods were developed for TDM of immunosuppressants. The configuration of the tandem quadrupole system was similar to that described by Keevil and his colleagues [72]. On-line sample clean-up was performed on a short extraction column at 60° with a 50% methanolic mobile phase. The compounds of interest were then eluted into the mass spectrometer by stepping the organic content to 100% for 0.4 minutes. The run time was 2.0 minutes with a 45-second injection cycle. For sirolimus, each sample required addition of a column clean-up step with 100% methanol to remove from the column more tightly retained compounds that interfered with quantitation of subsequent samples: this step effectively increased the run time to 3.0 minutes. Using electrospray in the positive ionization mode, ammoniated adducts were promoted. By washing the column overnight with 90% methanol, a lifetime of approximately three weeks was achieved. As with the single quadrupole system, eluent flow was diverted from entering the mass spectrometer except during data acquisition. These two systems, described in more detail in published works [43,87], have provided a seven-days-a-week clinical service for several years in the author's laboratory.

Calibration standard as well as quality control materials were prepared in house with the rationale that performance of using materials prepared fresh whole blood would best mimic that of clinical specimens. The original cyclosporine, sirolimus and tacrolimus drug compounds sourced through the manufacturers and used to prepare the calibration and quality control materials were stable for several years when stored as recommended. Later a commercial preparation of tacrolimus was successfully utilized.

One of the early techniques the author developed was a liquid-liquid extraction for tacrolimus for analysis using a single quadrupole system. Protein precipitation was achieved with zinc sulfate and methanol. The steps included addition of the internal standard (ascomycin) and then sodium carbonate buffer to whole blood. However, the presence of a high concentration of sodium ions made the sample extracts unsuitable for application to the tandem quadrupole system that became available later. A simple and effective protein precipitation method with zinc sulfate and acetonitrile supplemented with internal standard [72] proved acceptable for that LC-MS system. We later validated this technique for the single quadrupole system; however because of pressure for a faster turnaround time for tacrolimus levels, the single quadrupole system was used rarely for tacrolimus determination. The procedure has performed satisfactorily over several years, only failing the IPTS challenges when issues with stability of ascomycin in solution arose [166].

Figure 14.3 illustrates typical mass transition ion traces routinely observed on the tandem quadrupole system when a methanol/water blank, the low calibration standard (0.5 ng tacrolimus/ mL) and the high calibration standard (40 ng/mL) are analyzed. The amount of internal standard added to each sample was selected so that the highest peak area ratio would be approximately one. The last panel demonstrates interference in the ascomycin channel that occurs when a methanol/water blank is injected immediately subsequent to a previously frozen sample: the interference that appears

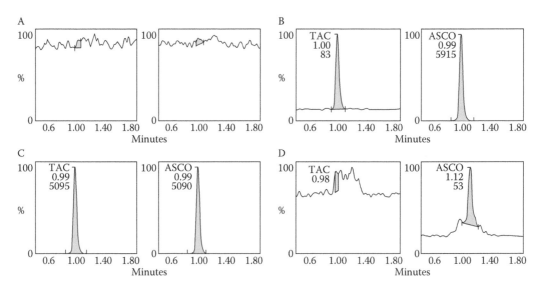

FIGURE 14.3 Multiple exaction monitoring signal traces during tacrolimus analysis on a tandem quadrupole system, detection at m/z 821.5 > 768.0 (tacrolimus), 809.5 > 756.1 (ascomycin). The tacrolimus peak (TAC) apex is at 0.99–1.00 min, internal standard (ascomycin, ASCO) at 0.99 minutes. The values beneath the retention times represent peak area. No data is collected before 0.4 minutes or after 1.9 minutes as eluent before and after those times is diverted to waste. Panel A: a methanol/water blank injected immediately prior to a tacrolimus analysis; Panel B: lowest tacrolimus whole blood standard (0.5 ng/mL); Panel C: highest tacrolimus whole blood standard (40 ng/mL); Panel D: insignificant carryover of tacrolimus and ascomycin and presence of a late-eluting compound (1.12 minutes) in the internal standard channel illustrated by injection of a methanol/water blank immediately following a previously frozen sample (32 ng/mL). The late-eluting compound appears only following injections of samples that have been previously frozen.

0.13 minutes later than ascomycin is due to a substance in the extract of frozen blood that was retained on the extraction column. In order to avoid any potential for inaccuracy in clinical samples, it is a routine practice to inject a blank following any sample that has been previously frozen. An alternative might be to add a second 100% organic step to the gradient program as is used for sirolimus.

Following implementation of the tacrolimus procedures into clinical service, development of a sample treatment for cyclosporine was initiated by the author. The criteria set at that time were for a technique that was suitable also for analysis of sirolimus and tacrolimus so that all three eventually could be assayed together. An initial attempt with the simple zinc sulfate and acetonitrile protein precipitation technique did not produce good results, as the performance of the quality control samples was poor. The author followed the procedure published by Annesley and his colleagues [40] where more effective cell lysis, resulting in release of the analyte from whole blood was achieved by mixing whole blood with water before the addition of zinc sulfate solution and acetonitrile. This procedure was ultimately modified by replacement of water with 10% methanol in an ammonium bicarbonate solution use of methanol instead of acetonitrile as the final protein precipitating agent and carrier for the cyclosporin D internal standard produced more accurate and precise results. This cyclosporine specimen preparation procedure worked equally well on both the single and tandem quadrupole systems. However, ensuring that whole blood was supplemented with cyclosporine solution accurately during preparation of calibration standards proved to be important because the analytical range for analysis of cyclosporine was wide. Figure 14.4 illustrates the ion traces routinely observed on the single quadrupole system when a methanol/water blank, the low calibration standard (10 ng cyclosporine/mL) and the high calibration standard (1200 ng/mL) were injected. The last panel demonstrates lack of carryover in an injection of a methanol/water blank made immediately following that of a high quality control sample (1000 ng/mL).

Figure 14.5 illustrates the mass transition ion traces observed on the tandem quadrupole system with the low calibration standard (10 ng cyclosporine/mL), the high calibration standard (1200 ng/mL). Because the source material for cyclosporin D used for the internal standard was contaminated with approximately 1% of cyclosporine, the amount of cyclosporin D added to each sample was chosen so the peak area ratio of the lowest standard would be about 0.03. A methanol/water blank injected immediately after a high quality control sample (1000 ng/mL) evidences a small amount of carryover. Because of this situation, when a clinical sample with a cyclosporine concentration <10% of that in a preceding sample is analyzed, the sample with the lower concentration is reinjected and the latter result is reported. The last panel shows a unique occurrence with clinical samples where, in the cyclosporin D channel a small peak precedes that of the internal standard. The size of this peak seems to parallel the concentration of the parent compound. Such interference has been observed by others [148,149] but perhaps because the concentration of cyclosporine in most of the clinical samples received by the laboratory is quite low, there has been insignificant interference in this procedure. If the interference becomes significant, of cyclosporin-d_{12} as the internal standard may circumvent this issue [149].

Later the author developed a procedure for LC-MS analysis of sirolimus. In this procedure, a 20-minute clock was started and then to each whole blood specimen 10% methanol in ammonium bicarbonate solution was added to as many as 24 samples followed by vigorous mixing of specimens. At the end of the time period, a 15-minute clock was set and then zinc sulfate was added and, after mixing, ascomycin in acetonitrile solution added to each specimen followed by final mixing. At the end of the time period the samples were centrifuged. Ascomycin was added to each sample to produce approximately 10^6 height units and peak height ratios between 0.03 and 0.75 on the single quadrupole system. Height was chosen rather than area for quantitation purposes because of the baseline can be quite noisy at low sirolimus concentrations (Figure 14.6, panel B). The success of this procedure on the single quadrupole system required washing of the extraction column with 60% rather than 40% methanol. Any higher percentage of methanol caused elution of ascomycin.

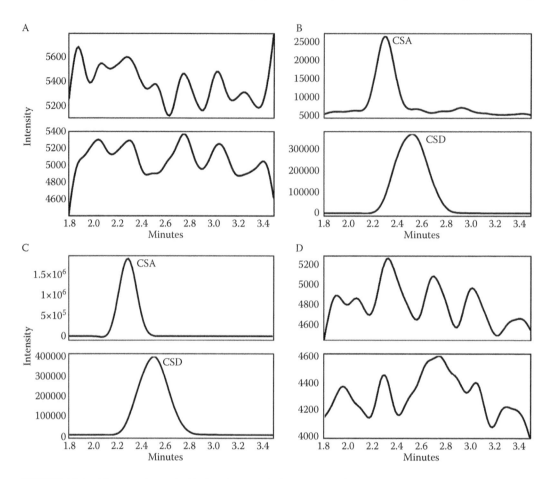

FIGURE 14.4   Mass-to-charge (m/z) signal traces during cyclosporine analysis on a single quadrupole system, detection at m/z 1225.2 (cyclosporine), *m/z* 1239.2 (cyclosporin D). The cyclosporine peak (CSA) is maximal at 2.3 min, internal standard (CSD, cyclosporin D) at 2.5 minutes. The values on the vertical axes indicate peak height. No data is collected before 1.75 minutes as eluent before that time is diverted to waste. Panel A: a methanol/water blank injected immediately prior to a cyclosporine analysis; Panel B: lowest cyclosporine whole blood standard (10 ng/mL); Panel C: highest cyclosporine whole blood standard (1200 ng/mL); Panel D: lack of carryover illustrated by a methanol/water blank injected immediately following a high quality control sample (1000 ng/mL).

On the tandem quadrupole system no more than 50% organic solvent could be used for the initial wash and a second 100% organic step was needed to sufficiently clean the column between sample injections. If this was not done, increasing deterioration in performance was always observed throughout an analytical run.

Figure 14.6 illustrates the ion traces routinely observed on the single quadrupole system when a methanol/water blank, the low calibration standard (2 ng sirolimus/mL), the high calibration standard (50 ng/mL) were injected. Ion suppression that occured in both the ascomycin and sirolimus channels between 2.1 and 2.6 minutes is observed clearly in the first panel. The small peak that precedes that of ascomycin is present in all extracted samples, but does not interfere with quantitation. The last panel shows an effect of frozen blood, the tail of a large peak is observed in the ascomycin channel of a methanol/water blank injected immediately after previously frozen sample (32 ng/mL). As with tacrolimus, it is routine to inject a methanol/water blank after any extract that has been prepared from frozen blood.

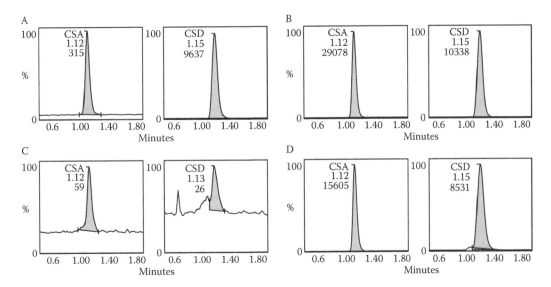

FIGURE 14.5 Multiple reaction monitoring (MRM) signal traces during cyclosporine analysis on a tandem quadrupole system, detection at m/z 1220.0>1202.5 (cyclosporine), m/z 1234.0>1216.5 (cyclosporin D). The cyclosporine peak (CSA) is centered at 1.12 minutes, internal standard (cyclosporin D, CSD) at 1.15 minutes. The values below the retention times represent peak area. No data is collected before 0.4 or after 1.9 minutes as elute is diverted to waste before and after those times. Panel A: lowest cyclosporine whole blood standard (10 ng/mL); Panel B: highest cyclosporine whole blood standard (1200 ng/mL); Panel C: carryover of approximately 0.3% of cyclosporine and cyclosporin D illustrated by injection of a methanol/water blank immediately following a high quality control sample (1000 ng/mL); Panel D: a clinical sample (cyclosporine=145 ng/mL) illustrating a small peak likely due to a metabolite or breakdown product that precedes the cyclosporin D peak.

Figure 14.7 illustrates the mass transition ion traces on the tandem quadrupole system for the low (2 ng sirolimus/mL) and high calibration standards (50 ng/mL). Traces from a quality control sample (32 ng/mL) show a small peak that appears after the internal standard ascomycin, this occurs only with samples that have been previously frozen. This interference is probably similar to that observed with the tacrolimus procedure, except in this case, the peak appears in the same, not subsequent, sample because a different gradient program has been used. Lack of carryover is shown in the last panel.

More recently, the author developed a procedure for total mycophenolic acid analysis using an HPLC-UV system because, based on the available literature, the author believed that HPLC-UV procedure should be accurate for TDM of mycophenolic acid. Mycophenolic acid, the phenol glucuronide metabolite, acyl glucuronide metabolite and internal standard materials were obtained from the drug manufacturer. Moreover, commercial mycophenolic acid material proved to be of equally good quality. The gradient chromatographic conditions [50,108] allowed for quantification of the metabolites to accommodate future requests of transplant physicians for determination of metabolites. Moreover, the 21-minute run time permitted decent turn around time. The author selected an acid-stable chromatographic column (Sunfire™ C_{18}, Waters Corporation) and this proved be a very good choice. The original column has been in service for over two years with no loss of resolution. Methanol and 10 mM phosphate buffer were used as the mobile phase. The buffer was prepared from proportional volumes of ortho-phosphoric acid and monobasic potassium phosphate solutions to provide a pH of 3. With the column at 40°C and a linear gradient from 35 to 60% methanol between 7 and 17 minutes, the compounds of interest were well resolved. The compounds were detected at 254 nm: although this is not the extinction maximum for mycophenolic acid, there were fewer interfering peaks at this wavelength. When the system was not in use over the short period, a 90% methanol mobile phase is applied, whereas the long term, water or a water/methanol mixture has been substituted for the buffer.

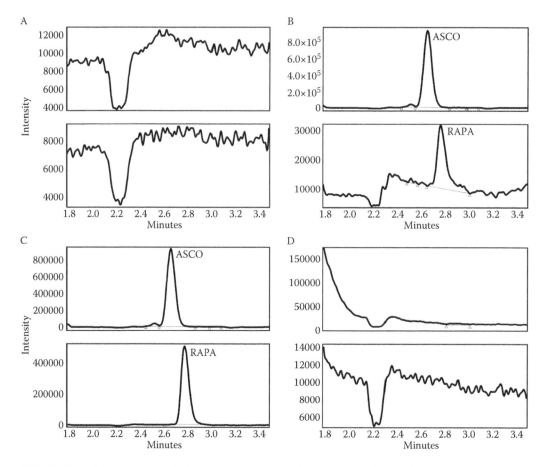

FIGURE 14.6 Mass-to-charge (m/z) signal traces during sirolimus analysis on a single quadrupole system, detection at m/z 814.8 (ascomycin), m/z 936.9 (sirolimus). The sirolimus peak (RAPA) apex is at 2.8 minutes, internal standard (ascomycin, ASCO) at 2.7 minutes. The values on the vertical axes indicate peak height. No data is collected before 1.75 minutes as eluent before that time is diverted to waste. Panel A: a methanol/water blank injected immediately prior to a sirolimus analysis (ion suppression occurs between 2.1 and 2.6 minutes); Panel B: lowest sirolimus whole blood standard (2 ng/mL); Panel C: highest sirolimus whole blood standard (50 ng/mL); Panel D: carryover especially in the internal standard channel between 1.8 and 2.4 minutes as the result of a previously injected frozen blood sample illustrated during the run cycle of a methanol/water blank.

As with the other immunosuppressants, calibration standards and quality control materials were prepared in the matrix of choice (in this case, plasma). Calibration curves prepared by supplementation of plasma with mycophenolic acid solution were stable for up to 6 weeks under refrigerated conditions. Quality control materials were prepared in batch and kept frozen until use ($-20°C$); these materials were stable for at least 6 months.

A simple protein precipitation with acetonitrile [49] provided extracts that were clean enough for accurate quantitation of mycophenolic acid but not the phenol glucuronide metabolite. A solid-phase extraction procedure [50,108] would be needed if the metabolites were to be quantified. There were no clinical plasma specimens available for testing during method development, so plasma was recovered from residuals of whole blood samples collected for sirolimus determination. It was not known whether the patients were receiving mycophenolic acid therapy or not. We observed peaks that interfered with resolution of the internal standard in some samples. Not knowing if this would occur in actual clinical specimens collected for mycophenolic acid determination, we decided to

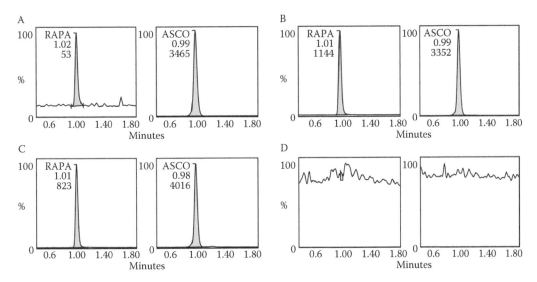

FIGURE 14.7   Multiple reaction monitoring signal traces during sirolimus analysis on a tandem quadrupole system, detection at m/z 931.6 > 864.1 (sirolimus), 809.5 > 756.1 (ascomycin). The sirolimus peak (RAPA) is maximal at 1.01 to 1.02 min, internal standard (ascomycin, ASCO) at 0.98 to 0.99 minutes. The values below the retention times represent peak area. No data is collected before 0.4 or after 1.9 minutes as elute is diverted to waste before and after those times. Panel A: lowest sirolimus whole blood standard (2.0 ng/mL); Panel B: Highest sirolimus whole blood standard (50 ng/mL); Panel C: high quality control sample (32 ng/mL) illustrating a small late eluting peak at approximately 1.2 min in the internal standard channel that occurs only with samples that have been previously frozen; Panel D: lack of carryover illustrated by a methanol/water blank injected immediately following a high quality control sample.

validate the procedure with the carboxy butoxy ether of mycophenolic acid as the primary internal standard and suprofen as a secondary choice. This proved to be useful occasionally when interference with the primary internal standard did occur. Unfortunately, under the established conditions the retention time for suprofen is nearly identical to that of the acyl glucuronide metabolite.

Figure 14.8 illustrates typical chromatograms for the low (0.2 μg mycophenolic acid/mL) and high calibration standards (20 μg/mL) and a clinical sample. The unidentified peak at 13 minutes is suprofen, the alternative internal standard. The glucuronide metabolite of mycophenolic acid that appears at 7 minutes (before the gradient is applied) is incompletely resolved from a coeluting interference. This interfering substance can be removed by using to solid-phase extraction. Challenge samples from the IPTS for mycophenolic acid have been received and stored at −40°C for up to several years. As for the other immunosuppressants, such challenge samples were invaluable for assessing method accuracy during development and for troubleshooting purposes after the procedures were put into clinical practice. We observed that the concentration of mycophenolic acid in challenge samples prepared by pooling clinical specimens increased over time, while that in plasma that has been supplemented with the drug remain relatively constant. This may be due to decomposition of the metabolites to mycophenolic acid during long term storage.

14.9   FUTURE DEVELOPMENTS

There are many possibilities for improvement and innovation with regard to therapeutic drug monitoring practices for immunosuppressant drugs, especially in the area of standardization of materials and methods. As has been shown, LC-MS seems to be the technology for the future, however, at this time neither the procedures nor the interpretation of data is simplistic and requires well-trained, specialized technologists to competently perform these assays. Meanwhile, new techniques

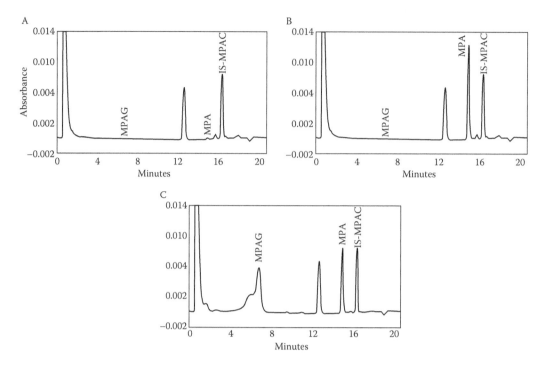

FIGURE 14.8 Chromatograms for mycophenolic acid analysis using a gradient HPLC procedure, UV detection at 254 nm. The mycophenolic acid peak (MPA) is centered at 15.2 minutes, internal standard (IS; MPA carboxy butoxy ether, MPAC) at 16.7 minutes. The retention time for the phenolic glucuronide metabolite of MPA (MPAG) is 6.9 minutes. The secondary internal standard, suprofen, peaks at approximately 13 minutes, similar to the acyl glucuronide metabolite (AcMPAG). Panel A: lowest mycophenolic acid standard (0. 2 µg/mL); Panel B: highest mycophenolic acid standard (20 µg/mL); Panel C: a clinical sample illustrating incomplete resolution of the phenolic glucuronide metabolite from an interfering substance (mycophenolic acid=13.2 µg/mL).

continue to be advanced. Using tacrolimus as an example, surface-activated chemical ionization in combination with high-flow gradient chromatography has been purported to reduce matrix effects and to increase efficiency of ionization [167]. This new type of mass spectrometer interface offers an increase in sensitivity by a factor of ten over electrospray that can be attributed to a decrease in chemical noise. The tedious but necessary sample treatment step cannot be eliminated but has been automated, including mechanized transfer of blood from collection tubes, without sacrificing performance [168]. One approach to increasing efficiency while decreasing cost is to determine multiple immunosuppressant agents from the same sample simultaneously. If the analysis can be optimized, analytes other than immunosuppressants can also be measured accurately. Recently commonly coprescribed glucocorticoids, methyl prednisolone and dexamethasone were analyzed along with mycophenolic acid and its phenol glucuronide metabolite [169].

Use of alternative matrices such as saliva may lead to more accurate diagnoses, in part because salivary drug concentrations represent the unbound fraction. Moreover, noninvasive collection of saliva is a preferred alternative to blood collection especially for children. Protein aggregates in salivary specimens must be disrupted by sonication prior to analysis. After that, saliva can be treated in a fashion similar to whole blood [170]. For determination of salivary cyclosporine, several obstacles were overcome, including extension of the limit of quantitation down to 1 ng/mL. Initial salivary cyclosporine concentrations were only in general agreement with whole blood levels (r=0.695), although weakness in this correlation might be expected as total cyclosporine is measured in whole blood while only unbound drug was measured in saliva. Later an LC-MS procedure for determination of mycophenolic acid in saliva was developed [171]. Mycophenolic glucuronide metabolites were separated chromatographically from mycophenolic acid prior to detection in the negative ionization mode on a triple quadrupole mass spectrometer. In this case levels of salivary mycophenolic acid closely paralleled plasma free mycophenolic acid levels over a 12-hour dosing interval. These observations suggested that saliva may serve as a better alternative than whole blood or plasma in the determination of unbound cyclosporine or mycophenolic acid.

Other than analysis of immunosuppressants in whole blood, an LC-MS procedure was developed using an ion trap mass spectrometer (in the positive ionization mode of atmospheric pressure chemical ionization) for determination of concentrations of cyclosporine and six metabolites simultaneously in isolated T-lymphocytes. The authors used solid phase extraction [172]. Cyclosporine, its metabolites and internal standard (cyclosporin C) were well-separated over a 35-minute per sample chromatographic run time. Superior resolution allowed for separation of isobaric compounds (e.g., metabolites AM1 and AM9) and division of the chromatogram into three segments, each with only two or more mass transition scanning events. This procedure was used to assess intracellular cyclosporine concentrations in twenty kidney transplant recipients, seven of which experienced acute rejection over the first three months' post-transplant period [173]. Interestingly lymphocyte cyclosporine levels declined during the week prior to acute rejection; the difference was significant three days before rejection was diagnosed clinically and remained low during the rejection episode. A 12-hour area-under-the-concentration-time curve measured in the stable phase was almost two-fold higher in the rejection-free patients, although there was no difference between C2 levels. A major drawback to the analytical method was the requirement of significant amount of whole blood (7 mL).

The superior sensitivity of LC-MS technology also proved advantageous for determination of the very low levels of mycophenolic acid in peripheral blood mononuclear cells [174]. The utility of TDM of mycophenolic acid in plasma is still under debate and it is thought that addressing drug concentration in the target cells may provide better prediction of clinical events. Complete cell lysis was achieved by an organic solvent-free Tris-hydrochloric acid buffer and manual scraping of the extraction tubes. Elution of the compounds of interest (e.g., mycophenolic acid and internal standard) from a cyano HPLC column was observed after five minutes using an isocratic ammonium acetate/acetonitrile mobile phase. Cleanliness of the mass spectrometer source was maintained using a water/acetonitrile/formic acid mixture applied before and after the analysis. Mycophenolic acid concentrations as low as 0.24 ng/sample were quantitated.

An initial investigation of intracellular tacrolimus levels in predose samples from 65 kidney transplant recipients using an LC-MS procedure indicated that, while whole blood concentrations varied only three-fold (4.9–14.8 ng/mL), levels in extracts of peripheral blood mononuclear cells ranged between 6 and 179 $pg/10^6$ cells, a thirty-fold difference [175]. As with the previous procedure for cyclosporine, seven milliliters of whole blood were required for isolation of an adequate number of peripheral blood mononuclear cells. Thereafter a time-consuming (1 hour) liquid-liquid extraction using 1-chlorobutane in the presence of ammonium hydroxide and the ascomycin internal standard lead to 75–87% recovery of tacrolimus. The compounds of interest were eluted quickly, within 0.8 minutes, when a 90% acetonitrile-based mobile phase was passed isocratically through a 50 mm reverse phase HPLC column. Detection of the mass transitions of the ammonium adducts was achieved using positive mode electrospray ionization. Because of the 5–6 hours required to prepare and analyze ten samples, this technique may not be applicable for a routine clinical TDM service but, if necessary for a particular patient, results may assist in elucidation of the pharmacokinetic and genetic variables that affect clinical outcome.

The utility of any analytical procedure is limited ultimately by the value of the information it provides. Although application of TDM has been integral to the successful clinical management of organ transplant recipients and others with auto-immune disease, it is becoming evident that quantification of the level of each individual agent in blood or plasma matrices may be an insufficient measure of overall immunosuppression, especially in the context of cocktail regimens. Determination of intracellular drug levels, made possible with LC-MS technology, may be useful in some circumstances but will only be available at research-based enterprises in the near term. However, the future is focused on biomarkers, pharmacodynamic measures of drug activity, some of which are related directly to the drug targets: they are calcineurin by cyclosporine and tacrolimus, inosine monophosphate dehydrogenase by mycophenolic acid and the mammalian target of rapamycin by sirolimus and everolimus. The only potential biomarker assayed so far using a chromatographic technique has been xanthine monophosphate, the product of the purine biosynthetic pathway reaction catalyzed by the enzyme inosine monophosphate dehydrogenase to form xanthine monophosphate from inosine monophosphate [176,177]. Using analysis by HPLC-UV, these procedures required as much as 5 mL of whole blood as the source of a sufficient number of cells to assess accurately inhibition of the enzyme, long incubation (120–150 min) and chromatographic cycles (20–25 min).

14.10 CONCLUSIONS

The immunosuppressants tacrolimus, cyclosporine, sirolimus and everolimus are analyzed in whole blood while mycophenolic acid can be analyzed using serum or plasma. In less than one decade LC-MS instrumentation has moved from the laboratories of the few pioneers into widespread use in the clinical setting for determination of immunosuppressive agents and a variety of other drugs. This trend has been due, in part, to recognition of the performance of LC-MS technology and to the limitations of commerical immunoassay procedures, such as metabolite cross-reactivities, insufficient precision and to matrix influence. Although LC-MS methods are superior to HPLC-UV methods, HPLC-UV methods may provide sufficient precision for analysis of mycophenolic acid.

REFERENCES

1. Shaw LM, Bowers L, Demers L, et al. 1987. Critical issues in cyclosporine monitoring: report of the task force on cyclosporin monitoring. *Clin Chem* 33:1269–88.
2. No authors. 1990. Consensus document: Hawk's Cay meeting on therapeutic drug monitoring of cyclosporine. *Transplant Proc* 22:1357–61.
3. Kahan BD, Shaw LM, Holt D, et al. 1990. Consensus document: Hawk's Cay meeting on therapeutic drug monitoring of cyclosporine. *Clin Chem* 36:1510–16.
4. Shaw LM, Yatscoff RW, Bowers LD, et al. 1990. Canadian consensus meeting on cyclosporine monitoring: report of the consensus panel. *Clin Chem* 36:1841–46.
5. Morris RG, Tett SE, Jay JE. 1994. Cyclosporin-A monitoring in Australia: consensus recommendations. *Ther Drug Monit* 16:570–76.
6. Jusko WJ, Thomson AW, Fung J, et al. 1995. Consensus document: therapeutic monitoring of tacrolimus (FK-506). *Ther Drug Monit* 17:606–14.
7. Oellerich M, Armstrong VW, Kahan B, et al. 1995. Lake Louise consensus conference on cyclosporin monitoring in organ transplantation: report of the consensus panel. *Ther Drug Monit* 17:642–54.
8. Yatscoff RW, Boeckx R, Holt DW, et al. 1995. Consensus guidelines of therapeutic drug monitoring of rapamycin: report of the consensus panel. *Ther Drug Monit* 17:676–80.
9. Oellerich M, Armstrong VW, Schütz E, et al. 1998. Therapeutic drug monitoring of cyclosporine and tacrolimus. Update on Lake Louise consensus conference on cyclosporin and tacrolimus. *Clin Biochem* 31:309–16.
10. Shaw LM, Nicholls A, Hale M, et al. 1998. Therapeutic monitoring of mycophenolic acid. A consensus panel report. *Clin Biochem* 31:317–22.
11. Morris RG, Ilett KF, Tett SE, et al. 2002. Cyclosporin monitoring in Australasia: 2002 update of consensus guidelines. *Ther Drug Monit* 24:677–88.
12. Holt DW, Armstrong VW, Griesmacher A, et al. 2002. International Federation of Clinical Chemistry/International Association of Therapeutic Drug Monitoring and Clinical Toxicology Working Group on immunosuppressive drug monitoring. *Ther Drug Monit* 24:59–67.
13. Morris RG, Holt DW, Armstrong VW, et al. 2004. Analytic aspects of cyclosporine monitoring, on behalf of the IFCC/IATDMCT Joint Working Group. *Ther Drug Monit* 26:227–30.

14. Chemistry and Toxicology Branch, Division of Clinical Laboratory Devices, Office of Device Evaluation; Center for Devices and Radiological Health, Food and Drug Administration, US Department of Health and Human Services. *Class II Special Controls Guidance Document: Cyclosporine and Tacrolimus Assays; Guidance for Industry and FDA*. At www.fda.gov/cdrh/ode/guidance/1380.pdf (accessed September 29, 2008).

15. Division of Chemistry and Toxicology Devices, Office of In Vitro Diagnostic Device Evaluation and Safety; Center for Devices and Radiological Health, US Food and Drug Administration, US Department of Health and Human Services. *Guidance for Industry and FDA Staff, Class II Special Controls Guidance Document: Sirolimus Test Systems*. At www.fda.gov/cdrh/oivd/guidance/1300.pdf (accessed September 29, 2008).

16. Sawchuk RJ, Cartier LL. 1981. Liquid chromatographic determination of cyclosporin A in blood and plasma. *Clin Chem* 27:1368–71.

17. Terrell AR, Daly TM, Hock KG, et al. 2002. Evaluation of a no-pretreatment cyclosporin A assay on the Dade Behring Dimension RxL clinical chemistry analyzer. *Clin Chem* 48:1059–65.

18. Huet E, Morand K, Blanchet B, et al. 2004. Evaluation of the new heterogeneous ACMIA immunoassay for the determination of whole-blood cyclosporine concentrations in bone marrow, kidney, heart, and liver transplant recipients. *Transplant Proc* 36:1317–20.

19. 510(k) Substantial Equivalence Determination Decision Summary for Dimension® Cyclosporine Extended Range Assay (CSAE) Flex® reagent cartridge. At http://www.fda.gov/cdrh/REVIEWS/K052017.pdf (accessed June 23, 2008).

20. CEDIA® Cyclosporine PLUS Assay Package Insert. Fremont, CA: Microgenics Corporation; 2006.

21. Architect System Cyclosporine Package Insert. Abbott Park, IL: Abbott Diagnostics; 2008.

22. Dasgupta A, Saldana S, Desai M. 1991. Analytical performance of EMIT™ cyclosporine assay evaluated. *Clin Chem* 37:2130–33.

23. Beresini MH, Davalian D, Alexander S, et al. 1993. Evaluation of EMIT® cyclosporine assay for use with whole blood. *Clin Chem* 39:2235–41.

24. Steimer W. 1999. Performance and specificity of monoclonal immunoassays for cyclosporine monitoring: how specific is specific? *Clin Chem* 45:371–81.

25. Kimura S, Iyama S, Yamaguchi Y, et al. 2001. Homogenous enzyme immunoassay for cyclosporine in whole blood using the EMIT® 2000 cyclosporine specific assay with the COBAS Mira-Plus analyzer. *J Clin Lab Anal* 15:319–23.

26. Butch W, Fukuchi AM. 2003. Evaluation of a new pretreatment reagent for use with the EMIT® 2000 cyclosporine assay. *Clin Biochem* 36:313–6.

27. 510(k) Substantial Equivalence Determination Decision Summary for EMIT® 2000 CSAE Cyclosporine Specific Assay. At http://www.fda.gov/cdrh/REVIEWS/K053061.pdf (accessed June 23, 2008).

28. COBAS Integra 400/700/800 Cyclosporine II Package Insert. Indianapolis, IN: Roche Diagnostics; 2004.

29. News Release. *Roche Diagnostics Introduces Cyclosporine Assay for the COBAS Integra® 400 Plus Chemistry System*. At http://www.roche-diagnostics.us/press_room/2002/031202.htm (accessed June 23, 2008).

30. TDx®/TDxFLx® Cyclosporine Monoclonal Whole Blood Package Insert. Abbott Park, IL: Abbott Diagnostics; 2005.

31. TDx®/TDxFLx® Cyclosporine and Metabolites Whole Blood Package Insert. Abbott Park, IL: Abbott Diagnostics; 2007.

32. AxSYM System Cyclosporine Package Insert. Abbott Park, IL: Abbott Diagnostics; 2007.

33. Wolf BA, Daft MC, Koenig JW, et al. 1989. Measurement of cyclosporine concentrations in whole blood: HPLC and radioimmunoassay with a specific monoclonal antibody and ^{3}H- or ^{125}I-labeled ligand compared. *Clin Chem* 35:120–24.

34. Wong PY, Ma J. 1990. Specific and nonspecific monoclonal ^{125}I-Incstar assays. *Transplant Proc* 22:1166–70.

35. Kahn GC, Shaw LM, Kane MD. 1986. Routine monitoring of cyclosporine in whole blood and in kidney tissue using high performance liquid chromatography. *J Anal Toxicol* 10:27–34.

36. Kabra PM, Wall JH, Dimson P. 1987. Automated solid-phase extraction and liquid chromatography for assay of cyclosporine in whole blood. *Clin Chem* 33:2272–74.

37. Christians U, Zimmer KO, Wonigeit K, et al. 1987. Measurement of cyclosporin A and of four metabolites in whole blood by high-performance liquid chromatography. *J Chromatogr* 23:121–29.

38. Christians U, Jacobsen W, Serkova N, et al. 2000. Automated, fast and sensitive quantification of drugs in blood by liquid chromatography – mass spectrometry with on-line extraction: immunosuppressants. *J Chromatog B* 748:41–53.

39. Keevil BG, Tierney DP, Cooper DP, et al. 2002. Rapid liquid chromatography-tandem mass spectrometry method for routine analysis of cyclosporin A over an extended concentration range. *Clin Chem* 48:69–76.

40. Annesley TM, 2004. Clayton L. Simple extraction protocol for analysis of immunosuppressants in whole blood. *Clin Chem* 50:1845–48.

41. Poquette MA, Lensmeyer GL, Doran TC. 2005. Effective use of liquid chromatography-mass spectrometry (LC-MS) in the routine clinical laboratory for monitoring sirolimus, tacrolimus, and cyclosporine. *Ther Drug Monit* 27:144–50.

42. Salm P, Taylor PJ, Lynch SV, et al. 2005. A rapid HPLC-mass spectrometry cyclosporin method suitable for current monitoring practices. *Clin Biochem* 38:667–73.

43. Napoli KL. 2006. 12-Hour area under the curve cyclosporine concentrations determined by a validated liquid chromatography-mass spectrometry procedure compared with fluorescence polarization immunoassay reveals sirolimus effect on cyclosporine pharmacokinetics. *Ther Drug Monit* 28:726–36.

44. CEDIA® Mycophenolic Acid Assay Package Insert. Fremont, CA: Microgenics Corporation; 2006.

45. EMIT® 2000 Mycophenolic Acid Assay Package Insert. Newark, DE: Dade Behring, Inc.; 2007

46. Shipkova M, Schütz E, Armstrong VW, et al. 2000. Determination of the acyl glucuronide metabolite of mycophenolic acid in human plasma by HPLC and EMIT. *Clin Chem* 46:365–72.

47. Hosotsubo H, Takahara S, Imamura R, et al. 2001. Analytic validation of the enzyme multiplied immunoassay technique for the determination of mycophenolic acid in plasma from renal transplant recipients compared with a high-performance liquid chromatographic assay. *Ther Drug Monit* 23:669–74.

48. COBAS INTEGRA 400/700/800 Mycophenolic Acid Package Insert. Indianapolis, IN: Roche Diagnostics; 2007.

49. Westley IS, Sallustio BC, Morris RG. 2005. Validation of a high-performance liquid chromatography method for the measurement of mycophenolic acid and its glucuronide metabolites in plasma. *Clin Biochem* 38:824–29.

50. Patel CG, Akhlaghi F. 2006. High-performance liquid chromatography method for the determination of mycophenolic acid and its acyl and phenol glucuronide metabolites in human plasma. *Ther Drug Monit* 28:116–22.

51. Streit F, Shipkova M, Armstrong VW, et al. 2004. Validation of a rapid and sensitive liquid chromatography-tandem mass spectrometry method for free and total mycophenolic acid. *Clin Chem* 50:152–59.

52. Prémaud A, Rousseau A, Le Meur Y, et al. 2004. Comparison of liquid chromatography-tandem mass spectrometry with a commercial enzyme-multiplied immunoassay for the determination of plasma MPA in renal transplant recipients and consequences for therapeutic drug monitoring. *Ther Drug Monit* 26:609–19.

53. Brandhorst G, Streit F, Goetze S, et al. 2006. Quantification by liquid chromatography tandem mass spectrometry of mycophenolic acid and its phenol and acyl glucuronide metabolites. *Clin Chem* 52:1962–64.

54. CEDIA® Sirolimus Assay Package Insert. Fremont, CA: Microgenics Corporation; 2004.

55. Architect System Sirolimus Package Insert. Abbott Park, IL: Abbott Diagnostics; 2007.

56. IMx® System Sirolimus Package Insert. Abbott Park, IL: Abbott Diagnostics; 2006.

57. Napoli KL. 2000. A practical guide to the analysis of sirolimus using high-performance liquid chromatography with ultraviolet detection. *Clin Ther* 22(Suppl B):B14–24.

58. French DC, Saltzgueber M, Hicks DR, et al. 2001. HPLC assay with ultraviolet detection for therapeutic drug monitoring of sirolimus. *Clin Chem* 47:1316–19.

59. Holt DW, Lee T, Jones K, et al. 2000. Validation of an assay for routine monitoring of sirolimus using HPLC with mass spectrometry. *Clin Chem* 46:1179–83.

60. Vogeser M, Fleischer C, Meiser B, et al. 2002. Quantification of sirolimus by liquid chromatography-tandem mass spectrometry using on-line solid-phase extraction. *Clin Chem Lab Med* 40:40–45.

61. Streit F, Armstrong VW, Oellerich M. 2002. Rapid liquid chromatography-tandem mass spectrometry routine method for simultaneous determination of sirolimus, everolimus, tacrolimus and cyclosporin A in whole blood. *Clin Chem* 48:955–58.

62. Wallemacq PE, Vanbinst R, Asta S, et al. 2003. High-throughput liquid chromatography–tandem mass spectrometric analysis of sirolimus in whole blood. *Clin Chem Lab Med* 41:921–25.

63. Dimension® clinical chemistry system TACR Flex® Reagent Cartridge Package Insert. Newark, DE: Dade Behring, Inc.; 2006.

64. CEDIA® Tacrolimus Assay Package Insert. Fremont, CA: Microgenics Corporation; 2005.

65. 510(k) Substantial Equivalence Determination Decision Summary for CEDIA® Tacrolimus Assay. At http://www.fda.gov/cdrh/REVIEWS/K050206.pdf (accessed June 23, 2008).

66. Architect System Tacrolimus Package Insert. Abbott Park, IL: Abbott Diagnostics; 2007.

67. MacFarlane GD, Scheller DG, Ersfeld DL, et al. 1999. Analytical validation of the PRO-Trac II ELISA for the determination of tacrolimus (FK506) in whole blood. *Clin Chem* 45:1449–58.

68. 510(k) Substantial Equivalence Determination Decision Summary for EMIT Tacrolimus Assay. At http://www.fda.gov/cdrh/REVIEWS/K060385.pdf (accessed June 23, 2008).

69. IMx® System Tacrolimus II Package Insert. Abbott Park, IL: Abbott Diagnostics; 2007.

70. Taylor PJ, Salm P, Lynch SV, et al. 2000. Simultaneous quantification of tacrolimus and sirolimus, in human blood, by high-performance liquid chromatography-tandem mass spectrometry. *Ther Drug Monit* 22:608–12.

71. Lensmeyer GL, Poquette MA. 2001. Therapeutic monitoring of tacrolimus concentrations in blood: semi-automated extraction and liquid chromatography-electrospray ionization mass spectrometry. *Ther Drug Monit* 23:239–49.

72. Keevil BG, McCann SJ, Cooper DP, et al. 2002. Evaluation of a rapid micro-scale assay for tacrolimus by liquid chromatography-tandem mass spectrometry. *Ann Clin Biochem* 39:487–92.

73. 510(k) Substantial Equivalence Determination Decision Summary for MassTrak Immunosuppressants Kit, LC/MS/MS Analysis for Tacrolimus in Whole Blood. At http://www.fda.gov/cdrh/REVIEWS/K063868.pdf (accessed June 23, 2008).

74. Seradyn Innofluor® Certican® Assay System Package Insert. Indianapolis, IN: Seradyn, Inc.; 2005.

75. Baldelli S, Crippa A, Gabrieli R, et al. 2006. Comparison of the Innofluor® Certican assays with HPLC-UV for the determination of everolimus concentrations in heart transplantation. *Clin Biochem* 39:1152–59.

76. Boudennaia TY, Napoli KL. 2005. Validation of a practical liquid chromatography with ultraviolet detection method for quantification of whole-blood everolimus in a clinical TDM laboratory. *Ther Drug Monit* 27:171–77.

77. Khoschorur GA. 2005. Simultaneous measurement of sirolimus and everolimus in whole blood by HPLC with ultraviolet detection. *Clin Chem* 51:1721–24.

78. Baldelli S, Zenoni S, Merlini S, et al. 2006. Simultaneous determination of everolimus and cyclosporine concentrations by HPLC with ultraviolet detection. *Clin Chim Acta* 364:354–58.

79. Korecka M, Solari SG, Shaw LM. 2006. Sensitive, high throughput HPLC-MS/MS method with on-line sample clean-up for everolimus measurement. *Ther Drug Monit* 28:484–90.

80. Taylor PJ, Franklin ME, Graham KS, et al. 2007. A HPLC-mass spectrometric method suitable for the therapeutic drug monitoring of everolimus. *J Chromatog B* 848:208–14.

81. Garrido MJ, Hermida J, Tutor CJ. 2002. Relationship between cyclosporine concentrations obtained using the Roche Cobas Integra and Abbott TDx monoclonal immunoassays in pre-dose and two hour post-dose blood samples from kidney transplant recipients. *Ther Drug Monit* 24:785–88.

82. Kuzuya T, Ogura Y, Motegi Y, et al. 2002. Interference of hematocrit in the tacrolimus II microparticle enzyme immunoassay. *Ther Drug Monit* 24:507–11.

83. Tomita T, Homma M, Yuzawa K, et al. 2005. Effect of hematocrit value on microparticle enzyme immunoassay of tacrolimus concentration in therapeutic drug monitoring. *Ther Drug Monit* 27:94–97.

84. Homma M, Tomita T, Yuzawa K, et al. 2002. False positive blood tacrolimus concentration in microparticle enzyme immunoassay. *Biol Pharm Bull* 25:1119–20.

85. Hermida J, Fernandez MC, Tutor JC. 2005. Clinical significance of hematocrit interference in the tacrolimus II microparticle enzyme immunoassay: a tentative approach. *Clin Lab* 51:43–45.

86. Brown NW, Gonde CE, Adams JE, et al. 2005. Low hematocrit and serum albumin concentrations underlie the overestimation of tacrolimus concentrations by microparticle enzyme immunoassay versus liquid chromatography-tandem mass spectrometry. *Clin Chem* 51:586–92.

87. Napoli KL. 2006. Is microparticle enzyme-linked immunoassay (MEIA) reliable for use in tacrolimus TDM? Comparison of MEIA to liquid chromatography with mass spectrometric detection using longitudinal trough samples from transplant recipients. *Ther Drug Monit* 28:491–504.

88. Dorizzi RM, Cocco C, Rizzotti P. 2008. Tacrolimus assays; new tools for new tests and for old problems. *Clin Chem Acta* 387:177–78.

89. Wilson DH, Sepe D, Barnwe G. 2005. Letter to the editor. Inter-laboratory differences in sirolimus results from six sirolimus testing centers using HPLC tandem mass spectrometry (LC/MS/MS). *Clin Chim Acta* 355:211–13.

90. Bowers LD, Canafax DM. 1984. Cyclosporine: experience with therapeutic monitoring. *Ther Drug Monit* 6:142–47.

91. Carruthers SG, Freeman DJ, Koegler JC, et al. 1983. Simplified liquid-chromatographic analysis for cyclosporin A, and comparison with radioimmunoassay. *Clin Chem* 29:180–83.

92. Annesley T, Matz K, Balough L, et al. 1986. Liquid-chromatographic analysis for cyclosporine with use of a microbore column and small sample volume. *Clin Chem* 32:1407–9.

93. Yee GC, Gmur DJ, Kennedy MS. 1982. Liquid-chromatographic determination of cyclosporine in serum with use of a rapid extraction procedure. *Clin Chem* 28:2269–71.

94. Furlanut M, Plebani M, Burlina A. 1989. Cyclosporin monitoring: methodological considerations. *J Liquid Chromatogr* 12:1759–89.

95. Poonkuzhali B, Victoria J, Selvakumar R, et al. 1995. Comparison of HPLC & EMIT methods of cyclosporine assay in blood after bone marrow transplantation. *Indian J Med Res* 102:39–41.

96. Brandhorst G, Marquet P, Shaw LM, et al. 2008. Multicenter evaluation of a new inosine monophosphate dehydrogenase inhibition assay for quantification of total mycophenolic acid in plasma. *Ther Drug Monit* 30:428–33.

97. Holt DW. 2002. Monitoring mycophenolic acid. *Ann Clin Biochem* 39:173–83.

98. Shipkova M, Armstrong VW, Wieland E, et al. 1999. Identification of glucoside and carboxyl-linked glucuronide conjugates of mycophenolic acid in plasma of transplant recipients treated with mycophenolic acid. *Brit J Pharmacol* 126:1075–82.

99. Tsina I, Chu F, Hama K, et al. 1996. Manual and automated (robotic) high-performance liquid chromatography methods for the determination of mycophenolic acid and its glucuronide conjugate in human plasma. *J Chromatog B* 675:119–29.

100. Shipkova M, Niedmann PD, Armstrong VW, et al. 1998. Simultaneous determination of mycophenolic acid and its glucuronide in human plasma using a simple high-performance liquid chromatography procedure. *Clin Chem* 44:1481–88.

101. Jones CE, Taylor PJ, Johnson AG. 1998. High-performance liquid chromatography determination of mycophenolic acid and its glucuronide metabolite in human plasma. *J Chromatog B* 708:229–34.

102. Hosotsubo H, Takahara S, Kokado Y, et al. 2001. Rapid and simultaneous determination of mycophenolic acid and its glucuronide conjugate in human plasma by ion-pair reversed-phase high-performance liquid chromatography using isocratic elution. *J Chromatog B* 753:315–20.

103. Bolon M, Jeanpierre L, El Barkil M, et al. 2004. HPLC determination of mycophenolic acid and mycophenolic acid glucuronide in human plasma with hybrid material. *J Pharm Biomed Anal* 36:649–51.

104. Teshima D, Otsubo K, Kitagawa N, et al. 2003. High-performance liquid chromatographic method for mycophenolic aid and its glucuronide in serum and urine. *J Clin Pharm Ther* 28:17–22.

105. Wiwattanawongsa K, Heinzen EL, Kemp DC, et al. 2001. Determination of mycophenolic acid and its phenol metabolite in human plasma and urine by high-performance liquid chromatography. *J Chromatog B* 763:35–45.

106. Khoschsorur GA, Erwa W. 2004. Liquid chromatographic method for simultaneous determination of mycophenolic acid and its phenol-and acylglucuronide metabolites in plasma. *J Chromatog B* 799:355–60.

107. Watson DG, Araya FG, Galloway PJ, et al. 2004. Development of a high pressure liquid chromatography method for the determination of mycophenolic acid and its glucuronide metabolite in small volumes of plasma from paediatric patients. *J Pharm Biomed Anal* 35:87–92.

108. Patel CG, Mendonza AE, Akhlaghi F, et al. 2004. Determination of total mycophenolic acid and is glucuronide metabolite using liquid chromatography with ultraviolet detection and unbound mycophenolic acid using tandem mass spectrometry. *J Chromatog B* 813:287–94.

109. Seebacher G, Weigel G, Wolner E, et al. 1999. A simple HPLC method for monitoring mycophenolic acid and its glucuronidated metabolite in transplant recipients. *Clin Chem Lab Med* 37:509–15.

110. Daurel-Receveur M, Titier K, Picard S, et al. 2006. Fully automated analytical method for mycophenolic acid quantification in human plasma using on-line solid phase extraction and high performance liquid chromatography with diode array detection. *Ther Drug Monit* 28:505–11.

111. Mandla R, Line P-D, Midtvedt K, et al. 2003. Automated determination of free mycophenolic acid and its glucuronide in plasma from renal allograft recipients. *Ther Drug Monit* 25:407–14.

112. Yau W-P, Vathsala A, Lou H-X, et al. 2007. Simple reversed phase liquid chromatographic assay for simultaneous quantification of free mycophenolic acid and its glucuronide metabolite in human plasma. *J Chromatog B* 846:313–18.

113. Cussonneau X, Bolon-Lager M, Prunet-Spano C, et al. 2007. Relationship between MPA free fraction and free MPAG concentrations in heart transplant recipients based on simultaneous HPLC quantification of the target compounds in human plasma. *J Chromatog B* 852:674–78.

114. Atcheson B, Taylor PJ, Mudge DW, et al. 2004. Quantification of free mycophenolic acid and its glucuronide metabolite in human plasma by liquid chromatography using mass spectrometric and ultraviolet detection. *J Chromatog B* 799:157–63.

115. Ting LSL, Partovi N, Levy RD, et al. 2006. Pharmacokinetics of mycophenolic acid and its glucuronidated metabolites in stable lung transplant recipients. *Ann Pharmacother* 40:1509–16.
116. de Loor H, Naesens M, Verbeke K, et al. 2008. Stability of mycophenolic acid and glucuronide metabolites in human plasma and the impact of deproteinization methodology. *Clin Chem Acta* 389:87–92.
117. Carlucci F, Anzini M, Rovini M, et al. 2007. Development of a CE method for the determination of mycophenolic acid in human plasma: A comparison with HPLC. *Electrophoresis* 28:3908–14.
118. Ohyama K, Kishikawa N, Nakagawa H, et al. 2008. Simultaneous determination of mycophenolic acid and its acyl and phenol glucuronide metabolites in human serum by capillary zone electrophoresis. *J Pharm Biomed Anal* 47:201–6.
119. Yatscoff RW, Faraci C, Bolingbroke P. 1992. Measurement of rapamycin in whole blood using reverse-phase high-performance liquid chromatography. *Ther Drug Monit* 14:138–41.
120. Napoli KL, Kahan BD. 1994. Sample clean-up and high-performance liquid chromatographic techniques for measurement of whole blood rapamycin concentrations. *J Chromatog B* 654:111–20.
121. Napoli KL, Kahan BD. 1996. Routine clinical monitoring of sirolimus (rapamycin) whole blood concentrations by HPLC with ultraviolet detection. *Clin Chem* 42:1943–48.
122. Maleki S, Graves S, Becker S, et al. 2000. Therapeutic monitoring of sirolimus in human whole-blood samples by high-performance liquid chromatography. *Clin Ther* 22(Suppl B):B25–37.
123. Holt DW, Lee T, Johnston A. 2000. Measurement of sirolimus in whole blood using high-performance liquid chromatography with ultraviolet detection. *Clin Ther* 22(Suppl B):B38–48.
124. Cattaneo D, Perico N, Gaspari F. 2002. Assessment of sirolimus concentration in whole blood by high-performance liquid chromatography with ultraviolet detection. *J Chromatog B* 774:187–94.
125. Connor E, Sakamoto M, Fujikawa K, et al. 2002. Measurement of whole blood sirolimus by an HPLC assay using solid-phase extraction and UV detection. *Ther Drug Monit* 24:751–56.
126. de Andrade MC, Di Marco GS, Felipe CR, et al. 2005. Sirolimus quantification by high-performance liquid chromatography with ultraviolet detection. *Transpl Int* 18:354–59.
127. Baldelli S, Murgia S, Merlini S, et al. High-performance liquid chromatography with ultraviolet detection for therapeutic drug monitoring of everolimus. *J Chromatogr B* 2005;816:99–105.
128. Cech NB, Enke CG. 2001. Practical implications of some recent studies in electrospray ionization fundamentals. *Mass Spectrom Rev* 20:362–87.
129. Wu Z, Gao W, Phelps M, et al. 2004. Favorable effects of weak acids on negative-ion electrospray ionization mass spectrometry. *Anal Chem* 76:839–47.
130. Maurer HH. 2007. Current role of liquid chromatography-mass spectrometry in clinical and forensic toxicology. *Anal Bioanal Chem* 388:1315–25.
131. Saint-Marcoux F, Sauvage F-L, Marquet P. 2007. Current role of LC-MS in therapeutic drug monitoring. *Anal Bioanal Chem* 388:1327–49.
132. Kushnir MM, Rockwood AL, Nelson GJ, et al. 2005. Assessing analytical specificity in quantitative analysis using tandem mass spectrometry. *Clin Biochem* 38:319–27.
133. Marchi I, Rudaz S, Selman M, et al. 2007. Evaluation of the influence of protein precipitation prior to on-line SPE–LC–API/MS procedures using multivariate data analysis. *J Chromatog B* 845: 244–52.
134. Bonfiglio R, King RC, Olah TV, et al. 1999. The effects of sample preparation methods on the variability of the electrospray ionization response for model drug compounds. *Rapid Commun Mass Spectrom* 13:1175–85.
135. Matuszewski BK, Constanzer ML, Chavez-Eng CM. 1998. Matrix effect in quantitative LC/MS/MS analyses for biological fluids: a method for determination of finasteride in human plasma at picogram per milliliter concentrations. *Anal Chem* 70:882–89.
136. Mallet CR, Lu Z, Mazzeo JR. 2004. A study of ion suppression effects in electrospray ionization from mobile phase additives and solid-phase extracts. *Rapid Commun Mass Spectrom* 18:49–58.
137. Chambers E, Wagrowski-Diehl DM, Lu Z, et al. 2007. Systematic and comprehensive strategy for reducing matrix effects in LC/MS/MS analyses. *J Chromatog B* 852:22–34.
138. Mei H, Hsieh Y, Nardo C, et al. 2003. Investigation of matrix effects in bioanalytical high-performance liquid chromatography/tandem mass spectrometric assays: application to drug discovery. *Rapid Commun Mass Spectrom* 17:97–103.
139. Polson C, Sarker P, Incledon B, et al. 2003. Optimization of protein precipitation based upon effectiveness of protein removal and ionization effect in liquid chromatography-tandem mass spectrometry. *J Chromatog B* 785:263–75.
140. King R, Bonfiglio R, Fernandez-Metzler C, et al. 2000. Mechanistic investigation of ionization suppression in electrospray ionization. *J Am Soc Mass Spectrom* 11:942–50.

141. Jemal M. 2000. High-throughput quantitative bioanalysis by LC/MS/MS. *Biomed Chromatogr* 14:422–29.

142. Annesley TM. 2007. Methanol-associated matrix effects in electrospray ionization tandem mass spectrometry. *Clin Chem* 53:1827–34.

143. Annesley TM. 2005. Application of commercial calibrators for the analysis of immunosuppressant drugs in whole blood. *Clin Chem* 51:457–60.

144. Voseger M. 2008. Instrument specific matrix effects of calibration materials in the LC-MS/MS analysis of tacrolimus. *Clin Chem* 54:1406–8. [Letter to the Editor]

145. Matuszewski BK, Constanzer ML, Chevez-Eng CM. 2003. Strategies for the assessment of matrix effect in quantitative bioanalytical methods based on HPLC-MS/MS. *Anal Chem* 75:3019–30.

146. Taylor PJ, Jones CE, Martin PT, et al. 1998. Microscale high-performance liquid chromatography–electrospray tandem mass spectrometry for cyclosporin A in blood. *J Chromatog B* 705:289–94.

147. Voseger M, Spöhrer U. 2005. Pitfall in the high-throughput quantification of whole blood cyclosporin A using liquid chromatography-tandem mass spectrometry. *Clin Chem Lab Med* 43:400–2.

148. Streit F, Armstrong VW, Oellerich M. 2003. Mass interference in quantification of cyclosporine using tandem mass spectrometry without chromatography. *Ther Drug Monit* 25:506. [Abstract]

149. Taylor PJ, Brown SR, Cooper DP, et al. 2005. Evaluation of 3 internal standards for the measurement of cyclosporin by HPLC-mass spectrometry. *Clin Chem* 51:1890–3.

150. Voseger M, Zachoval R, Spöhrer U, et al. 2001. Potential lack of specificity using electrospray tandem-mass spectrometry for the analysis of mycophenolic acid in serum. *Ther Drug Monit* 23:722–24.

151. Ting LSL, Decarie D. 2007. Effect of acidification on protein binding on mycophenolic acid. *Ther Drug Monit* 29:132–33. [Letter to the Editor]

152. Annesley TM, Clayton LT. 2005. Quantification of mycophenolic acid and glucuronide metabolite in human serum by HPLC-tandem mass spectrometry. *Clin Chem* 51:872–77.

153. Benoit-Biancamano M-O, Caron P, Lévesque É, et al. 2007. Sensitive high-performance liquid chromatography-tandem mass spectrometry method for quantitative analysis of mycophenolic acid an its glucuronide metabolites in human plasma and urine. *J Chromatog B* 858:159–67.

154. Stokvis E, Rosing H, Beijnen JH. 2005. Stable isotopically labeled internal standards in quantitative bioanalysis using liquid chromatography/mass spectrometry: necessity or not? *Rapid Commun Mass Spectrom* 19:401–7.

155. Pieri M, Miraglia N, Castiglia L, et al. 2005. Determination of rapamycin quantification of the sodiated species by an ion trap mass spectrometer as an alternative to the ammoniated complex analysis by triple quadrupole. *Rapid Commun Mass Spectrom* 19:3042–50.

156. O'Halloran S, Ilett KF. 2008. Evaluation of a deuterium-labeled internal standard for the measurement of sirolimus by high-throughput HPLC electrospray ionization tandem mass spectrometry. *Clin Chem* 54:1386–89.

157. Taylor PJ, Jones A, Balderson GA, et al. 1996. Sensitive, specific quantitative analysis of tacrolimus (FK506) in blood by liquid chromatography-electrospray tandem mass spectrometry. *Clin Chem* 42:279–85.

158. Taylor PJ, Hogan NS, Lynch SV, et al. 1997. Improved therapeutic drug monitoring of tacrolimus (FK506) by tandem mass spectrometry. *Clin Chem* 43:2189–90.

159. Boernsen KO, Egge-Jacobsen W, Inverardi B, et al. 2007. Assessment and validation of the MS/MS fragmentation patterns of the macrolide immunosuppressant everolimus. *J Mass Spectrom* 42:793–802.

160. Hoogtanders K, van der Heijden, Stolk LML, et al. 2007. Internal standard selection for the high-performance liquid chromatography tandem mass spectrometry assay of everolimus in blood. *Ther Drug Monit* 29:673–74.

161. McMahon LM, Luo S, Hayes M, et al. 2000. High-throughput analysis of everolimus (RAD001) and cyclosporin A (CsA) in whole blood by liquid chromatography/mass spectrometry using a semi-automated 96-well solid-phase extraction system. *Rapid Commun Mass Spectrom* 14:1965–71.

162. Brignol N, McMahon LM, Luo S, et al. 2001. High-throughput semi-automated 96-well liquid/liquid extraction and liquid chromatography/mass spectrometric analysis of everolimus (RAD001) and cyclosporin a (CsA) in whole blood. *Rapid Commun Mass Spectrom* 15:898–907.

163. Koal T, Deters M, Bruno C, et al. 2004. Simultaneous determination of four immunosuppressants by means of high speed and robust on-line solid phase extraction–high performance liquid chromatography–tandem mass spectrometry. *J Chromatog B* 805:215–22.

164. Hatsis P, Volmer DA. 2004. Evaluation of a cyano stationary phase for the determination of tacrolimus, sirolimus and cyclosporin A in whole blood by high-performance liquid chromatography–tandem mass spectrometry. *J Chromatog B* 809:287–94.

165. Salm P, Taylor PJ, Rooney F. 2008. A high-performance liquid chromatography-mass spectrometry method using a novel atmospheric pressure chemical ionization approach for the rapid simultaneous measurement of tacrolimus and cyclosporin in whole blood. *Ther Drug Monit* 30:292–300.

166. Napoli KL. 2006. Organic solvents compromise performance of internal standard (ascomycin) in proficiency testing of mass spectrometry-based assays for tacrolimus. *Clin Chem* 52:765–66. [Letter to the Editor].

167. Cristoni S, Bernardi LR, Gerthoux P, et al. 2006. Surface-activated chemical ionization and high-flow gradient chromatography to reduce matrix effect. *Rapid Commun Mass Spectrom* 20:2376–82.

168. Voseger M, Spöhrer U. 2006. Automated processing of whole blood samples for the determination of immunosuppressants by liquid chromatography tandem-mass spectrometry. *Clin Chem Lab Med* 44:1126–30.

169. DiFrancesco R, Frerichs V, Donnelly J, et al. 2007. Simultaneous determination of cortisol, dexamethasone, methylprednisolone, prednisolone, mycophenolic acid and mycophenolic acid glucuronide in human plasma utilizing liquid chromatography–tandem mass spectrometry. *J Chromatog B* 859:42–51.

170. Mednonza A, Gohh R, Akhlaghi F. 2004. Determination of cyclosporine in saliva using liquid chromatography–tandem mass spectrometry. *Ther Drug Monit* 26:569–75.

171. Mendonza AE, Gohh RY, Akhlaghi F. 2006. Analysis of mycophenolic acid in saliva using liquid chromatography tandem mass spectrometry. *Ther Drug Mont* 28:402–6.

172. Falck P, Guldseth H, Åsberg A, et al. 2007. Determination of ciclosporin A and its six main metabolites in isolated T-lymphocytes and whole blood using liquid chromatography–tandem mass spectrometry. *J Chromatog B* 852:345–52.

173. Falck P, Åsberg A, Guldseth H, et al. 2008. Declining intracellular T-lymphocyte concentration of cyclosporine A precedes acute rejection in kidney transplant recipients. *Transplantation* 85:179–84.

174. Bénech H, Hascoët S, Furlan V, et al. 2007. Development and validation of an LC/MS/MS assay for mycophenolic acid in human peripheral blood mononuclear cells. *J Chromatog B* 853:168–74.

175. Capron A, Musuamba F, Latinne D, et al. 2009. Validation of a liquid-chromatography mass spectrometric assay for tacrolimus in peripheral blood mononuclear cells. *Ther Drug Monit* 31:178–86.

176. Glander P, Braun KP, Hambach P, et al. 2001. Non-radioactive determination of inosine 5'-monophosphate dehydrogenase (IMPDH) in peripheral mononuclear cells. *Clin Biochem* 34:543–49.

177. Vethe NT, Bergan S. 2006. Determination of inosine monophosphate dehydrogenase activity in human CD4+ cells isolated from whole blood during mycophenolic acid therapy. *Ther Drug Monit* 28:608–13.

15 Therapeutic Drug Monitoring in Cancer Patients: Application of Chromatographic Techniques

Amitava Dasgupta
University of Texas Medical School

CONTENTS

15.1   INTRODUCTION

Normally in all living organisms, cells grow and die with newly grown cells replacing dying cells. Sometimes this process can go wrong where new cells are being formed but old cells are not dying. This uncontrolled cell growth produces a mass which can be either benign or malignant. Cells in malignant tumors can invade nearby tissue and can eventually spread all over the body (metastasis). Treatment of cancer may include chemotherapy, radiation or surgery or a combination of any of these options.

Cancer chemotherapy is used to stop growth of cancer cells. However, due to the cytotoxic nature of many anticancer drugs they are also toxic to normal cells. Chemotherapy drugs can be grouped under several categories depending on the mechanism of action, chemical structure, and other factors. Alkylating agents (cyclophosphamide, busulfan, dacarbazine, etc.), directly damage DNA to prevent cancer cell growth and can interfere with all phases of cell growth. They are used in treating different types of cancer including leukemia, lymphoma, Hodgkin disease, multiple myeloma, sarcoma, lung and breast cancer as well as other types of cancer. Antimetabolites (5-fluorouracil, 6-marcaptopurine, methotrexate, etc.), interfere with DNA and RNA growth by causing structural modification and they interfere with the S-phase of the cell cycle. These drugs are used in treating leukemia, various tumors and carcinoma of breast, ovary and other types of cancer. Some anthracycline antibiotics such as doxorubicin, epirubicin, etc., also have anticancer properties because they interfere with enzymes involved in DNA replication and are used in treating a variety of cancers. Other antibiotics such as bleomycin also have anticancer properties. Irinotecan (CPT-11) is a topoisomerase inhibitor (which helps in the separation of strands of DNA) and is used in treating leukemias and many types of cancer. Drugs such as vinblastine, vincristine and paclitaxel are plant alkaloids which can stop mitosis by inhibiting enzymes from making proteins needed for cell division. Differentiating agents (bexarotene, arsenic trioxide, etc.), force cancer cells to mature like normal cells so that these cells eventually die. Corticosteroids, targeted therapy, hormone therapy and immunotherapy are also used for treating patients with cancer (Table 15.1) [1].

Targeted therapy is one of the newer therapies for treating cancer patients. These drugs attack a particular type of cancer cell and usually have lesser side effects than conventional anticancer drugs. For example, lapatinib is used in treating breast cancer if HER2/neu is positive. Monoclonal antibodies can be used to guide a drug directly to cancer cells or can be used as immunotherapy to increase the body's immune system against cancer cells. For example, rituximab and alemtuzumab are directed at certain

TABLE 15.1
Different Classes of Drugs used in Cancer Chemotherapy

Drug Class	Representative Drug		
Alkylating agents	Cyclophosphamide*	Busulfan*	Mechlorethamine
	Chlorambucil	Ifosfamide*	Streptozocin
	Lomustine	Carmustine	Dacarbazine
	Temozolomide	Thiotepa	Altretamine
	Treosulfan		
Antimetabolites	5-Fluorouracil*	6-Marcaptopurine*	Methotrexate*
	Gemcitabine	Cytosine arabinoside (ARA-C)*	
	Fludarabine	Pemetrexed	
Antibiotics	Doxorubicin*	Daunorubicin*	Epirubicin*
	Idarubicin*	Mitomycin	Bleomycin
Topoisomerase inhibitors	Irinotecan (CPT-11)*	Topotecan*	
Mitotic inhibitors	Paclitaxel*	Vincristine	Vinblastine
Corticosteroids	Dexamethasone	Methylprednisolon	
Hormone modulator	Tamoxifen*		
Targeted therapies	Imatinib	Geritonic	Erlotinib
Differentiating agents	Tretinoin	Bexarotene	Arsenic trioxide

* Therapeutic drug monitoring recommended.

lymphoma cells and can be used for treating certain types of non-Hodgkin lymphoma. Liposomal therapy is where an anticancer drug is trapped inside liposomes and such liposomes deliver the drug at target cancer and also help the drug in penetrating cells due to lipophilic nature of liposomes [1].

Selection of a particular drug or drug combination for treating a cancer patient depends upon many factors such as type of cancer, stage of cancer, health status and age of the patient, other health issues and any previous history of cancer chemotherapy. Moreover, side effects of a drug or drug combination are also important concerns for cancer chemotherapy and sometimes lower dosages of two drugs instead of a single drug are used to reduce side effects as well as to improve efficacy of the drugs. In addition, certain chemotherapy agents require routine monitoring such as methotrexate, cisplatin, 5-fluorouracil, etc. Methotrexate is also used in low dosage as a disease modifying agent to treat certain patients with rheumatoid arthritis. Low dosage methotrexate therapy may under certain conditions require TDM.

15.2 THERAPEUTIC DRUG MONITORING (TDM) OF ANTICANCER DRUGS

Therapeutic drug monitoring (TDM) is important for drugs with narrow therapeutic range and where serum drug condition is a better predictor of clinical outcome than dosage (also see Chapter 1). Although it is broadly applied for different therapeutic classes such as cardiovascular drugs, anti-epileptics, certain antibiotics, immunosuppressants, antidepressants, specific antiretroviral agents, antiasthmatic, etc., TDM has limited use for antineoplastic agents [2]. Anticancer drugs demonstrate wide interindividual pharmacokinetic variability. In addition, sometimes toxicity better correlates with serum drug level than dosage. Although, the pharmacokinetic behavior of many anticancer drugs such as cyclophosphamide, cisplatin, methotrexate, cytarabine, 5-fluorouracil, doxorubicin, daunorubicin, bleomycin, vincristine, and vinblastine in humans has been described, complexity of drug metabolism and lack of established therapeutic range for many anticancer drugs have limited applications of TDM of anticancer drugs [3]. Nevertheless several studies have shown a relation between plasma drug concentrations and dose-limiting toxicities for a number of anticancer drugs such as busulfan [4], carboplatin [5,6], etoposide [7] and methotrexate [8] and 5-fluoro-uracil [9]. Methotrexate is the most frequently monitored anticancer drug but 5-fluorouracil and busulfan are also often monitored (see Figure 15.1 for chemical structures of methotrexate, 5-fluorouracil, and busulfan). In general other anticancer drugs such as cyclophosphamide, ifosfamide, 6-mercaptopurine, and cytosine arabinoside, several anthracycline anticancer antibiotics, irinotecan, paclitaxel, docetaxel, and tamoxifen also may require TDM and chromatographic techniques are used for determination of serum concentrations of these drugs. In Table 15.2 methods for chromatographic monitoring of these drugs are summarized.

Interestingly, many anticancer drugs are good candidates for routine monitoring. Underdosing of cancer patients with chemotherapeutic agents is not acceptable. On the other hand certain serious side effects of cancer chemotherapy such as myelosuppression can be life threatening. Therefore, establishment of therapeutic ranges for anticancer drugs would be beneficial. Clinical trials demonstrate that treating patients with dosages of an anticancer drug that would produce serum concentrations at the upper end of the nontoxic range is beneficial. Use of TDM to individualize chemotherapy in order to improve efficacy of anticancer agents and at the same time to avoid serious drug toxicity would be very effective in patient management. Additional benefits of TDM in cancer patients include enhancement of compliance, minimization of pharmacokinetic variabilities among patients, detecting drug–drug interactions as well as dosage adjustments for patients with hepatic or renal failure [10,11]. Successful implementation of TDM in cancer patients requires more than establishment of therapeutic ranges for anticancer drugs. In order to achieve benefits from TDM, correct administration of the drug, proper collection and processing of specimens for drug analysis, precise measurement of serum drug level, and proper interpretation of results are required. Therefore, for successful implementation of TDM in cancer patients, a multidisciplinary approach involving nurse, phlebotomist, medical technologist, clinical chemist, and physician is essential [10].

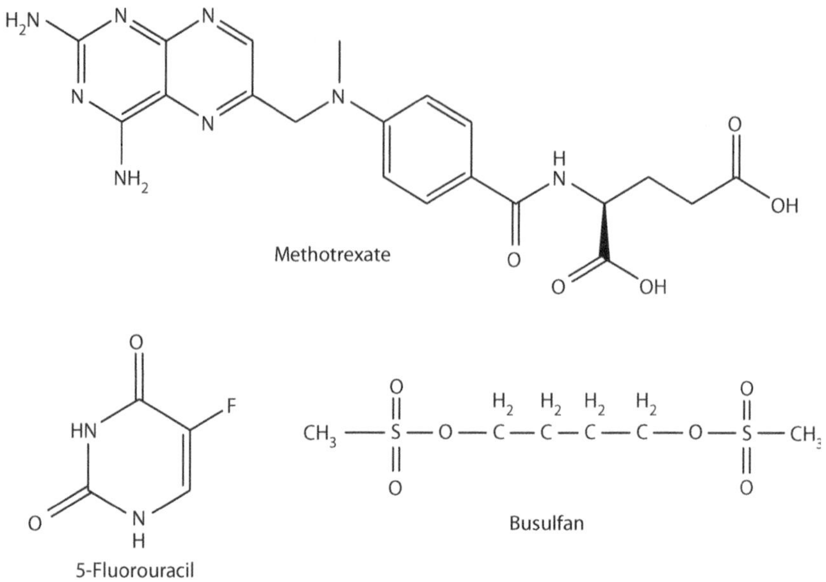

FIGURE 15.1   Chemical structures of frequently monitored anticancer drugs; methotrexate, 5-fluorouracil, and busulfan.

TABLE 15.2
Chromatographic Techniques for Monitoring of some Anticancer Drugs

Drug	Drug/Metabolite Monitored	Chromatographic Method
Busulfan	Parent drug	Both GC and HPLC
Cyclophosphamide	Parent drug and metabolites (4-hydroxycyclophosphamide)	Both GC and HPLC
Ifosfamide	Parent drug and metabolites (2 and 3 dechloroethylifosfamide)	Both GC and HPLC
Methotrexate	Parent drug and metabolite (7-Hydroxymethotrexate)	Only HPLC
5-Fluorouracil	Parent drug	Both GC and HPLC
6-Marcaptopurine	Parent drug and metabolites (6-methylmeracptopurine)	Only HPLC
Cytosine arabinoside (Ara-C)	Parent drug and metabolite Uridine arabinoside (Ara-U)	Only HPLC
Anthracyclines	Parent drugs and metabolites	Only HPLC
Irinotecan (CPT-11)	Parent drugs and metabolites 7-ethyl-10-hydroxycamptothecin (SN-38)	Only HPLC
Paclitaxel	Parent drug	Only HPLC
Docetaxel	Parent drug	Only HPLC
Tamoxifen	Parent drug and metabolite (4-hydroxytamoxifen)	Only HPLC

15.3   METHODOLOGIES USED FOR THERAPEUTIC DRUG MONITORING (TDM) IN CANCER PATIENTS

Methods of analysis for therapeutic drug in cancer patients include technologies that are often not found within routine clinical laboratories of many hospitals because immunoassays are commercially available for only a few anticancer drugs. The advanced technologies required for TDM of anticancer drugs include gas chromatography (GC) with numerous detection methods (FID: flame ionization detection, ECD: electron capture detection and MS: spectrometry) and high performance liquid chromatography

(HPLC) again with numerous detection methods (UV: ultraviolet; PDA: photodiode array detector, and MS or MS/MS; tandem mass spectrometry). These technologies demand both significant capital investment and higher level of expertise among medical technologists. Therefore, TDM of a few anticancer drugs such as methotrexate and 5-flurouracil are offered in most hospital laboratories while most specimens for TDM of other anticancer drugs are referred to large national reference laboratories.

15.4 THERAPEUTIC DRUG MONITORING (TDM) OF ALKYLATING AGENTS

Alkylating agents act by directly damaging DNA of cancer cells and prevent tumor growth. Alkylating agents are not phase specific and can act as inhibitors of cell growth at any stage of the cell cycle. Because these drugs are capable of damaging DNA, they have cytotoxic an effect on bone marrow and in a few cases may cause acute leukemia. The risk for developing leukemia is dose dependent and is highest 5–10 years after treatment.

15.4.1 THERAPEUTIC DRUG MONITORING (TDM) OF BUSULFAN

Busulfan (1, 4-butanediol dimethanesulfonate) is a bifunctional alkylating agent that acts in the cell cycle phase by alkylating DNA forming DNA–DNA and DNA protein cross-links, thus inhibiting DNA replication. It exhibits selective cytotoxicity for myeloid cells and also exhibits an ability to remove sulfur from other compounds, i.e., proteins, polypeptides and amino acids; but it is unclear how much this contributes to its cytotoxicity. The bone marrow depressive effect of busulfan is dose dependent. At low doses the drug depresses granulocytopoiesis and thrombocytopoiesis but has little effect on lymphocytes. Low dose busulfan is used to treat chronic myelogenous leukemia (CML), polycythemia vera, myelofibrosis, and primary thrombocythemia. The treatment of CML using busulfan does not result in a cure but is considered palliative. Patients who lack the Philadelphia chromosome or who are in a blast phase show a poor response to busulfan. At high doses, full bone marrow suppression is observed [11].

Busulfan can be administered orally or by intravenous administration. Absorption following oral administration is essentially complete. The drug is extensively metabolized in the liver such that < 2% of the drug is excreted unchanged. About 32% of busulfan is excreted in the urine as metabolic products. At lease 12 inactive metabolites have been identified among them tetrahydrothiophene, tetrahydrothiophene 12-oxide, sulfolane, 3-hydroxysulfolane, S-methanesulfonic acid, and 3-hydroxytetrahydrothiophene-1, 1-dioxide. In one study of the pharmacokinetics of high-dose therapy, the mean elimination half-life decreased from ~3.4 to ~2.3 hours after four days in which the patients received 1 mg/kg every six hours. While this suggests busulfan may induce its own metabolism, additional studies have not been performed. The remaining busulfan is thought to remain in the blood bound to functional groups on proteins and other biomolecules [12].

Adverse reactions to busulfan include nausea, vomiting, anorexia, weakness, anemia, infertility, hyperpigmentation, amenorrhea, and seizures. The most serious adverse effect reported is bone marrow suppression resulting in severe pancytopenia. The complication is reversible, but recovery may take one month to two years with supportive care. The development of bronchopulmonary dysplasia with pulmonary fibrosis is a rare and usually fatal complication. The histological findings associated with this condition are similar to those following pulmonary irradiation. Onset is varied with symptoms developing as rapidly as within eight months to as long as 10 years after initiation of therapy. Some patients receiving high-dose therapy have also experienced fatal cardiac tamponade and hepatic veno-occlusive disease. Busulfan is considered a mutagen and carcinogen and thus contraindicated in pregnancy.

Although TDM is not typically used for a patient undergoing low-dose therapies, but it is recommended for patients undergoing the high-dose regimens because TDM has proven beneficial for these patients. Pharmacokinetic and pharmacodynamic properties of busulfan have been well studied in order to establish therapeutic range and toxic range so that unwanted adverse effects can be avoided. Tran et al. studied whether adjusting oral busulfan dosage on the basis of early pharmacokinetic data in order to achieve a targeted drug exposure could reduce transplant related complications in children with advanced hematologic malignancies and observed that dosage adjustment based on serum level of busulfan is useful [13]. Dosage adjustment of oral busulfan based on TDM to bring exposure within established therapeutic range has been shown to reduce toxicity and improve clinical outcome [14]. Chandy and his colleagues have shown that the risk of graft rejection is higher when trough concentrations are below 150 ng/mL. [15,16] Patients whose serum drug concentrations exceeded 900 ng/mL had a greater risk of veno-occlusive disease compared to those whose concentrations were lower. Trough concentrations between 600 and 900 ng/mL are targeted. Concentrations have also been monitored in oral fluid and CSF [17,18]

A number of chromatography-based [17–21] methods with and without MS detection are described and an immunoassay method exists that can be performed as an ELISA or adapted to some automated platforms. Currently, the primary limitation of the chromatography-based methods is the lack of good internal standards. Specimens include serum and heparinized plasma. EDTA has been reported to interfere with at least one LCMS method [19] Samples should be processed immediately after collection as busulfan is reported to undergo in vitro hydrolysis with a degradation half-life of 8.7 hours in whole blood at 37°C, of 12 hours in plasma, and of 16 hours in phosphate buffer [1,21].

Erhsson and Hassan reported determination of busulfan in plasma using GC/MS after extracting the drug from plasma using methylene chloride followed by derivatization. The analysis of selected ion monitoring at *m/z* 183 produced good precision of analysis (CV: 4.3%) at busulfan plasma level of 10 ng/mL [22]. In another report Lai et al. used pusulfan (1,5-pentanediol dimethanesulfonate) as the internal standard for determination of busulfan in human plasma. The internal standard was added to 0.25 mL of plasma and then both busulfan and the internal standard were extracted from the plasma specimen using ethyl acetate. The organic phase was separated and sodium iodide was added to derivatize both busulfan and the internal standard. After iodination, the extract was treated with water to remove excess sodium iodide, followed by drying of the organic layer. The residue was reconstituted in 60 µL of ethyl acetate and 1 µL was injected into the GC/MS. Both derivatized busulfan and the derivatized internal standard were well separated in the chromatogram (Figure 15.2 shows overlay of a blank plasma and plasma of a child receiving busulfan, from Reference [23]). These compounds were identified by total ion monitoring using mass spectrometer and for quantitative analysis selected ion monitoring was used (*m/z* 183 from 1,4-diiodobutane derived from busulfan and m/z 197 from 1,5-diiodopentane derived from pusulfan) (Figure 15.3 shows mass spectra of both derivatized busulfan and the internal standard derivatized pusulfan). The assay was linear for plasma busulfan concentrations of up to 4000 ng/mL while the limit of quantitation was 40 ng/mL [23]. Abdel-Rehim also described analysis of busulfan in human plasma using GC/MS after solid phase microextraction of busulfan from human plasma and derivatization [20]. In another report the authors used deuterated busulfan (busulfan d8) for GC/MS determination of busulfan in plasma. Busulfan along with the internal standard were extracted from plasma using ethyl acetate and derivatized with 2,3,5,6-tetrafluorothiophenol prior to analysis by GC/MS using selected ion monitoring. The method was linear over the range of 10–2000 ng/mL of derivatized busulfan [20].

Methods for analysis of busulfan from human plasma using HPLC have also been reported. Quenrin et al. developed a HPLC method coupled with UV detection for determination of busulfan in plasma after extraction with toluene followed by derivatization with 2,3,5,6-tetrafluorothiophenol. Elution of peaks was monitored at 275 nm. The assay was linear for plasma busulfan concentrations between 50 and 2000 ng/mL [24]. Pichini used HPLC combined with mass spectrometry for determination of busulfan concentrations in serum and cerebrospinal fluid of children undergoing bone marrow autotransplantation. After two liquid-liquid extraction steps with dichloromethane, the separation of busulfan was carried out by isocratic reverse phase chromatography. The mass spectrometer was operated in electron impact mode and principal ions at m/z 175, 111 and 79 were observed for busulfan. However, the authors selected only *m/z* 175 for quantitation of busulfan. The

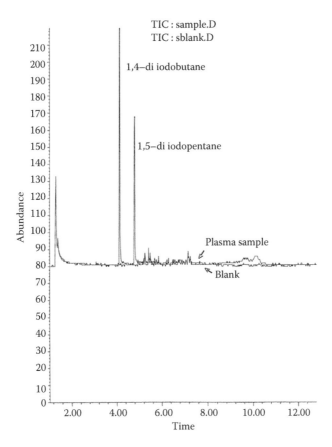

TIC : sample.D
TIC : sblank.D

1,4–di iodobutane

1,5–di iodopentane

Plasma sample

Blank

FIGURE 15.2 GC-MS analysis of BU and PU by total ion monitoring of their iodinated alkane derivatives, 1,4-diiodobutane (from BU) and 1,5-diiodopentane (from PU), presented as an overlay of a blank plasma and plasma sample of a child receiving busulfan. Retention times were in minutes. The amount of internal standard was 0.22 μg and amount of busulfan in patient's specimen was 0. 4 μg. (From Lai WK, Pang CP, Law LK, Wong R et al., *Clin Chem,* 44, 2506–2510, 1998. Copyright © 1998 American Association for Clinical Chemistry, reprinted with permission.)

retention time of busulfan was 2.5 min and the detection limit was 100 ng/mL [25]. Kellogg et al. described a liquid chromatography coupled with tandem mass spectrometric method (LC/MS/MS) for determination of busulfan concentrations in plasma. Plasma specimen (50 μL) was extracted with 1 mL of methanol containing the internal standard; 1,6-bis(methanesulfonyloxy)hexane. The supernatant was dried under nitrogen then reconstituted in methanol for analysis using LC/MS/MS. The total analysis time was 5 min and Q1/Q3 transition for busulfan was monitored at m/z 369/55 while Q1/Q3 transition of the internal standard was monitored at 297.1/55.1 [19].

15.4.2 Therapeutic Drug Monitoring (TDM) of Treosulfan

Treosulfan (L-threitol-1, 4-di-methanesulfonate) is a prodrug of a bifunctional alkylating agent with a structure similar to busulfan. This drug shows a broad spectrum antitumor activity and is indicated for treatment of ovarian carcinoma and other solid tumors. Due to limited non-hematological toxicity of treosulfan, it is a promising candidate in myeloablative therapy for hematopoietic transplantation in children [26,27]. There are only a few methods reported in the literature for determination of treosulfan concentrations in human plasma and urine. In one report, HPLC with refractometric detection was used for analysis of treosulfan. Barbital was used as the internal standard [28].

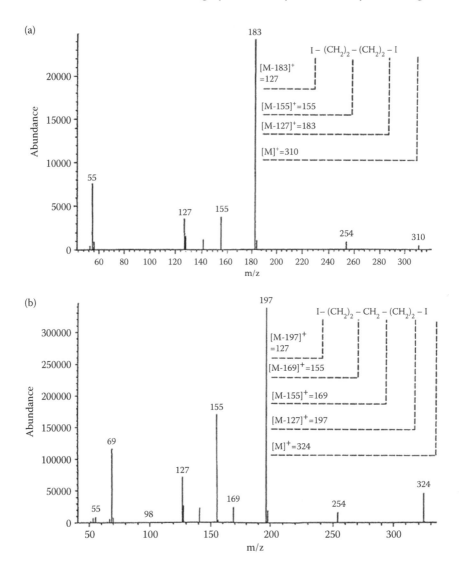

FIGURE 15.3 The mass spectra and major fragment ions of 1,4-diiodobutane (a) and 1,5-diiodopentane (b). (From Lai WK, Pang CP, Law LK, Wong R et al., *Clin Chem,* 44, 2506–2510, 1998. Copyright © 1998 American Association for Clinical Chemistry, reprinted with permission.)

15.4.3 THERAPEUTIC DRUG MONITORING (TDM) OF CYCLOPHOSPHAMIDE

Cyclophosphamide is a prodrug and is one of the most widely used antineoplastic agents. Cyclophosphamide is first converted into 4-hydroxycyclophosphamide that exists in equilibrium with its ring opened tautomeric form aldophosphamide. Inside the cell 4-hydroxyphosphamide spontaneously decomposes into the alkylating moiety phosphoramide mustard and urotoxic acrolein. Activation of cyclophosphamide is carried out by cytochrome P-450 mixed function oxidase and CYP2B6 is responsible for 45% conversion to 4-hydroxycyclophosphamide, CYP3QA4 for 25% conversion and CYP2C9 for 12% conversion (29). In general CYP2C9, CYP2C19, CYP3A4, and CYP2B6 are involved in cyclophosphamide metabolism and polymorphism of CYP2C19, CYP2B6, CYP3A4 and CYP3A5 have been implicated to correlate with altered pharmacokinetics of cyclophosphamide and or outcome of therapy [30].

Concentrations of cyclophosphamide and its metabolite 4-hydroxycyclophosphamide can be determined in human serum or urine using both GC and liquid chromatographic techniques. Because 4-hydroxycyclophosphamide is inherently unstable in blood (four minutes at 37°C) this compound must be converted to a stable derivative prior to analysis. Indirect estimation of 4-hydroxycyclophosphamide by measuring its degradation product acrolein has also been reported [31]. Sessinik et al. determined cyclophosphamide concentration in urine using GC/MS after liquid-liquid extraction with diethyl ether and derivatization with trifluoroacetic anhydride. The detection limit was 0.25 ng/mL [32]. In another report the authors determined concentrations of cyclophosphamide and its structural isomer iphosphamide (also used in cancer chemotherapy) using GC and tandem mass spectrometry with trophosphamide as the internal standard. The authors extracted the drugs from human urine using diethyl ether and derivatization was carried out using heptafluorobutyric anhydride. Quantification of derivatized cyclophosphamide was performed on product ions at m/z 150, 212, and 214 and for the internal standard product ions at m/z 118 and m/z 120 with the ions at m/z 273 and m/z 275 as precursors [33].

Baumann et al. described a sensitive HPLC protocol for determination of cyclophosphamide and its four metabolites (4-hydroxycyclophosphamide, 4-keto-cyclophosphamide, carboxyphosphamide and 3-dechloroethylifosfamide) in human plasma after converting 4-hydroxycyclophosphamide with methyl hydroxylamine to its stable methyloxime form. The authors used solid phase extraction and reverse phase HPLC with a C-18 column for analysis of cyclophosphamide and its four metabolites. The detection limit was 15 ng/mL except for 4-hydroxycyclophosphamide which had a detection limit of 30 ng/mL [34]. In another report the authors used liquid-liquid extraction with protein precipitation in one stage using acetonitrile to determine concentration of 4-hydroxycyclophosphamide in human plasma. The 4-hydroxycyclophosphamide was stabilized and converted into a fluorescent dansylhydrazone derivative which was chromatographed on a reverse phase column using fluorometric determination at excitation 350 nm and emission 550 nm. The limit of quantitation was 60 ng/mL [35]. Huitema et al. determined phosphoramide mustard metabolite of cyclophosphamide in human plasma using HPLC and UV detection at 276 nm wavelength after derivatization of phosphoramide mustard with diethyldithiocarbamate (at 70°C for 10 min) followed by extraction using acetonitrile. The authors used C-8 column and a mobile phase composition of acetonitrile/0.025 M potassium phosphate buffer at pH 8.0 (32:68 by vol). The calibration curve was linear from 50 to 10000 ng/mL [36].

15.4.4 THERAPEUTIC DRUG MONITORING (TDM) OF IFOSFAMIDE

Ifosfamide, a structural isomer of cyclophosphamide is also widely used in cancer chemotherapy to treat various solid tumors, soft tissue sarcoma and hematological malignancies in both adult and children. Ifosfamide is a drug which requires activation by cytochrome P-450. It is deactivated to various compounds such as 2-dechloroethylifosafamide and 3-dechloroethylifosafamide. Ifosfamide and its metabolites may cause dose limiting central neurotoxicity and at high dose ifosfamide therapy may even produce coma and death [37]. Therefore monitoring ifosfamide and its metabolites in plasma for dosage adjustment may reduce toxicity of this drug.

Kerbusch et al. described a protocol for simultaneous determination of ifosfamide and its 2 and 3-dechloroethylifosafamide in human plasma using GC combined with either mass spectrometer or nitrogen–phosphorus detector. The authors used trofosfamide as the internal standard. The drug, its metabolites and the internal standard were extracted using ethyl acetate and analyzed by either GC coupled with nitrogen–phosphorus detector (NPD) or ion trap mass spectrometer. The authors concluded that GC coupled with NPD was capable of analysis of ifosfamide along with its metabolites without derivatization [38]. Granville et al. determined enantiomers of ifosfamide and its metabolites in human plasma, urine and animal plasma using chiral column in a GC followed by mass spectrometric determination with selected ion monitoring. Enantiomers of ifosfamide and its two metabolites were extracted using chloroform and analyzed by GC using a chiral stationary phase heptakis (2,6-di-O-methyl-3-O-pentyl)-beta-cyclodextrin. The method can detect enantiomers concentrations as low as 250 ng/mL in plasma and urine [39].

The concentrations of ifosfamide and its metabolites in human plasma can also be determined by HPLC combined with mass spectrometry. Oliveira et al. described enantioselective analysis of ifosfamide and its two dechloroethylated metabolites from human plasma after solid phase extraction followed by analysis using a chiral column (Chirabiotic T chiral stationary phase). The mobile phase composition was 2-propanol/methanol (60:40 by by vol) and the flow rate was 0.5 mL/min. The lower limit of detection was 5.0 ng/mL [40].

15.5 THERAPEUTIC DRUG MONITORING (TDM) OF ANTIMETABOLITES

Antimetabolites interfere with DNA and RNA growth because they can interfere with S-phase of cell cycle and are widely used in cancer chemotherapy. All of these antineoplastic agents inhibit one or more critical steps of synthesis of DNA. Antimetabolites can be folic acid antagonist, purine antagonist, pyrimidine antagonist or can be antibiotics such as doxorubicin and bleomycin. Several drugs in this category require routine TDM.

15.5.1 THERAPEUTIC DRUG MONITORING (TDM) OF METHOTREXATE

Methotrexate is a competitive inhibitor of dihydrofolate reductase, a key enzyme for biosynthesis of nucleic acid. The cytotoxic activity of this drug was discovered in 1955. The use of leucovorin to rescue normal host cells has permitted the higher doses of methotrexate therapy in clinical practice. Methotrexate is used in the treatment of acute lymphoblastic leukemia (ALL), osteogenic sarcoma, brain tumors, and carcinomas of the lung. Most of the toxicities of this drug are related to serum concentrations of methotrexate as well as other pharmacokinetic parameters. Methotrexate is also approved for the treatment of refractory rheumatoid arthritis. Usually low doses of methotrexate are used for treating rheumatoid arthritis (5–25 mg once weekly). One study found that splitting a weekly dose of 25–35 mg of methotrexate into spilt doses separated by eight hours improved the bioavailability of the drug [41]. Although toxicity from low dose treatment is rare, toxic manifestation with low dose methotrexate has been reported. Izzedine et al. commented that permanent discontinuation of methotrexate therapy in one out of ten patients occurs due to toxicity. Moreover nephrotoxicity, which is common with high doses of methotrexate, may also occur with low doses of therapy in patients receiving methotrexate [42]. A frequent adverse reaction seen is myelosuppression which manifests as leucopenia and thrombocytopenia. TDM is strongly recommended during high dose treatment of methotrexate and may also be useful for certain patient populations with low dose methotrexate therapy.

The elimination half-life of methotrexate is 7–11 hours and on administration less than 10% is oxidized to 7-hydroxymethotrexate irrespective of the route of administration. The protein binding ranges varies from 30 to 70% and albumin is the major binding protein in the serum [43]. Peak serum concentration of methotrexate correlates with the outcome in the treatment of osteosarcoma. Modification of the dosage to achieve a peak serum concentration between 700 and 1000 μmol/L has been recommended [44]. Omeprazole may delay elimination of methotrexate and therefore when prescribing methotrexate to a patient, an alternative to omeprazole should be used [45]. One case study reported that amoxicillin decreased the renal clearance of methotrexate probably by competition at common tubular secretion system and by secondary methotrexate induced renal impairment [46].

Methotrexate is a widely monitored drug in many hospital laboratories because immunoassays are commercially available and analysis can be automated using automated analyzers. Moreover, TDM of methotrexate is also crucial in patient management. However, immunoassays suffer from cross-reactivity due to the presence of methotrexate metabolites as well as various endogenous compounds. In one report, authors compared concentrations of methotrexate determined in human plasma using HPLC and immunoassays and observed that all immunoassay procedures were subjected to interferences from metabolites and the main metabolite 7-hydroxymethotrexate interfered more with polyclonal fluorescence polarization immunoassay (FPIA: Abbott Laboratories, Abbott Park, IL) than monoclonal FPIA assay [47]. Fotoohi et al. determined accuracy of enzyme-multiplied immunoassay (EMIT) and FPIA (monoclonal antibody) for determination of methotrexate in human plasma (420 specimens analyzed) after high dose therapy in children with ALL by comparing values obtained by these immunoassay with concentrations determined by a specific HPLC method. The major metabolite of methotrexate; 7-hydroxymethotrexate can be detected in plasma in high concentrations for a long period of time after methotrexate infusion. The authors observed that 42 and 66 hours after infusion of methotrexate the plasma methotrexate was overestimated in 2 and 3% of specimens using FPIA and in 5% and 31% specimens using EMIT assay. The authors concluded that the presence of 7-hydroxymethotrexate exerted a highly significant interference with methotrexate measurement using EMIT assay [48]. Therefore, for more specific determination of serum or plasma methotrexate concentrations after high dose therapy in cancer patients, chromatographic techniques are preferred methods.

There are many published methods for determination of methotrexate along with its metabolites in human plasma and urine using HPLC. In one report the authors used solid phase extraction of methotrexate and its metabolite 7-hydroxymethotrexate from human serum and cerebrospinal fluid using solid phase (using C18 cartridge) extraction after deproteinization of the specimen. The HPLC analysis was carried out using reverse phase C-18 column and the elution of peaks were detected at 313 nm using UV detector [49]. Buice and Sidhu also reported HPLC analysis coupled with UV detection at 313 nm for determination of concentrations of methotrexate and 7-hydroxymethotrexate in serum after solid phase extraction. The mobile phase composition was acetate buffer (0.2 M, pH 5.5 with 0,03 M ethylenediamine tetraacetate), methanol, and acetonitrile (85.3:8.4:6.3 by vol) [50]. McCrudden and Tett developed a protocol where methotrexate along with its 7-hydroxymethotrexate metabolite was extracted from plasma using solid phase extraction. The authors used aminopterin as the internal standard. The chromatographic separation was achieved using a 15-cm poly (styrenedivinyl benzene) column and a mobile phase composition of 0.1 M phosphate buffer (pH 6.5), with 6% N,N-dimethylformamide and 0.2% of 30% hydrogen peroxide. Postcolumn, the eluent was irradiated with UV light producing a fluorescence photolytic degradation product of both methotrexate and its metabolite. The excitation and emission wavelengths for fluorescence detection were 350 nm and 435 nm, respectively [51]. In another report the authors used HPLC combined with field desorption mass spectrometry for quantitative determination of methotrexate and its metabolite using synthetic methotrexate-gamma-(2-hydrox)ethyl amide as the internal standard. HPLC analysis of methotrexate and its metabolites were carried out on a reverse phase C-18 column using a volatile ammonium bicarbonate/acetate containing mobile phase that suited well for mass spectrometric analysis of the compounds eluting from the column [52]. Steinborner and Henion described a semi-robotic liquid-liquid extraction using deep well 96-well plates for analysis of methotrexate and 7-hydroxymethotrexate using LC/MS. The extraction time for sample preparation was relatively short and one person was capable of preparing 384 samples using all 96-well plates in 90 min. The extracted specimen was analyzed within 1.2 min using a positive ion turbo-ionspray selected reaction monitoring liquid chromatography/mass spectrometric method (LC/MS) where 768 specimens can be analyzed within 22 h. The detection limit for methotrexate was 0.05 ng/mL while the detection limit for 7-hydroxymethotrexate was 0.1 ng/mL [53].

15.5.2 THERAPEUTIC DRUG MONITORING (TDM) OF 5-FLUOROURACIL

5-Fluorouracil is an antineoplastic antimetabolite discovered in the 1950s and 5-fluorouracil has been used to treat a vast array of neoplasms including carcinomas of the breast, colon, head and neck, pancreas, rectum, and stomach. 5-Fluorouracil is also used topically for the management of actinic or solar keratoses and superficial basal cell carcinomas. 5-Fluorouracil is a halogenated pyrimidine that interferes with DNA and RNA synthesis and processing. 5-Fluorouracil is a prodrug that is enzymatically converted to the active metabolite 5-fluorodeoxyuridine monophosphate. This active metabolite binds to thymidylate synthase preventing production of thymidine triphosphate thus causes thymidine triphosphate deficiency resulting in cytotoxicity. Several mechanisms of drug resistance have been reported. These include the loss of enzymes required to activate 5-fluorouracil, amplification of the target enzyme (thymidylate synthase), or production of altered thymidylate synthase that is unaffected by the drug. To minimize resistance and enhance drug efficacy, 5-fluorouracil is often used in combination with other chemotherapeutic agents such as cisplatin, leucovorin and methotrexate. The bioavailability of oral drug can vary significantly (0–80%) depending on saturable first pass effects. Because of this variability, 5-fluorouracil is typically administered intravenously. When administered by IV (intravenously), 5-fluorouracil is rapidly distributed yielding peak plasma concentrations ranging from 0.1 to 1 mM depending on the bolus dose. Continuous IV injection of 5-fluorouracil for 1–5 days results in steady state plasma concentrations of 0.5–0.8 μM. 5-Fluorouracil is metabolized in a variety of tissues, but is predominately processed by the liver. 5-Fluorouracil is inactivated by the enzyme dihydropyrimidine dehydrogenase (DPD). Approximately 8% of patients are DPD deficient, resulting in significantly increased drug sensitivity. In rare instances of complete deficiency, a typical dose can result in severe toxicity. DPD deficiencies can be detected using either enzyme assays or molecular techniques, or ratios of 5-fluorouracil to the degraded metabolite fluoro-β-alanine. Toxicity of 5-fluorouracil is typically delayed due to the lag time between treatment and the corresponding effect on cell division. Early symptoms of toxicity include nausea and anorexia followed by abdominal pain and diarrhea. In severe instances, mucosal ulcerations caused by 5-fluorouracil treatment can result in shock and death. The predominant toxic effect due to bolus injection of 5-fluorouracil is pancytopenia caused by the myelosuppressive effect of the drug. Common toxic manifestations include anemia, leukopenia, thrombocytopenia, as well as alopecia and nail loss. Additional toxic effects include skin alterations, such as hyperpigmentation or skin atrophy [54–56]. Therefore, TDM of 5-dluorouracil may be beneficial in patient management. Pharmacokinetic studies showed that clinical response as well as toxicity of 5-fluorouracil are related to area under the curve (AUC). Individual dosage adjustments based on pharmacokinetic monitoring lead to higher response rate of this drug as well as survival rates associated with tolerability. A limited sampling strategy using just two plasma concentrations can be used to predict AUC of 5-fluorouracil [57]. Santani et al. concluded based on a four-year study that therapeutic monitoring of 5-fluorouracil with dosage adjustment lead to an improved therapeutic index in patients with head and neck cancer [58].

Both GC and HPLC methods are reported in the literature for determination of 5-fluorouracil in human serum or plasma. Bates et al. analyzed 5-fluorouracil in human plasma using GC and negative ion chemical ionization mass spectrometry. The authors converted 5-fluorouracil to its N-ditrifluoromethylbenzyl derivative after extraction from human plasma followed by analysis using GC/MS. In the negative ionization mode, molecular ion (carrying a negative charge) was observed at m/z 355. The authors used [15N2]-5-fluorouracil as the internal standard which produced mass ion at m/z 357 and quantitation of 5-fluorouracil was achieved by comparison the ion ratio (m/z 355 and m/z 357) [59]. Anderson et al. reported a GC/MS method for simultaneous determination of alpha-fluoro-beta-alanine (FBA), the major end metabolite of 5-fluorouracil. The authors used 5-chlorouracil as the internal standard. After precipitation of protein in plasma specimen, derivatization was carried out using pentafluorobenzyl bromide followed by purification of sample with a C18 column. The ions measured for 5-fluorouracil, 5-chlorouracil and FBA were m/z 490, m/z 506 and m/z 390, respectively. Detection limits were < 1 ng/mL for 5-fluorouracil and < 5 ng/mL for FBA [60]. Recently, Kosovec et al. described a protocol for quantification of 5-fluorouracil in human plasma using liquid chromatography combined with electrospray ionization tandem mass spectrometry. The assay used an isotopically labeled 5-fluorouracil as the internal standard and ethyl acetate was used for extraction of the drug from human plasma. Hydrophilic interaction chromatographic separation was carried out using an amino column and an isocratic mobile phase composition of 0.1 % formic acid in acetonitrile/water (97:3 by vol) followed by a wash. Detection of peaks was achieved by electrospray, negative ionization tandem mass spectrometry in multiple reactions monitoring mode [61].

15.5.3 THERAPEUTIC DRUG MONITORING (TDM) OF THIOPURINE MEDICATIONS

The thiopurine drugs 6-marcaptopurine, 6-thioguanine, and azathioprine are used in treating several diseases including childhood ALL, Hodgkin disease, inflammatory bowl disease, severe rheumatoid arthritis and autoimmune disease. Azathioprine is also used as an immunosuppressant in transplant recipients along with other immunosuppressants to prevent host versus graft disease. Azathioprine is rapidly converted into 6-mercaptopurine. The cytotoxic effects of these drugs are mediated in part through their conversion to intercellular thioguanine nucleotides which are active inhibitors of a number of critical reactions involving nucleotide synthesis. This process is called "lethal synthesis." 6-mercaptopurine must first be metabolized to 6-thioinosine monophosphate which is then further metabolized to 6-thioguanisone monophosphate. However, 6-thioguanine can be converted directly into 6-thioguanisone monophosphate. Alternative metabolic path for these drugs is to get converted into thiouric acid by xanthine oxidase or S-methylation catalyzed by cytosolic enzyme thiopurine S-methyltransferase (TPMT). TPMT exhibits a wide interindividual variation due to genetic polymorphism. Lack of functional TPMT (one in 300 Caucasian populations) is associated with profound life threatening myelosuppression [62]. Both TPMT phenotypic activity and 6-thioguanine nucleotide (TGN) concentrations can be measured in red blood cells (erythrocytes). In the early 1980s Lennard et al showed that higher erythrocyte TGN concentrations were associated with development of neutropenia in children suffering from ALL and also in adults receiving azathioprine (a prodrug of 6-mercaptopurine) [63]. The erythrocyte TPMT activity correlated inversely with TGN concentration as expected and although patients with TPMT deficiency are at high risk of hematopoietic toxicity if treated with routine dose of 6-mercaptopurine or azathioprine, these patients can be safely treated with these drugs if dosages are reduced. Therefore, TDM of these drugs and phenotyping of TMPT are beneficial [64].

TPMT phenotype is measured in erythrocytes using either radioimmunoassay (RIA) or HPLC. The quantitation of 6-mercaptopurine and intercellular metabolites are measured using HPLC. An alternative to RIA, TPMT activity in erythrocytes can also be measured by incubating erythrocyte extract of TPMT with the substrate 6-mercaptopurine and then after 1 h incubation determining the concentration of 6-mercaptopurine using liquid chromatography couple with tandem mass spectrometry [65].

There are several reported HPLC methods for determination of 6-marcaptourin and its metabolites in erythrocytes as well as in blood. However, acid hydrolysis is needed to convert these nucleotides moiety to free base prior to analysis. Oliveira et al. described a protocol for rapid determination of the intra-erythrocyte concentrations of 6-mercaptopurine (6-MP), and its metabolite 6-thioguanine nucleotide (6-TGN) and 6-methyl mercaptopurine (Me6-MP) using reverse phase HPLC with a C-18 column and UV detection. Erythrocyte cells (in presence of dithiothreitol) were treated with 70% perchloric acid and after removing the precipitate, the supernatant was hydrolyzed at 100°C for 45 min. After cooling, the specimen was analyzed by HPLC and peaks were eluted with a mobile phase consisting of methanol-water (7.5:92.5 by vol) containing 100 mM triethylamine. The 6-thioguanine (6-TG), 6-MP and hydrolysis product of Me6-MP; 4-amino-5-(methylthio) carbonyl imidazole were monitored at 342, 322, and 303 nm using photo diode array UV detector [66].

In another report, the authors analyzed concentrations of Me-6-MP, 6-TGN and the two major metabolites of azathioprine in erythrocytes using HPLC. The authors hydrolyzed nucleotides using perchloric acid to liberate the free base but Me-6-MP was derivatized under this acidic hydrolysis condition by ring opening. The HPLC analysis was carried out using a C-18 reverse phase column and compounds were eluted with 0.02 mol/L dihydrogen phosphate buffer-methanol. Detection of eluting compound was achieved by UV detection (341 nm for 6-TG and 304 nm for derivatized Me-6-MP). Later the authors described LC/MS method for analysis of these compounds [67,68]. In Figure 15.4 chromatographic separation of 6-methylmercaptopurine (Me6-MP) and the derivative formed by treatment with perchloric acid is shown. The separation was achieved by using a C-18 reverse, gradient elution and detection of peaks by photodiode detector (291 nm wavelength). In Figure 15.5 UV spectrum of both Me-6-MP and derivatized Me-6-MP are shown justifying measuring both compounds at 292 nm because both demonstrate similar absorption peak. In Figure 15.6 mass spectrum of Me-6-MP is given (electron ionization mode) as described in Reference [68]. Erb et al. described a protocol for determination of concentration of the major metabolite of thioguanine and 6-mercaptopurine in capillary blood. The metabolite 6-methyl mercaptopurine (Me-6-MP) along with 6-TGN were extracted and hydrolyzed with perchloric acid to liberate free base while Me-6-MP was derivatized under such condition and transformed into 4-amino-5 -(methylthio) carbonyl imidazole. Chromatographic separation was carried out using an isocratic mobile phase. Because levels of erythrocytes in capillary blood (obtained from finger tip) was similar to those obtained in separated RBC, this analysis provides similar information obtained by analyzing levels of these metabolites in isolated erythrocytes [69].

15.5.4   TDM OF 1-β-D-ARABINOFURANOSYLCYTOSINE (CYTARABINE: CYTOSINE ARABINOSIDE; ARA-C)

Ara-C is a prodrug which is activated via cytidine kinase to pharmacologically active cytosine arabinose triphosphate which is then incorporated into DNA and inhibits cell cycle by inhibiting DNA

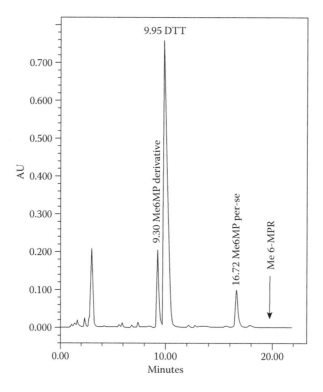

FIGURE 15.4   Chromatographic separation of Me6-MP and the Me6-MP derivative using reverse phase chromatography and photodiode array, detection at 291 nm. (From Dervieux T, Boulieu R, *Clin Chem*, 44, 2511–2515, 1998. Copyright © 1998 American Association for Clinical Chemistry, reprinted with permission.)

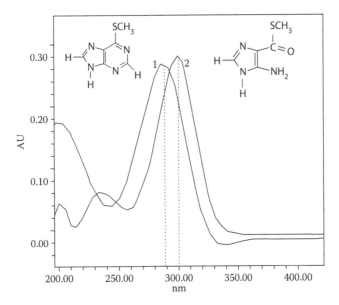

FIGURE 15.5 Ultraviolet spectra of Me6-MP (1) and the Me6-MP derivative (2). (From Dervieux T, Boulieu R, *Clin Chem*, 44, 2511–2515, 1998. Copyright © 1998 American Association for Clinical Chemistry, reprinted with permission.)

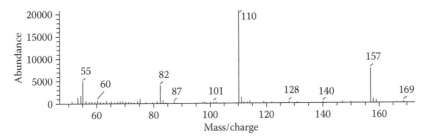

FIGURE 15.6 Mass spectrum of the Me6-MP derivative after electron ionization. (From Dervieux T, Boulieu R, *Clin Chem*, 44, 2511–2515, 1998. Copyright © 1998 American Association for Clinical Chemistry, reprinted with permission.)

polymerase. This drug is then inactivated by cytidine deaminase into uridine arabinoside (Ara-U). The plasma ratio of Ara-U/Ara-C has been used to analyze the phenotype for Ara-C deamination (ratio < 14 slow deamination while ratio > 14 fast deamination). In leukemic patients treated with a combination of Ara-C plus other conventional drugs, a tendency toward positive response (complete remission and partial response) was found for those showing low Ara-U/Ara-C ratio (slow deaminators) [70]. Concentrations of both Ara-U and Ara-C in human plasma can be determined by HPLC. Breithaupt and Schick used HPLC for determination of both Ara-U and Ara-C in human plasma and cerebrospinal fluid by isocratic reverse phase chromatography with phosphate buffer (0.05 M, pH 7.0) as the mobile phase. The limit of detection was 50 ng/mL [71]. In another report, the authors determined concentrations of Ara-U and Ara-C in human plasma using C-18 reverse phase column and ammonium acetate (0.5 mol/L, pH 6.5) as the mobile phase. The authors used tetrahydrouridine as the internal standard. The elution of peaks was monitored at 280 nm [72]. In Figure 15.7 HPLC chromatogram of Ara-C serum standards are shown as described by Wemelling et al. [72].

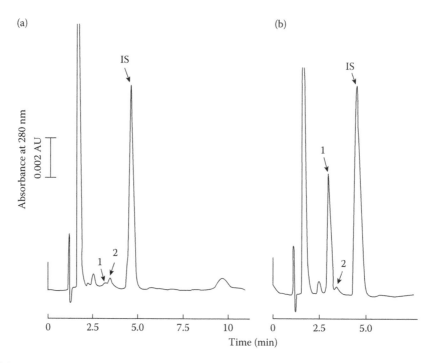

FIGURE 15.7   HPLC chromatogram of Ara-C serum standards. ARC-C serum concentration in (a) is 0 mg/L and in (b) 20 mg/L. Peak 1 represents ARA-C, peak 2 unknown endogenous compound and IS is the peak for Internal standard. (From Wermeling JR, Pruemer JM, Hassan FM, Warner A, *Clin Chem,* 35, 1011–1015, 1989. Copyright © 1989 American Association for Clinical Chemistry, reprinted with permission.)

In Figure 15.8. HPLC chromatograms of serum from a 67-year-old man with leukemia receiving Ara-C are shown and Figure 15.9 HPLC chromatograms of serum from a 67-year-old woman with leukemia receiving Ara-C are shown. The patient experienced fatal toxicity to this treatment [72].

15.6   THERAPEUTIC DRUG MONITORING (TDM) OF ANTICANCER ANTIBIOTICS

Anthracycline antibiotics isolated from streptomycin are also anticancer and are used widely in clinical practice for treating various types of cancers including carcinomas, sarcomas, and hematological malignancies. The first anthracycline antibiotics are daunorubicin and doxorubicin. Doxorubicin and epirubicin (4-epimer of doxorubicin) are highly potent agents to treat solid tumors including breast tumors. Idarubicin and daunorubicin are also used in treating acute leukemia. Valrubicin is used in treating patients with bladder cancer. Anthracyclines act by inhibiting DNA and RNA synthesis by intercalating between base pairs thus blocking replication of rapidly growing cancer cells and also inhibit topoisomerase II enzyme thus further preventing transcription and replication of DNA. In addition, these drugs also alter membrane fluidity and ion transport and may also generate oxygen free radicals. Cardiotoxicity is a serious problem of therapy with anthracyclines which may range from benign arrhythmia to potentially fatal myocardial ischemia or heart failure. However, not only anthracyclines but also other anticancer drugs such as mitomycin, monoclonal antibodies such as trastuzumab, 5-fluorouracil, cyclophosphamide, interferons and interleukin-2, all can produce cardiac toxicity [73]. Other anticancer antibiotics such as mitomycin, bleomycin, dactinomycin and plicamycin also have widespread use in cancer therapy.

A substantial pharmacokinetic/pharmacodynamic relationship with respect to bone marrow toxicity and therapeutic efficacy has been demonstrated. Moreover, there are significant interindividual variations in

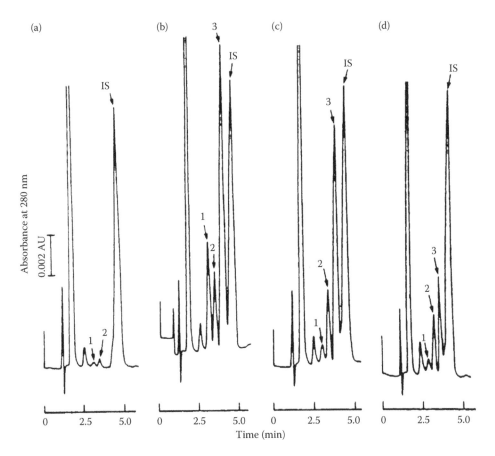

FIGURE 15.8 HPLC chromatograms of serum from a 67-year-old man with leukemia receiving-C, 2gm/m², infused over one hour every 12 hours. Peak 1 represents ARA-C, peak 2 unknown endogenous compound, peak 3; Aar-U (metabolite of Ara-C) and IS is the peak for internal standard. (a) Predose blank containing only internal standard, (b) end of infusion sample, (c) 2 hour postinfusion, and (d) trough specimen. (From Wermeling JR, Pruemer JM, Hassan FM, Warner A, *Clin Chem*, 35, 1011–1015, 1989. Copyright © 1989 American Association for Clinical Chemistry, reprinted with permission.)

pharmacokinetics of anthracyclines, making these drugs good candidates for TDM for treatment optimization [74]. Fogil et al. reported a HPLC method with fluorescence detection for TDM of daunorubicin, idarubicin, doxorubicin and epirubicin and their 13 dihydro metabolites in human plasma after first extracting with chloroform/1-heptanol (9:L1 by vol) and then re-extraction with orthophosphoric acid 0.1 M. The chromatographic analysis was carried out with a Supleco cyano column (LC-CN column; 25 cm × 4.6 mm internal diameter) and detection was achieved spectrofluorometry at excitation wavelength of 480 nm and emission wavelength of 560 nm. This protocol allows analysis of all anthracyclines in clinical practice along with their metabolites in single run thereby simplifying their monitoring in chemotherapeutic regimens of cancer patients [74]. In another report, the authors determined concentrations of doxorubicin, daunorubicin, epirubicin and idarubicin and their respective active metabolites in human serum by liquid chromatography combined with electrospray mass spectrometry. They used aclarubicin as the internal standard. After solid phase extraction of these drugs and metabolites from human serum using C-18 Bond Elut cartridges (Varian Corporation) using Zymark Rapid-Trace robot (compounds were eluted from solid phase extraction column using chloroform/2-propanol; 4:1 by vol), drugs and their metabolites were analyzed (after evaporation organic phase and reconstituting dry residue in a mixture of 5 mM ammonium formate buffer (pH 4.5)/acetonitrile

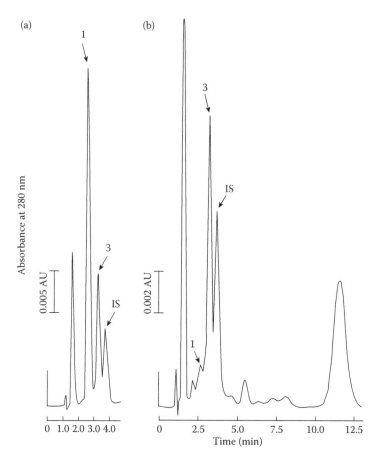

FIGURE 15.9   HPLC chromatograms of serum from a 67-year-old woman with leukemia receiving Ara-C, 1.25 gm/m2, infused over one hour every 12 hours. Peak 1 represents Ara-C, peak 2 unknown endogenous compound, peak 3 Aar-U (metabolite of Ara-C) and IS is the peak for internal standard. (a) End of infusion sample, and (b) trough specimen. The patient experienced fatal toxicity from the treatment. (From Wermeling JR, Pruemer JM, Hassan FM, Warner A, *Clin Chem*, 35, 1011–1015, 1989. Copyright © 1989 American Association for Clinical Chemistry, reprinted with permission.)

(60:40 by vol)), by a reverse phase C-18 column. The mobile phase composition was 5 mM ammonium formate (pH: 3)/acetonitrile (70:30 by vol). The eluting compounds were detected in selected ion monitoring mode, using as quantitation ions, m/z 291 for idarubicin and idarubicinol (metabolite), m/z 321 for daunorubicin and daunorubicinol (metabolite), m/z 361 for epirubicin and doxorubicin, m/z 363 for doxorubicinol and m/z 812 for aclarubicin (internal standard). The limit of quantitation was 2.5 ng/mL for doxorubicin, epirubicin and daunorubicinol and 5 ng/mL for daunorubicin, idarubicin, doxorubicinol and idarubicinol [75].

15.7   THERAPEUTIC DRUG MONITORING (TDM) OF TOPOISOMERASE INHIBITORS

Irinotecan (CPT-11) is a semisynthetic derivative of natural product camptothecin which exerts its anticancer effect by inhibiting DNA topoisomerase, thus causing cell death. CPR-11 is extensively metabolized in the liver by carboxylesterase to form 7-ethyl-10-hydroxycamptothecin (SN-38) and its cytotoxic activity is 100–1000 times greater than the parent drug [76]. Eventually SN-38 is conjugated with glucuronic acid (SN-38G). There are also other known metabolites of CPT-11. Poujol et al. described a HPLC method coupled with fluorescence detection for determination of CPT-11, SN-38, SN-38G and two other metabolites in human plasma and saliva using C-18 reverse phase column. The authors used camptothecin as the internal standard [77].

15.8   THERAPEUTIC DRUG MONITORING (TDM) OF MITOTIC INHIBITOR

Anticancer drugs that are mitotic inhibitors (paclitaxel, vincristine, vinblastine, etc.), are derived from plants (plant alkaloids) that exert their anticancer activities by inhibiting mitosis in cancer cells leading to apoptosis through inhibition of the depolymerization of microtubules [78]. The TDM of taxanes (paclitaxel and docetaxel) is useful because paclitaxel induced toxicity is dose dependent. In addition, the CYP2C8 enzyme is responsible for metabolism of paclitaxel to its metabolite which has 30 fold lesser activity than the parent compound. Polymorphism of CYP2C8 affects metabolism of paclitaxel [79].

Anderson et al. described HPLC assay with UV detection for determination of concentrations of paclitaxel and docetaxel in human plasma. The author extracted these drugs from plasma by solid phase extraction and analyzed them by reverse phase chromatography with UV detection at 227 nm (limit of quantitation was 1.2 nM for paclitaxel and 1.0 nM for docetaxel) [80]. Praise et al. used liquid chromatography combined with mass spectrometry for quantitation of docetaxel and paclitaxel in human plasma after solid phase extraction and analysis by reverse phase C-18 analytical column. The mobile phase composition was 0.1% formic acid in methanol/water (70:30 by vol). The lower limit of quantitation was 0.3 nM. The mass spectrometer (electrospray) was operated in positive single ion mode detection m/z 808.1 for docetaxel and m/z 854.0 for paclitaxel [81].

15.9   THERAPEUTIC DRUG MONITORING (TDM) OF HORMONE MODULATOR

The treatment of breast cancer with selective estrogen receptor modulators such as tamoxifen and with aromatase inhibitors is useful. Tamoxifen acts by binding to estrogen receptors in breast cancer cells thus blocking estrogen from reaching cancer cells causing prevention of cell growth. Aromatase inhibitors block estrogen production by binding to the enzyme responsible for estrogen production. TDM is crucial due to genetic polymorphism of CYP2D6, responsible for metabolic activation of tamoxifen.

15.9.1   THERAPEUTIC DRUG MONITORING (TDM) OF TAMOXIFEN

Tamoxifen requires metabolic activation to 4-hydroxytamoxifen and endoxifen (N-desmethyl-4-hydroxytamoxufen) by liver cytochrome P-450 enzymes especially CYP2D6. Because CYP2D6 is genetically polymorphic and 5–8% of Caucasian population are poor metabolizers (relatively poor activity of CYP2D6), these subjects are relatively unable to convert tamoxifen to its active metabolites and appear to have poor outcome compared to subjects who are extensive metabolizers (high enzyme activity). In 2006 the United States Food and Drug Administration (FDA) held a public hearing on the inclusion of this pharmacogenomics information in tamoxifen labeling [82]. The active metabolites of tamoxifen are then conjugated by sulfotransferase (SULT)1A1. Both CYP2D6 and SULT1A1 genotype may partly explain wide interindividual variations in serum levels of tamoxifen and its metabolites and TDM should be helpful to determine clinical outcome of therapy [83].

Zhu et al. described a HPLC protocol with fluorescence determination for quantification of tamoxifen and its two metabolites in human plasma using a reverse phase C-18 column which was set at 65°C and a mobile phase of methanol/1%-triethylamine aqueous solution (82:18 by vol, pH; 11). The detection system utilized off-line UV irradiation to convert analytes to their respective photo-cyclization products followed by fluorescence detection (excitation; 260 nm, emission; 375 nm).

Mexiletine was used as the internal standard [84]. In another report, the authors after protein precipitation in serum containing tamoxifen and four of its metabolites added deuterated tamoxifen (D5-tamoxifen; internal standard) and analyzed the supernatant using C-18 analytical column. Analytes were detected by tandem mass spectrometry [85].

15.10 THERAPEUTIC DRUG MONITORING (TDM) OF MISCELLANEOUS ANTINEOPLASTIC AND NONANTICANCER DRUGS

The platinum derivative cisplatin and carboplatin (both DNA alkylating agents) have been used in the treatment of various types of cancer including testicular cancer. In most studies determining pharmacokinetic parameters of cisplatin, free fractions were measured in plasma or tumor. There is a high variability between individual patients and the therapeutic window is narrow. Dosage is often based on body surface area. Salas et al described TDM of cisplatin using total platinum measurement in plasma [86]. Gietema et al. reported that platinum was detectable in plasma in patients twenty years after being cured from metastatic testicular cancer following cisplatin therapy [87]. Impaired bioavailability of phenytoin in a 24-year-old woman treated with cisplatin, vinblastine and bleomycin has been reported. Data revealed mean phenytoin absorption of 32% (normal greater than 80%) establishing malabsorption of phenytoin due to cancer chemotherapy [88]. TDM of carboplatin using atomic absorption spectrometry is also useful [89].

There are other anticancer drugs which may be candidates for TDM. In addition, there are many reported methods in the literature where more than one class of drugs can be determined in a single chromatographic method. For example, recently Sottani et al. described a method for simultaneous determination of cyclophosphamide, ifosfamide, doxorubicin, epirubicin and daunorubicin in human urine using HPLC coupled with electrospray ionization tandem mass spectrometry [90]. In addition, bone marrow transplant recipients and transplant recipients with cancer require monitoring of immunosuppressants. Cancer patients may also suffer from other chronic conditions where routine monitoring of anticonvulsants, cardioactive drugs or other classed of drugs may also be necessary.

15.11 CONCLUSIONS

Despite use of many anticancer drugs, relatively few drugs are routinely monitored in clinical laboratories. Methotrexate is the most frequently monitored anticancer drug. One difficulty of therapeutic monitoring of anticancer drugs is the lack of commercially available immunoassays and chromatographic techniques especially HPLC combined with mass spectrometry require big capital budget expenditure and specially trained personnel for operations. Nevertheless, more and more anticancer drugs are being monitored today because of better clinical outcome and more drugs will be added in this list in the near future.

REFERENCES

1. Website of American Cancer Society (http://www.cancer.org accessed November 1, 2008).
2. Alnaim L. 2007. Therapeutic drug monitoring of cancer chemotherapy. *J Oncol Pharm Practice* 13: 207–221.
3. Balis FM, Holcenberg JS, Bleyer WA. 1983. Clinical pharmacokinetics of commonly used anticancer drugs. *Clin Pharmacokinet* 8: 202–232.
4. Slattery JT, Sanders JE, Buckner CD, Schaffer RL et al. 1995. Graft-rejection and toxicity following bone marrow transplantation in relation to busulfan pharmacokinetics. *Bone Marrow Trans* 16: 31–42.
5. Newell DR, Pearson ADJ, Balmanno K, Price L et al. 1993. Carboplatin pharmacokinetics in children: the development of a pediatric dosing formula. *J Clin Oncol* 11: 2314–2323.
6. Chatelut E, Boddy AV, Peng B, Rubie H et al. 1996. Population pharmacokinetics of carboplatin in children. *Clin Pharmacol Ther* 59: 436–443.

7. Minami H, Shimokata K, Saka H, Satio H et al. 1993. Phase I clinical trial and pharmacokinetic study of a14 day infusion of etoposide in patients with lung cancer. *J Clin Oncol* 11: 1602–1608.
8. Cheng KK. 2008. Association of plasma methotrexate, neutropenia, hepatic dysfunction, nausea/vomiting and oral mucositis in children with cancer. *Eur J Cancer Care (Engl)* 17: 306–311.
9. Sanrini J, Milano G, Thyss A, Renee N et al. 1989. 5-FU therapeutic monitoring with dose adjustment leads to an improved therapeutic index in head and neck cancer. *Br J Cancer* 59: 287–190.
10. Hon YY, Evans WE. 1998. Making TDM work to optimize cancer chemotherapy: a multidisciplinary team approach. *Clin Chem* 44: 388–400.
11. Moore AJ, Erlichman C. 1987. Therapeutic drug monitoring in oncology. Problems and potential in antineoplastic therapy. *Clin Pharmacokinet* 13: 205–227.
12. Baselt RC. 2004. *Busulfan in Disposition of Toxic Drugs and Chemicals in Man*, 7th ed. Biomedical Publications, Foster City, CA, 142–143.
13. Tran HT, Maffen T, Petropoulos D, Worth LL et al. 2000. Individualized high dose oral busulfan: prospective dose adjustment in a pediatric population undergoing allogenic stem cell transplantation for advanced hematologic malignancies. *Bone Marrow Transplant* 26: 463–470.
14. Russell JA, Kangarloo SB. 2008. Therapeutic drug monitoring of busulfan in transplantation. *Curr Pharm Des* 14: 1936–1949.
15. Chandy M, Balasubramanian P, Ramachandran SV, Mathews V, et al. 2005. Randomized trial of two different condition regimens for bone marrow transplantation in thalassemia—the role of busulfan pharmacokinetics in determining outcome. *Bone Marrow Transplant* 36: 839–45.
16. Lindley C, Shea T, McCune J, Shord S, et al. 2004. Intraindividual variability in busulfan pharmacokinetics in patients undergoing a bone marrow transplant: assessment of a test dose and first dose strategy. *Anticancer Drugs* 15: 453–459.
17. Pichini S, Altieri I, Bacosi A, Di Carlo S, 1992. High-performance liquid chromatographic-mass spectrometric assay of busulfan in serum and cerebrospinal fluid. *J Chromatogr* 581: 143–146.
18. Rauh M, Stachel D, Kuhlen M, Groschl M, et al. 2006. Quantification of busulfan in saliva and plasma in hematopoietic stem cell transplantation in children: validation of liquid chromatography tandem mass spectrometry method. *Clin Pharmacokinet* 45: 305–316.
19. Kellogg MD, Law T, Sakamoto M, Rifai N. 2005. Tandem mass spectrometry method for the quantification of serum busulfan. *Ther Drug Monit* 27: 625–629.
20. Abdel-Rehim M, Hassan Z, Blomberg L, Hassan M. 2003. On-line derivatization utilizing solid-phase microextraction (SPME) for determination of busulphan in plasma using gas chromatography-mass spectrometry (GC-MS). *Ther Drug Monit* 25: 400–406.
21. Balasubramanian P, Srivastava A, Chandy M. 2001. Stability of busulfan in frozen plasma and whole blood samples. *Clin Chem* 47: 766–768.
22. Ehrsson H, Hassan M. 1983. Determination of busulfan in plasma by GC-MS with selected ion monitoring. *J Pharm Sci* 72: 1203–1205.
23. Lai WK, Pang CP, Law LK, Wong R et al. 1998. Routine analysis of plasma busulfan by gas chromatography-mass fragmentography. *Clin Chem* 44: 2506–2510.
24. Quernin MH, Poonkuzhali, Medard Y, Dennison D et al. 1999. High performance liquid chromatographic method for quantification of busulfan in plasma after derivatization by tetrafluorothiophenol. *J Chromatogr B Biomed Sci Appl* 721: 147–152.
25. Pichini S, Altieri I, Bacosi A, Di Carlo S et al. 1992. High-performance liquid chromatographic-mass spectrometric assay of busulfan in serum and cerebrospinal fluid. *J Chromatogr* 581: 143–146.
26. Breitbach GP, Meden H, Schmid H, Kuhn W et al. 2002. Treosulfan in the treatment of advanced ovarian cancer: a randomized co-operative multicenter phase III study. *Anticancer Res* 22: 2923–2932.
27. Munkelt D, Koehl U, Kloess S, Zimmermann SY et al. 2008. Cytotoxic effects of treosulfan and busulfan against leukemia cells of pediatric patients. *Cancer Chemother Pharmacol* 62: 821–830.
28. Glowka FK, Lada MK, Grund G, Wachowiak J.2007. Determination of treosulfan in plasma by HPLC with refractometric detection: pharmacokinetic studies in children undergoing myeloablative treatment prior to hematopoietic stem cell transplantation. *J Chromatogr B Analyt Technol Biomed Life Sci* 850: 569–574.
29. Huang Z, Roy P, Waxman DJ. 2000. Role of human liver microsomal CYP3A4 and CYP2B6 in catalyzing N-dechloroethylation of cyclophosphamide and ifosfamide. *Biochem Pharmacol* 59: 961–972.
30. van Schail RH. 2008. CYP450 pharmacogenomics for personalized cancer therapy. *Drug Resist Updat* 11: 77–98.

31. Bohnenstengel F, Eichelbaum M, Golbs E et al. 1997. High performance liquid chromatographic deter-mination of acrolein, as a marker for cyclophosphamide bioactivation in human liver microsome. *J Chromatogr B; Biomed Sci Appl* 692: 163–168.

32. Sessink PJ, Scholtes MM, Anzion RB, Bos RP. 1993. Determination of cyclophosphamide in urine by gas chromatography-mass spectrometry. *J Chromatogr* 616: 333–337.

33. Sannolo N, Miraglia N, Biglietto M, Acampora A et al. 1999. Determination of cyclophosphamide and ifosfamide in urine at trace level by gas chromatography/tandem mass spectrometry. *J Mass Spectrom* 34: 845–849.

34. Bauman F, Lorenz C, Jaehde U, Preiss R. 1999. Determination of cyclophosphamide and its metabo-lites in human plasma by high performance liquid chromatography-mass spectrometry. *J Chromatogr B Biomed Sci Appl* 729: 297–305.

35. Griskevicius L, Meurling L, Hassan M 2002. Simple method for determination on fluorescent detection for the determination of 4-hydroxycyclophosphamide in plasma. *Ther Drug Monit* 24: 405–409.

36. Huitema AED, Tibben MM, Kerbusch T, Kattenes-vad der Bosch JJ et al. 2000. Simple and selective determination of the cyclophosphamide metabolite phosphoramide mustard in human plasma using high performance liquid chromatography. *J Chromatogr B Biomed Sci Appl* 745: 345–355.

37. Cerny T, Kupfer A. 1992. The enigma of ifosfamide encephalopathy. *Ann Oncology* 3: 679–681.

38. Kerbusch T, Jeuken MJ, Derraz J, van Putten JW et al. 2000. Determination of ifosfamide, 2 and 3-dechlo-roethylifosafamide using gas chromatography with nitrogen-phosphorus or mass spectrometry detection. *Ther Drug Monit* 22: 613–620.

39. Granville CP, Gehrcke B, Konig WA, Wainer IW. 1993. Determination of enantiomers of ifosfamide and its 2 and 3 –N-dechloroethylated metabolites in plasma and urine using enantioselective gas chromatog-raphy with mass spectrometric detection. *J Chromatogr* 622: 21–31.

40. Oliveira RV, Onorato JM, Siluk D, Waljo CM. 2007. Enantioselective liquid chromatography-mass spec-trometry assay for the determination of ifosfamide and identification of the N-dechloroethylated metabo-lites of ifosfamide in human plasma. *J Pharm Biomed Appl* 45: 295–303.

41. Hoekstra M, Haagsma C, Neef C, Proost J et al. 2006. Splitting high dose oral methotrexate improves bioavailability: a pharmacokinetic study with rheumatoid arthritis. *J Rheumatol* 33: 481–485.

42. Izzedine H, Launay-Vacher V, Karie S, Caramella C et al. 2005. Is low dose methotrexate nephrotoxic? Case report and review of literature. *Clin Nephrol* 64: 315–319.

43. Endo L, Bressolle F, Gomeni R, Bologna C et al. 1996. Total and free methotrexate pharmacokinetics in rheumatoid arthritis patients. *Ther Drug Monit* 18: 128–134.

44. Zelcer S, Kellick M, Wexler LH, Shi w et al. 2002. Methotrexate levels and outcome in osteosarcoma. *Pediatr Blood Cancer* 44: 638–642.

45. Beorlegui B, Aldaz A, Ortega A, Aquerreta I et al. Potential interaction between methotrexate and omeprazole. Ann Pharmacother 2002; 34: 1024–1027.

46. Ronchera CL, Hernandez T, Peris JE, Torres F et al. 1993. Pharmacokinetic interaction between high dose methotrexate and amoxicillin. *Ther Drug Monit* 15: 375–379.

47. Albertioni F, Rask C, Eksborg S, Poulsen JH et al. 1996. Evaluation of clinical assays for measuring high-dose methotrexate in plasma. *Clin Chem* 42: 39–44.

48. Fotoohi K, Skarby T, Peterson C, Albertioni G. 2005. Interference of 7-hydroxymethotrexate with the determination of methotrexate in plasma from children with acute lymphoblastic leukemia employing routine clinical assay. *J Chromatogr B Analyt Technol Biomed Life Sci* 817: 139–144.

49. So N, Chandra DP, Alexander IS, Webster VJ et al. 1985. Determination of serum methotrexate and 7-hydroxymethotrexate concentrations. Method evaluation showing advantage of high performance liq-uid chromatography. *J Chromatogr* 337: 81–90.

50. Buice RG, Sindhu P. 1982. Reverse phase high pressure liquid chromatographic determination of serum methotrexate and 7-hydroxymethotrexate. *J Pharm Sci* 71: 74–77.

51. McCrudden EA, Tett SE. 1999. Improved high performance liquid chromatography determination of methotrexate and its major metabolite in plasma using a poly(styrene-divinyl benzene) column. *J Chromatogr B Biomed Sci Appl* 721: 87–92.

52. Przybylski M, Preiss J, Dennebaum R, Fischer J. 1982. Identification of methotrexate and methotrexate metabolites in clinical high dose therapy by high pressure liquid chromatography and field desorption mass spectrometry. *Biomed Mass Spectrom* 9: 22–32.

53. Steinborner S, Henion J. 1999. Liquid-liquid extraction in the 96 well plate formats with SRM LC/MS quantitative determination of methotrexate and its major metabolite in human plasma. *Anal Chem* 71: 2340–2345.

54. Diasio RB, Harris BE. 1989. Clinical pharmacology of 5-fluorouracil. *Clin Pharmacokinet* 16(4): 215–237. Review.

55. Joulia JM, Pinguet F, Grosse PY, Astre C, Bressolle F. 1997. Determination of 5-fluorouracil and its main metabolites in plasma by high-performance liquid chromatography: application to a pharmacokinetic study. *J Chromatogr B Biomed Sci Appl* 692(2): 427–435.

56. Hardman JG, Limbird LE, Gilman AG. 2001. *Goodman & Gilman's The Pharmacological Basis of Therapeutics*, 10th ed. New York, McGraw-Hill.

57. Gusella M, Ferrazzi E, Ferrari M, Padrini R. 2002. New limited sampling strategy for determination of 5-fluorouracil area under the concentration curve-time curve after rapid intravenous bolus. *Ther Drug Monit* 24:425–431.

58. Santani J, Milano G, Thyss A, Renee N et al. 1989. 5-FU monitoring with dose adjustment lead to an improved therapeutic index in head and neck cancer. *Br J Cancer* 59: 287–290.

59. Bates CD, Watson DG, Willmott N, Logan H et al. 1991. The analysis of 5-Fluorouracil in human plasma by gas chromatography-negative ion chemical ionization mass spectrometry (GC-NICIMS) with stable isotope dilution. *J Pharm Biomed Anal* 9: 19–21.

60. Anderson D, Kerr DJ, Blesing C, Seymour LW. 1997. Simultaneous gas chromatographic-mass spectrometric determination of alpha-fluoro-beta alanine and 5-Fluorouracil in plasma. *J Chromatogr B Biomed Sci Appl* 688: 87–93.

61. Kosovec JE, Egorin MJ, Gjurich S, Beumer JH. 2008. Quantitation of 5-Fluorouracil in human plasma by liquid chromatography/electrospray ionization tandem mass spectrometry. *Rapid Commun Mass Spectrom* 22: 224–230.

62. Lennard L, Lilleyman JS, Van Loon JA, Weinshilboum RM. 1990. Genetic variation in response to 6-mercaptopurine for childhood acute lymphoblastic leukemia. *Lancet* 336: 225–229.

63. Lenard K, Keen D, Lilleyman JS. 1986. Oral 6-mercaptopurine in childhood leukemia: parent drug pharmacokinetics and active metabolite concentrations. *Clin Pharmacol* 40: 287–292.

64. Evans WE, Horner M, Chu YQ, Kalwinsky D et al. 1991. Altered mercaptopurine metabolism, toxic effects and dosage requirement in thiopurine methyltransferase deficient child with acute lymphoblastic leukemia. *J Pediatr* 119: 985–989.

65. Kalsi K, Marinaki AM, Yacoub MH, Smolenski RT. 2006. HPLC/tandem ion trap mass detector methods for determination of inosine monophosphate dehydrogenase(IMPDH) and thiopurine methyltransferase (TPMT). *Nucleosides Nucelotides Nucleic Acids* 25: 1241–1244.

66. Oliverira BM, Romanha AJ, Alves TM, Viana MB et al. 2004. An improved HPLC method for the quantitation of 6-mercaptopurine and its metabolites in red blood cells. *Braz J Med Biol Res* 37: 649–658.

67. Dervieux T, Boulieu R. 1998. Simultaneous determination of 6-thioguanine and methyl 6-mercaptopurine nucleotides of azathioprine in red blood cells by HPLC. *Clin Chem* 44: 551–555.

68. Dervieux T, Boulieu R. 1998. Identification of 6-metcaptopurine derivative formed during acid hydrolysis of thiopurine nucleotides in erythrocytes, using liquid chromatography-mass spectrometry, infrared spectroscopy and nuclear magnetic resonance assay. *Clin Chem* 44: 2511–2515.

69. Erb N, Haverland U, Harms DO, Escherich G et al. 2003. High performance liquid chromatographic assay of metabolites of thioguanine and mercaptopurine in capillary blood. *J Chromatogr B Analyt Technol Biomed Life Sci* 796: 87–94.

70. Kries W, Lesser M, Budman DR, Arkin Z et al. 1992. Phenotypic analysis of 1-β-D-arabinofuranosylcytosine deamination in patients treated with high doses and correlation with response. *Cancer Chemother Pharmacol* 30: 126–130.

71. Breithaupt H, Schick J. 1981. Determination of cytarabine and uracil arabinoside in human plasma and cerebrospinal fluid by high-performance liquid chromatography. *J Chromatogr* 225: 99–106.

72. Wermeling JR, Pruemer JM, Hassan FM, Warner A. 1989. Liquid chromatographic monitoring of cytosine arabinoside and its metabolite, uracil arabinoside in serum. *Clin Chem* 35: 1011–1015.

73. Viale PH, Yamamoto DS. 2008. Cardiac toxicity associated with cancer treatment. *Clin J Oncol Nurs* 12: 627–638.

74. Fogli S, Danesi R, Innocenti F, Di Paolo A et al. 1999. An improved HPLC method for therapeutic drug monitoring of daunorubicin, idarubicin, doxorubicin, epirubicin and their 13 metabolites in human plasma. *Ther Drug Monit* 21: 365–375.

75. Lachatre F, Marquet P, Ragot S, Gaulier JM et al. 2000. Simultaneous determination of four anthracyclines and three metabolites in human serum by liquid chromatography-electrospray mass spectrometry. *J Chromatogr B Biomed Sci Appl* 738: 281–291.

76. Mathijssen RH, van Alphen RJ, Verweij J, Loos WJ et al. 2001. Clinical pharmacokinetics and metabolism of irinotecan (CPT-11). *Clin Cancer Res* 7: 2182–2194.

77. Poujol S, Pinguet F, Malosse F, Astre C et al. 2003. Sensitive HPLC-fluorescence method for irinotecan and four major metabolites in human plasma and saliva: application to pharmacokinetic studies. *Clin Chem* 49: 1900–1908.

78. Jordan MA. 2002. Mechanism of action of antitumor drugs that interact with microtubules and tubulin. *Curr Med Chem Anticancer Agents* 2: 1–17.

79. van Schaik RH. 2004. Implications of cytochrome P 450 genetic polymorphisms on the toxicity of anti-tumor agents. *Ther Drug Monit* 26: 236–240.

80. Anderson A, Warren DJ, Brunsvig PF, Asmdal S et al. 2006. High sensitivity assays for docetaxel and paclitaxel in plasma using solid phase extraction and high performance liquid chromatography with UV detection. *BMC Clin Pharmacol* January 13, 6: 2.

81. Praise RA, Ramanathan RK, Zamboni WC, Egorin MJ. 2003. Sensitive liquid chromatography-mass spectrometry assay for quantitation of docetaxel and paclitaxel in human plasma. *Chromatogr B Biomed Sci Appl* 783: 231–236.

82. Weinshilboum R. 2008. Pharmacogenomics of endocrine therapy in breast cancer. *Adv Exp Med Biol* 630: 220–231.

83. Gjerde J, Hauglid M, Breilid H, Lundgren S et al. 2008. Effects of CYP2D6 and SULT1A1 genotypes including SULT1A1 gene copy number on tamoxifen metabolism. *Ann Oncol* 19: 56–61.

84. Zhu YB, Zhang Q, Zou JJ, Yu CX et al. 2008. Optimizing high performance liquid chromatography method with fluorescence detection for quantification of tamoxifen and their two metabolites in human plasma: application to a clinical study. *J Pharm Biomed Appl* 46: 349–355.

85. Gjerde J, Kisanga ER, Hauglid M, Holm PI et al. 2005. Identification and quantification of tamoxifen and four metabolites in serum by liquid chromatography-tandem mass spectrometry. *J Chromatogr A* 1082: 6–14.

86. Salas S, Mercier C, Cicccolini J, Pourroy B et al. 2006. Therapeutic drug monitoring for dose individualization of cisplatin in testicular cancer patients based upon total platinum measurement. *Ther Drug Monit* 28: 532–539.

87. Gietema JA, Meinardi MT, Messerschmidt J, Gelevert T et al. 2000. Circulating plasma platinum more than 10 years after cisplatin treatment for testicular cancer. *Lancer* 355 (9209): 1075–1076.

88. Sylvester RK, Lewis FB, Caldwell KC, Lobell M et al. 1984. Impaired bioavailability secondary to cis-platinum, vinblastine, and bleomycin. *Ther Drug Monit* 6: 302–305.

89. Picton SV, Keeble J, Holden V, Errington J et al. 2008. Therapeutic drug monitoring of carboplatin dosing in a premature infant with retinoblastoma. *Cancer Chemother Pharmacol* July 8 [E-pub ahead of print].

90. Sottani C, Rinaldi O, Leoni E, Poggi G et al. 2008. Simultaneous determination of cyclophosphamide, ifosfamide, doxorubicin, epirubicin and daunorubicin in human urine by using high performance liquid chromatography/electrospray ionization tandem mass spectrometry: bioanalytical method validation. *Rapid Commun Mass Spectrom* 22: 2645–2659.

16 Therapeutic Drug Monitoring of Vancomycin and Aminoglycosides with Guidelines

Roger Dean
University of Washington Medical Center

Amitava Dasgupta
University of Texas Medical School

CONTENTS

16.1   INTRODUCTION

The worldwide development of bacterial resistance to beta-lactam antibiotics and the increasing incidence of methicillin-resistant *Staphylococcus aureus* (MRSA) infections in hospitalized and ambulatory patients have required the reassessment and use of older antibiotics. Although the aminoglycoside antibiotics and vancomycin have been available for over 50 years they remain important therapeutic agents in hospitalized patients. Even before much was understood about antibiotic pharmacokinetics and pharmacodynamics, investigators studied antibiotic serum concentrations with the purpose of optimizing efficacy and minimizing toxicity. Since introduction of the aminoglycosides and vancomycin much has been learned to change our practices of how to dose and monitor these antibiotics.

16.2 VANCOMYCIN: AN INTRODUCTION

Vancomycin is a glycopeptide antibiotic isolated from *Streptomyces orientalis*. It has only activity against gram-positive bacteria, including viridans streptococcus, Streptococcus species, methicillin-sensitive *Staphylococcus aureus*, methicillin-resistant *Staphylococcus aureus*, coagulase-negative staphylococcus, and Enterococcus species [1]. However, over the last 10–15 years the sensitivity of gram-positive bacteria to antibiotics has been decreasing. In 1992 the National Nosocomial Infection Surveillance System reported that 29% of hospital acquired enterococcal clinical isolates were vancomycin resistant [2]. The incidence of MRSA has increased to 45–50% in many U.S. hospitals [3]. As of 2002 18.4% of *Streptococcus pneumoniae* were resistant to penicillin [4]. Furthermore, the Clinical and Laboratory Standards Institute (CLSI) has recently lowered the breakpoint for *Staphylococcus aureus* sensitivity to vancomycin from 4 µg/mL to 2 µg/mL. This was required because of high vancomycin failure rates when treating infections caused by "susceptible" bacteria with MIC's of 4 µg/mL. Vancomycin produces time-dependent bacteriocidal activity against susceptible gram-positive bacteria. However, both *in vitro* and clinical trials have demonstrated that vancomycin may have slower bacteriocidal activity and be less effective in infections with large bacterial inoculum than linezolid, and daptomycin [5].

16.2.1 VANCOMYCIN PHARMACOKINETICS

Vancomycin is a large molecule having a molecular weight of 1456 daltons [6]. This large size (Figure 16.1) may help to understand a number of pharmacokinetic variables to be discussed. Vancomycin is thought to be primarily bound to serum albumin and not to acid-1-α glycoprotein, IgM or IgG [7]. Mean vancomycin protein binding, usually determined by ultrafiltration, has been reported to be 55%, however the range of reported values is 10–82% and percent bound vancomycin correlates with serum albumin concentrations [8,9]. Because only free vancomycin is considered to be active, interpatient vancomycin response and interpretation of serum concentrations may be dependent on protein binding. Vancomycin also binds to immunoglobulins (IgA). However, IgA binding that would affect free vancomycin concentrations and efficacy is only significant at very high IgA concentrations such as those seen in patients with IgA myeloma [10].

Oral vancomycin is generally poorly absorbed. However, patients with severe colonic inflammation due to pseudomembranous colitis may absorb substantial amounts of vancomycin [11,12]. Significant vancomycin serum concentrations have been reported in patients with end-stage renal disease given oral vancomycin 1000–2000 mg daily with *Clostridium difficile* pseudomembranous colitis [11]. In contrast to oral absorption, vancomycin absorption from the peritoneal cavity is good. Intraperitoneal vancomycin doses, when left to dwell for 6 hours, have a bioavailability of 52–66% and can produce therapeutic serum concentrations [13,14].

Vancomycin distribution is complex. Although one compartment model has been clinically used to monitor serum concentrations and adjust doses, two and three compartment pharmacokinetic models best described the concentration–time profile. The distribution half-life is 0.5–1 hours and may be longer in renal failure patients. The reported volume of distribution is 0.39–0.9 L/kg [15–17]. Many factors including the molecular weight of vancomycin, protein binding, tissue perfusion, diabetes, and degree of tissue inflammation affect vancomycin penetration into tissues and fluids [18,19]. Vancomycin penetrates relatively well into umbilical cord blood, skin, tissue interstitium, synovial fluid, bile, feces, pleural fluid, ascites, and peritoneal dialysate. Vancomycin penetrates poorly into cortical and cancellous bone, aqueous humor, and CSF without inflamed meninges [18–22]. Penetration into pulmonary epithelial lining fluid is highly variable and poor, averaging 19% of plasma concentrations. Furthermore, absolute concentrations ranged from 0.4 to 8.1 µg/mL. Penetration was found to be dependent on lung inflammation [23]. Although penetration into many of these sites and fluids is good, it may often be quite variable and at or below staphylococcal MIC_{90} values.

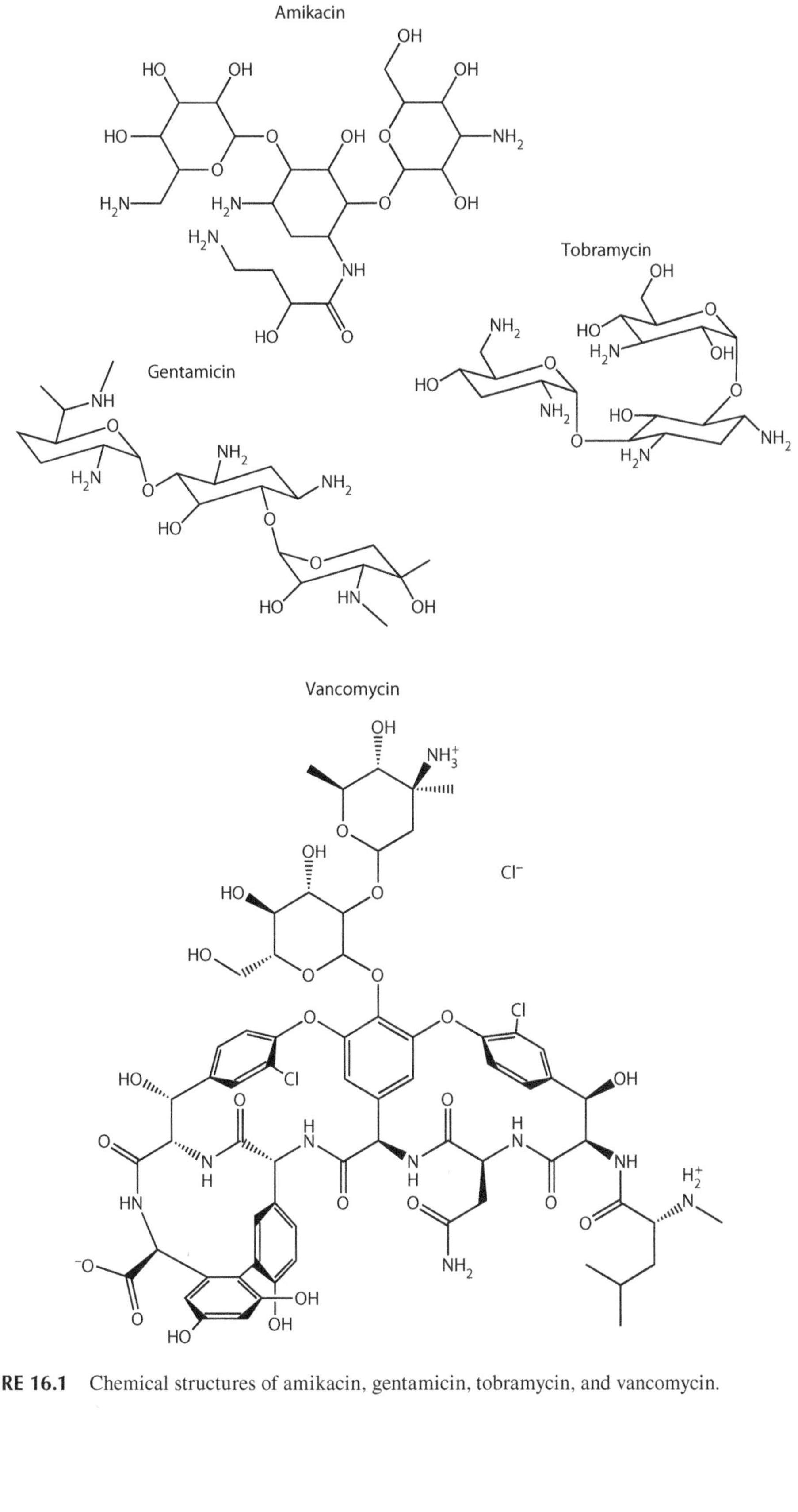

FIGURE 16.1   Chemical structures of amikacin, gentamicin, tobramycin, and vancomycin.

Vancomycin is primarily eliminated by glomerular filtration, and vancomycin clearance correlates with creatinine clearance. Some vancomycin is eliminated by renal tubular secretion [15,18]. However, some small percentage of vancomycin is eliminated by nonrenal mechanisms including biliary elimination and degradation to an inactive antibacterial compound called crystal degradation product [15,24,25]. As such vancomycin serum concentrations are affected by decreasing renal function and require dosage adjustment. The half-life increases and clearance decreases as glomerular filtration declines (Table 16.1) As the table shows these is some variability in vancomycin elimination pharmacokinetic parameters within ranges of creatinine clearance. This may be due to the methods of estimating creatinine clearance or the pharmacokinetic model chosen to study the vancomycin serum concentrations.

The elimination of vancomycin by extracorporeal devices has been studied in depth because of the frequent use of vancomycin in renal failure patients. Critical to predicting vancomycin elimination is an understanding the type of extracorporeal therapy being delivered. Vancomycin is minimally removed by plasmapheresis or peritoneal dialysis [26–28]. A single plasma volume plasmapheresis removed only about 6.3% of total body vancomycin [26]. Conventional low-flux hemodialysis with cellulose acetate or cuprophane membranes also removes little vancomycin, regardless of blood or dialysate flow. However, dialysis utilizing high-flux membranes composed of polysulfone, polyamide, polyacrylonitrile or polymethylmethacrylate can allow a significant amount of vancomycin elimination [29,30]. During high-flux dialysis with these membranes vancomycin clearance is increased to 40–152 mL/min as compared with vancomycin clearance of 9.6–15 mL/min during low-flux dialysis [30]. Furthermore, during high-flux dialysis 26–50% of total body vancomycin can be removed within four hours [29].

Pharmacokinetic studies have been performed in unique patient populations that frequently required vancomycin therapy. The pharmacokinetic differences that exist among these populations and otherwise normal patient populations are largely a manifestation of how the disease processes affect the vancomycin volume of distribution and renal clearance. Neonates, particularly premature

TABLE 16.1
Vancomycin Clearance and Half-Life and Renal Function

Creatinine Clearance	Vancomycin Clearance	Vancomycin Half-Life	Reference
117 mL/min	72.7 mL/min	5.2 hours	56
115 mL/min/1.73 m^2	114 mL/min/1.73 m^2	NA	57
110 mL/min/1.73 m^2	84.8–86.1 mL/min/m^2	7.7–8.1 hours	16
> 100 mL/min	88.7 mL/min	5.6 hours	17
93.4 mL/min/1.73 m^2	98.4 mL/min/1.73m^2	5.2 hours	15
94.2 mL/min	89.2 mL/min	5.1 hours	58
56–98 mL/min	88.7 mL/min	6.1 hours	17
83.1 mL/min	67.8 mL/min	12.7 hours	59
79.1 mL/min	76.7 mL/min	6.5 hours	58
51 mL/min/1.73 m^2	52.6 mL/min/1.73m^2	10.5 hours	15
47 mL/min	54.4 mL/min	10.5 hours	58
17–43 mL/min	60 mL/min	8.7 hours	17
37.4 mL/min	28.3 mL/min	32.3 hours	54
23.0 mL/min/1.73 m^2	31.3 mL/min/1.73m^2	19.9 hours	15
ESRD (3.9 mL/min)	5.4 mL/min	142.6 hours	60
ESRD on dialysis	4.87 mL/min	146.7 hours	54
ESRD on dialysis	NA	178 hours	29

Note: ESRD, end stage renal disease.

neonates have prolonged half-lives of 5.9–11.9 hours due to immature renal function and gestational age. Their volumes of distribution are 0.49–0.74 L/kg. In contrast infants and children may have shorter elimination half-lives, 2.2–6.6 hours and total body clearance values that are two to three times faster than adults [21,31] The pharmacokinetics of vancomycin is not different in cystic fibrosis patients than normal patients [32]. Burn patients have significantly greater renal and total vancomycin clearance than normal patients. As a result, burn patients may require larger daily dosages administered at shorter dosing intervals than usual vancomycin regimens given to normal subjects [33,34]. Lastly, vancomycin pharmacokinetics in obese patients is characterized by large volumes of distribution that correlate with total body weight [35].

16.2.2   VANCOMYCIN PHARMACODYNAMICS

Although basic vancomycin pharmacodynamics has been known for 20 years, it is within the last decade that these principles have begun to be clinically applied. Furthermore, changes in *Staphylococcus aureus* responses to vancomycin therapy have required further investigations into factors affecting vancomycin efficacy. Vancomycin exhibits time-dependent bacteria killing. Thus keeping vancomycin concentrations at the site of infection above the MIC will optimize killing [36,37]. In fact, maximal bacterial killing is obtained by keeping free vancomycin concentrations in the serum at four times the vancomycin bacterial MIC. Vancomycin, in contrast to nafcillin or daptomycin, *in vitro* demonstrates reduced bacteriocidal effects with increased bacterial inoculum [6]. Vancomycin also has a modest postantibiotic effect against gram-positive bacteria. The reported vancomycin MIC values in the United States are summarized in Table 16.2. Although vancomycin is thought of as a potent rescue antibiotic, its bacteriocidal effects are slower than beta-lactam antibiotics. Retrospective pharmacodynamics studies have found that maintaining an area under the concentration curve above the MIC (AUC_{24}/MIC) of 400 or 125 are associated with a greater chance of success in treating *Staphylococcus aureus* pneumonia or *Enterococcus faecium* infections, respectively [38,39]. The AUC_{24}/MIC suggests that as bacterial vancomycin MIC rises, the patient will need to be exposed to higher vancomycin concentrations. This pharmacodynamics

TABLE 16.2
Vancomycin MIC against Gram-Positive Bacteria

Gram-Positive Bacteria	Vancomycin MIC90	Vancomycin MIC Range
Methicillin-sensitive *Staphylococcus aureus*	1 µg/mL	≤ 0.25–2 µg/mL
Methicillin-resistant *Staphylococcus aureus*	1 µg/mL	0.25–4 µg/mL
Coagulase negative staphylococcus methicillin-sensitive	2 µg/mL	≤ 0.25–4 µg/Ll
Coagulase negative staphylococcus methicillin-resistant	2 µg/mL	0.25–4 µg/mL
Enterococcus faecalis vancomycin-sensitive	2 µg/mL	0.25–4 µg/mL
Enterococcus faecium vancomycin-sensitive	1 µg/mL	0.25–2 µg/mL
Streptococcus pyogenes	0.5 µg/mL	0.25–1 µg/mL
Streptococcus agalactiae	0.5 µg/mL	0.12–1 µg/mL
Penicillin-susceptible *Streptococcus pneumoniae*	0.5 µg/mL	≤ 0.06–1 µg/mL
Penicillin-nonsusceptible *Streptococcus pneumoniae*	0.5 µg/mL	0.25–0.5 µg/mL
Viridans group streptococcus	0.5 µg/mL	0.12–1 µg/mL

Sources: Draghi DC, Benton BM, Krause KM, Thronsberry C, Pillar C, Sahm DF, *Antimicrob Agents Chemother,* 52, 2383–2388, 2008 and Castanheira M, Jones RN, Sader HS, *Diagn Microbiol Infect Dis,* 61, 235–239, 2008.

relationship may also explain why it may not be possible to administer enough vancomycin to a patient infected with a *Staphylococcus aureus* (with a MIC of greater than or equal to 2 µg/mL) that will produce a desired AUC_{24}/MIC, so that infection can be eradicated without nephrotoxicity [40,41]. Similarly, infections caused by *Staphylococcus aureus* with increasing vancomycin MIC values, particularly those greater than or equal to 1.5 µg/mL, do not respond as well to vancomycin even with aggressive vancomycin dosing [38,42,43].

16.2.3 THERAPEUTIC DRUG MONITORING OF VANCOMYCIN

For years the standard of practice, for monitoring vancomycin serum concentrations was to measure both peak and trough vancomycin concentrations during intermittent vancomycin dosing. The desired range for peak concentrations was imprecise but commonly reportedly as 20–40 µg/mL and the desired range for trough concentrations was 5–10 µg/mL [16,44]. These desired concentrations were based less on clinical trials defining vancomycin efficacy and more on attainable serum concentrations using standard doses [16]. Furthermore, these serum concentrations were developed prior to the marketing of the purified vancomycin product. The elimination of the impurities in the 1970s has been associated with a reduction in nephrotoxicity and ototoxicity [44,45]. The red-man's syndrome, although commonly reported with vancomycin, is a vancomycin infusion rate related toxicity and is not associated with specific serum concentrations [16,46]. The two most cited vancomycin toxicities possibly associated with serum concentrations are ototoxicity and nephrotoxicity. The case for monitoring peak vancomycin concentrations to prevent toxicity or improve efficacy is weak. First, vancomycin does not exhibit concentration-dependent bacteriocidal effects so the peak concentration would not be expected to predict efficacy. Secondly, the original case reports of vancomycin induced ototoxicity were in patients with serum concentrations greater than 80 µg/mL. This toxicity-concentration association did not clearly define the desired upper limit of 20–40 µg/mL. Thirdly, after a dose is infused the peak concentration is difficult to accurately characterize for several reasons (first, the distribution phase can be rather long and variable and secondly, the recommended time for drawing peak concentrations is not established, but ranges from 0.5 to 2 hours after completion of an infused dose) [16,47]. Given the variable distribution phase, the time at which the peak concentration is drawn after the end of an infusion can greatly influence the measured peak concentration, adequacy of a dosing regimen and the potential for toxicity. As a result, peak concentrations do not reliably predict tissue concentrations or toxicity. Furthermore, utilizing this variable peak serum vancomycin to calculate one-compartment pharmacokinetic parameters and then use the parameters to adjusting therapy may result in overdosing or underdosing vancomycin. This may explain why clinical efficacy trials and reviews have not been able to correlate efficacy with peak concentrations of vancomycin [6,48].

Clinical trials have focused on monitoring vancomycin serum trough concentrations for efficacy and the risk of nephrotoxicity. Depending on the definition of nephrotoxicity the reported incidence is less than 5% [49–51]. However, vancomycin trough concentrations greater than 10–15 µg/mL, total vancomycin daily dose greater than 4 g, and prolonged therapy have been associated with higher incidences of nephrotoxicity [49,50]. In addition, the concurrent use of vancomycin with an aminoglycoside, amphotericin B, vasopressors and sepsis may increase nephrotoxicity regardless of the trough vancomycin serum concentration [51].

Based on known vancomycin pharmacokinetics and pharmacodynamics, optimal trough vancomycin serum concentrations maybe predicted. If most gram-positive pathogens have vancomycin MIC values of 1 µg/mL or less, vancomycin protein binding is about 50%, and optimal bacteriocidal activity is attained at free serum drug concentrations of about four times the MIC, then the minimally desired trough vancomycin concentration for bacteremias should be at least 8–10 µg/mL. If optimal serum concentrations are needed at a site not easily penetrated by vancomycin then higher troughs concentrations might be desired. The American Thoracic Society has recommended trough vancomycin concentrations of 15–20 µg/mL for *Staphylococcus aureus* pneumonia [52]. Similarly, for endocarditis, osteomyelitis, and meningitis higher trough concentrations, 10–15 µg/mL might be desired to optimize vancomycin penetration into the infection site [51]. Because vancomycin exhibits time-dependent bacteriocidal activity several clinical trials have investigated the administration of vancomycin in a continuous infusion to treat staphylococcal infections [51,53]. The desired vancomycin steady state concentrations during an infusion have not been well defined but values such as 15–25 µg/mL have been reported.

16.2.4   Recommended Monitoring of Vancomycin

The recommendations for routine monitoring of vancomycin have changed over the last decade. The types of serum concentrations, frequency of monitoring and desired ranges have changed. Not all patients receiving vancomycin need to have serum concentrations monitored if they are started using one of several vancomycin dosing methods [54,55]. Patients receiving vancomycin for less than five days or receiving oral vancomycin therapy do not need monitoring of vancomycin serum concentrations.

Vancomycin therapy warrants monitoring if the patient receives five or more days of treatment, receives vancomycin concurrently with aminoglycosides or other nephrotoxic medications, receives high dose vancomycin (greater than 4 g/day), creatinine clearance less than 60 mL/min, is infected with a relatively insensitive bacteria or methicillin-resistant *Staphylococcus aureus* with MIC values greater than 1.5 µg/mL, is infected in a difficult to penetrate site, or is on hemodialysis, peritoneal dialysis or renal replacement therapy. If the patient is receiving a regularly scheduled vancomycin dose, only trough serum concentrations are indicated. For most infections a trough concentration of 5–15 µg/mL will be sufficient. For endocarditis a trough concentration is 10–15 µg/mL is desired. Lastly, the American Thoracic Society now recommends trough vancomycin concentrations for *Staphylococcus aureus* ventilator-associated pneumonia to be 15–20 µg/mL [52]. Monitoring vancomycin therapy in patients on dialysis, peritoneal dialysis or renal replacement therapy is more complicated. After the first vancomycin dose it is important to verify the patient has attained a desired vancomycin serum concentration. The most critical factor for monitoring vancomycin therapy is to determine the type of therapy a patient is receiving. If the patient receives low-flux dialysis they require less monitoring than if the patient is receiving high-flux dialysis. The latter removes much more vancomycin and requires more frequent dosing. Similarly monitoring can be infrequent in patients receiving only peritoneal dialysis. Patients receiving renal replacement therapy involving high blood flows and a dialysis component will need close monitoring. In all patients, administration of vancomycin should occur when random serum concentrations are below 15 µg/mL.

16.3   AMINOGLYCOSIDES

The aminoglycoside antibiotics consist of two or more aminosugar joined by a glycosidic linkage to a hexose or aminocyclitol. Streptomycin was the first aminoglycoside discovered in 1914 but later many other aminoglycosides such as amikacin, gentamicin, isepamicin, kanamycin, netilmicin, sisomicin, streptomycin, tobramycin, etc., have become available for treating serious bacterial infections. Out of all aminoglycoside antibiotics approved for use in the United States, amikacin, gentamicin, and tobramycin (see Figure 16.1 for chemical structures) are the three most commonly monitored drugs. These drugs are used to treat infections with *Escherichia coli* and *Pseudomonas aeruginosa* in addition to infections with susceptible organisms such as *Pseudomonas*, *Enterobacteria*, *Serratia*, *Proteus*, *Acinetobacter*, and *Klebsiella*. These drugs are used alone or in combination with another antibiotic when treating more serious gram-negative infections and some gram-positive infections. These drugs are bactericidal but must first be transported into the cell in order to elicit their killing action. Once internalized, the drugs bind to the bacterial ribosomal 30S subunit causing misreading of mRNA. This inhibits protein synthesis or leads to the production of defective proteins, and subsequently the microorganism dies. Alterations by the microorganism to this region contribute to the development of resistant strains as can be seen by the following example. To elicit its action on a specific organism, gentamicin binds to the aminoacyl-tRNA site (A site) of 16S rRNA on the ribosomal 30S subunit causing inhibition of translocation. Methylation of the ribosomal 16S target causes resistance to most aminoglycosides [63,64].

Therefore, aminoglycosides are highly active antimicrobial agents in treating bacteriemia caused by aerobic gram-negative bacilli. These drugs cause rapid concentration-dependent death and their activity is not affected by the size of the bacterial inoculum. In addition, the emergence of drug resistance during therapy is uncommon. The outcome of therapy is strongly associated with a high peak serum aminoglycoside concentration. After a few hours of bacterial death, a bacteriostatic phase without any regrowth (postantibiotic effect) may be observed which is reinforced by the presence of leucocytes [65]. However, due to their toxicity, the use of aminoglycosides is somewhat restrained and as a result resistance has remained at low levels for many pathogens. The major toxicities of aminoglycosides are similar to vancomycin i.e., ototoxicity and nephrotoxicity.

16.3.1 Pharmacokinetics of Aminoglycosides

All of the aminoglycosides are poorly absorbed from the gut and for this reason are administered parenterally for treating systematic infections. Interestingly, aminoglycosides demonstrate very similar kinetics and elimination half-lives generally vary between two and three hours, in otherwise healthy subjects. Volumes of distribution are also similar in aminoglycosides [66]. Volumes of distribution are low which are consistent with the distribution of aminoglycosides in extracellular water. Penetration of these drugs into peritoneal, ascitic, pleural and synovial fluid is good but these drugs are distributed rather slowly into bile, feces, prostate, and amniotic fluid [67]. Volumes of distribution are higher (causing lower peak levels) in patients with sepsis [68].

Aminoglycosides are rapidly absorbed after intramuscular administration with peak concentrations usually achieved within one hour. Following intravenous administration, peak concentrations are usually observed immediately following the completion of the infusion. Aminoglycosides can be administered in a single daily dose or divided doses. Nebulized forms of amikacin and tobramycin are also used for patients with cystic fibrosis as a means of treating chronic infections of *Pseudomonas aeruginosa* [69].

Aminoglycosides are poorly protein bound (<10%). The major route of elimination is through the kidney where 85–95% of the drugs are recovered unchanged. Patients with impaired renal function have lower aminoglycoside elimination rates and longer half-lives compared to patients with normal renal function. Moreover, elimination of aminoglycosides is slower in elderly patients and many patients require prolonged dosing interval. Children have a higher clearance of aminoglycosides. Siber et al. reported that after 1 mg/kg dose of gentamicin, the mean peak plasma concentration was 1.58 µg/mL in children with age between 6 months and 5 years, 2.03 µg/mL in children between 5 and 10 years old and 2.81 µg/mL in children older than 10 years. Patients with fever showed shorter half-life and lower plasma concentrations of gentamicin [70].

Patients with cystic fibrosis usually exhibit an altered pharmacokinetics of the antibiotics. After a conventional dose of an aminoglycoside, a patient with cystic fibrosis shows a lower serum concentration compared to a patient not suffering from cystic fibrosis. The lower serum concentrations of aminoglycoside in patients with cystic fibrosis may be due to increased total body clearance of these drugs combined with a larger volume of distribution [71]. Bosso et al. reported that mean clearance of netilmicin was higher in patients with cystic fibrosis compared to patients with no cystic fibrosis. Therefore, patients with cystic fibrosis required larger than normal dosages of netilmicin on a weight basis. The study also showed that the serum concentrations of netilmicin should be monitored carefully to individualize dosage in these patients [72]. Another study indicated that the major route of elimination of gentamicin in patients with mild cystic fibrosis is through renal excretion but aminoglycoside pharmacokinetics was changed with progression of disease [73]. Mann et al. reported increased dosage requirement for tobramycin and gentamicin for treating *Pseudomonas pneumonia* in patients with cystic fibrosis [74]. Dupuis et al. observed significant differences in pharmacokinetics of tobramycin in patients with cystic fibrosis before and after lung transplantation using 29 patients who received at least one dosage of tobramycin before and after lung transplant. The clearance of tobramycin was decreased by 40% and the half-life was increased by 141% after transplant compared to pretransplant values [75]. Patients with cystic fibrosis are also susceptible to renal impairment from repeated intravenous use of aminoglycosides and these drugs should be cautiously used in these patients with regular monitoring of renal function [76].

The two major toxicities associated with aminoglycoside therapy are nephrotoxicity and ototoxicity. Nephrotoxicity is encountered in 15–17% of patients treated with conventional divided dose regimen while ototoxicity is encountered in 20–25% patients. The drugs are taken-up by the epithelial cells of the renal proximal tubules where they bind to acidic phospholipids and megalin in the brush border membrane, and accumulate. Megalin is a receptor expressed at the apical membrane of renal proximal tubules. Animal studies suggest that by blocking the binding to the megalin receptor, nephrotoxicity can be prevented [77]. Peak serum concentrations for amikacin and kanamycin above 32–34 µg/mL are associated with a higher risk of nephrotoxicity and ototoxicity [78]. Sustained peak concentrations above 12–15 µg/mL are associated with an increased risk of developing nephrotoxicity and ototoxicity for gentamicin, tobramycin and sisomicin. For netilmicin, the toxicity is encountered at a peak concentration above 16 µg/mL. Peak concentration of streptomycin should not exceed 30 µg/mL [79].

The risk of amikacin-induced nephrotoxicity is increased for patients with chronic liver disease and hypoalbuminemia. Though the proximal tubules are the target of the drugs' toxicities, serum creatinine is monitored before and after initiating therapy to assess or define nephrotoxicity. The criteria used, i.e., the change in the serum creatinine measured before aminoglycoside dosing versus after, varies between institutions. The following are considered significant indicators for nephrotoxicity: an increase in serum creatinine of 5 mg/dL or above when the baseline creatinine is 1.9 mg/dL or lower; an increase of 1 mg/dL or higher when the baseline is between 2.0 and 4.9 mg/dL; and an increase of 1.5 mg/dL or more when the baseline is above 5 mg/dL. Glomerular filtration rate and cystatin C are also used as indicators of nephrotoxicity [80]. Variations in clearance and half-life of aminoglycosides due to renal function are listed in Table 16.3.

Unfortunately, aminoglycoside induced ototoxicity is often irreversible. Vestibular and cochlear sensory cells are damaged resulting in both auditory loss and vestibular dysfunction. Initial symptoms include tinnitus, decreased perception of high frequency sound, headache, and vertigo. Total dose, total area under the curve (AUC) and duration of therapy seem to correlate better with ototoxicity than peak and trough concentrations. In animal models, ototoxicity is enhanced when amikacin is coadministered with the herbal product ginkgo. Other toxicities of aminoglycosides such as neuromuscular blockage and hypersensitivity are less common. The most important drug interactions occur with other drugs that are nephrotoxic or ototoxic: for example, cyclosporine, tacrolimus, cisplatin, ethacrynic acid, furosemide, and cephalosporin antibiotics. Neuromuscular blockade has been reported with the coadministration of an aminoglycoside and a calcium channel blocker. This can lead to respiratory depression and neuromuscular blockage and is a particular problem with verapamil. When given with rocuronium, a neuromuscular blocking agent used in intubation, the action of rocuronium has been prolonged. Therefore neuromuscular blockade should be closely monitored for patients also receiving aminoglycosides [101].

16.3.2 PHARMACODYNAMICS OF AMINOGLYCOSIDES

Aminoglycoside exhibit rapid bactericidal activity in vitro and demonstrate concentration dependent killing. In addition, aminoglycosides also show post-antibiotic effect where a delayed period of bacterial regrowth can be observed after a brief exposure. In human model, Moore et al. demonstrated efficacy to the ratio of peak aminoglycoside concentration (Cmax) to MIC [102]. It appears that aminoglycosides have two predictors for efficacy; AUC of 24 hours (AUC-24) to MIC ratio as

TABLE 16.3
Aminoglycoside Clearance and Half-Life and Renal Function

Creatinine Clearance	Gentamicin Clearance	Gentamicin Half-Life	Tobramycin Clearance	Tobramycin Half-Life	Amikacin Clearance	Amikacin Half-Life	Reference
172.1 mL/kg/ 1.73m^2	NA	0.85 hours					99
142.5 mL/min	118.5 mL/ min	1.8 hours					98
140.7 mL/ kg/1.73m^2					129.7 mL/ kg/1.73m^2	NA	88
125 mL/ kg/1.73m^2	NA	1.13 hours					99
119 mL/min	95.9 mL/ min	2.2 hours					93
111 mL/min			101.5 mL/ min	2.1 hours	78.6 mL/ kg/1.73m^2	1.4 hours	89,93
110 mL/kg/ 1.73m^2					NA	2.9 hours	91
99–109 mL/ min	79 mL/min	2.63 hours	67 mL/min	3.2	99 mL/min	2.2 hours	93,94,100
98–105 mL/kg/ 1.73m^2			43.5 mL/ kg/1.73m^2	3.0 hours	86–95 mL/ min	2.1–2.5	85,92
101 mL/ kg/1.73m^2					NA	2.1 hours	90
> 100 mL/min	110.6 mL/ min	1.6 hours					97
> 80 mL/min/ 1.73m^2					NA	1.4 hours	86,87
80.8 mL/kg/ 1.73m^2	91.8 mL/ kg/1.73m^2	3.4 hours					95
69.2 mL/min	92.3 mL/ min	3.4 hours					98
63 mL/min	75.9 mL/ kg/1.73m^2	4.2 hours	44 mL/min	4.3 hours			94,96
59.8 mL/ kg/1.73m^2	75.3 mL/ kg/1.73m^2	4.8 hours					95
55–55.5 mL/ kg/1.73m^2					NA	4.7– 5.8 hours	90,91
51.2 mL/min	36.9 mL/ min	5.8 hours					100
45 mL/min	29.85 mL/ min	3.85 hrs			33.45 mL/ min	6.93 hours	83
33.3 mL/ kg/1.73m^2			26.4 mL/ kg/1.73m^2	5.2 hours			85
31 mL/min			18 mL/min	9.9 hours			94
15 mL/kg/ 1.73m^2					NA	29.6 hours	90
13 mL/kg/ 1.73m^2					13.7 mL/ kg/1.73m^2	18.4 hours	91
12.9 mL/kg/ 1.73m^2					NA	16.3 hours	91

(Continued)

TABLE 16.3   (Continued)

ARF on dialysis (4.1 mL/min)			7.31 mL/min	53.3 hours	82
ESRD on dialysis			1.6 mL/min/1.73 m²	86.5 hours	84
ESRD on dialysis			4.6 mL/kg/1.73m²	37.2 hours	89
ESRD on PD	2.9 mL/min	36 hours	3.9 mL/min/1.73m²	42.2 hours	81

Notes: ARF, acute renal failure; PD, peritoneal dialysis.

well as Cmax to MIC ratio. Kashuba et al. demonstrated that the first time an aminoglycoside was given to a patient with nosocomial pneumonia, the chances of resolution of remission of fever and resolution of white blood cells within seven days of therapy was over 90% with a Cmax/MIC ratio of equal to or greater than 10 [103]. In Table 16.4 aminoglycoside MIC against selected gram-negative bacteria are listed with references.

16.3.3   MONITORING AMINOGLYCOSIDE ANTIBIOTICS

The aminoglycosides are generally used in one of three different scenarios, traditional dosing, once-daily dosing or extended interval dosing, and synergy dosing. Each use has different methods of monitoring. Serum concentrations are readily available and turnaround of serum concentration information is usually within hours, allowing for rapid dosage adjustments to optimize therapy. The purpose of monitoring serum concentrations is to attain desired therapeutic concentrations and to try to avoid toxic serum concentrations. As a result, if aminoglycoside therapy is needed only for three or less days, monitoring serum concentrations is probably not necessary [108].

Traditional dosing is the intermittent dosing of aminoglycoside, usually two or three times each day, with the goal of attaining traditional serum concentrations (Table 16.5) Although controversial and requiring more study, the desired serum concentrations are based on known bacterial MIC values, concentration-dependent bacterial killing, and toxicity–concentration relationships [108–110]. During traditional dosing peak concentrations should be drawn 30 to 60 minutes after each dose is infused over 30 minutes. The trough concentration is drawn within 30 minutes of next dose. The serum concentrations should be drawn at steady state, which occurs after the patient has received a single regimen for at least four to five half-lives. Aminoglycoside therapy should be individualized, optimally utilizing pharmacokinetic parameters determined from serum concentration data to adjust aminoglycoside regimens [111–113]. Once the desired serum concentrations are achieved, trough concentrations should be monitored once weekly unless renal function is unstable or other nephrotoxic drugs are started.

Once-daily dosing or extended interval dosing involves administering large aminoglycoside doses, 5–7 mg/kg, once each day. This method takes advantage of ease of administration, reduced cost of therapy, aminoglycoside concentration-dependent killing, optimizes peak concentration to MIC ratios of eight to ten, postantibiotic effects, saturable kidney proximal tubule reuptake, and prolonged low serum concentrations allowing for drug redistribution out of tissues [109,110,114] Although once-daily dosing is commonly used it has not been extensively studied or is contraindicated, and thus not recommended for use, in patients with endocarditis, greater than 20% burns, cystic fibrosis, children less than 12 years of age, creatinine clearance less than 20 mL/minute, ascites, enterococcal infections, or surgical prophylaxis [114,115]. However, as this method is

TABLE 16.4
Aminoglycoside MIC against Selected Gram-Negative Bacteria

Bacteria	Gentamicin MIC50 (μg/mL)	Gentamicin MIC90 (μg/mL)	Tobramycin MIC50 (μg/mL)	Tobramycin MIC90 (μg/mL)	Amikacin MIC50 (μg/mL)	Amikacin MIC90 (μg/mL)
Acinetobacter species	0.5–≤2	>8	≤1	>8	NA	32
Citrobacter species	≤0.25–≤2	≤1–8	≤1	2	NA	NA
Enterobacter species	≤0.25–≤2	0.5–≤2	≤1	≤1–2	NA	4
Escherichia coli	0.5–≤2	2	≤1	≤1	NA	4
Klebsiella species	≤0.25–≤2	0.5–≤2	≤1	≤1	NA	2
Proteus mirabilis	0.5–≤2	≤2–4	≤1	≤1	NA	NA
Pseudomonas aeruginosa	2–4	>8	≤1	4–8	NA	8
Serratia species	≤0.25–≤2	1–≤2	2	4	NA	4

Sources: Kashuba AD, Nafziger AN, Drusano GL, Bertino JS, *Antimicrob Agents Chemother,* 43, 623–629, 1999; Rhomberg PR, Jones RN, Sader HS, Fritsche TR, The MYSTIC Programme Study Group, *Diagn Microbiol Infect Dis,* 49, 273–281, 2004; Zhanel GG, DeCorby M, Nichol KA, Wierzbowski A, Baudry PJ, Karlowsky JA, Lagace-Weins P, Walkty A, Mulvey MR, Hoban DJ, *Diagn Microbiol Infect Dis,* 62, 67–80, 2008; Rhomberg PR, Jones RN, Sader HS, The MYSTIC Programme (US) Study Group, *Int J Antimicrob Agents,* 23, 52–59, 2004; and Reinert RR, Low DE, Rossi F, Zhang X, Wattal C, Dowzicky MJ, *J Antimicrob Chemother,* 60, 1018–1029, 2007.
Note: NA, not available.

TABLE 16.5
Aminoglycoside Desired Serum Concentrations with Traditional Dosing Methods

Aminoglycoside Antibiotic	Gentamicin (μg/mL)	Tobramycin (μg/mL)	Amikacin (μg/mL)
Peak concentrations			
Infections	6–10	6–10	20–35
Urinary tract infection	4–6	4–6	15–20
Gram-positive synergy	3–4	None	None
Cystic fibrosis	6–12	6–12	30–40
Trough concentrations	<2	<2	5–10

studied further it may be adapted to these patient populations. Although there are no guidelines for monitoring serum concentrations, use of the Hartford Nomogram is commonly used for dosing and monitoring [115]. In this nomogram serum concentrations are drawn 6–14 hours after the first dose to determine the appropriate dosing interval.

The TOPIC study applied the once-daily dosing approach to cystic fibrosis patients [116]. Because of enhanced aminoglycoside elimination in cystic fibrosis patients, the once daily dose is 10 mg/kg given once daily. Serum concentrations are drawn at 30 minutes after and immediately before a dose. Although the study's efficacy was not defined by serum concentrations, some have tried to attain a target AUC of 80–120 μg hour/mL.

Aminoglycosides can be used synergistically with other antibiotics when treating either gram-negative or gram-positive bacterial infections. When the aminoglycosides are used synergistically for treating gram-negative infections, full therapy and monitoring should occur as outlined above. When gentamicin is used for synergy with other cell wall active antibiotics for treatment of gram-positive infections, minimal monitoring is required. In general gentamicin synergy dosing, typically 1 mg/kg per dose, for gram-positive bacterial infections will not produce excessive peak concentrations. Therefore, only trough gentamicin concentrations should be monitored to detect gentamicin accumulation. Optimally the trough concentration should be 0.5–1 µg/mL.

During aminoglycoside therapy several other tests, besides aminoglycoside serum concentrations, should be monitored. Serum creatinine values should be monitored twice a week until they are constantly changing. Clinical assessments of vestibular function should be monitored at baseline and at least once a week, especially during prolonged therapy of more than seven days [108,117] Lastly, hearing test should be monitored at baseline and weekly if the aminoglycoside course of therapy is expected to be greater than two weeks [108,111,117].

16.4 TECHNIQUES FOR THERAPEUTIC DRUG MONITORING OF VANCOMYCIN AND AMINOGLYCOSIDE

Serum is the preferred specimen for monitoring vancomycin and aminoglycosides. Immunoassays are commercially available for routine monitoring of these drugs and these assays usually produce reliable results. However, immunoassays are subjected to interferences. For example, crystalline decomposition product of vancomycin (CDP-1) which may accumulate in patients with renal failure may interfere with the fluorescence polarization immunoassay for vancomycin (Abbott Laboratories, Abbott Park, IL). Chromatographic techniques are very analyte specific for determination of vancomycin and aminoglycosides in serum or other biological matrix. For in depth discussion on this subject please see Chapter 17.

16.5 CONCLUSIONS

Vancomycin and aminoglycosides are important antibiotics which are used for treating life threatening bacterial infections. Ototoxicity which may be irreversible and nephrotoxicity are two major concerns for treating patients with these antibiotics. Careful monitoring of serum levels of these drugs are indicated to improve clinical outcomes as well as reducing toxicities especially if the therapy is continued for more than three days in most patients receiving these antibiotics.

REFERENCES

1. Biedenbach DJ, Bell JM, Sader HS, Fritsche TR, Jones RN, Turnidge JD. 2007. Antimicrobial susceptibility of Gram-positive bacterial isolates from the Asia-Pacific region and an in vitro evaluation of the bacteriocidal activity of daptomycin, vancomycin, and teicoplanin: A SENTRY Program Report (2003–2004). *Int J Antimicrob Agents* 30: 143–149.
2. National Nosocomial Infections Surveillance (NNIS) System Report, data summary from January 1992 through June 2004, issued October 2004. 2004. *Am J Infect Control* 32: 470–485.
3. Rybak MJ. 2004. Resistance to antimicrobial agents: an update. *Pharmacotherapy* 24 (Pt 2): 203S–215S.
4. Karlowsky JA, Thornsberry C, Jones ME; Evangelista AT, Critchley IA, Sahm DF. 2003. Factors associated with relative rates of antimicrobial resistance among Streptococcus pneumoniae in the United States: results from the TRUST Surveillance Program (1998–2002). *Clin Infect Dis* 36: 963–970.
5. LaPlante KL, Rybak MJ. 2004. Impact of high-inoculum Staphylococcus aureus on the activities of nafcillin, vancomycin, linezolid, and daptomycin, alone and in combination with gentamicin in an *in vitro* pharmacodynamics model. *Antimicrob Agents Chemother* 48: 4665–4672.
6. Rybak MJ. 2006. The pharmacokinetic and pharmacodynamics properties of vancomycin. *Clin Infect Dis* 42 (Suppl 1): S35–S39.
7. Sun H, Maderazo EG, Krusell AR. 1993. Serum protein-binding characteristics of vancomycin. *Antimicrob Agents Chemother* 37: 1132–1136.

8. Zokufa HZ, Solem LD, Rodvold KA, Crossley KB, Fischer JH, Rotschager JC. 1989. The influence of serum albumin and α_1-acid glycoprotein on vancomycin protein binding in patients with burn injuries. *J Burn Care Rehabil* 10: 425–428.

9. Ackerman BH, Taylor EH, Olsen KM, Abdel-Malak W, Pappas AA. 1988. Vancomycin serum protein binding determination by ultrafiltration. *Drug Intell Clin Pharm* 22: 300–303.

10. Cantu TG, Dick JD, Elliott RL, Humphrey RL, Kornhauser DM. 1990. Protein binding of vancomycin in a patient with immunoglobulin A myeloma. *Antimicrob Agents Chemother* 34: 1459–1461.

11. Aradhyula S, Manian FA, Hafidh SAS, Bhutto SS, Alpert MA. 2006. Significant absorption of oral vancomycin in a patient with Clostridium difficile colitis and normal renal function. *South Med J* 99: 518–520.

12. Spitzer PG, Eliopoulos GM. 1984. Systemic absorption of enteral vancomycin in a patient with pseudomembranous colitis. *Ann Intern Med* 100: 533–534.

13. Pancorbo S, Comty C. 1982. Peritoneal transport of vancomycin in 4 patients undergoing continuous ambulatory peritoneal dialysis. *Nephron* 31: 37–39.

14. Bailie GR, Eisele G, Venezia RA, Yocum D, Hollister A. 1992. Prediction of serum vancomycin concentrations following intraperitoneal loading doses in continuous ambulatory peritoneal dialysis patients with peritonitis. *Clin Pharmacokinet* 22: 298–307.

15. Rodvold KA, Blum RA, Fischer JH, Zokufa HZ, Rotschafer JC, Crossley KB, Riff LJ. 1988. Vancomycin pharmacokinetics in patients with various degrees of renal function. *Antimicrob Agents Chemother* 32: 848–852.

16. Healy DP, Polk RE, Garson ML, Rock D, Comstock TJ. 1987. Comparison of steady-state pharmacokinetics of two dosage regimens of vancomycin in normal volunteers. *Antimicrob Agents Chemother* 31: 393–397.

17. Rotschafer JC, Crossley K, Zaske DE, Mead K, Sawchuk RJ, Solem LD. 1982. Pharmacokinetics of vancomycin: Observations in 28 patients and dosage recommendations. *Antimicrob Agents Chemother* 22: 391–394.

18. Rybak MJ. 2006. The pharmacokinetic and pharmacodynamic properties of vancomycin. *Clin Infect Dis* 42 (Supply): S35–S39.

19. Skhirtladze K, Hutschala D, Fleck T, Thalhammer F, Ehrlich M, Vukovich T, Muller M, Tschernko EM. 2006. Impaired target site penetration of vancomycin in diabetic patients following cardiac surgery. *Antimicrob Agents Chemother* 50: 1372–1375.

20. Laiprasert J, Klein K, Mueller BA, Pearlman MD. 2007. Transplacental passage of vancomycin in non-infected term pregnant women. *Obstet Gynecol* 109: 1105–1110.

21. Rodvold KA, Everett JA, Pryka RD, Kraus DM. 1997. Pharmacokinetics and administration regimens of vancomycin in neonates, infants and children. *Clin Pharmacokinet* 33: 32–51.

22. Moise-Broder PA, Forrest A, Birmingham MC, Schentag JJ. 2004. Pharmacodynamics of vancomycin and other antimicrobials in patients with *Staphylococcus aureus* lower respiratory tract infections. *Clin Pharmacokinet* 43: 925–942.

23. Lamer C, de Beco V, Soler P, Calvat S, Fagon JY, Dombret MC, Farinotti R, Chaste J, Gibert C. 1993. Analysis of vancomycin entry into pulmonary lining fluid by bronchoalveolar lavage in critically ill patients. *Antimicrob Agents Chemother* 37: 281–286.

24. Currie, BP, Lemos-Filho L. 2004. Evidence for biliary excretion of vancomycin into stool during intravenous therapy: potential implications for rectal colonization with vancomycin-resistant enterococci. *Antimicrob Agents Chemother* 48: 4427–4429.

25. Smith PF, Morse GD. 1999. Accuracy of measured vancomycin serum concentrations in patients with end-stage renal disease. *Ann Pharmacother* 33: 1329–1335.

26. McClellan SD, Whitaker CH, Friedberg RD. 1997. Removal of vancomycin during plasmapheresis. *Ann Pharmacother* 31(10): 1132–1136.

27. Morse GD, Faroline DF, Apicella MA, Walshe JJ. 1987. Comparative study of intraperitoneal and intravenous vancomycin pharmacokinetics during continuous ambulatory peritoneal dialysis. *Antimicrob Agents Chemother* 31: 173–177.

28. Blevins RD, Halstenson CE, Salem NG, Matzke GR. 1984. Pharmacokinetics of vancomycin in patients undergoing continuous ambulatory peritoneal dialysis. *Antimicrob Agents Chemother* 25: 603–606.

29. Ariano RE, Fine A, Sitar DS, Resrode S, Selenitsky SA. 2005. Adequacy of a vancomycin dosing regimen in patients receiving high-flux hemodialysis. *Am J Kid Dis* 46: 681–687.

30. Launay-Vacher V, Izzedine H, Mercada L, Deray G. 2002. Clinical review: Use of vancomycin in haemodialysis patients. *Crit Care* 6: 313–316.

31. de Hoog M, Mouton JW, van den Anker JN. 2004. Vancomycin: pharmacokinetics and administration regimens in neonates. *Clin Pharmacokinet* 43: 417–440.

32. Pleasants RA, Michalets EL, Williams DM, Samuelson WM, Rehm JR, Knowles MR. 1996. Pharmacokinetics of vancomycin in adult cystic fibrosis patients. *Antimicrob Agents Chemother* 40: 186–190.
33. Brater DC, Bawdon RE, Anderson SA, Purdue GF, Hunt JL. 1986. Vancomycin elimination in patients with burn injury. *Clin Pharmacol Ther* 39: 631–634.
34. Garrelts JC, Peterie JD. 1988. Altered vancomycin dose vs. serum concentration relationship in burn patients. *Clin Pharmacol Ther* 44: 9–13.
35. Vance-Bryan K, Guay DRP, Gilliland SS, Rodvold KA, Rotschafer JC. 1993. Effect of obesity on vancomycin pharmacokinetic parameters as determined by using a bayesian forecasting technique. *Antimicrob Agents Chemother* 37: 436–440.
36. Drusano GL. 2004. Antimicrobial pharmacodynamics: Critical interactions of "bug and drug". *Nature Rev* 2: 289–300.
37. Roberts JA, Lipman J, Blot S, Rello J. 2008. Better outcomes through continuous infusion of time-dependent antibiotics to critically ill patients? *Curr Opin Crit Care* 14: 390–396.
38. Moise-Broder PA, Forrest A, Birmingham MC, Schentag JJ. 2004. Pharmacodynamics of vancomycin and other antimicrobials in patients with *Staphylococcus aureus* lower respiratory tract infections. *Clin Pharmacokinet* 43: 925–942.
39. Hyatt JM, McKinnon PS, Zimmer GS, Schentag JJ. 1995. The importance of pharmacokinetic/pharmacodynamic surrogate markers to outcome: focus on antibacterial agents. *Clin Pharmacokinet* 28: 143–160.
40. Lodise TP, Lomaestro B, Graves J, Drusano GL. 2008. Larger vancomycin doses (at least four grams per day) are associated with an increased incidence of nephrotoxicity. *Antimicrob Agents Chemother* 52: 1330–1336.
41. Jeffres MN, Isakow W, Doherty JA, McKinnon PS, Ritchie DJ, Micek ST, Kollef MH. 2006. Predictors of mortality for methicillin-resistant *Staphylococcus aureus* health-care-associated pneumonia. *Chest* 130: 947–955.
42. Lodise TP, Graves J, Evans A, Graffunder E, Helmecke M, Lomaestro BM, Stellrecht K. 2008. Relationship between vancomycin MIC and failure among patients with methicillin-resistant *Staphylococcus aureus* bacteremia treatment with vancomycin. *Antimicrob Agents Chemother* 52: 3315–3320.
43. Sakoulas G, Moise-Broder PA, Schentag J, Forrest A, Moellering RC, Eliopooulos GM. 2004. Relationship of MIC and bacteriocidal activity to efficacy of vancomycin for treatment of methicillin-resistant *Staphylococcus aureus* bacteremia. *J Clin Microbiol* 42: 2398–2402.
44. Kitzis MD, Goldstein FW. 2006. Monitoring of vancomycin serum levels for the treatment of staphylococcal infections. *Clin Microbiol Infect* 12: 92–95.
45. Farber BF, Moellering RC. 1983. Retrospective study of the toxicity of preparations of vancomycin from 1974 to 1981. *Antimicrob Agents Chemother* 23: 138–141.
46. Renz CL, Thurn JD, Finn HA, Lynch JP, Moss J. 1998. Oral antihistamines reduce the side effects from rapid vancomycin infusion. *Anesth Analg* 87: 681–685.
47. Rodvold KA, Zokufa H, Rotschafer JC. 1987. Routine monitoring of serum vancomycin concentrations: can waiting be justified. *Clin Pharm* 6: 55–58.
48. Cantú TG, Yamanaka-Yuen NA, Lietman PS. 1994. Serum vancomycin concentrations: reappraisal of their clinical value. *Clin Infect Dis* 18: 533–543.
49. Hidayat LK, Hsu DI, Quist R, Shriner KA, Wong-Beringer A. 2006. High-dose vancomycin therapy for methicillin-resistant *Staphylococcus aureus* infections. *Arch Intern Med* 166: 2138–2144.
50. Rybak MJ, Albrecht LM, Boike SC, Chandrasekar PH. 1990. Nephrotoxicity of vancomycin, alone and with an aminoglycoside. *J Antimicrob Chemother* 25: 679–687.
51. Wysocki M, Delatour F, Faurisson F, Rauss A, Pean Y, Misset, B, Thomas F, Timsit JF, Similowski T, Mentec H, Mier L, Dreyfuss D, and The Study Group. 2001. Continuous versus intermittent infusion of vancomycin in severe staphylococcus infections: Prospective multicenter randomized study. *Antimicrob Agents Chemother* 45: 2460–2467.
52. American Thoracic Society, Infectious Diseases Society of America. 2005. Guidelines for the management of adults with hospital-acquired, ventilator-associated, and healthcare-associated pneumonia. *Am J Respir Crit Care Med* 171: 388–416.
53. Byl B, Jacobs F, Wallemacq P, Rossi C, de Francquen P, Cappello M, Leal T, Thys JP. 2003. Vancomycin penetration of uninfected pleural fluid exudate after continuous or intermittent infusion. *Antimicrob Agents Chemother* 47: 2015–2017.
54. Matzke GR, McGory RW, Halstenson CE, Keane WF. 1984. Pharmacokinetics of vancomycin in patients with various degrees of renal function. *Antimicrob Agents Chemother* 25: 433–437.

55. Moellering RC, Krogstad DJ, Greenblatt DJ. 1981. Vancomycin therapy in patients with impaired renal function: a nomogram for dosage. *Ann Intern Med* 94: 343–346.
56. Garrelts JC, Peterie JD. 1988. Altered vancomycin dose versus serum concentration relationship in burn patients. *Clin Pharmacol Ther* 44: 9–13.
57. Golper TA, Noonan HM, Elzinga L, Gilbert D, Brummett R, Anderson JL, Bennett WM. 1988. Vancomycin pharmacokinetics, renal handling, and nonrenal clearance in normal human subjects. *Clin Pharmacol Ther* 43: 565–570.
58. Ducharme MP, Slaughter RL, Edwards DJ. 1994. Vancomycin pharmacokinetics in a patient population: effect of age, gender, and body weight. *Ther Drug Monit* 16: 513–518.
59. Nakayama H, Echizen H, Tanaka M, Sato M, Orii T. 2008. Reduced vancomycin clearance despite unchanged creatinine clearance in patients treated with vancomycin for longer than 4 weeks. *Ther Drug Monit* 30: 103–107.
60. Tan CC, Lee HS, Ti TY, Lee EJ. 1990. Pharmacokinetics of intravenous vancomycin in patients with end-stage renal failure. *Ther Drug Monit* 12: 29–34.
61. Draghi DC, Benton BM, Krause KM, Thronsberry C, Pillar C, Sahm DF. 2008. Comparative surveillance study of telavancin activity against recently collected gram-positive clinical isolates from across the United States. *Antimicrob Agents Chemother* 52: 2383–2388.
62. Castanheira M, Jones RN, Sader HS. 2008. Update on the in vitro activity of daptomycin tested against 6710 gram-positive cocci isolated in North America (2006). *Diagn Microbiol Infect Dis* 61: 235–239.
63. Yoshizawa S, Fourmy D, Puglisi JD. 1998. Structural origins of gentamicin antibiotic action. *EMBO J* 17: 6437–6448.
64. Liou GF, Yoshizawa S, Courvalin P, Gailmand M. 2006. Aminoglycosides resistance by Arm A mediated ribosomal 16S methylation in human bacterial pathogens. *J Mol Biol* 359: 358–364.
65. Lortholary, O, Tod M, Cohen Y, Petitjean O. 1995. Aminoglycosides. *Med Clin North Am* 79: 761–787.
66. Turnidge J. 2003. Pharmacodynamics and dosing of aminoglycosides. *Infect Dis Clin North Am* 17: 503–528.
67. Zaske DE. 1986. Aminoglycosides. In Evans WE, Schentag JJ, Juska WJ editors. *Applies Pharmacokinetics.* 2nd edition. Applied Therapeutics, Spokane, WA, pp. 331–381.
68. Buijk SE, Mouton JW, Gyssens IC, Verbrugh HA et al. 2002. Experience with a once daily dosing program of aminoglycosides in critically ill patients. *Intensive Care Med* 28: 936–942.
69. Sermet-Gaudelus I, Le Cocguic Y, Ferroni A, Clairicia M et al. 2002. Nebulized antibiotics in cystic fibrosis. *Paediatr Drugs* 4: 455–467.
70. Siber GR, Echeverria P, Smith AL, Paisley JW et al. 1975. Pharmacokinetics of gentamicin in children and in adults. *J Infect Dis* 132: 637–651.
71. Horrevorts AM, Driessen OM, Michel MF, Kerrebijin KF. 1988. Pharmacokinetics of antimicrobial drugs in cystic fibrosis. Aminoglycoside antibiotics. *Chest* 94: 120S–125S.
72. Bosso J, Townsend PL, Herbst JJ, Masten JM. 1985. Pharmacokinetics and dosage requirements of netilmicin in cystic fibrosis patients. *Antimicrob Agent Chemother* 28: 829–831.
73. McDonald NE, Anas NG, Peterson RG, Schwartz RH et al. 1983. Renal clearance of gentamicin in cystic fibrosis. *J Pediatr* 103: 985–990.
74. Mann HJ, Canafax DM, Cipolle RJ, Daniels CE et al. 1985. Increased dosage requirement of tobramycin and gentamicin for treating Pseudomonas pneumonia in patients with cystic fibrosis. *Pediatr Pulmonol* 1: 238–243.
75. Dupuis RE, Sredzienski ES. 1999. Tobramycin pharmacokinetics in patients with cystic fibrosis preceding and following lung transplantation. *Ther Drug Monit* 21: 161–165.
76. Al-Aloul M, Miller H, Alapati S, Stockton PA et al. 2005. Renal impairment in cystic fibrosis patients due to repeated intravenous aminoglycoside use. *Pediatr Pulmonol* 39: 15–20.
77. Nagai J, Takano M. 2004. Molecular aspect of renal handling of aminoglycosides and strategies for preventing nephrotoxicity. *Drug Metab Pharmacokinetic* 19: 159–170.
78. Black RE, Lau WK, Weinstein RJ, Young LS, Hewitt WL. 1976. Ototoxicity of amikacin. *Antimicrob Ag Chemother* 9: 956–961.
79. Erlason P, Lundgren A. 1964. Ototoxicity side effects following treatment with streptomycin, dihydrostreptomycin and kanamycin. *Acta Med Scand* 176: 147–163.
80. Hermida J, Tutor JC. 2006. Serum cystatin C for the prediction of glomerular filtration rate with regard to the dose adjustment of amikacin, gentamicin, tobramycin and vancomycin. *Ther Drug Monit* 28: 326–331.
81. Smelzer BD, Schwartzman MS, Bertino JS. 1988. Amikacin pharmacokinetics during continuous ambulatory peritoneal dialysis. *Antimicrob Agents Chemother* 32: 236–240.

82. Armstrong DK, Hodgeman T, Visconti JA, Reilley TE, Garner WL, Dasta JF. 1988. Hemodialysis of amikacin in critically ill patients. *Crit Care Med* 16: 517–520.
83. French MA, Cerra FB, Plaut ME, Schentag JJ. 1981. Amikacin and gentamicin accumulation pharmacokinetics and nephrotoxicity in critically ill patients. *Antimicrob Agents Chemother* 19: 147–152.
84. Regeur L, Colding H, Jessen H, Kampmann JP. 1977. Pharmacokinetics of amikacin during hemodialysis and peritoneal dialysis. *Antimicrob Agents Chemother* 11: 214–218.
85. Naber KG Westenfelder SR, Madsen PO. 1973. Pharmacokinetics of the aminoglycoside antibiotic tobramycin in humans. *Antimicrob Agents Chemother* 3: 469–473.
86. Pechere JC, Dugal R. 1976. Pharmacokinetics of intravenous administered tobramycin in normal volunteers and in renal-impaired and hemodialyzed patients. *J Infect Dis* 134 (Suppl): S118–S124.
87. Malacoff RF, Finkelstein FO, Andriole VT. 1975. Effect of peritoneal dialysis on serum levels of tobramycin and clindamycin. *Antimicrob Agents Chemother* 8: 574–580.
88. Lode H, Grunert K, Koeppe P, Langmaack H. 1976. Pharmacokinetics and clinical studies with amikacin, a new aminoglycoside antibiotic. *J Infect Dis* 134 (Suppl): S316–S321.
89. Plantier J, Forrey AW, O'Neill MA, Blair AD, Christopher TG, Cutler RE. 1976. Pharmacokinetics of amikacin in patients with normal or impaired renal function: radioenzymatic acetylation assay. *J Infect Dis* 134 (Suppl): S323–S330.
90. McHenry MC, Wagner JG, Hall PM, Vidt DG, Gavan TL. 1976. Pharmacokinetics of amikacin in patients with impaired renal function. *J Infect Dis* 134 (Suppl): S343–S347.
91. Pijck J, Hallynck T, Soep H, Baert L, DAnneels R, Boelaert J. 1976. Pharmacokinetics of amikacin in patients with renal insufficiency: relation of half-life and creatinine clearance. *J Infect Dis* 134 (Suppl): S331–S3341.
92. Bauer LA, Blouin RA. 1983. Influence of age on amikacin pharmacokinetics in patients without renal disease, comparison with gentamicin and tobramycin. *Eur J Clin Pharmacol* 24: 639–642.
93. Bauer LA, Edwards WAD, Dellinger EP, Simonowitz DA. 1983. Influence of weight on aminoglycoside pharmacokinetics in normal weight and morbidly obese patients. *Eur J Clin Pharmacol* 24: 643–647.
94. Schentag JJ, Lasezkay G, Cumbo TJ, Plaut ME, Jusko WJ. 1978. Accumulation pharmacokinetics of tobramycin. *Antimicrob Agents Chemother* 13: 649–656.
95. Bertino JS, Booker LA, Franck P, Rybicki B. 1991. Gentamicin pharmacokinetics in patients with malignancies. Antimicrob Agents Chemother 35: 1501–1503.
96. Etzel JV, Nafziger AN, Bertino JS. 1992. Variation in the pharmacokinetics of gentamicin and tobramycin in patients with pleural effusion and hypoalbuminemia. *Antimicrob Agents Chemother* 36: 679–681.
97. Zaske DE, Cipolle RJ, Rotshafer JC, Solem LD, Mosier NR, Strate RG. 1982. Gentamicin pharmacokinetics in 1,640 patients: method for control of serum concentrations. *Antimicrob Agents Chemother* 21: 407–411.
98. Zaske DE, Chin T, Kohls PR, Solem LD, Strate RG. 1991. Initial dosage regimens of gentamicin in patients with burns. *J Burn Care Rehabil* 12: 46–50.
99. Loirat P, Rohan J, Baillet A, Beaufils F, David R, Chapman A. 1978. Increase glomerular filtration rate in patients with major burns and its effect on the pharmacokinetics of tobramycin. *N Engl J Med* 299: 915–919.
100. Matzke GR, Jameson JJ, Halstenson CE. 1987. Gentamicin disposition in young and elderly patients with various degrees of renal function. *J Clin Pharmacol* 27: 216–220.
101. Gilliard V, Delvaux B, Russell K, Dubois PE. 2006. Long lasting potentiation of a single dose of rocuronium by amikacin: a case report. *Acta Anaesthesiol Belg* 57: 157–159.
102. Moore RD, Lietman PS, Smith CR. 1987. Clinical response to aminoglycoside therapy: importance of the ratio of pick concentration to minimum inhibitory concentration. *J Infect Dis* 155: 93–99.
103. Kashuba AD, Nafziger AN, Drusano GL, Bertino JS. 1999. Optimizing aminoglycoside therapy for nosocomial pneumonia caused by gram negative bacteria. *Antimicrob Agents Chemother* 43: 623–629.
104. Rhomberg PR, Jones RN, Sader HS, Fritsche TR, The MYSTIC Programme Study Group. 2004. Antimicrobial resistance rates and clonality results from the meropenem yearly susceptibility test information collection (MYSTIC) programme: report of year five (2003). *Diagn Microbiol Infect Dis* 49: 273–281.
105. Zhanel GG, DeCorby M, Nichol KA, Wierzbowski A, Baudry PJ, Karlowsky JA, Lagace-Weins P, Walkty A, Mulvey MR, Hoban DJ. 2008. The Canadian Antimicrobial Resistance Alliance. *Diagn Microbiol Infect Dis* 62: 67–80.
106. Rhomberg PR, Jones RN, Sader HS, The MYSTIC Programme (US) Study Group. 2004. Results from the meropenem yearly susceptibility test information collections (MYSTIC) programme: report of the 2001 data from 15 United States medical centers. *Int J Antimicrob Agents* 23: 52–59.

107. Reinert RR, Low DE, Rossi F, Zhang X, Wattal C, Dowzicky MJ. 2007. Antimicrobial susceptibility among organisms from the Asia/Pacific Rim, Europe, and Latin and North America collected as part of TEST and the *in vitro* activity of tigecycline. *J Antimicrob Chemother* 60: 1018–1029.
108. McCormack JP, Jewesson PJ. 1992. A critical reevaluation of the "therapeutic range" of aminoglycosides. *Clin Infect Dis* 14: 320–339.
109. Drusano GL, Ambrose PG, Bhavnani SM, Bertino JS, Nafzinger AN, Louie A. 2007. Back to the future: using aminoglycosides again and how to dose them optimally. *Clin Infect Dis* 45: 753–760.
110. Moore RD, Leitman PS, Smith CR. 1987. Clinical response to aminoglycoside therapy: Importance of the ratio of peak concentration to minimal inhibitory concentration. *J Infect Dis* 155: 93–99.
111. Sawchuk RJ, Zaske DE, Cipolle RJ, Wargin WA, Strate RG. 1977. Kinetic model for gentamicin dosing with the use of individual patient parameters. *Clin Pharmacol Ther* 21: 362–369.
112. Kashuba ADM, Nafziger AN, Drusano GL, Bertino JS. 1999. Optimizing aminoglycoside therapy for nosocomial pneumonia caused by gram-negative bacteria. *Antimicrob Agents Chemother* 43: 623–629.
113. Zaske DE, Bootman JL, Solem LB, Strate RG.. 1982. Increased burn patient survival with individualized dosages of gentamicin. *Surgery* 91: 142–149.
114. Freeman CD, Nicolau DP, Belliveau PB, Nightingale CH. 1997. One-daily dosing of aminoglycosides: review and recommendations for clinical practice. *J Antimicrob Chemother* 39: 677–686.
115. Nicolau DP, Freeman CD, Belliveau PP, Nightingale CH, Ross JW, Quintiliani R. 1995. Experience with a once-daily aminoglycoside program administered to 2,184 patients. *Antimicrob Agents Chemother* 39: 650–655.
116. Smyth A, Tan KHV, Hyman-Taylor P, Mulheran M, Lewis S, Stableforth D, Know A, for the TOPIC Study Group. 2005. Once versus three-times daily regimens of tobramycin for pulmonary exacerbations of cystic fibrosis—The TOPIC study: a randomized controlled trial. *Lancet* 365: 573–578.
117. Ariano RE, Selenitsky SA, Kassum DA. 2008. Aminoglycoside-induced vestibular injury: maintaining a sense of balance. *Ann Pharmacother* 42: 1282–1289.

17 Chromatographic Methods for Analysis of Antibiotics

Ronald W. McLawhon
University of California, San Diego, School of Medicine

CONTENTS

17.1 INTRODUCTION

Antibiotics represent a diverse group of chemotherapeutic agents with activity against microorganisms such as bacteria, fungi or protozoa. This chapter will focus primarily on the current methods to analyze drugs that are used to treat bacterial infections. Antibacterial antibiotics may be categorized [1–3] based on their target specificity: narrow-spectrum antibiotics target particular types of bacteria, such as gram-negative or gram-positive bacteria, while broad-spectrum antibiotics affect a wide range of bacteria. In addition, antibiotics can be broadly classified as either bactericidal or bacteriostatic, based on their mechanism of action [1,4]. Bactericidal agents typically kill bacteria directly, whereas bacteriostatic agents prevent cell growth and division, although there can be considerable overlap these classifications depending on the drug and organism. Typically, minimum inhibitory concentration (MIC) and minimum bactericidal concentration are used to measure in vitro activity antimicrobial and is an excellent indicator of antimicrobial potency [2]. As such, antibiotics can be further characterized as either concentration-dependent (for which achieving a large postdose concentration to MIC ratio appears important) or concentration-independent/time-dependent (where efficacy is related to maintaining the overall concentration above the MIC). Therapeutic ranges and dosage regimen can be based theoretically on its known pharmacokinetics and pharmacodynamics [2,3–6]; thus, in some clinical situations, direct monitoring of drug concentrations within serum, plasma, or other body fluids may be warranted.

In general, antibiotics that target the bacterial cell wall and membrane, such as penicillins, cephalosporins, or vancomycin, or interfere with essential bacterial enzymes, such as the quinolones and sulfonamides, are usually bactericidal in nature. In contrast, those which target protein synthesis, such as the macrolides and tetracycline, tend to have bacteriostatic actions. Figure 17.1 shows the general chemical structures of representative antibiotics from all major classes currently prescribed.

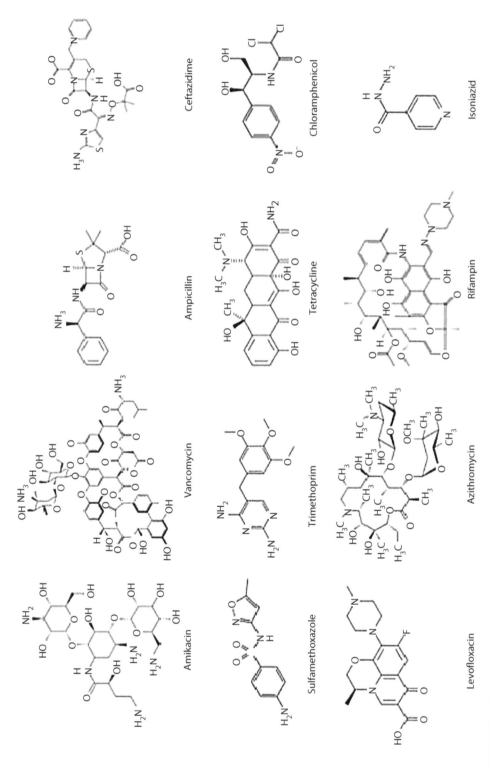

FIGURE 17.1 Chemical structures of representative major classes of antibiotics used in current medical practice.

Side effects and toxicity of antibiotic therapy [1,6,7] may range from fever nausea, vomiting and diarrhea to severe allergic reactions. In addition, serious and irreversible complications, such as nephrotoxicity and ototoxicity, can be observed with drugs like aminoglycosides and vancomycin. When these agents are used, peak and trough concentrations should be closely monitored due to their narrow therapeutic index and serious risks of toxicity [5,7]. Other antibiotics are rarely measured in routine clinical practice, due to wider therapeutic indices and lower toxicity risks and complications. However, these risks can increase considerably in certain clinical situations (e.g., decreased renal clearance with kidney failure) and therapeutic monitoring may be beneficial.

Currently, therapeutic drug monitoring of antibiotic concentrations in serum, plasma, or other body fluids may be performed to assess optimal therapy, toxicity, and patient compliance [5,7,8]. Aminoglycosides and vancomycin are most frequently performed in today's clinical laboratories, due to the need for close monitoring and widespread availability and application of commercially available immunoassays. Most other antibiotics require chromatographic methods—either gas liquid chromatography (GC) with or without mass spectrometry, high performance liquid chromatography (HPLC), or liquid chromatography/mass spectrometry (LC/MS) for quantitation of drug concentrations in serum or plasma. This chapter will review chromatographic techniques currently employed in the analyses of a wide range of antimicrobial agents used in medical practice.

17.2 AMINOGLYCOSIDES AND VANCOMYCIN

Therapeutic monitoring of antibiotics, such as aminoglycosides and vancomycin in serum or plasma, are well established in current medical practice [5,7,8]. Aminoglycoside antibiotics, such as gentamicin, amikacin, and tobramycin are polycationic inhibitors of the 30s ribosomal subunit that interferes with protein synthesis and disrupts cell membrane transport and cell permeability. These drugs are most commonly used [1] for the treatment of life threatening systemic infections with gram-negative bacilli, such as *Escherichia coli, Klebsiella pneumoniae, Proteus mirabilis,* and *Pseudomonas aeruginosa.* Other aminoglycosides, such as streptomycin and kanamycin, have been shown to be effective in the treatment of mycobacterial infections and will be discussed briefly elsewhere in this chapter.

Vancomycin is a tricyclic glycopeptide that interferes with cell well biosynthesis, which has also proven effective against both gram-negative and gram-cocci and currently is widely used to treat both sepsis and endocarditis [1]. In recent years, vancomycin has received consideration attention and has become the primary drug of choice against the growing problem of community and hospital acquired methicillin-resistant *Staphylococcus aureus* (MRSA).

Due to poor absorption, variable distribution and narrow therapeutic index, quantitative measurement of both trough and peak concentrations of bacteriocidal agents in these classes are routinely performed [5–7] to assess both therapeutic benefit and toxicity—most notably, nephrotoxicity (acute tubular necrosis) and ototoxicity (long-term vestibular and sensory damage). Reliable, inexpensive and easy to perform homogeneous and heterogeneous immunoassays [5,7,8] are commercially available in a variety of different formats which are readily adapted to existing instrumentation (including high throughput, random access, automated chemistry and immunoassay analyzers).

While HPLC methods for separation and quantitation of aminoglycosides and vancomycin have been developed [8,9], the availability of these sensitive and precise immunoassays have largely supplanted chromatographic methods as they rarely offer any additional analytical and clinical advantages for serum and plasma measurements in most patients. However, HPLC and, more recently, LC/MS applications are most widely used when analysis is required on a particular biological matrix of the specimen for which immunoassay is inappropriate or unsuitable, including human body fluid and tissue extracts as well as environmental and agricultural applications [8]. In addition, certain analytical biases and potential inaccuracies have been reported with some immunoassay methods in specific clinical situations, and chromatographic separation may be preferred as the method of choice to resolve such diagnostic dilemmas [10]. In renally impaired patients, the fluorescence polarization immunoassay (FPIA, Abbott Laboratories, Abbott Park, IL) for vancomycin may overestimate vancomycin concentration due to cross-reactivity of vancomycin crystalline degradation product (CDP-1 which is inactive) because this assay uses a polyclonal antibody against vancomycin. However, enzyme multiplied immunoassay techniques (EMIT) assay for vancomycin which uses a monoclonal antibody against vancomycin is not affected by CDP-1 [11].

Most HPLC methods for aminoglycosides and vancomycin use reverse phase, ion pair, ion exchange, and normal phase separation protocols, and employ either ultraviolet or fluorescent detection methods [8,9,11–16]. Additionally, some type of precolumn derivatization [12,13,16] is required which is labor-intensive and time consuming, although some methods do not require this step [9,17–20]. Most HPLC methods described in the literature also have excellent imprecision with coefficient of variation (CVs) in the range of 5–9% and limits of detection below 0.1 μg/mL.

Gentamicin, an aminoglycoside is not a single molecule but a complex of three major (C_1, C_{1a} and C_2) and several minor components Figure 17.2). In addition, the C_2 component is a mixture of stereoisomers. Therefore, immunoassay methods can measure total gentamicin concentration in serum or plasma but are not capable of measuring individual components. Animal data indicates that different components of gentamicin differ in their toxicities. Because of toxicity of gentamicin, therapeutic drug monitoring is recommended. Isoherranen and Soback described a HPLC protocol for determination of three major (C_1, C_{1a}, and C_2) components of gentamicin in plasma and urine [16]. Figure 17.3 shows a representative chromatogram illustrating quantitating gentamicin C_1, C_{1a}, and C_2 fractions from dog's plasma 2 h after an intravenous bolus of gentamicin. In this protocol gentamicin C_1, C_{1a}, and C_2 were determined as their 2 ,4-dinitrophenyl derivatives using a mobile phase of 680 mL/L acetonitrile-320 mL/L Tris buffer (8.3 mmol/L, titrated to pH 7.0 with HCl) at a flow rate 1.2 mL/min, on a Hewlett-Packard H-P 1100 low-pressure mixing gradient HPLC equipped with a diode array ultraviolet-visible detector, autosampler, and column oven. A Symmetry C18 reversed-phase column (100 3 4.6 mm; 3.5 mm particle size; Waters Corporation) connected to a C18 pre-column was used for separation. The injection volume was 20 μL, the column temperature was 25°C, and the chromatographic eluent was monitored at 365 nm wavelength. The authors also characterized gentamicin preparation by separating major components using silica column and components were further characterized by nuclear magnetic resonance spectroscopy and ion trap mass spectrometry with atmospheric pressure chemical ionization interface. The mass spectrum of C_1 showed [M+H] peak at m/z 478 Figure 17.4). The other components of gentamicin also showed distinct protonated molecular ion peak (m/z 450 and m/z 464 for C_{1a} and C_2 respectively) [16].

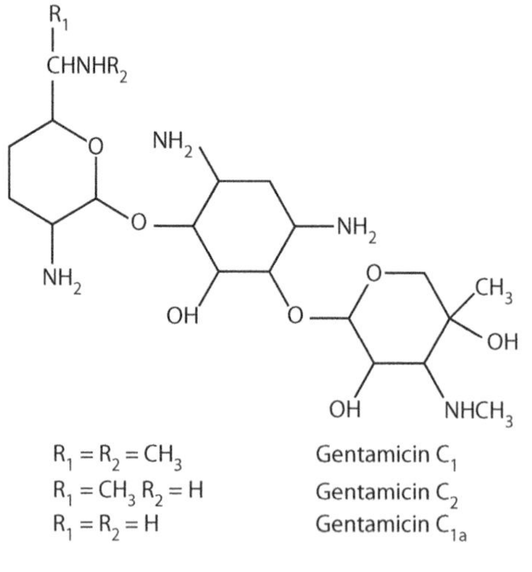

$R_1 = R_2 = CH_3$	Gentamicin C_1
$R_1 = CH_3 R_2 = H$	Gentamicin C_2
$R_1 = R_2 = H$	Gentamicin C_{1a}

FIGURE 17.2 Chemical structures of gentamicins C1, C1a, and C2. (From Isoherranen N, Soback S, *Clin chem,* 46, 837–842, 2000. Copyright © 2000 American Association for Clinical Chemistry. Reprinted with permision.)

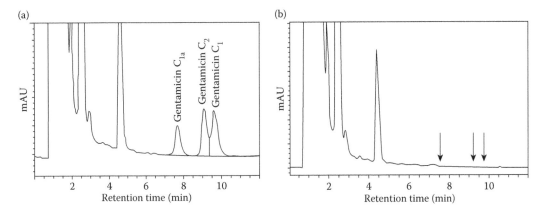

FIGURE 17.3 Representative chromatograms of gentamicin from dog plasma two hours after an intravenous bolus of gentamicin representing 0.39 mg/L C1a, 1.36 mg/L C2, and 0.74 mg/L C1 (a), and chromatogram of blank plasma (b). (From Isoherranen N, Soback S, *Clin chem,* 46, 837–842, 2000. Copyright © 2000 American Association for Clinical Chemistry. Reprinted with permission.)

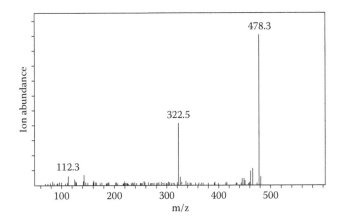

FIGURE 17.4 Mass spectrum of gentamicin C1. (From Isoherranen N, Soback S, *Clin chem,* 46, 837–842, 2000. Copyright © 2000 American Association for Clinical Chemistry. Reprinted with permission.)

Liquid chromatography-tandem mass spectrometry methods have been reported [21–23] in recent years for aminoglycosides and vancomycin, which demonstrate enhanced sensitivity, linearity, imprecision, and accuracy compared to either immunoassay or conventional HPLC. These LC/MS applications can be used for a wide range of biological matrices and eliminates the need for laborious and time consuming pretreatment and derivatization steps. For example, Zhang et al. reported a protocol for determination of vancomycin in serum by liquid chromatography with high resolution full scan mass spectrometry using electrospray ionization. The authors used atenolol as the internal standard and extracted vancomycin (after adding internal standard to the specimen) using strong cation exchange solid phase extraction followed by chromatographic analysis using a C-8 column, C-18 guard column and a mobile phase composition of 0.15 formic acid and acetonitrile (9:1 by vol). The temperature of the column was maintained at 40°C. The mass spectrometer was operated in full scan mode (*m/z* 200–800 amu). A strong molecular ion at *m/z* 267.17 was observed for atenolol, but for vancomycin instead of a molecular peak (molecular weight 1499.22), a group of ions was observed at *m/z* 725.72 [22]. Although LC/MS methods are more precise and do not require derivatization, these methods are adopted slowly in clinical laboratories due to the investment costs associated with the acquisition of instrumentation and operation compared to other available methods HPLC-UV methods.

17.3   BETA-LACTAM ANTIBIOTICS (PENICILLINS AND CEPHALOSPORINS)

Penicillins and cephalosporins are part of a broad classes of antimicrobial agents know as beta-lactam antibiotics [1] and are named as such because they share a beta-lactam ring nucleus as part of their core molecular structure. They are currently the most widely-used group of antibiotics available, with penicillin being one of the oldest commercially available antibiotics that revolutionized the management of infectious diseases during the 1930–1940s. Penicillins and cephalosporins [1,4] are bactericidal and have the same mode of action, namely to disrupt the synthesis of the peptidoglycan layer of bacterial cell walls and cell wall structural integrity. Beta-lactam antibiotics interfere with the final transpeptidation step and competitively inhibit crosslinking of peptidoglycan.

Penicillins, such as Penicillin G, Penicillin V, amoxicillin, nafcillin and ampicillin, are used for treatment of gram-positive infections [1,5,7] such as Staphylococcus species, *Streptococcus pneumoniae*, beta-hemolytic strains of Streptococcus, and *Enterococcus faecalis*. They may be used alone or in preparations that include beta-lactamase inhibitors, such as clavulanic acid, tazobactam, sulbactam, for treatment of penicillin-resistant organisms.

Cephalosporins are indicated for the prophylaxis and treatment of infections caused by bacteria susceptible to this particular form of antibiotic. Several generations (first through fifth) of cephalosporin antibiotics have now been developed and are widely prescribed, with an increasingly broader spectrum of action against both gram-negative and gram-positive organisms [1]. First-generation cephalosporins (e.g., cephazolin) are predominantly active against gram-positive bacteria, and successive generations have increased activity against gram-negative bacteria (albeit often with reduced activity against gram-positive organisms). Later generations of cephalosporins, such as cefaclor, ceftazidime, ceftriaxone, and cefazolin are effective against organisms including *Proteus mirabilis*, Klebsiella species, *Enterobacter aerogenes*, *Haemophilus influenzae,* and *Pseudomonas aeruginosa*. Adverse drug reactions [1] with beta-lactam antibiotics include diarrhea, nausea, rash, urticaria fever, vomiting, erythema, and dermatitis. Allergic hypersensitivity occurs in up to 10% patients, with anaphylaxis as a rare complication (most frequently with penicillins).

Because beta-lactam antibiotics (both penicillins and cephalosporins) have wide therapeutic indices and dose-dependent toxicity, routine therapeutic drug monitoring is not indicated in all patients [5–7,25]. Monitoring adequacy of blood concentration may be beneficial especially in patients with kidney failure, where renal clearance of the drug is compromised or to assess overall patience compliance. In general, antibiotic levels for these will need to be above a certain minimum concentration (e.g., 3 μg/mL), but no additional benefit will be derived with concentrations even slightly above that range (e.g., 6–9 μg/mL), depending on the drug used.

Currently, the common methods used in clinical and reference laboratories employ HPLC techniques, as no immunoassay is commercially available. These methods [24–28] use simple liquid-liquid extraction in combination with reversed phase HPLC and employ either ultraviolet or fluorescent (with postcolumn derivatization) techniques for detection. Annesley et al. described simultaneous determination of penicillin and cephalosporin antibiotics in human serum using HPLC, after acidification of specimen, followed by extraction of drugs along with internal standard (cephalothin as the internal standard for most analysis but when cefoperazone or cephalothin were assayed, cefazolin was used as the internal standard) using chloroform/butanol (3:1 by vol). Using gradient mobile phase (solution A; 10 mmol/L ammonium acetate at pH 4.2 in distilled water and solution B: 10 mmol/L ammonium acetate at pH 4.2 in an equivolume mixture of methanol and water), the authors were able to analyze a number of antibiotics (carbenicillin, cefazolin, cephalothin, cefaclor, cefoperazone, cefotaxime, cefamandole, nafcillin, moxalactam, piperacillin, and ticarcillin). The elution of peaks was monitored at 250 nm wavelength [29]. All these methods are robust with analytical detection down to 0.1 μg/mL, excellent recovery and accuracy, and between day imprecision of <7%.

Newer LC/MS methods with electrospray ionization [30–33] have been developed not only to quantitate various penicillins and cephalosporins in serum or plasma, but can also applications for a wide range of fluids including breast milk and can provide reliable and reproducible analysis of drug concentrations in tissue extracts. LC/MS analysis of beta-lactam antibiotics is extremely powerful, resolving multiple drugs in a single analytical run, with limits of quantitation reported down to 0.1 ng/mL and improved precision with CVs of 3%.

17.4 SULFONAMIDES AND TRIMETHOPRIM

Sulfonamides (sometimes called simply sulfa drugs) are synthetic antimicrobial agents that contain the sulfonamide group. Sulfa drugs, along with penicillin, are among the oldest and, historically, most widely prescribed chemotherapeutic agents for the treatment of infectious diseases. This large and diverse group of antimicrobial agents (which include sulfamethoxazole, sulfisoxazole, sulfadiazine, and many others) act as competitive inhibitors of dihydropteroic synthetase, a key enzymatic key step in folate synthesis [1,7]. Folate is required for nucleic acids (DNA and RNA) synthesis and, as such, sulfonamides block normal cell division and exhibit a bacteriostatic rather than bactericidal effect [1,4].

Sulfonamides are most frequently used in the prophylaxis and treatment of urinary tract infections and, in some cases (sulfapyridine), have been found effective in the treatment of dermatitis herpetiformis and inflammatory bowel disease [1,7]. The spectrums of activity of these drugs are similar for all. Susceptible organisms include group A streptococcus, *Streptococcus pneumoniae*, *Haemophilus influenzae*, *Haemophilus ducreyi*, *Vibrio cholerae*, *Chlamydia trachomatis*, some strains of *Bacillus anthracis* and *Corynebacterium diphtheriae*, and Brucella, Yersinia, Nocardia, and Actinomyces species.

Trimethoprim is another bacteriostatic antibiotic, mainly used in the prophylaxis and treatment of urinary tract infections that acts by interfering with the action of bacterial dihydrofolate reductase [1]. By inhibiting synthesis of tetrahydrofolic acid, it also deprives nucleotides necessary for DNA replication and cell division. Although it may be used as a monotherapy, trimethoprim has been commonly used in prescription combination (Bactrim, Septra) with the sulfonamide antibiotic, sulfamethoxazole. This cotrimoxazole therapy results in an in a synergistic antibacterial effect by inhibiting successive steps in the pathway of folate synthesis. When used in conjunction with sulfamethoxazole, trimethoprim has proven effective for treatment of infections due to chlamydia, susceptible strains of *Enterobacteriaceae* species such as *Escherichia coli*, Klebsiella species, *Morganella morganii*, *Proteus mirabilis, and Proteus vulgaris*, in addition to gram-positive cocci such as *Staphylococcus pyogenes*, *Streptococcus pyogenes*, *Streptococcus pneumoniae*, and *Streptococci viridans*.

In general, sulfonamides do not distribute at high concentrations [6,7] outside the serum, but are effective against infections located in deep tissue sites because high serum concentrations can be achieved relatively safely. Toxicity is expressed as renal disease characterized by formation of sulfonamide crystals [1,7] in the kidney resulting in calculi development, and is concentration dependent (usually with prolonged serum concentrations in excess of 125 μg/mL). Thus, the primary indication for therapeutic monitoring is to assess therapeutic dosing to prevent crystal formation, particularly in patients with renal disease. Some drugs in this class, like sulfapyridine, can also cause agranulocytosis and leukopenia. Trimethoprim, when used as monotherapy or cotrimoxazole therapy, has a wide therapeutic index and dose-dependent toxicity [1,5]. Accordingly, routine drug monitoring is not indicated in all patients. Trimethoprim also accumulates in patients with renal failure.

The most commonly used method for assaying sulfonamides, either alone or in combination with trimethoprim, is HPLC [34,35]. Following simple protein precipitation of serum or plasma with acetonitrile and centrifugation, the supernatant is dried and reconstituted with mobile phase and analyzed by HPLC with UV detection [32]. An internal standard (appropriate for each sulfa drug) is added to the specimen prior to analysis to account for losses during precipitation and chromatography. More recently, a sold phase extraction LC/MS method has been developed for simultaneous quantitation of sulfonamides and trimethoprim that is six-times more sensitive than conventional HPLC-UV and has broader applications for use a wide range of biological fluids [35]. In this study, comparing HPLC-UV protocol for determination of sulfamethoxazole and trimethoprim in biological fluids with liquid chromatography coupled with tandem mass spectrometry, the authors used benznidazole as the internal standard. For HPL-UV analysis, the authors analyzed these drugs and internal standard after solid phase extraction from human plasma using reverse phase C-18 column and the isocratic mobile phase composition of 20 mM sodium hydrogen phosphate buffer (adjusted to pH 3.0 with phosphoric acid) and acetonitrile (89:11 by vol) and the column temperature was maintained at 40°C. The elution of peaks was detected with photodiode array ultraviolet detector at 230 nm wavelength. For liquid chromatography combined with tandem mass spectrometric analysis, the isocratic mobile phase composition was acetonitrile/water (50:50 by vol) and the reverse phase C-18 column was kept at the room temperature. The mass spectrometer was operated in positive ionization mode and positive ion electrospray mass spectra of sulfamethoxazole, trimethoprim, and the internal standard all produced protonated molecular ions [M+H, parent ion] at m/z 254, 291, and 261, respectively. The base peak of sulfamethoxazole, trimethoprim, and the internal standard as observed from their respective daughter ion spectra were at m/z 108, 230 and 91 [35].

17.5   CHLORAMPHENICOL AND TETRACYCLINE

Chloramphenicol and tetracycline are bactericidal agents that inhibit protein synthesis [1,7]. Chloramphenicol acts by binding to the 50S ribosomal subunit of bacteria mRNA and inhibits protein synthesis in prokaryotic organisms. In contrast, tetracycline (and related drugs such as doxycycline) inhibits the action of the prokaryotic 30S ribosome, by binding the 16S rRNA, thereby, blocking the aminoacyl-tRNA. In eukaryotic cells, toxicity of tetracycline and its analogs may be related to inactivation of mitochondrial 30S ribosomes.

Use of chloramphenicol and drugs in the tetracycline family are dependent on its relative toxicity against the microorganism versus the host [1,5–7]. Chloramphenicol is used [1,7] against gram-negative bacteria such as *Haemophilus influenzae, Neisseria meningitidis, Neisseria gonorrhoeae, Salmonella typhi,* Brucella species, *Bordetella pertussis, Vibrio cholerae,* and Shigella. Tetracycline's primary use is now limited for the treatment of acne vulgaris and rosacea. In contrast, doxycycline is frequently used to treat chronic prostatitis, sinusitis, syphilis, chlamydia, pelvic inflammatory disease, acne, and rosacea, as well as *Yersinia pestis* (the infectious agent of bubonic plague), Lyme disease, ehrlichiosis, and Rocky Mountain spotted fever.

Host toxicity displayed after chloramphenicol therapy [1,7] includes blood dyscrasias and cardiovascular collapse; both show a modest relationship to blood concentration [2,6]. Anemia, characterized by maturation arrest in the marrow is seen with serum concentrations in excess of 25 μg/mL. Cardiovascular collapse, which occurs primarily in newborns, has been observed with serum chloramphenicol concentrations >50 μg/mL. Tetracycline and doxycycline adverse side effects are skin photosensitivity, drug-induced lupus, and hepatitis, tinnitus, and staining of developing teeth [1].

The primary goal of therapeutic monitoring of both of these antibiotics is assess adequacy of blood concentrations while balancing potential risks of host toxicity. These drugs are currently only rarely monitored using reversed phase HPLC techniques using simple organic extraction in the presence of an internal standard and ultraviolet detection [36,37]. A solid phase LC/MS method for separation and quantitation various tetracycline analogs, but has largely been applied to environmental monitoring [38] and has not been proven for clinical applications.

17.6 QUINOLONES

Quinolones, also known as fluoroquinolones, are a group of broad-spectrum bactericidal antibiotics that are active against both gram-positive and gram-negative bacteria [1]. Drugs in this group include levofloxacin and ciprofloxacin. These agents function by inhibiting DNA gyrase, a type II topoisomerase, and topoisomerase, which is an enzyme necessary to separate replicated DNA and, thereby, interferes with cell division. Levofloxacin and ciprofloxacin are effective [1] in treating infections (particularly tenacious and recurring respiratory tract infections) caused by gram-positive pathogens (*Streptococcus pneumoniae* and *Streptococcus pyogeneses* and some activity against *Staphylococcus aureus* and *Enterococcus faecalis*), gram-negative pathogens (*Escherichia coli, Haemophilus influenzae, Moraxella catarrhalis, Klebsiella pneumoniae,* and *Pseudomonas aeruginosa*), and atypical pathogens (*Chlamydia pneumoniae, Mycoplasma pneumoniae,* and *Legionella pneumophila*).

Toxicities [1] may include diarrhea, gastrointestinal upset, allergic reactions, and phototoxicity. Central nervous system (CNS) effects such as agitation, restlessness, anxiety, and nightmares can also occur. QT prolongation has also been observed and rare cases of *torsades de pointes*, an uncommon type of ventricular tachycardia, have been reported. Achilles tendon rupture due to fluoroquinolone use is typically associated with renal failure. Current methods for quantitation of quinolones in serum and plasma involve simple liquid-liquid extraction techniques followed by HPLC-UV analysis. These methods [39,40] typically span the clinically relevant range of 10–1000 ng/mL. Kamberi et al. analyzed ciprofloxacin in human plasma and urine using HPLC and UV detection using lomefloxacin as the internal standard. For analysis of plasma sample, acetonitrile was used for protein precipitation and extraction of ciprofloxacin. After centrifugation, clear supernatant was dried under nitrogen at 500°C and residue was reconstituted with internal standard and 200 µl of 50 mL/L of acetic acid followed by analysis using C-18 reverse phase column and a mobile phase composition of 50 mL/L acetic acid/acetonitrile/methanol (90:5:5 by volume) and elution of peaks was monitored at 280 nm wavelength [40]. In Figure 17.5, representative chromatograms of plasma and urine specimens analyzed for ciprofloxacin using this protocol are shown.

17.7 MACROLIDES

The macrolides are a unique class of antibiotics whose activity stems from the presence of a macrolide ring, a large macrocyclic lactone ring to which one or more deoxysugar, usually cladinose and desosamine, may be attached. Like chloramphenicol, the site of action of these antimicrobial agents is inhibiting bacterial protein biosynthesis by binding reversibly to the subunit 50S of the bacterial ribosome and preventing translocation of peptidyl tRNA [1]. Drugs in this class are primarily bacteriostatic, but can also be bacteriocidal in high concentrations. Erythromycin was one of the first drugs of this type used in clinical practice, but subsequent broader spectrum drugs, such as clarithromycin and azithromycin, have been developed more recently and are widely utilized.

Macrolide antibiotics are most frequently used to treat infections of the upper and lower respiratory tract and skin and soft tissue infections [1]. The antimicrobial spectrum of macrolides is broader than that of penicillins (and comparable to many late generation cephalosporins); therefore, macrolide antibiotics have been successfully used as a substitute in treating patients with known penicillin allergy. They are effective against beta-hemolytic streptococci, pneumococci, staphylococci, and enterococci, in addition to many atypical respiratory pathogens such as *Mycoplasma pneumoniae* and *Legionella pneumophila*. Macrolides have also used to treat chlamydia, syphilis, acne, gonorrhea, and nongonococcal cystitis. Many have also proven effective against some types of mycobacterial and rickettsial infections.

Adverse reactions with macrolide antibiotics are relatively rare, and most do not require discontinuance of drug or routine therapeutic monitoring of drug concentrations in serum or plasma

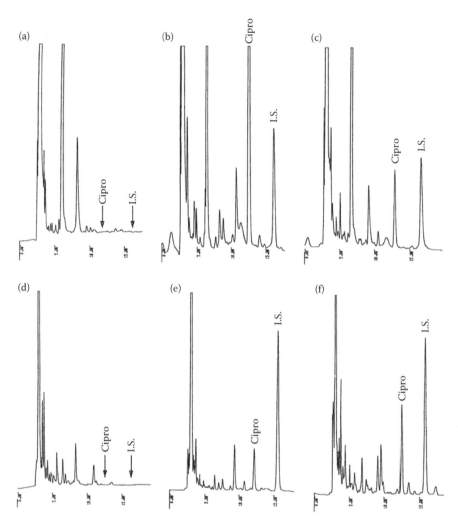

FIGURE 17.5 Representative chromatograms of (a) plasma blank, (b) plasma standard (0.5 mg/L), (c) plasma sample collected 6 hours after a 200-mg oral dose of ciprofloxacin, (d) urine blank, (e) urine standard (5 mg/L), and (f) urine sample collected 24 h after a 200-mg oral dose of ciprofloxacin. (From Kamberi M, Tsutsumi K, Kotegawa T, Nakamura K, Nakano S, *Clin Chem,* 44: 1251–1255, 1998. Copyright © 1998 American Association for Clinical Chemistry. Reprinted with permission.)

[1,5]. Most common side-effects involve gastrointestinal symptoms (diarrhea, nausea, abdominal pain, and vomiting) and occasional facial swelling. Less common side-effects include headaches, dizziness, nervousness, rashes, and alteration in senses of smell and taste. Serious allergic and dermatologic reactions have been reported with some drugs in this class, with the most serious and potentially life-threatening cases being toxic epidermal necrolysis and Stevens–Johnson syndrome (clarithromycin).

Macrolide antibiotics, such as erythromycin, azithromycin, and clarithromycin, can be readily analyzed using HPLC techniques with solid phase or liquid–liquid extraction [41–43]. Ultraviolet, electrochemical, and fluorescence (following derivatization with agents like 9-fluorenylmethyl chloroformate) detection methods have been used successfully. Sensitive methods using liquid chromatography-tandem mass spectrometry have also been introduced in recent years [43,44], which eliminates time consuming pretreatment and derivatization steps and show greater reproducibility and less interferences than the conventional HPLC methods.

17.8 ANTIMYCOBACTERIAL AGENTS

Antimycobacterial, or antituberculosis, agents represent a diverse group of compounds, when used alone or in combination, to treat *Mycobacterium* infections, including tuberculosis and leprosy. Several drugs currently fall into this broad category [1,5], including rifampin, isoniazid, ethambutol, streptomycin, and kanamycin. Each of these agents has different and unique biological mechanisms of biological actions [1]. Rifampin inhibits DNA-dependent RNA polymerase in bacterial cells by binding its beta-subunit and, thus, prevents RNA transcription and subsequent translation to proteins. Both isoniazid and ethambutol exert their bacteriostatic effects, by interfering with the synthesis of the mycobacterial cell wall. Isoniazid is actually a probiotic drug that must be activated by bacterial catalase to inhibits the synthesis of mycolic acid, whereas ethambutol inhibits the enzyme, arabinosyl transferase; both are essential for successful formation of the mycolic acid-peptidoglycan complex of the cell wall, and treatment with either of these drugs has the net effect of increasing cell permeability. Streptomycin and kanamycin are aminoglycoside antibiotics that interfere with protein synthesis and alter cell membrane transport and increase overall cell permeability as well.

Currently, antimycobacterial agents are most commonly prescribed [1] as multidrug combinations due to the emergence of tuberculosis resistance, which is often seen as a consequence of poor patient compliance and incomplete treatment of active infections during the long course of most therapeutic regimens. The most serious adverse and toxic side effects have been observed [1,5] with rifampin and isoniazid—most notably, hepatitis and jaundice (with liver failure in severe cases) and sideroblastic anemia. Other milder side effects include flushing, pruritus, rash, redness and watering of eyes, as well as gastrointestinal and CNS disturbances, and general flu-like symptoms. As with observed with most other bacteriostatic agents, toxicity with these drugs is concentration independent.

Antimycobacterial agents are generally monitored [45–50] using reversed phased HPLC, with no pretreatment following deproteinization of serum or plasma, or by gas chromatography/mass spectometry (GC/MS) techniques. Both methods appear to provide acceptable reproducibility, accuracy, and limits of quantitation. For example LoDico et al. described a GC/MS analysis of isoniazid after extraction followed by derivatization with trifluoroacetic anhydride in a person died of isoniazid overdose. The concentration of isoniazid in heart blood, subclavian blood, urine and bile were 43 mg/L, 94 mg/L, 470 mg/L, and 900 mg/L, respectively while the liver and kidney levels were 650 mg/kg and 110 mg/kg, respectively [47]. Um et al. determined low serum concentrations of antituberculosis drugs (isoniazid, rifampicin, ethambutol, pyrazinamide and two metabolites aetyl-isonizid and 25-desacetyl rifampicin) in human serum using liquid chromatography coupled with tandem mass spectrometry because low levels of these drugs have been associated with treatment failures. Interestingly, among 69 patients studied, the prevalence of a low 2 h serum concentration of at least one antituberculosis drug was 46.4%. The authors concluded that low levels of antituberculosis drugs among patients suffering from tuberculosis are common and it may be necessary to optimize drug dosages with therapeutic drug monitoring especially in patients with an inadequate clinical response [50].

17.9 CONCLUSIONS

Therapeutic monitoring of antibiotic concentrations in blood and other body fluids is only rarely indicated due to the efficacy and clinical safety of most commonly prescribed antimicrobial agents. Notably, exceptions include the aminoglycosides and vancomycin, which have narrow therapeutic indices and drug levels have to be closely followed to optimize therapy and to prevent the serious and irreversible complications of nephrotoxicity and ototoxicity. In the majority of patients, immunoassays will suffice, reserving more specific chromatographic techniques for special clinical situations or unique biological matrices. The majority of other antibiotics have wider therapeutic margins and lower toxicity risks as the dosages prescribed and do not require routine monitoring of drug concentrations in serum or plasma for patient management. When other clinical conditions warrant (e.g., kidney failure, crystalluria, etc), a wide range of antibiotics can be easily and reliably monitored using established chromatographic techniques—most commonly, HPLC and, more recently, liquid chromatography coupled with tandem mass spectrometry. In the majority of cases, chromatography is used to optimize drug concentrations and dosing while balancing potential risks of toxicity and adverse side effects. All methods appear to perform acceptably both analytically and clinically, although newer LC/MS methods may have a distinct advantage from a sensitivity standpoint when applied to other body fluid and tissue specimens where concentrations may be significantly lower than found in human serum or plasma.

REFERENCES

1. Section VIII. Chemotherapy of microbial diseases. In: *Goodman & Gilman's The Pharmacological Basis of Therapeutics*, 11th Edition (Brunton L, Lazo J, Parker K, eds). McGraw-Hill Professional, New York, NY, 1141–1294.
2. Dawson SJ, Reeves DS. 1997. Therapeutic monitoring, the concentration-effect relationship and impact on the clinical efficacy of antibiotic agents. *J Chemother* 9(Suppl1): 84–92.
3. Spanu T, Santangelo R, Andreotti F, Cascio GL, Velardi G, Fadda G. 2004. Antibiotic therapy for severe bacterial infections: correlation between the inhibitory quotient and outcome. *Int J Antimicrob Agents* 23: 120–128.
4. Rhee KY, Gardiner DF. 2004. Clinical relevance of bacteriostatic versus bactericidal activity in the treatment of gram-positive bacterial infections. *Clin Infec Dis* 39: 755–756.
5. Klein RD, Edberg SC. 2005. Applications, significance of, and methods for the measurement of antimicrobial concentrations in human body fluids. In: *Antibiotics in Laboratory Medicine*, 5th Edition (Lorian, V, ed). Lippincott Williams & Wilkins, Philadelphia, PA, 290–364.
6. Burton ME, Shaw LM, Schentag JJ, Evans WE, eds. 2006. *Applied Pharmacokinetics & Pharmacodynamics, Principles of Therapeutic Drug Monitoring*. Lippincott Williams & Wilkins, Baltimore, MD, 285–353.
7. Moyer TP. 2005. Therapeutic drug monitoring. In: *Tietz Textbook of Clinical Chemistry and Molecular Diagnostics*, 4th Edition (Burtis CA, Ashwood ER, eds). WB Saunders Company, Philadelphia, PA, 1237–1285.
8. Dasgupta A, Datta P. 2007. Analytical techniques for measuring concentrations of therapeutic drugs in biological fluids. In: *Handbook of Drug Monitoring Methods* (Dasgupta A, ed). Humana Press Inc., Totowa, NJ, 67–86.
9. Soltes L. 1999. Aminoglycoside antibiotics-two decades of their HPLC bioanalysis. *Biomed Chromatogr* 13: 3–10.
10. Tanaka M, Orii T, Tomoko T, Gomi T, Kobayashi H, Kanke M, Hironoe S. 2002. Clinical estimation of vancomycin measurement method on hemodialysis patient. *Yakugaku Zasshi* 122: 269–275.
11. Anne L, Hu M, Colin L, Gottwald K. 1989. Potential problem with fluorescence immunoassay cross-reactivity to vancomycin degradation productCDP-1; its detection in sera of renally impaired patients. *Ther Drug Monit* 11: 585–591.
12. Isoherrane N, Soback S. 1999. Chromatographic methods for analysis of aminoglycoside antibiotics. *J AOAC Int* 82: 1017–1045.
13. Lai F, Sheehan T. 1992. Enhanced of detection sensitivity and cleanup selectivity for tobramycin through pre-column derivatization. *J Chromatogr* 609: 173–179.
14. Ovalles JF, Brunetto Mdel R, Gallignani M. 2005. A new method for the analysis of amikacin using 6-aminoquinolyl-N-hydroxysuccinimidyl carbamate (AQC) derivatization and high performance liquid chromatography with UV detection. *J Pharm Biomed Anal* 39: 294–298.
15. Nicoli S, Santi P. 2006. Assay of amikacin in the skin by high performance liquid chromatography. *J Pharm Biomed Anal* 41: 994–997.
16. Isoherrane N, Soback S. 2000. Determination of gentamicin C1, C1a, and C2 in plasma and urine by HPLC. *Clin Chem* 46: 837–842.
17. Kim BH, Lee SC, Lee HJ, Ok JH. 2003. Reversed-phase liquid chromatographic method for the analysis of aminoglycoside antibiotics using pre-column derivatization with phenylisocyanate. *Biomed Chromatogr* 17: 396–403.

18. Galanakis EG, Megoulas NC, Solich P, Koupparis MA. 2006. Development and validation of a novel LC nonderivatization method for the determination of amikacin in pharmaceuticals based on evaporative light scattering detection. *J Pharm Biomed Appl* 40: 1114–1120.

19. Jehl F, Corinne Gallion C, Robert C. Thierry RC, Monteil H. 1985. Determination of vancomycin in human serum by high-pressure liquid chromatography. *Antimicrob Agents Chemother* 27: 503–507.

20. Furuta I, Kitahashi T, Kuroda T, Nishio H, Oka C, Morishima Y. 2000. Rapid serum vancomycin assay by high-performance liquid chromatography using a semipermeable surface packing material column. *Clin Chim Acta* 301: 31–39.

21. Concepcion Lecaroz C, Miguel A, Campanero MA, Gamazo C, Blanco-Prieto MJ. 2006. Determination of gentamicin in different matrices by a new sensitive high-performance liquid chromatography-mass spectrometric method. *J Antimicrob Chemother* 58: 557–563.

22. Zhang T, Watson DG, Azike C, Tettey JN, Stearns AT, Binning AR, Payne CJ. 2007. Determination of vancomycin in serum by liquid chromatography-high resolution full scan mass spectrometry. *J Chromatogr B Analyt Technol Biomed Life Sci* 857: 352–356.

23. Cass RT, Villa JS, Karr DE, Schmidt Jr, DE. 2001. Rapid bioanalysis of vancomycin in serum and urine by high-performance liquid chromatography tandem mass spectrometry using on-line sample extraction and parallel analytical columns. *Rapid Commun Mass Spectrom* 15: 406–412.

24. Gerson B, Anhalt JP. 1980. *High Pressure Liquid Chromatography and Therapeutic Drug Monitoring.* American Society of Clinical Pathologists, Chicago, IL, 172.

25. Moyer TP. 2001. Therapeutic drug monitoring. In: *Tietz Fundamentals of Clinical Chemistry*, 5th Edition (Burtis CA, Ashwood AR, eds). WB Saunders Company, Philadelphia, PA, 608–635.

26. Pires de Abreu LR, Agustin R, Mas Ortiz M. 2003. HPLC determination of amoxicillin comparative bioavailability in healthy volunteers after a single dose administration. *J Pharm Pharmaceut Sci* 6: 223–230.

27. Mascher HJ, Kikuta C. 1998. Determination of amoxicillin in human serum and plasma by high-performance liquid chromatography and on-line postcolumn derivatization. *J Chromatogr A* 812: 221–226.

28. Bompadre S, Ferrante L, Leone L. 1998. On-line solid-phase extraction of cephalosporins. *J Chromatogr A* 812: 191–196.

29. Annesley T, Wilkerson K, Matz K, Glacherlo D. 1984. Simultaneous determination of penicillin and cephalosporin antibiotics in serum gradient liquid chromatography. *Clin Chem* 30: 908–910.

30. Viberg A, Sandström M, Britt S, Jansson B. 2008. Determination of cefuroxime in human serum or plasma by liquid chromatography with electrospray tandem mass spectrometry. *Rapid Commun Mass Spectrom* 18: 707–710.

31. Heller DN, Smith ML, Chiesa OA. 2005. LC/MS/MS measurement of penicillin G in bovine plasma, urine, and biopsy samples taken from kidneys of standing animals. *J Chromatogr B Analyt Technol Biomed Life Sci* 830: 91–99.

32. Becker M, Erhard Z, Petz M. 2004. Residue analysis of 15 penicillins and cephalosporins in bovine muscle, kidney and milk by liquid chromatography-tandem mass spectrometry. *Analyt Chimica Acta* 520: 19–32.

33. Heller DN, Smith ML, Albert CO. 2000. Confirmatory assay for the simultaneous detection of penicillins and cephalosporins in milk using liquid chromatography/tandem mass spectrometry. *Rapid Commun Mass Spectrom* 15: 1404–1409.

34. DeAngelis DV, Wooley JL, Sigel CW. 1990. High performance liquid chromatographic assay for the simultaneous measurement of trimethoprim and sulfamethoxazole in plasma or urine. *Ther Drug Monit* 12: 382–392.

35. Bedor DC, Gonçalvesa TM, Ferreira ML, de Sousa CE, Menezesa AL, Oliveira EJ, de Santana DP. 2008. Simultaneous determination of sulfamethoxazole and trimethoprim in biological fluids for high-throughput analysis: comparison of HPLC with ultraviolet and tandem mass spectrometric detection. *J Chromatogr B* 863: 46–54.

36. Moyer TP. 1999 Therapeutic drug monitoring. In: *Tietz Textbook of Clinical Chemistry,* 3rd Edition (Burtis CA, Ashwood ER, eds). WB Saunders Company, Philadelphia, PA, 862–905.

37. Koup R, Brodsky B, Alan Lau A, Beam Jr. TR. 1978. High-Performance Liquid chromatographic assay of chloramphenicol in serum. *Antimicrob Agents Chemother* 14: 439–443.

38. Zhu J, Snow DD, Cassada DA, Monson SJ, Spalding RF. 2001. Analysis of oxytetracycline, tetracycline, and chlortetracycline in water using solid-phase extraction and liquid chromatography–tandem mass spectrometry. *J Chromatogr A* 928: 177–186.

39. Srinivas N, Narasu L, Shankar BP, Mullangi R. 2008. Development and validation of a HPLC method for simultaneous quantitation of gatifloxacin, sparfloxacin and moxifloxacin using levofloxacin as internal standard in human plasma: application to a clinical pharmacokinetic study. *Biomed Chromatogr* 22: 1288–1295.
40. Stubbs C, Haigh JM, Kanfer I. 2006. Determination of erythromycin in serum and urine by high-performance liquid chromatography with ultraviolet detection. *J Pharmaceut Sci* 74: 1126–1128.
41. Kamberi M, Tsutsumi K, Kotegawa T, Nakamura K, Nakano S. 1998. Determination of ciprofloxacin in plasma and urine by HPLC with ultraviolet detection. *Clin Chem* 44L: 1251–1255.
42. Bahramia G, Mirzaeeib S, Kiania A. 2005. High performance liquid chromatographic determination of azithromycin in serum using fluorescence detection and its application in human pharmacokinetic studies. *J Chromatogr B* 820: 277–281.
43. Fouda HG, Schneider RP. 1995. Quantitative determination of the antibiotic azithromycin in human serum by high performance liquid chromatography (HPLC)-atmospheric pressure chemical ionization mass spectrometry: correlation with a standard HPLC electrochemical method. *Ther Drug Monit* 17: 179–183.
44. Barrett B, Bořek-Dohalský V, Fejt P, Vaingátová S, Huclová J, Němec B, Jelínek I. 2005. Validated HPLC–MS–MS method for determination of azithromycin in human plasma. *Anal Bioanal Chem* 383: 210–217.
45. Holdiness MR. 1985. Chromatographic analysis of antituberculosis drugs in biological samples. *J Chromatogr* 340: 321–359.
46. Malone RS, Fish DN, Spiegel DM, Childs JM, Peloquin CA. 1999. The effect of hemodialysis on isoniazid, rifampin, pyrazinamide, and ethambutol. *Am J Respir Crit Care Med* 159: 1580–1584.
47. LoDico CP, Levine BS, Goldberger BA, Caplan YH. 1992. Distribution of isoniazid in an overdose death. *J Anal Toxicol* 16: 57–59.
48. Chen X, Song B, Jiang H, Yu K, Zhong D. 2005. A liquid chromatography/tandem mass spectrometry method for simultaneous quantification of isoniazid and ethambutol in human plasma. *Rapid Commum Mass Spectrom* 19: 2591–2596.
49. Calleri E, De Lorenzi E, Furlanetto S, Massolini G, Caccialanza G. 2002. Validation of a RP-LC method for the simultaneous determination of isoniazid, pyrazinamide and rifampicin in a pharmaceutical formulation. *J Pharm Biomed Anal* 29: 1089–1096.
50. Um SW, Lee SW, Kwon SY, Yoon HI et al. 2007. Low serum concentrations of anti-tuberculosis drugs and determinants of their serum levels. *Int J Tuberc Lung Dis* 11: 972–978.

18 Need for Therapeutic Drug Monitoring of Antiretroviral Medications in HIV Infection

Natella Y. Rakhmanina and John N. van den Anker
Children's National Medical Center, The George Washington
University School of Medicine and Health Sciences

CONTENTS

18.1 INTRODUCTION

Five classes of drugs are used today to treat people with human immunodeficiency virus (HIV) infection including nucleoside and nucleotide analog reverse transcriptase inhibitors (NRTIs), non-nucleoside reverse transcriptase inhibitors (NNRTIs), protease inhibitors (PIs), entry and fusion inhibitors, and integrase inhibitors [1–3]. Three or more antiretroviral medications are administered concomitantly as antiretroviral treatment (ART). ART is designed to provide durable virologic suppression with immunologic recovery while preventing and minimizing toxicities and resistance [1]. By identifying and adjusting ART exposures that are suboptimal, therapeutic drug monitoring (TDM) can help prev––ent the development of viral resistance. In addition, TDM of ART might be instrumental in overcoming moderately decreased viral susceptibilities by allowing controlled increase of the antiretroviral (ARV) exposure [4]. More specifically, TDM may prevent suboptimal ARV drug concentrations which limit the response to ART even in the absence of HIV resistance [5]. It is helpful in management of drug-drug interactions and in identifying nonadherence, both of which are major

355

challenges in the successful treatment of HIV infection [6,7]. In addition, by identifying patients who are noncompliant or by reducing high drug concentrations based on TDM, it is possible to prevent nonadherence or avoidable toxicity [8,9]. TDM of ART has therefore been proposed as a tool to optimize response to ART in HIV infection [10–12]. Sensitive and specific assays are available to measure serum and bodily fluids (saliva, spinal fluid, semen, vaginal secretions, and urine) concentrations of ARV drugs. The most used analytical methods to determine plasma levels of ARV drugs are high performance liquid chromatography with ultraviolet detection (HPLC-UV) and HPLC combined with mass spectrometry or tandem mass spectrometry (MS/MS), while MALDI (matrix assisted laser desorption/ionization, a soft ionization technique in mass spectrometry)-based methods and enzyme immunoassay (EIA) technologies have also been employed for TDM of ARV drugs [13–18].

18.2 CURRENT APPLICATION OF THERAPEUTIC DRUG MONITORING (TDM) IN ANTIRETROVIRAL (ARV) THERAPY

A number of clinical trials have demonstrated that serum concentrations of ARV drugs are an important factor in response to therapy for HIV, and TDM of ART has become an accepted clinical tool in the management of HIV infection in children [3,19–22], pregnant women [23,24] and patients with renal or liver dysfunction [25,26]. In addition, current applications of TDM in ART include monitoring of adherence, multiple drug–food and drug–drug interactions, and virologic failure in the absence of viral resistance and nonadherence to medications.

18.2.1 RATIONALE FOR THERAPEUTIC DRUG MONITORING (TDM)

Large interindividual differences in drug disposition have been observed with the use of many ARV agents, which makes dose based prediction of plasma concentrations unreliable [9,27,28]. The cause of such significant interpatient pharmacokinetic (PK) variability is multifactorial and includes drug–drug and drug–food interactions, drug binding to plasma proteins, hepatic and renal impairment, sex, age and developmental stage, pregnancy, and host genetic factors including polymorphism of genes expressing various cytochrome P450 liver enzymes (CYPP450) as well as multi-drug resistance 1 (MDR1) polymorphisms [11,29] which affect ARV drug metabolism and bioavailability. The wide interpatient variability in ARV drug pharmacokinetics supports the application of TDM to the clinical management of HIV-infected patients [2,3,9,30,31].

18.2.2 TOXICITIES AND DRUG INTERACTIONS

The toxicities of ART range from nausea and vomiting to pancreatitis, nephrolithiasis, and neurologic side effects [30,32,33]. Studies have shown, that some of these toxicities might be prevented with the appropriate use of TDM [34,35]. In addition to the direct ART related toxicities the metabolism of the NNRTIs and PIs predisposes them to multiple drug–drug and drug–food interactions. NNRTIs (efavirenz (EFV) and nevirapine) are substrate of the CYPP450 metabolic pathway (primarily CYP2B6 with addition of the CYP3A and CYP2A pathways) [29,36–38]. The PIs are metabolized by CYP2B6, CYP2C19, CYP2D6 and by the 3A family, creating a solid base for multiple drug-drug interactions [27,28,39]. Many drugs used in the treatment of infections associated with HIV disease (ketoconazole, fluconazole, rifampin, rifabutin, methadone) as well as herbal supplements (garlic, St John's wort) have shown significant interactions with PIs leading to toxicity-related complications and subtherapeutic concentrations [40–43]. The interactions between PIs and NNRTIs, and among different PIs have also become clinical issues with the growing resistance pattern of HIV. The application of TDM in the patients who are using two and more drugs CYPP450 liver enzymes interacting agents is a proven and useful tool to optimize therapy of HIV and associated comorbidities, such as tuberculosis, malaria, fungal, and opportunistic infections [43–45].

18.2.3　Genetic Factors

The difference in host genetic factors such as drug metabolizing capacity is an additional indication for the application of TDM in ART. For example, the polymorphic expression of CYP2B6 has been associated with significant changes in the pharmacokinetics of EFV in HIV-infected adults and children [46–49].

The CYP2B6 G to T polymorphism at position 516 produces elevated EFV plasma concentrations and an increase in neurotoxicity of EFV [4,37], while up to 20% of subjects with wild-type genotype have sub-therapeutic concentrations of EFV [50]. The CYP2B6 G516T polymorphism has also been associated with a prolonged elimination serum half-life and an increased risk of developing drug resistance after discontinuation of an EFV based regimen [51] While genotyping of the patients on EFV for the CYP2B6 polymorphisms has limited application due to the cost and availability considerations, TDM can serve as an useful tool in identifying the patients at risk for toxic and subtherapeutic EFV concentrations.

18.2.4　Association of Drug Concentrations with Viral Loads

Applying TDM to enhance treatment outcome is much more complex and difficult to achieve. Multiple studies have demonstrated an association between plasma ARV drugs concentrations and virologic response especially in treatment-naïve patients [52–55]. In addition, it has been reported that the rate at which ARV resistance mutations appear is inversely related to plasma ARV concentrations [56]. The pharmacokinetic (PK) data from the Viradapt study have shown a significant correlation between suboptimal drug concentrations and the risk of virologic failure [57]. This is of particular importance because preliminary studies from centers that offer TDM have been reporting that a substantial proportion of patients may have sub-therapeutic levels of antiretroviral agents [53,58]. Adverse events, nonadherence, and drug interactions are frequently responsible for subtherapeutic drug levels. A study by De Maat et al. [59], however, demonstrated a high number of subtherapeutic drug concentrations without an identifiable cause, which may increase the potential of ARV drug resistance and treatment failure.

Studies of virologic efficacy have found a significant correlation both with trough (C_{min}) plasma concentrations and area under the curve (AUC) of many ARV medications with HIV RNA viral load [4,5,8,18,60,61]. Since feasibility of obtaining AUCs in clinical settings is limited the C_{min} became the point of interest for further investigation. The ratio of C_{min} to inhibitory concentration at 50% (IC_{50}), defined as inhibitory quotient (IQ), is used by many researchers and is believed to be the parameter most likely to predict efficacy. The phenotypic inhibitory quotient (PIQ) is calculated as the trough (C_{min}) concentration divided by the IC_{50} or IC_{90} [5,34]. The IC_{50} for a specific patient is measured by a phenotypic resistance test. Because there are differences in the efficacy of plasma concentrations in vitro and in vivo, the IC_{50} for the PIs needs to be corrected for protein binding. While PIQ values are frequently reported with correction for protein binding, it is important to understand that the correction for protein binding differs from assay to assay. Genotypic inhibitory quotient (GIQ), defined as the trough (C_{min}) plasma drug concentration divided by the number of primary, PI associated, genotypic mutations in the HIV, assumes an equal importance for each resistance mutation included. However, in reality there might be differences [61–63]. To date, no gold standard to weigh the importance of different mutations has been agreed upon. The established cutoff values for GIQ are accompanied by a list of mutations that were used in the GIQ model as well as median trough concentrations that can be expected for a certain drug. These data are designed to help make a clinical decision on the feasibility of the trough concentrations that need to be achieved in order to ensure an adequate GIQ in the patient.

18.2.5　Patient Noncompliance and Therapeutic Drug Monitoring (TDM)

TDM of ARV drugs is also being used to monitor patient adherence to the regimen [7]. Poor adherence has been identified as a leading cause of treatment failure by many authors [64]. Nonadherence is a serious problem and is reported in 33–69% of this patient population [40,65]. Common reasons for missing doses include clinical toxicity, forgetfulness, sleeping through the time of prescribed dose, and being away from home. TDM can help identify nonadherence, although a drug concentration only reflects the last few drug doses taken by the patient. It is crucial that any TDM results are incorporated with careful adherence assessment to facilitate interpretation of the results and adherence counseling should be established as part of clinical care in the centers practicing TDM.

18.2.6   LIMITATION OF THERAPEUTIC DRUG MONITORING (TDM) FOR ANTIRETROVIRAL TREATMENT (ART)

Several important limitations to the application of TDM for ART should be recognized, including uncertainty about the best PK predictor of response and insufficient validation of target concentrations for individual PIs and NNRTIs.

A high degree of the intraindividual variability in virologically suppressed HIV patients has been reported and has been cited as a valuable argument in usefulness of the TDM [66]. TDM results are also confounded by nonadherence. Adequate in-clinic measurements of ARV drugs may not reflect out-of-clinic concentrations, considering that patients may adhere more to their dosages schedules before appointments with their physicians. Conversely, an inadequate drug concentration may not reflect an insufficient dose for a particular patient, but rather represent nonadherence prior to the sampling in the clinic. TDM measures total concentrations of ARV drugs, and protein binding adjustment needs to be applied to estimate the free ARV drug concentrations. The lack of standards on the importance of different viral factors such as the weight of different mutations in the overall resistance development is another serious limitation in applying IQ driven TDM. On the practical side, the scheduling of the clinic appointments around the trough times for ARV doses, particularly for the PI with shorter half-life and the lack of data on diurnal variations in PK of those drugs represent another limitation for the application of TDM in clinical practice.

In 2003, a guideline regarding TDM for ARV drugs was published [67]. Three years later, new drugs have been licensed and the guidelines have been updated in 2006 [61]. In line with DHHS United States Department of Health and Humans services) and British HIV Association (BHIVA) guidelines, updates with indications for TDM were provided [2,3,31,68]. The updates included concentration-based cutoff values for efficacy and toxicity and cutoff values for PIQ and GIQ. The PIQ and GIQ values are not directly comparable across family of PIs, as the plasma concentrations and resistance profiles of different PIs are not the same. The guidelines can be accessed on the web www.hivpharmacology.com and are continuously updated with new information. The website provides information and references to the TDM laboratories that participate in the external quality programs such as Asqualab, KKGT, International Interlaboratory Quality Control Programs for TDM in HIV Infection and International Interlaboratory Quality Control Program for Measurement of Antiretroviral Drugs in Plasma.

The guidelines recommend using trough samples to monitor virologic efficacy and peak samples for toxicity management. Two weeks of established ART are recommended prior to TDM to evaluate the ARV concentrations at steady state. Trough samples need to be measured at eight hours postdose (PD) for the medications administered three times daily, 12 hours PD for medications administered twice daily and 24 hours PD for once daily medications. Peak samples vary according to the PK of the particular ARV drugs. The guidelines stress the importance of treating the patient and not his/her plasma ARV levels. The ARV concentrations should never be used in isolation, but have to be interpreted in the context of a specific patient [6,61,67]. In addition of the routinely obtained TDM information such as the dose and frequency of the drug, time of the last medication intake and the time of blood sampling, and coadministration of other medications, the ART TDM sample must also incorporate information about previous ART and present phenotypic or genotypic resistance of HIV.

There are only a few randomized prospective studies that have examined the utility of TDM in the treatment of HIV, which showed mixed results. The ATHENA study conducted in The Netherlands included two clinical trials using TDM in treatment-naïve patients who started indinavir- (IDV) or nelfinavir- (NFV) based regimens. TDM of NFV improved viral load effects but did not reduce toxicity, while dose adjustment for IDV reduced toxicity did not improve antiviral effect [53,69]. TDM did prevent either virologic failure (presumably by preventing development of resistance) or treatment discontinuation because of concentration related toxicities. These findings are even more impressive, taking into consideration that only 20% of the physicians responded to the dosing recommendations of the intervention group. This protocol, however, did not incorporate resistance data in the dosage adjustment calculation. Another study conducted in France (PharmAdapt) was a prospective study comparing the use of TDM versus non TDM in treatment experience patients failing therapy [70,71]. The study failed to find a significant benefit of TDM versus standard care [70]. However, there were numerous concerns regarding the study design, such as dosage adjustment at week 8 which may have been too late to prevent genotypic evaluation of the virus and lack of power analysis. In summary, only limited data from randomized clinical trials have been reported to date. Many study protocols evaluating the PK and pharmacodynamics of ARV therapies in children and pregnant women have incorporated the ARV dose adjustment into the study design, which allowed to achieve high rates of full virologic suppression in the patients who otherwise were at risk of treatment failure [28]. Additional clinical trials with improved design are needed to investigate if routine TDM as standard of care for the treatment of HIV infection are warranted. The availability of a large TDM database may facilitate the establishment of expected concentration ranges for a variety of antiretroviral drugs. A logistical problem remains with regard to its feasibility, and theoretical issues such as protein binding, variability, and the appropriate time of sampling continue to be debated. Available technology allows setting target inhibitory concentrations for a particular virus isolate based on genotypic and phenotypic sensitivity; however it is expensive and requires highly specialized assistance. With the emergence of newer ART agents in recent years, ongoing research in the field of the HIV pharmacology is necessary for the future improvement of ART.

18.3 THERAPEUTIC DRUG MONITORING (TDM) OF DIFFERENT CLASSES OF ANTIRETROVIRAL DRUGS

In this section TDM of different classes of antiretroviral drugs where TDM may be useful will be addressed. There are three classes of antiretroviral drugs, including NRTIs, NNRTIs, and PIs where TDM may be useful. No data on target therapeutic concentrations of fusion inhibitors, and novel integrase inhibitor and CC chemokine receptor 5 (CCR5) antagonists are available to date.

18.3.1 THERAPEUTIC DRUG MONITORING (TDM) OF NUCLEOTIDE ANALOG REVERSE TRANSCRIPTASE INHIBITORS (NRTIs)

The NRTIs are active as intracellular triphosphates, and there is little evidence to suggest that their measurement would be helpful other than to assess adherence to the drug regimen. Several studies have established a relationship between plasma concentrations of NRTI and virologic and immunologic outcomes [72,73]. The usefulness of NRTI plasma concentration in predicting the intracellular levels of their triphosphate metabolites for TDM remains unclear. The relationship between the intracellular drug levels and outcome parameters for zidovudine and lamivudine has been shown to be significant [73], but the methodology of intracellular triphosphate metabolites is expensive and labor-intensive and is limited to highly specialized centers. Currently, the monitoring of the NRTIs is considered to be useful for the evaluation and management of drug-drug interactions that affect the plasma concentrations of NRTIs only [61] (Table 18.1).

18.3.2 THERAPEUTIC DRUG MONITORING (TDM) OF NON NUCLEOSIDE REVERSE TRANSCRIPTASE INHIBITORS (NNRTIs)

For the NNRTIs, the relationship between plasma drug concentrations and their efficacy and toxicity has been identified [74,75]. The patients taking NNRTIs (EFV, nevirapine) are at the greatest risk for developing resistance due to the low threshold to the high level virological resistance requiring

TABLE 18.1
Plasma Half-Life and Efficacy Concentrations of Antiretroviral Medications

Drug	Mean Plasma Half-Life ($t_{1/2} = h$)*	Efficacy C_{trough} (mg/L)**
Nucleoside and Nucleotide Reverse Transriptase Inhibitors		
Abacavir (ABC, Ziagen®)	1.5	NA[a]
Didanosine (dideoxinosine, ddI, Videx®)	1.5	NA
Delavirdine (DLV, Rescriptor®)	6.0	NA
Emtricitabine (FTC, Emtriva™)	10.0	NA
Lamivudine (3TC, Epivir®, Epivir HBV)	6.0	NA
Stavudine (d4T, Zerit®)	1.4	NA
Tenofovir (TDF, Viread®)	17.0	NA
Zalcitabine (ddC, Hivid®)	2.0	NA
Zidovudine (ZDV, AZT, Retrovir®)	1.1	NA
Non-nucleoside Reverse Transcriptase Inhibitors		
Efavirenz (DMP-266EFV, Sustiva™)	45.0	1.0
Etravirine (ETR, Intelence™, TMC125)	41.0	NR[b]
Nevirapine (NVP, Viramune®)	28.0	3.0
Protease Inhibitors		
Amprenavir (AMP, Agenerase®)	8.8	NR
Atazanavir (ATV, Reyataz™)	12.0	0.15
Darunavir (DRV, TMC114, Prezista®)	15.0	NR
Fosamprenavir (f-AMP, Lexiva™)	7.7	0.40
Indinavir (IDV, Crixivan®)	2.0	0.10
Lopinavir/Ritonavir (LPV/RTV, Kaletra, ABT 378)	5.5	1.0
Nelfinavir (NFV, Viracept®)	4.0	0.80
Ritonavir (RTV, Norvir®)	4.0	2.1
Saquinavir (SQV, Invirase®)	9.5	0.1
Tipranavir (TPV, Aptivus®)	5.4	20.5
Entry and Fusion Inhibitors		
Maraviroc (MVC, Selzentry®)	16.0	NR
Enfuvirtide (Fuzeon™, T-20)	3.8	NR
Integrase Inhibitors		
Raltegravir (MK-0518, RGV, RAL, Insentress®)	9.0	NR

[a] Not applicable.
[b] Not reported.
* The information about half-life was obtained from the manufacturer (US) inserts. The half-lives of ATV, DRV, and TPV are reported following coadministration with the booster RTV dose.
** The information about efficacy C_{trough} was obtained from publications referenced in the text.

single codon mutation (K103N,Y188L, or V106M) in HIV. For that reason, no PIQ or GIQ model has been applied to the NNRTIs. Long term virologic suppression of HIV has been associated with maintenance of efficacy trough plasma concentrations above 1 mcg/mL for EFV and 3 mcg/mL for NVP in adult and pediatric patients with HIV infection [61]. Among the currently utilized ARV medications EFV has the smallest therapeutic window with concentrations exceeding 4 mcg/mL proven to increase the risk of adverse neuropsychiatric effects [9,76].

18.3.3   THERAPEUTIC DRUG MONITORING (TDM) OF PROTEASE INHIBITORS (PIs)

The PIs with established efficacy trough concentrations (C_{min}) include atazanavir, fosamprenavir, indinavir, lopinavir/ritonavir, nelfinavir, ritonavir, saquinavir and tipranavir [61]. The therapeutic window with toxicity range has been defined for indinavir only, with a high frequency of urological complications associated with peak (C_{max}) IDV concentrations of 10.0 mcg/mL [77]. The PIQ data has been studied in most commonly used PIs fosamprenavir, lopinavir/ritonavir, saquinavir, and tipranavir [5,63,78–82]. Because all PIs are strongly protein bound, and especially to α-1-acid glycoprotein (AAG), an acute phase protein [83], the PIQ for PIs have been corrected for protein binding. However, it is important to understand that the correction for protein binding differs from assay to assay. The GIQ (genotypic inhibitory quotient, a way to integrate drug exposure and genotypic resistance to protease inhibitors) data has been derived for all aforementioned PIs plus atazanavir (ATV). The expected trough concentrations have been calculated for all PIs in combination with a ritonavir booster, except for ATV, where the C_{min} for unboosted and ritonavir boosted ATV both have been reported [61]. It is important to note that the data presented in the guidelines were the most current to date, but the cutoff continues to evolve as other studies are published. This is particularly relevant to the measure of GIQ, as new insights gained regarding the value of specific mutations in the response to PIs will need to be incorporated into the older models. It is also important to note that, for IQ based TDM, no prospective studies have been conducted for the validation of cutoff values for the most commonly used PIs and the information on the strategy of IQ based TDM is very limited.

18.4   CONCLUSIONS

The concept of managing pharmacotherapy based on plasma drug concentrations has been used for decades in a variety of clinical settings. The interest in TDM of ARV medications has grown significantly since ART became a standard of care in clinical practice. While a number of clinical trials have demonstrated that TDM can improve the outcome of the HIV infection, the universal application of TDM as tool for the routine management of HIV infection remains to be determined. In order to be efficient, TDM of ART needs to be incorporated with other interventions such as resistance testing, adherence monitoring, and patient counseling. Optimal care in HIV requires individualized management and ongoing attention to relevant scientific and clinical information in the field [1,20]. Prospective randomized and double-blinded clinical trials are necessary to establish the role of concentration targeted therapy of HIV in routine clinical care. Properly applied TDM programs carry clear benefit for many HIV-infected patients on ART, especially those at risk for sub-therapeutic or toxic drug concentrations.

REFERENCES

1. Hammer SM, Eron JJ, Jr., Reiss P, Schooley RT, Thompson MA, Walmsley S, et al. 2008. Antiretroviral treatment of adult HIV infection: 2008 recommendations of the International AIDS Society-USA panel. *JAMA* 300(5):555–70.
2. Department of Health and Human Services. *Guidelines for the Use of Antiretroviral Agents in HIV-Infected Adults and Adolescents*. January 29, 2008. Available at http://www.aidsinfor.nih.gov. Accessed September 12, 2008.
3. Department of Health and Human Services. *Guidelines for the Use of Antiretroviral Agents in Pediatric HIV Infection*. July 29, 2008. Available at http://www.aidsinfor.nih.gov. Accessed September 12, 2008.
4. Haas DW. 2006. Can responses to antiretroviral therapy be improved by therapeutic drug monitoring? *Clin Infect Dis* 42(8):1197–99.
5. Hoefnagel JG, Koopmans PP, Burger DM, Schuurman R, Galama JM. 2005. Role of the inhibitory quotient in HIV therapy. *Antivir Ther* 10(8):879–92.
6. Gerber JG, Acosta EP. 2003. Therapeutic drug monitoring in the treatment of HIV-infection. *J Clin Virol* 27(2):117–28.

7. Hugen PW, Burger DM, Aarnoutse RE, Baede PA, Nieuwkerk PT, Koopmans PP, et al. 2002. Therapeutic drug monitoring of HIV-protease inhibitors to assess noncompliance. *Ther Drug Monit* 24(5):579–87.

8. Kappelhoff BS, Crommentuyn KM, de Maat MM, Mulder JW, Huitema AD, Beijnen JH. 2004. Practical guidelines to interpret plasma concentrations of antiretroviral drugs. *Clin Pharmacokinet* 43(13):845–53.

9. Marzolini C, Telenti A, Decosterd LA, Greub G, Biollaz J, Buclin T. 2001. Efavirenz plasma levels can predict treatment failure and central nervous system side effects in HIV-1-infected patients. *AIDS* 15(1):71–75.

10. Back D, Khoo S, Gibbons S. 2002. Therapeutic drug monitoring. *J Int Assoc Physicians AIDS Care* 1(3):84–85.

11. Acosta EP, Gerber JG.2002. Position paper on therapeutic drug monitoring of antiretroviral agents. *AIDS Res Hum Retroviruses* 18(12):825–34.

12. Aarnoutse RE, Schapiro JM, Boucher CA, Hekster YA, Burger DM. 2003. Therapeutic drug monitoring: an aid to optimizing response to antiretroviral drugs? *Drugs* 63(8):741–53.

13. Crommentuyn KM, Rosing H, Nan-Offeringa LG, Hillebrand MJ, Huitema AD, Beijnen JH. 2003. Rapid quantification of HIV protease inhibitors in human plasma by high-performance liquid chromatography coupled with electrospray ionization tandem mass spectrometry. *J Mass Spectrom* 38(2):157–66.

14. Ghoshal AK, Soldin SJ. 2003. Improved method for concurrent quantification of antiretrovirals by liquid chromatography-tandem mass spectrometry. *Ther Drug Monit* 25(5):541–43.

15. Titier K, Lagrange F, Pehourcq F, Edno-Mcheik L, Moore N, Molimard M. 2002. High-performance liquid chromatographic method for the simultaneous determination of the six HIV-protease inhibitors and two non-nucleoside reverse transcriptase inhibitors in human plasma. *Ther Drug Monit* 24(3):417–24.

16. Villani P, Feroggio M, Gianelli L, Bartoli A, Montagna M, Maserati R, et al. 2001. Antiretrovirals: simultaneous determination of five protease inhibitors and three nonnucleoside transcriptase inhibitors in human plasma by a rapid high-performance liquid chromatography--mass spectrometry assay. *Ther Drug Monit* 23(4):380–88.

17. Volosov A, Alexander C, Ting L, Soldin SJ. 2002. Simple rapid method for quantification of antiretrovirals by liquid chromatography-tandem mass-spectrometry. *Clin Biochem* 35(2):99–103.

18. Jelena I, Emanuele N, Paolo A, Rita B, Elisabetta de M, Stefania N, et al. 2008. Therapeutic drug monitoring in the management of HIV-infected patients. *Curr Med Chem* 15(19):1925–39.

19. Fraaij PL, Rakhmanina N, Burger DM, de Groot R. 2004. Therapeutic drug monitoring in children with HIV/AIDS. *Ther Drug Monit* 26(2):122–26.

20. Neely M, Jelliffe R. 2008. Practical therapeutic drug management in HIV-infected patients: use of population pharmacokinetic models supplemented by individualized Bayesian dose optimization. *J Clin Pharmacol* 48(9):1081–91.

21. Rosso R, Di Biagio A, Dentone C, Gattinara GC, Martino AM, Vigano A, et al. 2006. Lopinavir/ritonavir exposure in treatment-naive HIV-infected children following twice or once daily administration. *J Antimicrob Chemother* 57(6):1168–71.

22. Bunupuradah R, van der Lugt J, JKosalaraska P, et al. 2008. Therapeutic drug monitoring of lopinavir and saquinavir in Thai HIV-infected children. *15th Conference on Retroviruses and Opportunistic Infections. February 2008*. Boston, MA. Abstract 575.

23. Lyons F, Lechelt M, De Ruiter A. 2007. Steady-state lopinavir levels in third trimester of pregnancy. *AIDS* 21(8):1053–54.

24. Ripamonti D, Cattaneo D, Maggiolo F, Airoldi M, Frigerio L, Bertuletti P, et al. 2007. Atazanavir plus low-dose ritonavir in pregnancy: pharmacokinetics and placental transfer. *AIDS* 21(18):2409–15.

25. Kearney B, Liaw S, Yale K, et al. 2002. Pharmacokinetics following single-dose administration of tenofovir DF in patients with renal impairment. *6th International Congress of Drug Therapy in HIV Infection. November 2002*. Glasgow, Scotland. Abstract 4.

26. Seminari E, Gentilini M, De Bona A, et al. 2005. Liver cirrhosis but not chronic hepatitis is associated with higher amprenavir plasma levels in patients treated with amprenavir/ritonavir. *6th International Workshop on Clinicl Pharmacology of HIV Therapy. April, 2005*. Quebec City, Canada. Abstract 66.

27. Langmann P, Zilly M, Weissbrich B, Desch S, Vath T, Klinker H. 2002. Therapeutic drug monitoring of indinavir in HIV-infected patients undergoing HAART. *Infection* 30(1):13–16.

28. Fletcher CV, Anderson PL, Kakuda TN, Schacker TW, Henry K, Gross CR, et al. 2002. Concentration-controlled compared with conventional antiretroviral therapy for HIV infection. *AIDS* 16(4):551–60.

29. Burger D, van der Heiden I, la Porte C, van der Ende M, Groeneveld P, Richter C, et al. 2006. Interpatient variability in the pharmacokinetics of the HIV non-nucleoside reverse transcriptase inhibitor efavirenz: the effect of gender, race, and CYP2B6 polymorphism. *Br J Clin Pharmacol* 61(2):148–54.
30. Back DJ, Khoo SH, Gibbons SE, Barry MG, Merry C. 2000. Therapeutic drug monitoring of antiretrovirals in human immunodeficiency virus infection. *Ther Drug Monit* 22(1):122–26.
31. European AIDS Clinical Society (EACS). *Guidelines for the Clinical Management and Treatment of HIV-Infected Adults in Europe.* December 1, 2007. Available at http://www.eacs.eu/guide/index.htm. Accessed September 12, 2008.
32. Soldin OP, Elin RJ, Soldin SJ. 2003. Therapeutic drug monitoring in human immunodeficiency virus/ acquired immunodeficiency syndrome. Quo vadis? *Arch Pathol Lab Med* 127(1):102–5.
33. van Heeswijk RP, Veldkamp AI, Mulder JW, Meenhorst PL, Wit FW, Lange JM, et al. 2000. The steady-state pharmacokinetics of nevirapine during once daily and twice daily dosing in HIV-1-infected individuals. *AIDS* 14(8):F77–82.
34. Casado JL, Moreno A, Sabido R, Marti-Belda P, Antela A, Dronda F, et al. 2000. A clinical study of the combination of 100 mg ritonavir plus 800 mg indinavir as salvage therapy: influence of increased plasma drug levels in the rate of response. *HIV Clin Trials* 1(1):13–19.
35. Lamotte C, Peytavin G, Perre P, et al. 2001. Increasing adverse events with indinavir dosages and plasma concentrations in four different ritonavir-indinavir containing regimens in HIV-infected patients. *Eighth Conference on Retroviruses and Opportunistic Infections.* Chicago, IL. Abstract 738.
36. Khaliq Y, Gallicano K, Seguin I, Fyke K, Carignan G, Bulman D, et al. 2000. Single and multiple dose pharmacokinetics of nelfinavir and CYP2C19 activity in human immunodeficiency virus-infected patients with chronic liver disease. *Br J Clin Pharmacol* 50(2):108–15.
37. Desta Z, Saussele T, Ward B, Blievernicht J, Li L, Klein K, et al. 2007. Impact of CYP2B6 polymorphism on hepatic efavirenz metabolism in vitro. *Pharmacogenomics* 8(6):547–58.
38. Bumpus NN, Kent UM, Hollenberg PF. 2006. Metabolism of efavirenz and 8-hydroxyefavirenz by P450 2B6 leads to inactivation by two distinct mechanisms. *J Pharmacol Exp Ther* 318(1):345–51.
39. Flexner CW. 2003. Advances in HIV pharmacology: protein binding, pharmacogenomics, and therapeutic drug monitoring. *Top HIV Med* 11(2):40–44.
40. Dasgupta A, Okhuysen PC. 2001. Pharmacokinetic and other drug interactions in patients with AIDS. *Ther Drug Monit* 23(6):591–605.
41. Piscitelli SC, Burstein AH, Chaitt D, Alfaro RM, Falloon J. 2000. Indinavir concentrations and St John's wort. *Lancet* 355(9203):547–48.
42. Piscitelli SC, Burstein AH, Welden N, Gallicano KD, Falloon J. 2002. The effect of garlic supplements on the pharmacokinetics of saquinavir. *Clin Infect Dis* 34(2):234–38.
43. Cohen K, van Cutsem G, Boulle A, McIlleron H, Goemaere E, Smith PJ, et al. 2008. Effect of rifampicin-based antitubercular therapy on nevirapine plasma concentrations in South African adults with HIV-associated tuberculosis. *J Antimicrob Chemother* 61(2):389–93.
44. German P, Parikj S, Lawrence J, et al. 2008. Drug interactions between antimalarial drugs and lopinavir/ ritonavir. *15th Conference on Retroviruses and Opportunistic Infections. February 2008.* Boston, MA. Abstract 132.
45. Elsherbiny D, Cohen K, Jansson B, Smith P, McIlleron H, Simonsson US. 2009. Population pharmacokinetics of nevirapine in combination with rifampicin-based short course chemotherapy in HIV- and tuberculosis-infected South African patients. *Eur J Clin Pharmacol* 65(1):71–80.
46. Lang T, Klein K, Richter T, Zibat A, Kerb R, Eichelbaum M, et al. 2004. Multiple novel nonsynonymous CYP2B6 gene polymorphisms in Caucasians: demonstration of phenotypic null alleles. *J Pharmacol Exp Ther* 311(1):34–43.
47. Rotger M, Colombo S, Furrer H, Bleiber G, Buclin T, Lee BL, et al. 2005. Influence of CYP2B6 polymorphism on plasma and intracellular concentrations and toxicity of efavirenz and nevirapine in HIV-infected patients. *Pharmacogenet Genomics* 15(1):1–5.
48. Tsuchiya K, Gatanaga H, Tachikawa N, Teruya K, Kikuchi Y, Yoshino M, et al. 2004. Homozygous CYP2B6 *6 (Q172H and K262R) correlates with high plasma efavirenz concentrations in HIV-1 patients treated with standard efavirenz-containing regimens. *Biochem Biophys Res Commun* 319(4):1322–6.
49. Klein K, Lang T, Saussele T, Barbosa-Sicard E, Schunck WH, Eichelbaum M, et al. 2005. Genetic variability of CYP2B6 in populations of African and Asian origin: allele frequencies, novel functional variants, and possible implications for anti-HIV therapy with efavirenz. *Pharmacogenet Genomics* 15(12):861–73.

50. Barreiro P, Rodriguez-Novoa S, Labarga P, Ruiz A, Jimenez-Nacher I, Martin-Carbonero L, et al. 2007. Influence of liver fibrosis stage on plasma levels of antiretroviral drugs in HIV-infected patients with chronic hepatitis C. *J Infect Dis* 195(7):973–79.

51. Ribaudo HJ, Haas DW, Tierney C, Kim RB, Wilkinson GR, Gulick RM, et al. 2006. Pharmacogenetics of plasma efavirenz exposure after treatment discontinuation: an Adult AIDS Clinical Trials Group Study. *Clin Infect Dis* 42(3):401–7.

52. Fiorante S, Rodriguez Novoa S, Gasco PG, et al. 2008. Association between blips and subtherapeutic antiretroviral plasma levels. *15th Conference on Retroviruses and Opportunistic Infections. February 2008*. Boston, MA. Abstract 772.

53. Burger DM, Hugen PW, Aarnoutse RE, Hoetelmans RM, Jambroes M, Nieuwkerk PT, et al. 2003. Treatment failure of nelfinavir-containing triple therapy can largely be explained by low nelfinavir plasma concentrations. *Ther Drug Monit* 25(1):73–80.

54. Alexander CS, Asselin JJ, Ting LS, Montaner JS, Hogg RS, Yip B, et al. 2003. Antiretroviral concentrations in untimed plasma samples predict therapy outcome in a population with advanced disease. *J Infect Dis* 188(4):541–48.

55. Best BM, Goicoechea M, Witt MD, Miller L, Daar ES, Diamond C, et al. 2007. A randomized controlled trial of therapeutic drug monitoring in treatment-naive and -experienced HIV-1-infected patients. *J Acquir Immune Defic Syndr* 46(4):433–42.

56. Hoetelmans RM, Reijers MH, Weverling GJ, ten Kate RW, Wit FW, Mulder JW, et al. 1998. The effect of plasma drug concentrations on HIV-1 clearance rate during quadruple drug therapy. *AIDS* 12(11):F111–15.

57. Durant J, Clevenbergh P, Garraffo R, Halfon P, Icard S, Del Giudice P, et al. 2000. Importance of protease inhibitor plasma levels in HIV-infected patients treated with genotypic-guided therapy: pharmacological data from the Viradapt Study. *AIDS* 14(10):1333–39.

58. Gibbons ES, Reynolds H.E., Tija JF, et al. 2000. Therapeutic drug monitoring in the management of subjects on the protease inhibitors nelfinavir and saquinavir: results of the Roche UK TDM service. *5th International Congress on Drug Therapy in HIV Infection*. Glasgow, Scotland. Abstract P259.

59. de Maat MM, Huitema AD, Mulder JW, Meenhorst PL, van Gorp EC, Mairuhu AT, et al. 2003. Subtherapeutic antiretroviral plasma concentrations in routine clinical outpatient HIV care. *Ther Drug Monit* 25(3):367–73.

60. Park-Wyllie LY, Levine MA, Holbrook A, Thabane L, Antoniou T, Yoong D, et al. 2007. Outcomes of dosage adjustments used to manage antiretroviral drug interactions. *Clin Infect Dis* 45(7):933–36.

61. Back D, Gibbons S, Khoo S. 2006. An update on therapeutic drug monitoring for antiretroviral drugs. *Ther Drug Monit* 28(3):468–73.

62. Molto J, Santos J, Perez-Alvarez N, et al. 2008. Inhibitory quotient as a predictor of virological response to darunavir-based salvage regimens. *15th Conference on Retroviruses and Opportunistic Infections. February 2008*. Boston, MA. Abstract 768.

63. Marcelin AG, Lamotte C, Delaugerre C, Ktorza N, Ait Mohand H, Cacace R, et al. 2003. Genotypic inhibitory quotient as predictor of virological response to ritonavir-amprenavir in human immunodeficiency virus type 1 protease inhibitor-experienced patients. Antimicrob Agents Chemother 47(2):594–600.

64. Descamps D, Flandre P, Calvez V, Peytavin G, Meiffredy V, Collin G, et al. 2000. Mechanisms of virologic failure in previously untreated HIV-infected patients from a trial of induction-maintenance therapy. Trilege (Agence Nationale de Recherches sur le SIDA 072) Study Team). *JAMA* 283(2):205–11.

65. Van Heeswijk RP. 2002. Critical issues in therapeutic drug monitoring of antiretroviral drugs. *Ther Drug Monit* 24(3):323–31.

66. Nettles RE, Kieffer TL, Parsons T, Johnson J, Cofrancesco J, Jr., Gallant JE, et al. 2006. Marked intraindividual variability in antiretroviral concentrations may limit the utility of therapeutic drug monitoring. *Clin Infect Dis* 42(8):1189–96.

67. Back DJ, Blanschke T, Boucher CA, et al. 2003. *Optimizing TDM in HIV Clinical Care*. A practical guide to perform therapeutic drug monitoring (TDM) for antiretroviral agents, version 1.0. Available at www.hivpharmacology.com. Accessed September 12, 2008.

68. Gazzard B. 2005. British HIV Association (BHIVA) guidelines for the treatment of HIV-infected adults with antiretroviral therapy. *HIV Med* (6 Suppl 2):1–61.

69. Burger D, Hugen P, Reiss P, Gyssens I, Schneider M, Kroon F, et al. 2003. Therapeutic drug monitoring of nelfinavir and indinavir in treatment-naive HIV-1-infected individuals. *AIDS* 17(8):1157–65.

70. Clevenbergh P, Garraffo R, Durant J, Dellamonica P. 2002. PharmAdapt: a randomized prospective study to evaluate the benefit of therapeutic monitoring of protease inhibitors: 12 week results. *AIDS* 16(17):2311–15.

71. Clevenbergh P, Garraffo R, Dellamonica P. 2003. Impact of various antiretroviral drugs and their plasma concentrations on plasma lipids in heavily pretreated HIV-infected patients. *HIV Clin Trials* 4(5):330–36.

72. Fletcher CV, Acosta EP, Henry K, Page LM, Gross CR, Kawle SP, et al. 1998. Concentration-controlled zidovudine therapy. *Clin Pharmacol Ther* 64(3):331–38.

73. Fletcher CV, Kawle SP, Kakuda TN, Anderson PL, Weller D, Bushman LR, et al. 2000. Zidovudine triphosphate and lamivudine triphosphate concentration-response relationships in HIV-infected persons. *AIDS* 14(14):2137–44.

74. Leth FV, Kappelhoff BS, Johnson D, Losso MH, Boron-Kaczmarska A, Saag MS, et al. 2006. Pharmacokinetic parameters of nevirapine and efavirenz in relation to antiretroviral efficacy. *AIDS Res Hum Retroviruses* 22(3):232–39.

75. Duong M, Buisson M, Peytavin G, Kohli E, Piroth L, Martha B, et al. 2005. Low trough plasma concentrations of nevirapine associated with virologic rebounds in HIV-infected patients who switched from protease inhibitors. *Ann Pharmacother* 39(4):603–9.

76. Ren Y, Nuttall JJ, Egbers C, Eley BS, Meyers TM, Smith PJ, et al. 2007. High prevalence of subtherapeutic plasma concentrations of efavirenz in children. *J Acquir Immune Defic Syndr* 45(2):133–36.

77. Dieleman JP, Gyssens IC, van der Ende ME, de Marie S, Burger DM. 1999. Urological complaints in relation to indinavir plasma concentrations in HIV-infected patients. *AIDS* 13(4):473–78.

78. Valer L, Gonzalez de Requena D, de Mendoza C, Martin-Carbonero L, Gonzalez-Lahoz J, Soriano V. 2004. Impact of drug levels and baseline genotype and phenotype on the virologic response to amprenavir/ritonavir-based salvage regimens. *AIDS* Patient Care STDS 18(1):1–6.

79. Barrios A, Rendon AL, Gallego O, Martin-Carbonero L, Valer L, Rios P, et al. 2004. Predictors of virological response to atazanavir in protease inhibitor-experienced patients. *HIV Clin Trials* 5(4):201–5.

80. Pellegrin I, Breilh D, Ragnaud JM, Boucher S, Neau D, Fleury H, et al. 2006. Virological responses to atazanavir-ritonavir-based regimens: resistance-substitutions score and pharmacokinetic parameters (Reyaphar study). *Antivir Ther* 11(4):421–29.

81. Marcelin AG, Dalban C, Peytavin G, Lamotte C, Agher R, Delaugerre C, et al. 2004. Clinically relevant interpretation of genotype and relationship to plasma drug concentrations for resistance to saquinavir-ritonavir in human immunodeficiency virus type 1 protease inhibitor-experienced patients. *Antimicrob Agents Chemother* 48(12):4687–92.

82. Bonora S, Gonzalez de Requena D, Calcagno A, et al. 2006. Tipranavir genotypic inhibitory quotient predicts early virological response to TPV-based salvage regimens. *13th Conference on Retroviruses and Opportunistic Infections*. Denver, Colorado, Abstract 577.

83. Zhang XQ, Schooley RT, Gerber JG. 1999. The effect of increasing alpha1-acid glycoprotein concentration on the antiviral efficacy of human immunodeficiency virus protease inhibitors. *J Infect Dis* 180(6):1833–37.

19 Chromatographic Techniques for Therapeutic Drug Monitoring of Antiretroviral Drugs

Amitava Dasgupta
University of Texas Medical School

CONTENTS

19.1 INTRODUCTION

The year 2008 when this book chapter is being written marks the 27th anniversary of the discovery of the first reported case of a patient suffering from human immunodeficiency virus (HIV). In the beginning of reported HIV infections, only very few drugs were available in treating patients. Since then many new antiretroviral agents have been discovered and approved by the Federal Drug Administration (FDA) of the U.S. thus revolutionizing the antiretroviral therapy in treating patients with AIDS (Table 19.1). With the success of these medications in restoring immune function, now HIV infected patients can be managed like patients suffering from a chronic disease. Unfortunately, in developing countries only approximately 20% of patients have access to antiretroviral therapy, thus causing AIDS epidemic [1]. In highly active antiretroviral therapy (HAART); several drugs of

TABLE 19.1
Drugs that are Clinically Approved for Treating Patients with HIV Infection

Drug Class	Individual Drug	Year approved by FDA
Nucleoside/nucleotide reverse transcriptase inhibitors (eight total drugs in this class)	Zidovudine	1987
	Didanosine	1991
	Zalcitabine	1992
	Stavudine	1994
	Lamivudine	1995
	Abacavir	1998
	Tenofovir	2001
	Emtricitabine	2003
Nonnucleoside reverse transcriptase inhibitors (four total drugs in this class)	Nevirapine	1996
	Delavirdine	1997
	Efavirenz	1998
	Etravirine	2008
Protease inhibitors (10 total drugs in this class)	Indinavir	1996
	Ritonavir	1996
	Nelfinavir	1997
	Saquinavir	1997
	Amprenavir	1999
	Lopinavir	2000
	Atazanavir	2003
	Fosamprenavir	2003
	Tipranavir	2005
	Darunavir	2006
Entry inhibitor	Maraviroc	2007
Fusion inhibitor	Enfuvirtide	2003
Integrase inhibitor	Raltegravir	2007

different class are used in combination to treat patients with HIV. Currently there are 25 approved drugs belonging to six different classes are available for treating patients with HIV infection [2].

19.1.1 NUCLEOSIDE/NUCLEOTIDE REVERSE TRANSCRIPTASE INHIBITORS

These are the first antiretroviral agents available for treating HIV infection with the introduction of zidovudine in 1987. Since then seven other drug have been approved in this class and these drugs are used as the backbone of HAART therapy. These drugs after undergoing intracellular phosphorylation have a high affinity for HIV-1 reverse transcriptase. Then these phosphorylated drugs act as chain terminators for viral DNA replication [3].

19.1.2 NONNUCLEOSIDE REVERSE TRANSCRIPTASE INHIBITORS

Three drugs in this class are commonly available and all drugs are inhibitors of reverse transcriptase at a site distinct from the nucleoside reverse transcriptase inhibitors. The nonnucleoside reverse transcriptase inhibitors do not require intracellular phosphorylation for activation. Efavirenz is the most widely used drug in this class. These drugs are metabolized by the cytochrome P-450 mixed function oxidase [3].

19.1.3 Protease Inhibitors

Protease inhibitors were first available in 1995 and with the introduction of these drugs, immediate effect of decreased morbidity and mortality from HIV infection was noted [4]. Protease inhibitors block HIV replication by inhibiting protease, an enzyme needed by the HIV virus to cleave nascent proteins for final assembly of new virions. These drugs are metabolized by the cytochrome P-450 mixed function oxidase and most protease inhibitors also inhibit these enzymes. Therefore, these drugs interact pharmacokinetically with many other drugs that are metabolized by the cytochrome P-450 family of enzymes. These drugs or drug classes include azoles, opiates, oral contraceptives, rifamycin, statins, cyclosporine, tacrolimus, macrolide, and erectile dysfunction agents which may require dosage adjustments for both protease inhibitor and the interacting drug. Popular herbal antidepressant St. John's wort reduces efficacy of protease inhibitors due to induction of cytochrome P-450 mixed function oxidase and this herbal antidepressant should never be taken with protease inhibitors [2].

19.1.4 Entry Inhibitors

Maraviroc is the only entry inhibitor which is approved for clinical use by the FDA on 7th August 2007 [5]. Maraviroc inhibits chemokine (C-C motif) receptor 5 (CCR5) which is a receptor protein encoded by the human gene CCR5. CCR5 protein functions as a chemokine receptor and is predominately expressed on T cells, macrophages, dendritic cells and microglia. The HIV virus uses CCR5 and another protein CXCR4 as a coreceptor to enter target cells causing infection and immunodeficiency. CCR5 antagonist meraviroc does not interfere with any step of HIV viral replication [6].

The CCR5 coreceptor antagonists inhibit fusion of HIV virus with host cells by blocking the interaction between gp-120 viral protein and CCR5 chemokine receptor. Only four CCR5 inhibitors entered the clinical trial. The first drug aplaviroc showed promise but the trail was stopped in October 2005 because some patients developed severe toxicity. Currently only one drug is clinically approved [5].

19.1.5 Fusion Inhibitors

The only drug in this class is enfuvirtide, which is a 36 amino acid synthetic peptide. This drug binds to the gp^{4}1 envelop subunit of HIV and prevents the conformational change necessary for HIV virus to fuse with CD4+ cells. This drug is not absorbed orally, is given subcutaneously twice per day and it is the only injectable antiretroviral agent. Enfuvirtide is metabolized by hydrolysis, the only known pathway and its half-life is 3.6 h [3].

19.1.6 Integrase Inhibitors

The only FDA approved drug in this class is raltegravir which was approved for clinical use in 2007. In order for HIV to destroy immune function of the body, the HIV virus must take over function of CD4 cells. The RNA of HIV virus is converted into to DNA by reverse transcriptase enzyme and then after reverse transcription of RNA to DNA is complete, then viral DNA is incorporated into the DNA of CD4 cells and this process is called integration and is mediated by integrase enzyme. While nucleotide/nucleoside reverse transcriptase inhibitors block conversion of viral RNA to DNA, integrase inhibitor raltegravir blocks HIV replication by inhibiting integrase, a viral enzyme that inserts the viral genome to host cells. Therefore, replication of HIV virus is halted. This drug is rapidly absorbed and no dosage adjustment is needed in moderate hepatic or renal diseases. Adverse effects from this drug include nausea, headache, and diarrhea. This drug is not metabolized by cytochrome P-450 mixed function oxidase and no drug–drug interaction is expected from raltegravir and any drug which is a substrate for cytochrome P-450 mixed function oxidase [7].

19.1.7 MATURATION INHIBITORS

Currently, there is no maturation inhibitor that is approved by the FDA for clinical use. Bevirimat is under clinical trail and is a novel HIV-1 maturation inhibitor with a mechanism of action which is different from any antiretroviral drug used in treating HIV infected patients. Bevirimat inhibits replication of both wild type and drug resistant HIV-1 isolates in vitro. Specific inhibition of final rate limiting step in gag processing by this drug prevents release of mature capsids proteins from the precursor (CA-SP1), resulting in the production of non infective immature HIV viral particles. In healthy volunteers this drug was absorbed after oral administration and peak plasma concentration was observed between 1 and 3 h. The mean plasma elimination half-life is 50–80 h and due to long half-life this drug can be administered once daily [8].

19.2 RATIONALE FOR THERAPEUTIC DRUG MONITORING OF ANTIRETROVIRAL DRUGS

The rationales for therapeutic drug monitoring of specific antiretroviral drugs have been discussed in detail in Chapter 18. Briefly, low concentrations of antiretroviral agents in blood cause treatment failure and although many experts recommend routine therapeutic drug monitoring of antiretroviral drugs, there are still controversies regarding effects of drug monitoring on clinical outcomes. However, hepatic and renal insufficiency due to coinfection, diabetes mellitus, alcohol abuse, adverse effects of antiretroviral drugs, family history, and other factors commonly seen in HIV infected patients may alter pharmacokinetic parameters of antiretroviral drugs and clinicians must consider such parameters when prescribing HAART therapy for these patients [9]. HAART is recommended for pregnant mothers in order to prevent mother to fetus transmission of the HIV virus but potential variability in plasma concentrations of antiretroviral drugs during gestation lead to potential pharmacokinetic changes of these drugs during pregnancy requiring therapeutic drug monitoring of protease inhibitors and nonnucleoside reverse transcriptase inhibitors [10]. Suboptimal adherence to antiretroviral therapy is the most common cause of viral rebound and viral resistance causing treatment failure. Accurate and reliable adherence to therapy is vital in the transition from reactive response to the treatment to proactive prevention of rebound of HIV virus in patients infected with HIV [11]. Therapeutic drug monitoring is one of the tools available to clinicians in order to determine patient compliance with therapy. Suggested therapeutic ranges of several antiretroviral drugs are given in Table 19.2.

Although in some patients treatment with antiretroviral therapy is not effective and suppression of viral load is not achieved, in other patients the therapy has to be stopped or drug regime must be altered due to substantial toxicity. Several studies have demonstrated a relationship between plasma concentrations of protease inhibitors and nonnucleoside reverse transcriptase inhibitors and viral suppression and toxicity. Therapeutic drug monitoring uses plasma or serum drug concentrations to individualize and optimize therapy by dosage adjustments and many clinicians have advocated for routine therapeutic drug monitoring in patients receiving antiretroviral therapy [12]. In addition, antiretroviral drugs undergo numerous pharmacokinetic drug interactions with other drugs and herbal supplements and again therapeutic drug monitoring can alert clinicians by identifying potential clinically significant interactions between antiretroviral agents and another drug or herbal supplement [13]. In general, patients who have virological failure, show drug-drug interactions, pregnant women and the pediatric population with HIV infection, patients showing adverse effects from antiretroviral therapy and patients with hepatic or renal failure are benefited from therapeutic drug monitoring of antiretroviral drugs. Chemical structures of some commonly monitored antiretroviral drugs are given in Figure 19.1.

TABLE 19.2
Suggested Therapeutic Ranges of some of Antiretroviral Drugs

Drug	Specimen Requirement	Therapeutic Range* (trough)
Amprenavir	Serum/plasma	150–400 ng/ml
Atazanavir	Serum/plasma	100 ng/ml
Fosamprenavir	Serum/plasma	400 ng/ml
Indinavir	Serum/plasma	80–120 ng/ml
Lopinavir	Serum/plasma	700 ng/ml
Nelfinavir	Serum/plasma	700–1000 ng/ml
Saquinavir	Serum/plasma	100–250 ng/ml
Ritonavir	Serum/plasma	1000–2100 ng/ml
Nevirapine	Serum/plasma	150–400 ng/ml
Efavirenz	Serum/plasma	100 ng/ml
Delavirdine	Serum/plasma	2000–8000 ng/ml
Didanosine	Serum/plasma	100–300 ng/ml
Lamivudine	Serum/plasma	100–1000 ng/ml

* Reference ranges are recommended ranges only and may vary between institutions and based on published papers as well as scientific monographs.

19.3 CHROMATOGRAPHIC TECHNIQUES FOR MONITORING OF NUCLEOSIDE/NUCLEOTIDE REVERSE TRANSCRIPTASE INHIBITORS

Nucleoside/nucleotide reverse transcriptase inhibitors are the back bone of antiretroviral therapy and these drugs prevent replication of HIV virus by inhibiting synthesis of viral DNA. These drugs are prodrugs and must be phosphorylated intracellularly by endogenous kinase in order to obtain pharmacologically active triphosphate moieties. Therefore, these drugs are not routinely monitored because it may be difficult to establish correlation between plasma concentrations and antiretroviral effects of these drugs. Nevertheless, there is a clinical need for determining plasma concentrations of these drugs in case of poor response to therapy to determine whether virologic failure is due to noncompliance. In addition, there are some correlations between toxicity and plasma drug concentrations for these drugs. For example, zidovudine induced anemia is related to high zidovudine plasma concentration. In children the risk of anemia develops at zidovudine concentrations over 350 ng/ml [14]. Abacavir, a guanine analog could also be a good candidate for therapeutic drug monitoring because there is a correlation between viral load and CD4 count and serum drug level. Tenofovir, a nucleoside analog can cause tubular dysfunction leading to renal impairment in a limited number of patients. It was suggested that plasma concentrations over 200 ng/ml may cause renal dysfunction [15].

Only chromatographic methods are available for determination of serum concentrations of nucleoside/nucleotide reverse transcriptase inhibitors in serum and plasma. There are many reported methods in the literature. Uslu et al. developed a simple high performance liquid chromatography (HPLC) combined with ultraviolet (UV) detection method for determination of zalcitabine in bulk form, pharmaceutical dosage form and also in human serum. The mobile phase composition was methanol and 0.01 M sodium dihydrogen phosphate (85:15 by vol) after adjustment of pH using 1 M sodium hydroxide to 4.62. The elution of peaks was monitored at 265 nm wavelength [16]. In another report the authors simultaneously determined concentrations of zidovudine, lamivudine and the nonnucleoside reverse transcriptase inhibitor nevirapine in human plasma after solid phase

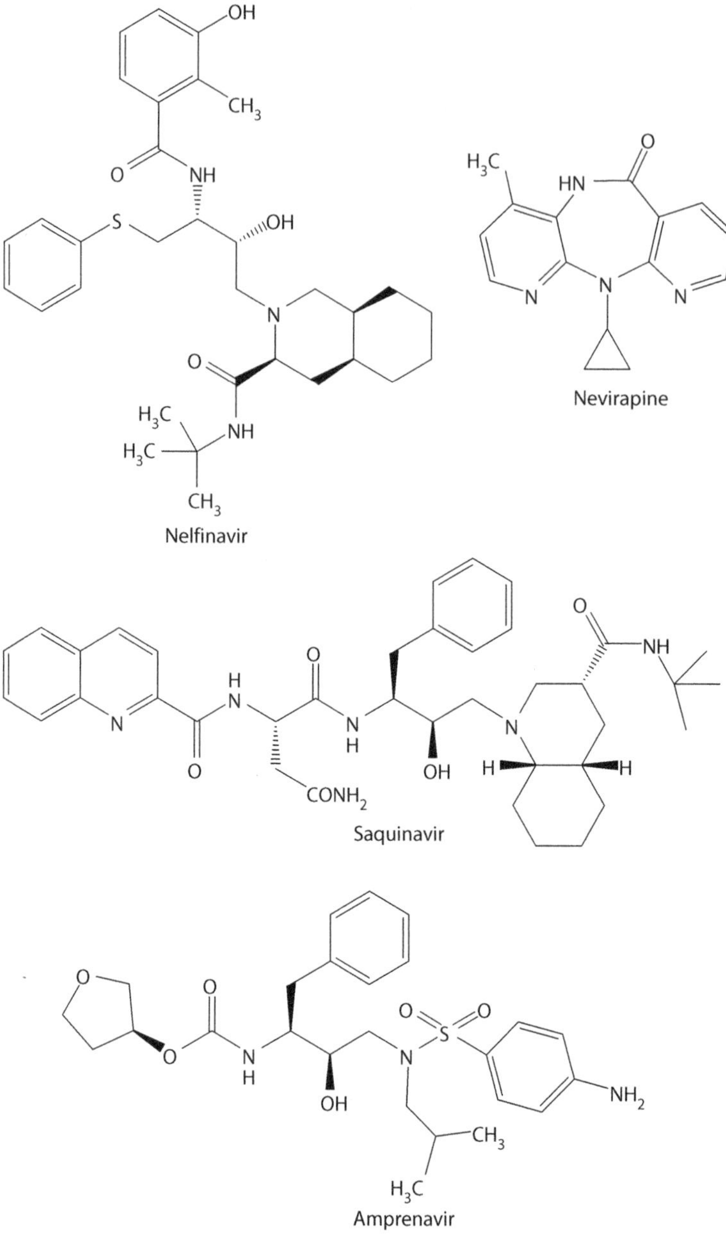

FIGURE 19.1 Chemical structures of nelfinavir, nevirapine, saquinavir, amprenavir, indinavir, and ritonavir.

extraction and using a mobile phase composition of 20 mM sodium phosphate buffer (containing 8 mM 1-octanesulfonic acid sodium salt) and acetonitrile (86:14 by vol). The pH of the mobile phase was adjusted to 3.2 with phosphoric acid. The chromatographic separation was achieved by using an octylsilane column (150 mm × 3.9 mm internal diameter) and elution of peak was monitored at 265 nm wavelength using a UV detector. Apobarbital was selected as the internal standard. The extraction recoveries of drugs and the internal standard were over 92% and the method was validated over a range of 57.6–2880 ng/ml for zidovudine, 59.0–17650 ng/ml for lamivudine and 53.2–13300 ng/ml for nevirapine [17]. Marchei et al. developed a simple HPLC method for simultaneous determination of zidovudine and nevirapine in human plasma after solid phase extraction and

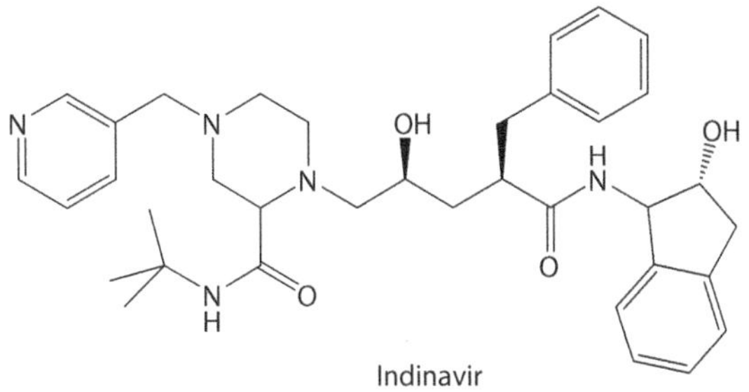

Indinavir

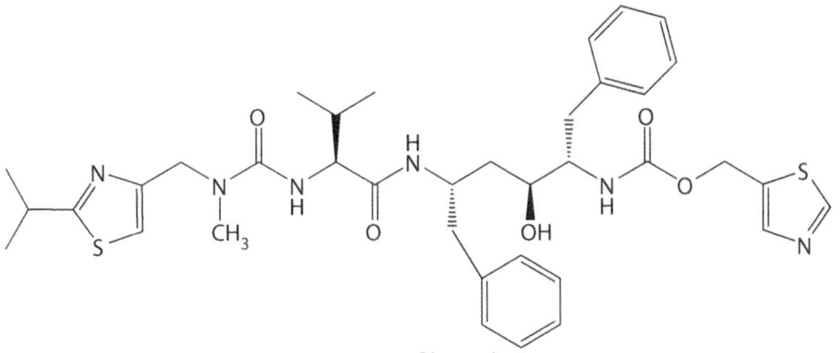

Ritonavir

FIGURE 19.1   (Continued)

chromatography using a C-18 reverse phase column and a mobile phase composition of potassium dihydrogen phosphate (10 mM, pH 6.5) and acetonitrile (83:17 by vol). The elution of peaks was monitored at 265 nm [18].

In addition to many HPLC-UV methods for determination of concentrations of nucleoside/nucleotide reverse transcriptase inhibitors in human serum, numerous methods combining HPLC with mass spectrometry have also been reported in the literature for determination of concentrations of these drugs in human serum or plasma. Usually mass spectrometric determination can results in much higher sensitivity as well as specificity compared to HPLC-UV methods. Kenney et al. simultaneously determined concentrations of zidovudine and lamivudine in human serum using ultrafiltration step instead of the solid phase extraction method commonly used in HPLC-UV methods. The sensitivity of the method was 2.5 ng/ml for each drug and the analysis can be performed using only 0.25 ml of human serum. The assay was linear from 2.5 to 2500 ng/ml for zidovudine and from 2.5 to 5000 ng/ml for lamivudine [19]. Quantitation of tenofovir in human plasma is important due to rise in use of this drug and the potential of renal dysfunction with higher drug levels. This drug can not be analyzed easily using HPLC and UV detection due to the presence of interfering peaks. D'Avolio et al. simultaneously determined concentrations of tenofovir and emtricitabine in plasma of HIV infected patients using liquid chromatography combined with electrospray ionization mass spectrometry (positive ionization mode). The mobile phase composition was acetonitrile in water gradient containing 0.05% formic acid. Calibration ranged from 15.6 to 4000 ng/ml for tenofovir and from 11.7 to 3000 ng/ml for emtricitabine. The limit of detection was 2 ng/ml for tenofovir and 1.5 ng/ml for emtricitabine. The method did not show any interference from other retroviral agents or drugs used by HIV patients. Moreover, there was no interference from the matrix [20]. Takahasi et al. determined concentration of tenofovir in human plasma using liquid chromatography combined with mass spectrometry and the assay was linear for tenofovir concentration of 19–1567 ng/ml and the recovery of tenofovir was more than 80.2% [21].

In another method authors determined concentrations of six nucleoside reverse transcriptase inhibitors (abacavir, didanosine, emtricitabine, lamivudine, stavudine, and zidovudine) and one nucleotide reverse transcriptase inhibitor (tenofovir) in human plasma using only 0.1 ml of specimen and liquid chromatography combined with mass spectrometry (LC-MS). The authors used 6-beta-hydroxy theophylline as the internal standard. Plasma proteins were precipitated with 0.5 ml acetonitrile and the supernatant was evaporated to dryness. The residues was reconstituted with 0.5 ml of water and only 10 µl was injected into LC-MS. The chromatographic analysis was carried out using a C-18 reverse phase column and a gradient of mobile phase using water and methanol, both containing 0.05% formic acid. After separation analytes were introduced into the mass spectrometer (triple quadrupole) through a heated electrospray ionization source (50°C) operating in the positive mode at a constant voltage of 5000 V. The temperature of the capillary transfer column was 270°C. The analytes were analyzed using selected reaction mode (SEM) and one precursor ion and one product ion were determined for each drug (Table 19.3). Ion suppression was negligible in the analysis. The run time of the assay was 14 min which was longer than the run time necessary for quantification of one or two drugs in this class but shorter than analysis of seven antiretroviral drugs when compared with other published methods. The detection limit varied from 5 to 20 ng/ml [22].

There are also numerous methods reported in the literature where the authors determined active phosphorylated metabolites of nucleoside reverse transcriptase inhibitors in human matrices. These methods involve liquid chromatography with UV detection, liquid chromatography with tandem mass spectrometric detection, capillary electrophoresis/electrochromatography with UV as well as mass spectrometric detection. Because of extremely low concentrations of these phosphorylated metabolites, specimen pretreatment using protein precipitation, liquid-liquid extraction and solid phase extraction have played important roles in developing successful methodologies for analysis of these active metabolites [23]. Moore et al. determined 5′-triphosphate metabolites of zidovudine, lamivudine and stavudine in peripheral mononuclear blood cells from HIV infected patients using HPLC combined with tandem mass spectrometry. These metabolites were extracted from peripheral mononuclear cells which are the site of HIV replication and drug action. The authors used ion exchange solid phase extraction followed by enzymatic digestion with alkaline phosphatase to yield measurable nucleoside forms of the nucleotides. The authors used 3′-azido-2, 3′-dideoxyuridine as the internal standard and reverse phase HPLC with a C-18 column for indirect measurement of original 5′-triphosphate metabolites and authors concluded that this method can be used for indirect determination of active metabolites of these drugs in patients infected with HIV [24]. Font et al. determined concentration of zidovudine triphosphate, the active metabolite of zidovudine in peripheral blood mononuclear cells in HIV infected patients indirectly using solid phase extraction and HPLC combined with tandem mass spectrometry using azidodeoxyuridine (3′-azido-3′-deoxyuridine) as the internal standard. Peripheral blood mononuclear cells were separated from erythrocytes by centrifugation and mononuclear cells were recovered and counted in an analyzer

TABLE 19.3
Ions used for Determination of Seven Nucleoside/Nucleotide Reverse Transcriptase Inhibitors and Linearity Ranges of each Drug

Drug	Precursor Ion	Product Ion	Calibration Curve
Abacavir	287.1	190.0	20–3000 ng/ml
Didanosine	237.1	137.0	10–1500 ng/ml
Emtricitabine	248.0	129.9	10–1500 ng/ml
Lamivudine	230.1	112.0	10–1500 ng/ml
Stavudine	225.1	126.9	20–3000 ng/ml
Tenofovir	288.1	176.1	5–750 ng/ml
Zidovudine	268.1	127.0	20–2500 ng/ml

Source: Takahasi M, Kudaka Y, Okumura N, Hirano A et al., *Biol Pharm Bull*, 30, 1784–1786, 2007.

(Coulter, Hialeah, FL) and metabolites were extracted from cells using 70% methanol. Then zidovudine triphosphate was finally extracted using solid phase extraction and then alkaline phosphates was for enzymatic digestion of triphosphate metabolite to liberate zidovudine and then the internal standard was added and recovered simultaneously with zidovudine using another solid phase extraction. The HPLC analysis was carried out using a C-18 reverse phase column and mobile phase consisted of acetonitrile/methanol (10:30 by vol) with 0.25% acetic acid with a flow rate of 0.2 ml/min. The zidovudine showed a protonated molecular ion at m/z 268 and a daughter ion at m/z 127 due to fragmentation of the glycoside bond. The internal standard showed a protonated molecular ion at m/z 254 and a daughter ion at m/z 113. The limit of detection of the assay was 4.0 fmol/10^6 cells. In a Hispanic population zidovudine triphosphate was detectable even 15 h after therapy and intracellular zidovudine triphosphate concentrations in these patients ranged from 41 to 193 fmol/10^6 cells [25].

19.4 CHROMATOGRAPHIC TECHNIQUES FOR MONITORING OF NONNUCLEOSIDE REVERSE TRANSCRIPTASE INHIBITORS

Nonnucleotide reverse transcriptase inhibitors do not require cellular activation for their pharmacological activities. Moreover, therapeutic efficacy as well as toxicity correlates with serum drug concentrations thus indicating benefits of therapeutic drug monitoring. There are several HPLC combined with UV methods for determination of serum or plasma concentrations of these drugs in patients infected with HIV virus. Pav et al. described a HPLC-UV method for the determination of nevirapine in human plasma, milk and cerebrospinal fluid using solid phase extraction followed by chromatographic analysis using a Supelco LC-8 analytic column. The authors used isocratic mobile phase consisting of 63% phosphate buffer (0.025 M, pH: 6.0) with 1-butanesulfonic acid as an anion pair reagent, 21.5% methanol and 15.5% acetonitrile. The elution of peaks was detected at 280 nm and the run time was 10 min. The assay was linear from 25 to 10,000 ng/ml [26]. Lopez et al. also used HPLC combined with UV detection for rapid determination of nevirapine in human plasma after deproteinization of 0.2 ml plasma with 50% trichloroacetic acid. The supernatant was directly injected into the HPLC instrument consisting of a C-18 reverse phase column. The mobile phase composition was 10 mM phosphate buffer (pH:5.0) and acetonitrile (82:18 by vol). The elution of peak was monitored at 240 nm. The retention time of nevirapine was only 2 min. The limit of detection was 100 ng/ml [27]. Langman et al. determined concentration of efavirenz in human plasma after liquid–liquid extraction of the drug from 0.2 ml specimen using diethyl ether. The authors used a C-18 reverse phase column and a guard column for HPLC analysis and the mobile phase composition was 67 mM potassium dihydrogen phosphate/acetonitrile. The elution of peak was detected at 246 nm wavelength and the assay was linear from plasma efavirenz concentration of 25–15,000 ng/ml [28].

There are also several published methods for determination of plasma concentrations of non-nucleotide reverse transcriptase inhibitors in human plasma using liquid chromatography combined with mass spectrometry. Gas chromatography combined with mass spectrometry (GC/MS) can also be used for analysis of these drugs. Lemmer et al. determined concentration of efavirenz and nevirapine in human plasma using GC/MS. The authors used hexobarbital as the internal standard. Before extraction, 0.8 ml ammonium buffer (pH: 9.5) and internal standard were added to 0.2 ml of specimen. Drugs along with the internal standard were extracted using solid phase extraction column and were finally eluted from the column with 2 ml methanol. The extract was evaporated to dryness and reconstituted with ethyl acetate/methanol (90:10 by vol) for analysis using GC/MS without derivatization. Baseline separation was achieved where hexobarbital was eluted from gas chromatographic capillary column first followed by efavirenz and nevirapine was eluted last. The mass spectrometer was operated under selected ion monitoring mode. The ions monitored for efavirenz were m/z 315, the molecular peak, 246, the base peak and 243 while m/z 266 (molecular ion), 265 (base peak) and 251 were monitored for efavirenz. For the internal standard m/z 221 (both molecular ion and base peak), 157 and 81 were monitored. The lower limit of detection was 26 ng/ml for efavirenz and 27 ng/ml for nevirapine while lower limit of quantitation was 54 ng/ml for nevirapine and 72 ng/ml for efavirenz [29].

There are also many liquid chromatography combined with mass spectrometric methods for determination of concentrations of nonnucleoside reverse transcriptase inhibitors in human serum or plasma. Laurito et al. determined concentrations of nevirapine in human plasma using HPLC coupled with electrospray tandem mass spectrometry after liquid-liquid extraction and chromatographic separation using a reverse phase C-18 column. The tandem mass spectrometric analysis was carried out using multiple reaction mode and the chromatographic run time was 5 min. The range of calibration curve was 10–5000 ng/ml [30].

19.5 CHROMATOGRAPHIC TECHNIQUES FOR MONITORING OF PROTEASE INHIBITORS

Therapeutic drug monitoring of protease inhibitors are highly recommended and not surprisingly numerous methods have been reported in the literature describing determination of concentrations of various protease inhibitors in human serum or plasma. In addition, there are also some indications for therapeutic drug monitoring of nonnucleoside reverse transcriptase inhibitors and many methods also describe simultaneous analysis of both protease inhibitors and nonnucleoside reverse transcriptase inhibitors in human serum or plasma. Both ultraviolet detection and mass spectrometric detection methods have been described for a analysis of these drugs. Although HPLC-UV methods can achieve adequate sensitivity for routine therapeutic drug monitoring of these antiretroviral agents, HPLC combined with mass spectrometric detection offers higher sensitivity and better specificity than HPLC-UV methods.

A reverse phase HPLC assay for simultaneous determination of five protease inhibitors (amprenavir, indinavir, nelfinavir, ritonavir, and saquinavir) in human plasma has been described where the authors used solid phase extraction followed by ion-pair reverse phase chromatography with UV detection at 210 nm for amprenavir, indinavir and nelfinavir and 239 nm for saquinavir and ritonavir. For amprenavir, indinavir and saquinavir, the assay was validated over the range of 25–25,000 ng/ml, using 0.6 ml plasma for analysis. For nelfinavir and ritonavir, the method was validated over the range of 50–25,000 ng/ml [31]. Sarasa-Nacenta et al. also described a HPLC-UV method for determination of five protease inhibitors; indinavir, amprenavir, ritonavir, saquinavir, and nelfinavir in human plasma after solid phase extraction and using verapamil as the internal standard. The chromatographic separation of these five drugs was achieved by using a C-18 column and a gradient mobile phase consisting of 15 mM phosphate buffer (pH: 5.75) and acetonitrile and elution of peaks was detected by a UV detector [32].

Remmel et al. described a HPLC-UV method for simultaneous quantification of indinavir, nelfinavir, ritonavir and saquinavir in human plasma. The authors used A-86093 {(5S, 8S,10S,11S)-9-hydroxy2-cyclopropyl-5-(1-methylethyl)-1-[(2-1-methylethyl)-4-thiazolyl]-3,6-dioxy-8,11-bis(phenylmethyl)-2,4,7, 12-tetraazatridecan-13-oic acid, 5-thiazolylmethyl ester}which they obtained from the Abbott Laboratories (Abbott Park, IL) as the internal standard. After adding the internal standard into a 0.25 ml plasma specimen, 0.25 ml of 0.05 mol/L of sodium hydroxide was added to make the specimen basic and then the drugs along with the internal standard were extracted using 2 ml methyl-tert-butyl ether. The organic layer was dried, then reconstituted with 0.2 ml of mobile phase and 50 μl was injected into the HPLC. The drugs along with the internal standards were separated using a C-4 column (250 mm × 3 mm internal diameter, 5 μm particle size) and a mobile phase composition of acetonitrile/50 mmol/L sodium formate buffer (52: 48 by vol, pH adjusted to 4.10 with 2 mmol/L sodium hydroxide). The flow rate was 0.5 ml/min and UV detection wavelength was set at 218 nm for indinavir, nelfinavir, ritonavir, and the internal standard while the detection wavelength for saquinavir was 235 nm. Representative chromatograms showing separation of drugs and internal standards obtained by this protocol are shown in Figure 19.2.

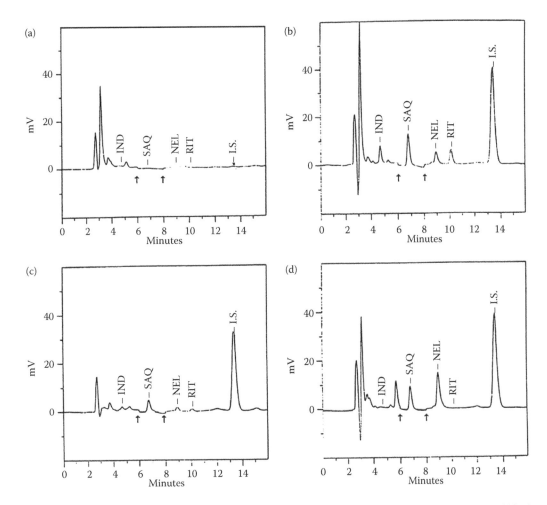

FIGURE 19.2 Chromatograms from simultaneous HPLC assay of HIV protease inhibitors. (a) extracted blank EDTA-derived plasma; (b) extracted plasma calibrator containing 964 µg/L indinavir (IND), 438 µg/L saquinavir (SAQ), 428 µg/L nelfinavir (NEL) and 1000 µg/L ritonavir (RTI), (c) extracted low concentration quality control sample containing 194 µg/L indinavir (IND), 175 µg/L saquinavir (SAQ), 171 µg/L of nelfinavir (NEL) and 200 µg/L ritonavir (RIT), (d) patient's sample containing 309 µg/L saquinavir (SAQ) and 1253 µg/L nelfinavir (NEL). The peak eluting before saquinavir is M-8 metabolite of nelfinavir. The arrows indicate the time the detector wavelength switch. IS, internal standard. (From Remmel R, Kawle S, Weller D, Fletcher C., *Clin Chem*, 46, 73–81, 2000. Reprinted with permission. Copyright: 2000: American Association for Clinical Chemistry.)

The limits of quantification were 40–50 ng/ml for indinavir, nelfinavir and ritonavir while the limit of quantification was 20 ng/ml for saquinavir. Extraction recoveries were between 87 and 92%. No interference in this method was observed from drugs commonly used in patients with HIV infection [33]. Verbesselt et al. also used A-86093 available from the Abbott Laboratories as the internal standard for simultaneous determination of several HIV proteose inhibitors in human plasma by isocratic HPLC with combined UV and fluorescence detection: amprenavir, indinavir, atazanavir, ritonavir, lopinavir, saquinavir, and nelfinavir along with M8-nelfanivir metabolite. The authors extracted these drugs from 0.5 ml human plasma after adding the internal standard and borate buffer (pH: 9.0) and then extracting drugs along with the internal standard using liquid–liquid extraction using hexane and ethyl acetate. Isocratic chromatographic separation was achieved by using a hexyl column with combined UV and fluorescence detection. Calibration curves ranged from 25 to 10,000 ng/ml. The authors concluded that their method can be applied for routine therapeutic drug monitoring of protease inhibitors [34].

The concentrations of protease inhibitors in human plasma can also be determined by using liquid chromatography combined with mass spectrometry or tandem mass spectrometry. In one report simultaneous determination of five HIV protease inhibitors (nelfinavir, indinavir, ritonavir, saquinavir, and amprenavir) in human plasma was carried out by liquid chromatography combined with tandem mass spectrometry after a simple acetonitrile protein precipitation step. The mass spectrometer was operated in positive mode using ion pairs at m/z 568.4/330.0, 614.3/421.2, 720.9/296.0, 671.1/570.2, and 505.9/245.0 for nelfinavir, indinavir, ritonavir, saquinavir, and amprenavir, respectively. The ion pair 628/421 was used for the internal standard. The overall recoveries of all drugs were over 87% [35]. Crommentuyn et al. reported liquid chromatography coupled with electrospray ionization tandem mass spectrometric method for rapid determination of six protease inhibitors (amprenavir, indinavir, lopinavir, nelfinavir, ritonavir and saquinavir) in human plasma using deuterated saquinavir (saquinavir d5) and indinavir (indinavir-d6) as the internal standards. The sample pretreatment consisted of a protein precipitation step using a mixture of methanol and acetonitrile, using only 0.1 ml of specimen. The chromatographic separation was achieved using a reverse phase column (Inertsil ODS3 column; 50X 2.0 mm internal diameter; particle size 5 µm) and a quick stepwise gradients using acetate buffer (pH: 5) and methanol at a flow rate of 0.5 ml/min. The analytical run time was 5.5 min. The mass spectrometer was operated in a positive ion mode and multiple reaction monitoring was used for quantification of drugs. The authors validated the method from 10 to 10,000 ng/ml for both indinavir and saquinavir, from 100 to 10,000 ng/ml for amprenavir, from 50 to 10,000 ng/ml for both nelfinavir and ritonavir and from 100 to 20,000 ng/ml for lopinavir and finally from 10 to 5000 ng/ml for M8 metabolite. The authors successfully applied this robust and fast method for therapeutic drug monitoring of protease inhibitors in their hospital [36]. In another report, Dickinson et al. described a protocol using liquid chromatography combined with tandem mass spectrometry for quantitation of amprenavir, atazanavir, indinavir, lopinavir, nelfinavir, ritonavir and saquinavir using Ro31-9564 (Roche Discovery, Welwyn, UK) as the internal standard. The chromatographic analysis of these seven protease inhibitors along with the internal standard was carried out using a reverse phase C-18 column after extraction of these drugs along with the internal standard from human plasma (using acetonitrile for protein precipitation followed by addition of ammonium formate buffer) and a gradient mobile phase composed of acetonitrile and ammonium formate buffer. Parent and daughter ion combination was used for mass spectrometric identification and quantification of each drug; for example ion pair 614.4 (parent) and 465.2 (daughter) was used for analysis of indinavir. The run time was 9 min. The intra and interassay variability was less than 11% and recovery of protease inhibitors from plasma was above 87% [37].

19.6 CHROMATOGRAPHIC TECHNIQUES FOR MONITORING OF FUSION INHIBITORS

There are few published methods for the measurement of concentrations of fusion inhibitors in human plasma. These polypeptides can not be analyzed by gas chromatography and liquid chromatography is the only available method. In one method, the authors determined concentrations of fusion inhibitors enfuvirtide and tifuvirtide along with M-20 metabolite of enfuvirtide using liquid chromatography combined with mass spectrometry. The authors used deuterated enfuvirtide (d60) and tifuvirtide (d50) as the internal standards. The analytes were extracted from 0.5 ml of plasma after addition of internal standards using solid phase extraction with vinyl-copolymer cartridges. Chromatographic separation was achieved by a reverse phase C-18 column (50 mm×2.1 mm internal diameter, particle size 3.5 µm) using a water-acetonitrile gradient mobile phase containing 0.25% formic acid. The triple quadrupole mass spectrometer was operated in the positive ion mode and the multiple reaction monitoring mode for identification and quantification of these fusion inhibitors. Enfuvirtide is a polypeptide with a molecular weight of 4492 daltons. For enfuvirtide the most abundant ion as at m/z 1123.8 representing $[M+4H]^{4+}$. The mass spectrum of tifuvirtide demonstrated two abundant peaks, corresponding to $[M+5H]^{5+}$ and $[M+4H]^{4+}$. The fragmentation of $[M+5H]^{5+}$ only yielded useful product ions. The transition m/z 1124.0–1343.5 was used for determination of both enfuvirtide and M-20 metabolite while transition m/z 1008.4–1219.0 was used for determination of tituvirtude. The assay was linear for a concentration range of 20–10,000 ng/ml for both enfuvirtide and tifuvirtide and from 20 to 2000 ng/ml for M-20 metabolite of enfuvirtide. This method can be applied for therapeutic drug monitoring of enfuvirtide in patients receiving this only clinically approved fusion inhibitor [38]. Enzymatic digestion technique using chymotrypsin has been applied for determination of enfuvirtide concentration in human plasma along with its M-20 metabolite. The authors used deuterated enfuvirtide (d60) as the internal standard. Enzyme digestion step was carried out after solid phase extraction of the drug and could use as much as four different chymotryptic fragments for the quantification of enfuvirtide in a concentration range from 100 to 10,000 ng/ml [39].

19.7 CHROMATOGRAPHIC TECHNIQUES FOR MONITORING OF INTEGRASE INHIBITORS

Raltegravir is the only fusion inhibitor approved for clinical use in treating HIV infected patients. There are several chromatographic methods described for determination of this drug in human plasma. Rezk et al. used HPLC combined with UV detection for rapid quantification of raltegravir in human plasma after solid phase extraction of the drug and the internal standard from the specimen. The method was validate over the range of 20–10,000 ng/ml. The recovery was over 90% [40]. Takahasi et al. developed a simple liquid chromatography combined with mass spectrometric method for determination of raltegravir in human plasma after liquid-liquid extraction of the drug along with the internal standard (A-86093, Abbott Laboratories) from 0.5 ml of specimen. Two milliliter of methylene chloride/hexane (50:50 by vol) containing the internal standard (328 ng/ml) and 0.3 ml 0.2 M ammonium acetate were added to 0.5 ml of plasma for extraction of the drug along with the internal standard. After drying the organic phase containing the drug and the internal standard, the dry residue was reconstituted with the mobile phase for chromatographic analysis using a reverse phase C-18 column and mobile phase consisting of 0.1 mM EDTA in 0.15 acetic acid (A), acetonitrile (B) and methanol (C). An isocartic mobile phase consisting of A, B and C (65:15:20) was used for the first 2 min of the analysis followed by a linear gradient of elution for next 8 min. The mass spectrometer was operated in positive ion electrospray mode and quantitative analysis was carried out in selected ion monitoring mode using m/z 445 for raltegravir and m/z 748 for the internal standard. The method was validated over the concentration range of 10–7680 ng/ml [41]. A sensitive method using liquid chromatography combine with tandem mass spectrometry has also been reported for analysis of raltegravir in human plasma [42].

19.8 CHROMATOGRAPHIC TECHNIQUES FOR MONITORING MULTIPLE CLASSES OF DRUGS IN A SINGLE RUN

There are numerous chromatographic methods published in the literature for simultaneous analysis of more than one class of antiretroviral agent using either UV detection or mass spectrometric analysis of these drugs [43–56]. Usually HAART therapy uses more than one class of drugs and there is an advantage in using chromatographic methods that are capable of analyzing multiple drug classes in a single run for therapeutic drug monitoring of patients receiving antiretroviral therapy.

In an earlier report, Moyer et al. using three different HPLC-UV methods determined concentrations peak of trough concentrations of seven antiretroviral agents (delavirdine, lamivudine, nevirapine, indinavir, nelfinavir, ritonavir, and saquinavir) as well as peak concentrations of stavudine, zidovudine and didanosine in human plasma. The authors used tegafur as the internal standard for the analysis of didanosine, lamivudine, and stavudine. Internal standard was added to the 1 ml serum and drugs along with the internal standard were extracted from serum using solid phase C-18 extraction column. After washing, drugs along with the internal standard were eluted from the extraction column using 1 ml methanol. After evaporation of methanol, the dry residue was reconstituted with the mobile phase and analyzed using a C-18 column and mobile phase composition of 40 ml/L of acetonitrile in 10 mmol/L phosphate at pH 6.9. Elution of peaks was monitored using a UV detector at 248 nm wavelength. For analysis of nevirapine and zidovudine, the authors used 3-isobutyl-1-methylxanthine as the internal standard and extracted these drugs along with the internal standard from human serum specimen using chloroform and isopropyl alcohol. Chromatographic separation was carried out using a C-8 column and elution of peaks was monitored at 266 nm wavelength. For analysis of delavirdine, indinavir, nelfinavir, ritonavir, and saquinavir, encainide was used as the internal standard and again chromatographic separation was achieved by a C-8 column. The elution of peak was monitored at 254 nm. Representative chromatograms showing analysis of these drugs are given in Figure 19.3. The limit of defection was 100 ng/ml, for delavirdine, nevirapine, indinavir, nelfinavir, ritonavir and lamivudine while limit of detection was 25 ng/ml, for stavudine. For three other drugs; didanosine, zidovudine, and saquinavir, the detection limit was 10 ng/ml. Using this method the authors reported that peak indinavir

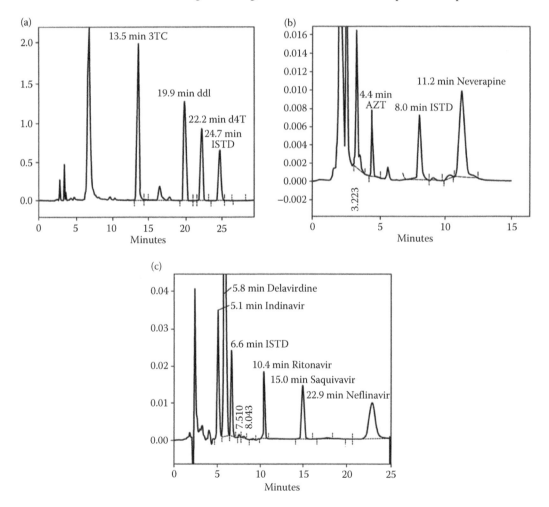

FIGURE 19.3 High performance liquid chromatograms of antiretrovirals at concentrations near Cmax. (a) didanosine (ddi), lamivudine (3TC), and stavudine (d4T); (b): nevirapine and zidovudine; (c); indinavir, delavirdine, ritonavir, saquinavir, and nelfinavir. ISTD; internal standard. (From Moyer TP, Temesgen Z, Enger R, et al., *Clin Chem,* 45, 1465–1476, 1999. Reprinted with permission. Copyright: 1999: American Association for Clinical Chemistry.)

serum concentration in most patients were in the range 1–10 mg/L and trough concentration sin the range 0.1–0.5 mg/L. Peak stavudine concentrations were in the range of 0.3–1.3 mg/L and trough concentrations were in the range of 0.1–0.5 mg/L. Peak zidovudine concentrations were in the range of 0.1–1.1 mg/L [43]. Notari et al. determined concentrations of 16 antiretroviral drugs simultaneously in human plasma using a simple HPLC-UV method. These drugs include seven protease inhibitors (amprenavir, atazanavir, indinavir, lopinavir, nelfinavir, ritonavir and saquinavir), seven nucleoside reverse transcriptase inhibitors (abacavir, didanosine, emtricitabine, lamivudine, stavudine, zalcitabine, and zidovudine) and two nonnucleoside reveres transcriptase inhibitors (efavirenz and nevirapine). The authors used 0.6 ml of specimen for the analysis and chromatographic separation was achieved by using a C-18 column. Elution of peaks was monitored at 240 nm and 260 nm [53].

Many authors also used liquid chromatography combined with mass spectrometry for analysis of different class of antiretroviral agents from human plasma or serum. Villani et al. using liquid chromatography coupled with electrospray mass spectrometry analyzed five protease inhibitors (saquinavir, indinavir, ritonavir, nelfinavir, and amprenavir) and three nonnucleoside reverse transcriptase inhibitors (nevirapine, delavirdine, and efavirenz) in a single run (10 min) using a linear gradient of mobile phase consisting of water and acetonitrile and a reverse phase C-18 column. The authors used 6,7-dimethyl-quinoxaline as the internal standard. The assay showed good linearity (20–10,000 ng/ml) for most drugs [47]. In another method the authors simultaneously determined concentrations of the new HIV protease inhibitor darunavir along with 11 other antiretroviral agents using liquid chromatography combined with mass spectrometry. A simple protein precipitation procedure was applied to 50 μl of specimen and quinoxaline was used as the internal standard and chromatographic separation was achieved by using a reverse phase C-18 column and a solvent gradient consisting of acetonitrile and water with 0.05% formic acid [52]. Volosov et al. used 80 μl of specimen for rapid quantification of 15 antiretroviral agents using protein precipitation with 200 μl acetonitrile. The authors used cimetidine as the internal standard [48]. Recently, a MALDI/TOF/TOF method has been described in the literature for determination of abacavir, didanosine, efavirenz, nevirapine and stavudine in human plasma [57].

19.9 CONCLUSIONS

Chromatographic techniques are the only available methods for therapeutic drug monitoring of antiretroviral agents. Although, HPLC-UV methods provide adequate sensitivity for determination of serum concentrations of these drugs, better sensitivity and specificity can be achieved by using liquid chromatography combined with mass spectrometry. However, liquid chromatography combined with mass spectrometry is expensive and the laboratories need to invest a large sum of money to acquire such instrumention. In contrast, HPLC-UV systems are relatively less expensive than liquid chromatography combined with mass spectrometry instruments.

REFERENCES

1. Greene WC, Debyser Z, Ikeda Y, Freed EO et al. 2008. Novel targets for HIV therapy. *Antiviral Res* 80: 251–265.
2. Hoffman RM, Currier JS. 2007. Management of antiretroviral treatment-related complications. *Infect Dis Clin North Am* 21: 103–132.
3. Kalkut G. 2005. Antiretroviral therapy: an update for non-AIDS specialist. *Curr Opin Oncol* 17: 479–484.
4. Palella FJ, Delaney KM, Moorman AC et al. 1998. Declining morbidity and mortality among patients with advanced human immunodeficiency virus infection. HIV outpatient study investigators. *N Eng J Med* 338: 853–860.
5. Emmelkamp JM, Rockstroh JK. 2007. CCR5 antagonists: comparison of efficacy, side effects, pharmacokinetics and interactions-review of the literature. *Eur J Med Res* 12: 409–417.

6. Bredeek UF, Harbour MJ. 2007. CCR5 antagonists in the treatment–naïve patients infected with CCR5 topic HIV-1. *Eur J Med Res* 12: 427–434.

7. Cocohoba J, Dong BJ. 2008. Raltegravir: the first HIV integrase inhibitor. *Clin Ther* 30: 1747–1765.

8. Martin DE, Salzwedel K, Allaway GP. 2008. Bevirimat: a novel maturation inhibitor for the treatment of HIV-1 infection. *Antivir Chem Chemother* 19: 107–113.

9. McCabe SM, Ma Q, Slish JC, Catanzaro LM et al. 2008. Antiretroviral therapy: pharmacokinetic considerations in patients with renal or hepatic impairment. *Clin Pharmacokinetic* 47: 153–172.

10. Roustit M, Jlaiel M, Leclercq P, Stanke-Labesque F. 2008. Pharmacokinetics and therapeutic drug monitoring of antiretroviral in pregnant women. *Br J Clin Pharamacol* 66: 179–195.

11. Bangsberg DR. 2008. Preventing HIV antiretroviral resistance through the better monitoring of treatment adherence. *J Infect Dis* 197 Suppl: S272–278.

12. Justesen US. 2006. Therapeutic drug monitoring and human immunodeficiency virus (HIV) antiretroviral therapy. *Basic Clin Pharmacol Toxicol* 98: 20–31.

13. Dasgupta A, Okhuysen PC. 2001. Pharmacokinetics and other drug interactions in patients with AIDS. *Ther Drug Monit* 23: 591–605.

14. Capparelli EV, Englund JA, Connor JD, Spector SA et al. 2003. Population pharmacokinetics and pharmacodynamics of zidovudine in HIV-infected infants and children. *J Clin Pharmacol* 43: 133–140.

15. Jullien V, Treluyer JM, Rey E, Jaffray P et al. 2005. Population pharmacokinetics of tenofovir in human immunodeficiency virus-infected patients taking highly active antiretroviral therapy. *Antimicrob Agents Chemother* 49: 3361–3366.

16. Uslu B, Savaser A, Ozkan SA, Ozkan Y. 2004. Validated RP-hPLC method for the assay of zalcitabine in drug substance, formulated products and human serum. *Pharmazzie* 59: 604–607.

17. Fan B, Stewart JT. 2002. Determination of zidovudine/lamivudine/nevirapine in human plasma using ion-pair HPLC. *J Pharm Biomed Anal* 28: 903–908.

18. Marchei E, Valvo L, Pacifici R, Pellegrini M et al. 2002. Simultaneous determination of zidovudine and nevirapine in human plasma by RP-LC. *J Pharm Biomed Anal* 29: 1081–1088.

19. Kenney KB, Wring SA, Carr RM, Wells GN et al. 2000. Simultaneous determination of zidovudine and lamivudine in human serum using HPLC and tandem mass spectrometry. *J Pharm Biomed Anal* 22: 967–983.

20. D'Avolio A, Sciandra M, Siccardi M, Baietto L et al. 2008. A new assay based on solid phase extraction procedure with LC-MS to measure plasmatic concentrations of tenofovir and emtricitabine in HIV infected patients. *J Chromatogr Sci* 46: 524–528.

21. Takahasi M, Kudaka Y, Okumura N, Hirano A et al. 2007. Determination of plasma tenofovir concentrations using a conventional LC-MS method. *Biol Pharm Bull* 30: 1784–1786.

22. Le saux T, Chhun S, Rey E, launay O et al. 2008. Quantification of seven nucleoside/nucleotide reverse phase transcriptase inhibitors in human plasma by high performance liquid chromatography with tandem mass spectrometry. *J Chromatogr B Analyt Technol Biomed Life Sci* 865: 81–90.

23. Lai J, wang J, Cai Z. 2008. Nucleoside reverse transcriptase inhibitors and their phosphorylated metabolites in human immunodeficiency virus-infected human matrices. *J Chromatogr B Analyst Technol Biomed Life Sci* 868: 1–12.

24. Moore JD, Valette G, Darque A, Zhou XJ et al. 2000. Simultaneous quantitation of the 5-triphosphate metabolites of zidovudine, lamivudine and stavudine in peripheral mononuclear blood cells of HIV infected patients by high performance liquid chromatography tandem mass spectrometry. *J Am Soc Mass Spectrom* 11: 1134–1143.

25. Font E, Rosario O, Santana J, Garcia H et al. 1999. Determination of zidovudine triphosphate intracellular concentrations in peripheral blood mononuclear cells from human immunodeficiency virus infected individuals by tandem mass spectrometry. *Antimicrob Agents Chemother* 43: 2964–2968.

26. Pav JW, Rowland LS, Korpalski DJ. 1999. HPLC-UV method for the quantitation of nevirapine in biological matrices following solid phase extraction. *J Pharm Biomed Anal* 20: 91–98.

27. Lopez RM, Pou L, GomezMR, Ruiz I et al. 2001. Simple and rapid determination of nevirapine in human serum by reverse-phase high-performance liquid chromatography. *J Chromatogr B Biomed Appl* 751: 371–376.

28. Langman P, Schirmer D, Vath T, Zilly M et al. 2001. High performance liquid chromatographic method for the determination of HIV-1 non nucleoside reverse transcriptase inhibitor efavirenz in plasma of patients during highly active antiretroviral therapy. *J Chromatogr B Biomed Appl* 755: 151–156.

29. Lemmer P, Schneider S, Schuman M, Omes C et al. 2005. Determination of nevirapine and efavirenz in plasma using GC/MS in selected ion monitoring mode. *Ther Drug Monit* 27: 521–525.

30. Laurito TL, Sanragada V, Caliendo G, Oliveira CH et al. 2002. Nevirapine quantification in human plasma by high performance liquid chromatography coupled to electrospray tandem mass spectrometry. Application to bioequivalence study. *J Mass Spectrom* 37: 434–441.
31. van Heeswijk RP, Hoetelmans RM, Harms R, Meenhorst PL et al. 1998. Simultaneous quantitative determination of HIV protease inhibitors amprenavir, indinavir, nelfinavir, ritonavir and saquinavir in human plasma by ion-pair high performance liquid chromatography with ultraviolet detection. *J Chromatogr B Biomed Sci Appl* 719: 159–168.
32. Sarasa-Nacenta M, Lopez-Pua Y, Mallolas J, Blanco JL et al. 2001. Simultaneous determination of HIV protease inhibitors indinavir, amprenavir, ritonavir, saquinavir and nelfinavir in human plasma by reverse phase high performance liquid chromatography. *J Chromatogr B Biomed Sci Appl* 757: 325–332.
33. Remmel R, Kawle S, Weller D, Fletcher C. 2000. Simultaneous HPLC assay for quantification of indinavir, nelfinavir, ritonavir and saquinavir in human plasma. *Clin Chem* 46: 73–81.
34. Verbesselt R, Van Wijngaerden E, de Hoon J. 2007. Simultaneous determination of 8 HIV proteose inhibitors in human plasma by isocratic high performance liquid chromatography with combined UV and fluorescence detection: amprenavir, indinavir, atazanavir, ritonavir, lopinavir, saquinavir, nelfinavir and M8-nelfanivir metabolite. *J Chromatogr B Analyt Technol Biomed Life Sci* 845: 51–60.
35. Chi J, Jayewardene AL, Stone JA, Motoya T et al. 2002. Simultaneous determination of five HIV protease inhibitors nelfinavir, indinavir, ritonavir, saquinavir and amprenavir in human plasma by LC/MS/MS. *J Phram Biomed Appl* 30: 675–684.
36. Crommentuyn KM, Rosing H, Nan-Offeringa LG, Hillebrand MJ et al. 2003. Rapid quantification of HIV protease inhibitors in human plasma by high performance liquid chromatography couples with electrospray ionization mass spectrometry. *J Mass Spectrom* 38: 157–166.
37. Dickinson L, Robinson L, Tjia J, Khoo S et al. 2005. Simultaneous determination of HIV protease inhibitors amprenavir, atazanavir, indinavir, lopinavir, nelfinavir, ritonavir and saquinavir in human plasma by high performance liquid chromatography-tandem mass spectrometry. *J Chromatogr B Analyt Technol Biomed Life Sci* 829: 82–90.
38. van den Broek I, Sparidans RW, Huitema ADR, Schellens JH et al. 2006. Development and validation of a quantitative assay for the measurement of two HIV fusion inhibitors, enfuvirtide and tifuvirtide and one metabolite enfuvirtide (M-20) in human plasma by liquid chromatography-tandem mass spectrometry. *J Chromatogr B Analyt Technol Biomed Life Sci* 837: 49–58.
39. van den Broek I, Sparidans RW, Schellens JH, Beijnen JH. 2007. Enzymatic digestion as a tool for the LC-MS/MS quantification of larger peptides in biological matrices: measurement of chymotryptic fragments from HIV-1 fusion inhibitor enfuvirtide and its metabolite M-20 in human plasma. *J Chromatogr B Analyt Technol Biomed Life Sci* 854: 245–259.
40. Rezk NL, White N, Kashuba AD. 2008. An accurate and precise high performance liquid chromatography method for the rapid quantification of the novel HIV integrase inhibitor raltegravir in human blood plasma after solid phase extraction. *Anal Chim Acta* 628: 204–213.
41. Takahasi M, Konishi M, Kudaka Y, Okumura N et al. 2008. A conventional LC-MS method developed for the determination of plasma raltegravir concentrations. *Biol Pharm Bull* 31: 1601–1604.
42. Long MC, Bennetto-Hood C, Acosta EP. 2008. A sensitive JPLC-MS-MS method for the determination of raltegravir in human plasma. *J Chromatogr B Analyt Technol Biomed Life Sci* 867: 165–171.
43. Moyer TP, Temesgen Z, Enger R, et al. 1999. Drug monitoring of antiretroviral therapy for HIV-1 infection: method validation and results of a pilot study. *Clin Chem* 45:1465–1476.
44. Elens L, Veriter S, Fazio VD, Vanbinst R et al. 2009. Quantification of 8 HIV protease inhibitors and 2 non-nucleoside reverse transcriptase inhibitors by ultra performance liquid chromatography with diode array detection. *Clin Chem* 55: 170–174.
45. Poirier JM, Robidou P, Jaillon P. 2005. Simple simultaneous determination of the HIV-protease inhibitors amprenavir, atazanavir, indinavir, lopinavir, nelfinavir, ritonavir and saquinavir plus M* nelfinavir metabolite and the two nonnucleoside reverse transcriptase inhibitors efavirenz and nevirapine in human plasma by reverse phase liquid chromatography. *Ther Drug Monit* 27: 186–192.
46. Titier K, Lagrange F, Pehourcq F, et al. 2002. High-performance liquid chromatographic method for the simultaneous determination of the six HIV-protease inhibitors and two non-nucleoside reverse transcriptase inhibitors in human plasma. *Ther Drug Monit* 24: 417–424.
47. Villani P, Feroggio M, Gianelli L, et al. 2002. Antiretrovirals: simultaneous determination of five protease inhibitors and three nonnucleoside transcriptase inhibitors in human plasma by a rapid high-performance liquid chromatography-mass spectrometry assay. *Ther Drug Monit* 24: 380–388.

48. Volosov A, Alexander C, Ting L, Soldin SJ. 2002. Simple rapid method for quantification of antiretrovi-rals by liquid chromatography-tandem mass-spectrometry. *Clin Biochem* 35: 99–103.

49. Ghoshal AK, Soldin SJ. 2003. Improved method for concurrent quantification of antiretrovirals by liquid chromatography-tandem mass spectrometry. *Ther Drug Monit* 25: 541–543.

50. ter Heine R, Alderden –Los CG, Rosing H, Hillebrand MJ et al. 2007. Fast and simultaneous determina-tion of daunavir and eleven other antiretroviral drugs for therapeutic drug monitoring: method develop-ment and validation for the determination of all currently approved HIV protease inhibitors and non nucleoside reverse transcriptase inhibitors in human plasma by liquid chromatography coupled with electrospray ionization mass spectrometry. *Rapid Commun Mass Spectrom* 21: 2505–2514.

51. Jung BH, Rezk NL, Bridges AS, Corbrett AH et al. 2007. Simultaneous determination of 17 antiretroviral drugs in the human plasma for quantitative analysis with liquid chromatography-tandem mass spectrom-etry. *Biomed Chromatogr* 21: 1095–1104.

52. D'Avolio A, Siccardi M, Sciandra M, Lorena B et al. 2007. HPLC-MS method for the simultaneous quantification of the new HIV protease inhibitor draunavir and 11 other antiretroviral agents in plasma of HIV infected patients. *J Chromatogr B Analyt Technol Biomed Life Sci* 859: 234–240.

53. Notari S, Bocedi A,Ippolito G, Narciso P et al. 2006. Simultaneous determination of 16 anti-HIV drugs in human plasma by high performance liquid chromatography. *J Chromatogr B Analyt Technol Biomed Life Sci* 831: 258–266.

54. Rouzes A, Berthoin K, Xuereb F, Djabarouti S. et al. 2004. Simultaneous determination of the antiretro-viral agents: amprenavir, lopinavir, ritonavir, saquinavir and efavirenz in human peripheral blood mono-nuclear cells by high performance liquid chromatography-mass spectrometry. *J Chromatogr B Analyt Technol Biomed Life Sci* 813: 209–216.

55. Koal T, Sibum M, Koster E, Resch K et al. 2006. Direct and fast determination of antiretroviral drugs by automated online solid phase extraction-liquid chromatography-tandem mass spectrometry in human plasma. *Clin Chem Lab Med* 44: 299–305.

56. D'Avolio A, Baietto L, Siccardi M, Sciandra M et al. 2008. An HPLC-PDA method for the simultaneous quantification of the HIV integrase inhibitor raltegravir and the new non-nucleoside reverse transcriptase inhibitor etravirine and 11 other antiretroviral agents in the plasma of HIV infected patients. *Ther Drug Monit* 30: 662–669.

57. Notari S, Mancone C, Alonzi T, Tripodi M et al. 2008. Determination of abacavir, didanosine, efavirenz, nevirapine and stavudine concentration in human plasma by MALDI/TOF/TOF. *J Chromatogr B Analyt Technol Biomed Life Sci* 863: 249–257.

20 Chromatography in Therapeutic Drug Monitoring of Nonnarcotic Analgesics and Antiinflammatory Drugs

Uttam Garg
Children's Mercy Hospitals and Clinics

CONTENTS

20.1 INTRODUCTION

Analgesics are a class of drugs used to relieve pain without causing loss of consciousness. They can be broadly divided into narcotic and nonnarcotic analgesics. In general narcotic analgesics do not have antiinflammatory properties, however many nonnarcotic analgesics have antiinflammatory properties and can be broadly categorized into steroidal and nonsteroidal antiinflammatory drugs (NSAIDs). In addition to analgesics and antiinflammatory properties, many NSAIDs have antipyretic properties. These nonnarcotic analgesics and antiinflammatory drugs are in widespread use and a number of them are available over-the-counter. These drugs are primarily used for the treatment of low to moderate pain, although a number of newer compounds can be used for management of severe pain also. The common indications for their use include soft tissue injury, strains, sprains, headaches, and arthritis. Although these drugs are relatively safe, toxicity from these compounds can also be encountered due to widespread use of these drugs. Furthermore, many of these compounds are available in combination with other drugs, thus adding to the toxicity profile of these compounds. This chapter discusses the therapeutic drug monitoring of several commonly used NSAIDs. Acetaminophen which mostly has analgesic and antipyretic with limited antiinflammatory properties is also discussed in this chapter. The chemical structures of some of these drugs are shown in Figure 20.1, and some pharmacokinetic properties of these drugs are shown in Table 20.1.

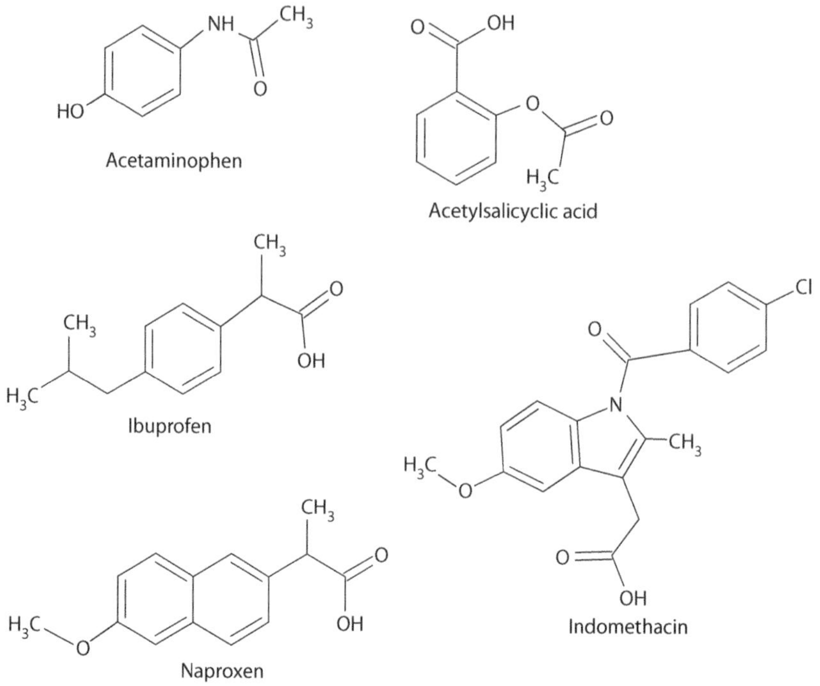

FIGURE 20.1 Chemical structure of some nonnarcotics analgesics and antiinflammatory drugs.

20.2 ACETAMINOPHEN

Acetaminophen (N-acetyl-p-amino phenol) is an analgesic and antipyretic drug which is in widespread use. It is available singly or in combination with number of medications such as opioid analgesics, diphenhydramine, pseudoephedrine, caffeine, codeine and acetylsalicylic acid. In the United States it is the most commonly ingested medication and is frequently seen in the deliberate overdose situations.

Acetaminophen acts by inhibiting the synthesis of prostaglandins in the central nervous system (CNS) and peripherally blocks pain impulse generation. Its antipyretic action is through inhibition of hypothalamic heat-regulating center. In contrast to NSAIDs, acetaminophen does not have notable antiinflammatory or antiplatelet aggregation properties and is thus not a NSAID. Acetaminophen is generally ingested orally and is almost completely absorbed in the intestinal tract reaching a peak plasma level in 30–60 minutes. Most of the drug is metabolized in the liver to glucuronide and sulfate conjugates which are relatively nontoxic. About 5–10% of the drug is metabolized by mixed function oxidases to a highly reactive intermediate N-acetyl-p-benzoquinoneimine which is inactivated by cysteine and mercapturic acid conjugation. Glutathione is required for formation of cysteine and mercapturic acid conjugates. If N-acetyl-p-benzoquinone imine is not detoxified, it covalently binds to critical intracellular molecules leading to cell toxicity and death. In overdose or prolonged use of acetaminophen, glutathione stores get depleted resulting in decreased capacity to detoxify N-acetyl-p-benzoquinone imine. The major toxic effect of acetaminophen overdose is liver toxicity and widespread liver cell necrosis [1].

Alcoholics are at higher risk of developing acetaminophen toxicity. This is due to depletion of glutathione stores and induction of mixed oxidases by ethanol. It has been noted that in alcoholics the toxic dose of acetaminophen may be five fold lower than nonalcoholics. In a famous court case a plaintiff was awarded millions of dollars due to acetaminophen related liver failure requiring liver transplant. The claim was that the drug manufacturer did not provide

TABLE 20.1

Pharmacokinetic Properties of some Nonnarcotic Analgesics and Antiinflammatory Drugs

Drug	Half-life (h)	Vd (L/kg)	Oral Bioavailability (%)	Average Protein Binding (%)	Therapeutic Range (µg/mL)	Toxic Level (µg/mL)
Acetaminophen	1–4	0.95	99	25	10–20	>150, 4 h postingestion. Use Rumack nomogram [37].
Salicylic acid	2–3	0.20	90	>90%	Analgesia—200–1000; Antiinflammatory—1000–3000	Impaired hemostasis: >1000; vertigo, tinnitus: 1500—3000; nausea, vomiting, hyperventilation: 2500—4000; intoxication: >5000
Ibuprofen	1–3	0.11	85	99	10–20	>200
Indomethacin	Adults: 2–6; Neonates: ~20	0.95	100; low in neonates	97	0.3–3.0	>5
Naproxen	Adults: 12–17; Child: 8–10	0.10	100	99	30–90	>400

Source: Adapted from Broussard LA, McCudden CR, Garg U, *Therapeutic drug monitoring data.* AACC Press, Washington, DC, 2007, 193–208.

adequate warning that wine would increase the risk of acetaminophen toxicity. Liver enzyme cytochrome-P450 inducers such as barbiturates, carbamazepine, phenytoin, rifampin and isoniazid increase acetaminophen toxicity.

20.2.1 MONITORING OF ACETAMINOPHEN

Acetaminophen is the most commonly used over-the-counter medication. It is generally not monitored except in the overdose situations. However, timely monitoring in overdose situations is very important as effective antidote, N-acetyl-L-cysteine (Mucomyst), is available for the treatment of acetaminophen toxicity. For its full benefit, the patient should be treated with the antidote early in the course of toxicity, generally <10 h after ingestion. The antidote increases the glutathione concentrations which in turn detoxifies the toxin N-acetyl-p-benzoquinone imine.

Most laboratories perform acetaminophen by immunoassays and the assays are available on stat basis on chemistry analyzers. These assays are fairly specific and compare well with HPLC methods [2,3]. Although immunoassays have improved with time, chromatographic methods remain the reference methods and are helpful when interference is suspected. Also chromatographic methods are essential for the study of acetaminophen metabolism. Several high performance liquid chromatography (HPLC) methods for the estimation of acetaminophen and its metabolites have been published. A reversed-phase HPLC method with UV (ultraviolet) detection has been described for the estimation of acetaminophen and its glucuronide, sulphate, cysteine, and mercapturate metabolites. The same method can be used to analyze both plasma and urine samples [4]. Another, sensitive, reverse phase HPLC method with electrochemical detection is available [5]. In recent years HPLC-tandem mass spectrometric methods have been developed for the determination of acetaminophen and its metabolites. As discussed earlier acetaminophen is relatively nontoxic, but its metabolite

N-acetyl-p-benzoquinone imine is responsible for most of its toxicity. The mechanism involves the formation covalent bonding between electrophilic N-acetyl-p-benzoquinone imine and various proteins. This area is of great interest in understanding the mechanism of acetaminophen toxicity. Also the estimation of drug-protein adducts may be very helpful in explaining drug toxicity when the parent drug has been cleared from the blood. It happens when an overdosed patient presents with late clinical symptoms such as liver failure and the drug is not detected in blood. A HPLC-tandem mass spectrometric method involving isolation of albumin from blood, its digestion to peptides by pronase E and the detection of adducts has been published. The method was tested for in vitro formation of acetaminophen-albumin adducts and albumin isolated from blood of patients exposed to acetaminophen [6].

20.3 ACETYLSALICYLIC ACID

Acetylsalicylic acid (aspirin) is a nonsteroidal antiinflammatory and analgesic drug used in the treatment of mild-to-moderate pain such as headache, myalgia, arthralgia, toothache, and dysmenorrhea, inflammation and fever. It is also frequently used as prophylaxis of myocardial infarction and stroke and/or transient ischemic episodes. Inflammatory conditions which are frequently treated with aspirin include rheumatoid arthritis, rheumatic fever and osteoarthritis. In the body, acetylsalicylic acid is rapidly converted to salicylic acid which is also active. Like other NSAIDs, aspirin acts through inhibition of the enzyme cyclooxygenase, resulting in impairing the conversion of arachidonic acid to prostaglandins, prostacyclin, and thromboxanes. Now it is known that there are two isoforms of cyclooxygenase (COX)—COX-1 and COX-2. COX-1 is expressed in most tissues and is involved in prostaglandin synthesis and functions. In contrast, COX-2 appears to be preferentially expressed in inflammatory tissues. Therefore, specific COX-2 inhibitors are preferred as antiinflammatory drugs as compared to aspirin. As aspirin inhibits both COX-1 and COX-2, and in stomach only COX-1 is expressed, it may lead to gastrointestinal bleeding and ulcerations. In addition to gastrointestinal toxicity, other side effects of aspirin include prolonged bleeding time and acute renal failure due to either renal vasoconstriction or acute interstitial nephritis. Aspirin is contraindicated in patients with bleeding problems, hepatic damage, vitamin K deficiency, hypoprothrombinemia, hemophilia, and peptic ulcer disease. Aspirin is also known to uncouple oxidative phosphorylation leading to ketoacidosis and stimulation of respiratory center to cause respiratory alkalosis. Prolonged higher doses of aspirin can lead to "salicylism" which is characterized by tinnitus, lassitude, deafness and other mental status changes. Aspirin is also associated with Reye's syndrome in children and is not a preferred pediatric antipyretic agent.

Salicylic acid therapeutic range for analgesia and fever is ~20–100 μg/mL, and for antiinflammation is ~100–300 μg/mL. The toxic concentrations are: >100 μg/mL, impaired homeostasis; 150–300 μg/mL, vertigo and tinnitus; 250–400 μg/mL, nausea, vomiting, and hyperventilation; >500 μg/mL, severe intoxication [7]. Salicylic acid monitoring is recommended in suspected toxicity, acute overdose, suspected noncompliance and changes in renal function, acid–base status, pulmonary function, and mental status.

20.3.1 MONITORING OF SALICYLIC ACID

A number of methods for monitoring of salicylic acid are available. Classical methods are based on the method of Trinder where reaction of salicylate with ferric ions produces a purple color that can be measured at 540 nm [8]. The method is prone to interference from proteins and many other metabolites and drugs. The interference can be reduced by precipitating proteins or including a serum or plasma blank. A qualitative spot urine test using 10% ferric chloride can detect the presence of salicylates by producing purple color. Ketoacids such as acetoacetic acid and phenylpyruvic acid give false positive reactions with ferric chloride. The other commonly and routinely used methods are immunoassays and enzymatic methods. Some immunoassays are subject to the same interference as the Trinder method. Enzymatic methods such as salicylate hydrolase are more specific [9].

Though not routinely used, chromatographic methods remain reference methods. These methods are used when interference is suspected or for drug metabolism studies. Gas [10] and liquid [11–13] chromatographic methods are available for the determination of salicylates. A HPLC method for the simultaneous determination of three salicylate glucuronide conjugates and other salicylate metabolites in human urine has been described [14]. The method involves hydrolysis step with beta-glucuronidase and sodium hydroxide. The study on volunteers found that >90% of aspirin was excreted in urine.

20.4 IBUPROFEN

Ibuprofen, a chiral compound derived from arylproprionic acid, is chemically related to fenoprofen and ketoprofen. It has been available with prescription since 1968 and without prescription since 1984. It is used for the treatment of mild-to-moderate pain, fever, and dysmenorrhea. It is also used to treat inflammatory diseases such as rheumatoid arthritis, gout, cystic fibrosis, osteoarthritis, and ankylosing spondylitis. Ibuprofen lysine is used in premature infants to induce closure patent ductus arteriosus (PDA). For PDA treatment, ibuprofen is preferred over indomethacin due to its lesser side effects. In children, ibuprofen is also used for the treatment of cystic fibrosis. Twice daily dosing adjusted to maintain serum levels of 50–100 µg/mL has been associated with slowing of disease progression in younger patients with mild lung disease.

Ibuprofen is available in number of formulations including oral, liquid and injection forms. It is available singly or in combination with other drugs such as diphenhydramine, pseudoephedrine and hydrocodone. Over the counter forms are generally 200 mg tablets or 200 mg/5 mL liquid. The general recommended dose is 200–800 mg two to four times a day. Higher doses are generally given under medical supervision.

When taken orally, approximately 80% of the drug is absorbed. It reaches peak plasma concentration in 1–2 h with maximum effect at 2–4 h. The half-life of ibuprofen is approximately 1–4 h, but is prolonged in patients with liver cirrhosis. In plasma, most of the drug is protein bond. Ibuprofen is extensively metabolized in the liver by oxidation of isobutyl group. The major metabolites are 2-hydroxyibuprofen and 2-carboxyibuprofen, and are excreted by the kidneys. Less than 10% of the drug is excreted unchanged.

Although the exact mechanism of action of ibuprofen is not known, it is believed to be through the inhibition of cyclooxygenase resulting in the inhibition of prostacyclin production. Ibuprofen is less toxic as compared to salicylates and acetaminophen. The side effects include nausea, epigastric pain, diarrhea, vomiting, dizziness, blurred vision, tinnitus, and edema. Severe anaphylactic reactions to ibuprofen have been reported. Severe but rare effects such as gastrointestinal bleeding, seizures, metabolic acidosis, hypotension, bradycardia, tachycardia, atrial fibrillation, coma, hepatic dysfunction, acute renal failure, and cardiac arrest have been reported. On the other hand there are reports of massive overdoses (>8 g) with little or no clinical effects. In a report, an adolescent who ingested 100 g of ibuprofen developed coma, metabolic acidosis, and mild thrombocytopenia but improved rapidly with supportive care. In this patient the renal functions remained normal and there was no gastrointestinal bleeding [15]. The studies indicate that ibuprofen overdose may result in highly variable picture of toxicity, and supportive care usually results in good outcome.

The treatment of ibuprofen toxicity is generally supportive. Gastric decontamination with activated charcoal or gastric lavage is used in severe cases. Emesis is not recommended and forced alkaline diuresis is of limited value. The drug levels are more useful in predicting the toxicity than a dose. The nomogram developed by Hall et al. [16] may be helpful in treating overdoses, though the levels may not correlate well with the symptoms.

Unlike acetaminophen and salicylates, testing of ibuprofen is not routinely available. This is due to unavailability of a rapid method such as immunoassay. Due to higher safety of the drug the manufacturers have not shown a great interest in the development of rapid tests on autoanalyzers. Nevertheless in overdose situations and in long term treatments the levels may be very helpful and may be needed for patient management. For example in a recent study on cystic fibrosis patients on high dose ibuprofen the authors concluded that some interindividual variation can be explained by variations in body weight, dose, fasting status and ibuprofen dosage form and therapeutic drug monitoring is essential to explain the unexplained variability and also in the better patient management [17].

Chromatometric methods including thin layer chromatography (TLC), HPLC and gas chromatography (GC) are available for the estimation of ibuprofen. TLC method such as ToxiLab (Varian Inc., Palo Alto, CA) can detect the presence of ibuprofen and provide qualitative results. HPLC methods involving liquid phase or solid phase extraction with ultraviolet detection have been described [18–21]. Reverse phase HPLC, as compared to normal phase, is a common method. A specific HPLC method, with spectrofluorometer detector, for the simultaneous determination of S-(+) ibuprofen and R-(−) ibuprofen enantiomers in human plasma has been described. In this study, the drugs were extracted from plasma in alcohol medium and were separated on C18 column, using acetonitrile-water-acetic acid-triethylamine as mobile phase [21]. In addition to the parent drug, the assay of metabolites is important in pharmacokinetic studies. A HPLC method for the simultaneous determination of the major phase I and II metabolites of ibuprofen in biological fluids is published [22]. Several GC-MS methods involving derivatization have been also described [23,24]. In general the methods involve the addition of internal standard such as meclofenamic acid in the sample followed by acidification and extraction of the drugs in organic solvent. Derivatization is necessary as underivatized ibuprofen does not chromatograph well. The derivatized extract is then injected onto a gas chromatograph/mass spectrometer (GC/MS) for analysis. Example of GC-MS chromatogram and ion selected monitoring are shown in Figure 20.2. The electron impact ionization mass spectrum of trimethylsilyl (TMS) derivative of ibuprofen is shown in Figure 20.3. GC-MS instrumentation and conditions used to generate this data are given in Table 20.2.

20.5   INDOMETHACIN

Indomethacin (Indocin) is a potent nonsteroidal antiinflammatory drug (NSAID) used for the management of inflammatory diseases such as rheumatoid disorders, ankylosing spondylitis, osteoarthritis and acute gouty arthritis. Intravenous form is used as an alternative to surgery for closure of PDA in neonates. The mechanism of action is through inhibition of prostaglandin synthesis by decreasing the activity of the enzyme cyclooxygenase and thus, decreasing the formation of prostaglandin precursors. Prostaglandins are the mediators of inflammation and are also known to sensitize afferent nerves to induce pain.

Indomethacin is available in several forms including oral, rectal and intravenous. Both oral and rectal forms are readily and completely absorbed in adults however in infants oral forms are poorly absorbed with bioavailability of only 15–20%. The peak plasma concentration is at ~2 h. Indomethacin undergoes enterohepatic recycling with one third of the drug excreted in feces as demethylated metabolites. Rest of the drug and its metabolites including glucuronidation conjugates are eliminated through kidneys. The mean half-life of indomethacin is 3–11 h in adults and ~20 h in infants.

Indomethacin carries the same risk as other NSAIDs. Also its use is contraindicated with the use of aspirin and other NSAIDs. In infants with untreated or suspected infection, the use of indomethacin lysine is contraindicated. Also in neonates, the contraindications include necrotizing enterocolitis, impaired renal functions, active bleeding, and thrombocytopenia. The use of suppositories are contraindicated in patients with a history of proctitis or recent rectal bleeding. Adverse reactions and symptoms to the overdose include gastritis, drowsiness, lethargy, nausea, vomiting, convulsions, paresthesia, headache, dizziness, hypertension, cerebral edema, tinnitus, disorientation, hepatitis, and renal failure. A number of drug interactions have been reported with

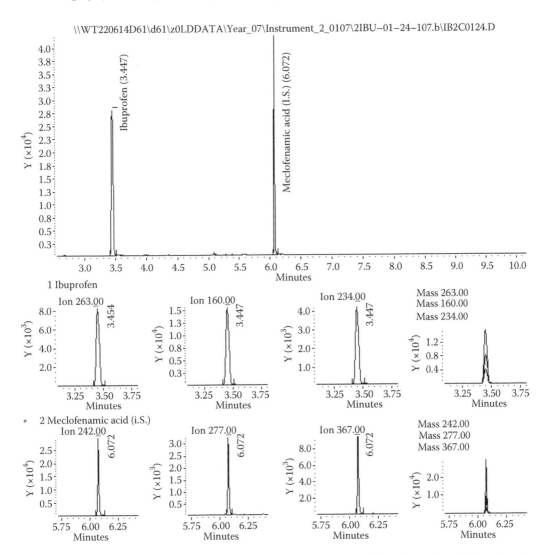

FIGURE 20.2 GC-MS selected ion chromatogram of ibuprofen. Plasma ibuprofen and meclofenamic acid (internal standard) were extracted in Toxi-Lab (Varian Inc., Palo Alto, CA) acidic tubes. The organic extract was dried at 45°C. To the residue BSTFA+1% TMCS were added to make trimethylsilyl (TMS) derivatives of ibuprofen. The derivatized drug was injected on the GC-MS.

indomethacin. Indomethacin may increase levels of digoxin, methotrexate, lithium, and aminoglycosides. Indomethacin may increase nephrotoxicity of cyclosporine; may decrease antihypertensive and diuretic effects of furosemide and thiazides; may increase serum potassium with potassium-sparing diuretics; may decrease antihypertensive effects of beta-blockers, hydralazine, ACE inhibitors and angiotensin II antagonists [25].

20.5.1 Monitoring of Indomethacin

There is no rapid test such as spot test or immunoassay available for the monitoring of indomethacin. The commonly used methods include HPLC and GC. Recently, a reverse phase HPLC method has been described for estimation of indomethacin in premature infants [26]. In this method methylester of indomethacin was used as an internal standard and the samples for HPLC analysis were prepared by plasma protein precipitation with acetonitrile. Column was C18 and the mobile phase

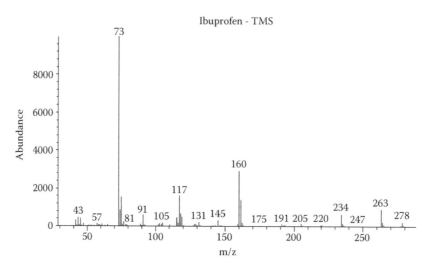

FIGURE 20.3 GC-MS electron impact ionization mass spectrum of TMS derivative of ibuprofen. The extraction conditions are given in legends for Figure 20.2.

TABLE 20.2
GC-MS Instrument and Conditions used to obtain
Data shown in the Figures

Instrument	Agilent 5890 GC/5972 MS
GC column	DB-1, 15 m × 0.25 mm × 0.25 μm
Initial oven temperature	120°C
Initial time	1.0 min
Temperature Ramp	30°C/min
Final temperature	270°C
Hold time	4 min
Injector temperature	250°C
Detector temperature	280°C
Purge time on	0.5 min
Column pressure	5 psi

---

was methanol, water and orthophosphoric acid (70:29.5:0.5, v/v, respectively). The measurement wavelength was 270 nm and the linearity was from 25 to 2500 μg/L. A HPLC-MS-MS method which uses small volume of sample, which is important for infants has been published [27]. In this paper 100 μL sample was used. After addition of internal standard, mefenamic acid, the sample was buffered to pH 3.5 and the drugs were extracted using solid phase extraction. The chromatography included C8 column and mobile phase of 80% methanol and 20% ammonium acetate buffer (40 mM, pH 5.1). Detection involved selected reaction monitoring with mass transitions of m/z 357.9 → 139.0 and m/z 242 → 209.0 for indomethacin and internal standard, respectively. The assay was linear from 5 to 2000 μg/L with analysis time of four minutes. In addition to analysis of parent drug, some times it is important to measure the metabolites. The drug is metabolized through demethylation and glucuronidation, and a HPLC method to measure both parent drug and its metabolites is available [28]. The authors reported that indomethacin, its metabolite O-desmethylindomethacin and their conjugates can be measured directly by gradient HPLC without enzymatic deglucuronidation. With this method, glucuronides were only detected in urine but not in plasma.

GC is also frequently used for the measurement of indomethacin. Capillary columns are the most commonly used columns. Various detectors including flame ionization, electron capture and mass spectrometry have been used [29–31]. In one GC-electron capture method the drug was extracted from serum or urine and the ethyl ester derivatives were prepared using diazoethane in diethyl ether and the derivatized drug was analyzed using electron-capture gas–liquid chromatography [31]. A sensitive GC-MS method involving negative ion chemical ionization has been described for estimation of indomethacin in plasma and synovial fluid. The limit of quantification of this GC-MS method was 0.1 ng/mL [30]. Example of GC-MS chromatogram and ion selected monitoring for indomethacin is shown in Figure 20.4. The electron impact ionization mass spectrum of TMS (trimethylsilyl) derivative of indomethacin is shown in Figure 20.5. GC-MS instrumentation and conditions used to generate this data are given in Table 20.2.

In addition to monitoring the levels of indomethacin, several other laboratory parameters such as renal functions, liver functions, electrolytes and CBC with differential are recommended. Infants

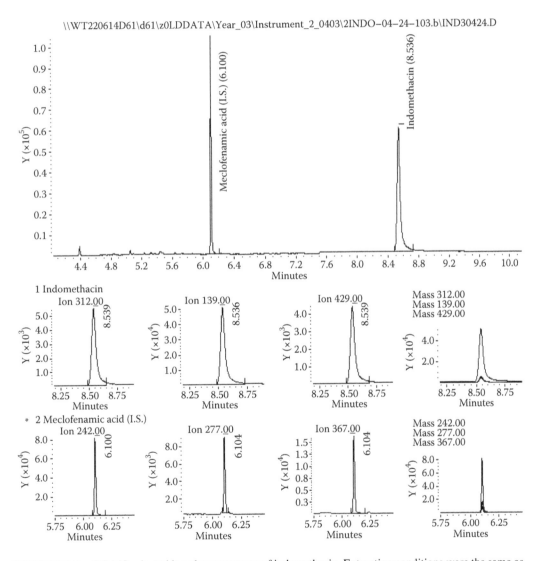

FIGURE 20.4 GC-MS selected ion chromatogram of indomethacin. Extraction conditions were the same as described in legends for Figure 20.2.

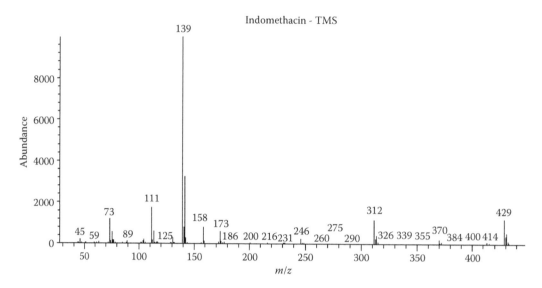

FIGURE 20.5 GC-MS electron impact ionization mass spectrum of TMS derivative of indomethacin. The extraction conditions are given in legends for Figure 20.2.

with PDA and being treated with indomethacin should be monitored for heart rate, heart murmur, blood pressure, urine output, echocardiogram, serum sodium and glucose, platelet count, and serum concentrations of concomitantly administered drugs such as aminoglycosides and digoxin which are cleared through kidneys [25].

20.6 NAPROXEN

Naproxen is another frequently used NSAID. In addition to antiinflammatory properties, it has analgesics and antipyretic properties. It is used in the management of various inflammatory diseases such as rheumatoid arthritis, juvenile rheumatoid arthritis, osteoarthritis, ankylosing spondylitis, tendonitis, and bursitis. It is also used in the treatment of acute gout, mild to moderate pain, primary dysmenorrheal and fever. Like other NSAIDs, the mechanism of action of the naproxen is believed to be related to the inhibition of cyclooxygenase and thus prostacyclin production. Patients treated with naproxen and other NSAIDs had decreased levels of IL-6 and substance P in both plasma and synovial fluid as compared to untreated patients [32]. Naproxen is available in several forms including delayed released formulations. Delayed release formulations release part of the drug immediately and the remaining drug as sustained release. Typical, over-the counter, naproxen dose vary from 500 to 1000 mg/day. The higher doses are given under medical supervision. When taken orally, naproxen is completely absorbed from the gastrointestinal tract with bioavailability of ~100%. Naproxen is extensively metabolized to O-desmethylnaproxen. Both parent and the metabolite are conjugated and eliminated in urine. In patients with renal failure, these metabolites may accumulate in the blood. Metabolites do not have a significant pharmacological activity.

Although naproxen is relatively safe, the higher doses and accumulation of drug can cause toxicity. The toxic effects include nausea, abdominal pain, constipation, headache, dizziness, drowsiness, tinnitus, and skin eruptions. Severe allergic reactions to naproxen have been reported. It is also contraindicated in patients who are receiving aspirin or other NSAIDs.

There is no commercial immunoassay or quick spot test for the estimation of naproxen. Although, naproxen levels may not correlate well with toxicity, they are useful in the patients who do not respond to therapy. HPLC and GC are the common methods for estimation of naproxen [33–36]. HPLC is more commonly used method as compared to GC. Other laboratory tests including CBC

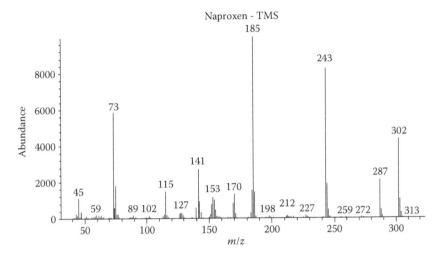

FIGURE 20.6 GC-MS electron impact ionization mass spectrum of TMS derivative of naproxen. The extraction conditions are given in legends for Figure 20.2.

with differential, platelets, BUN, serum creatinine, liver enzymes, and occult blood loss are useful in patients being treated with naproxen. GC-MS, electron impact ionization mass spectrum of TMS derivative of naproxen is shown in Figure 20.6.

20.7 GENERAL WARNING FOR NONSTEROIDAL ANTIINFLAMMATORY DRUGS (NSAIDs)

NSAIDs discussed above share many properties and common side effects. Food and Drug Administration issued number of warnings on NSAIDs and asked manufacturer to list some of these warnings on the product labels. These warnings include: [1] NSAIDs may cause an increased risk of serious cardiovascular thrombotic events, myocardial infarction, and stroke, which can be fatal. This risk may increase with duration of use. Patients with cardiovascular disease or risk factors for cardiovascular disease may be at greater risk. [2] NSAIDs cause an increased risk of serious gastrointestinal adverse events including bleeding, ulceration, and perforation of the stomach or intestines, which can be fatal. These events can occur at any time during use and without warning symptoms. Elderly patients are at greater risk for serious gastrointestinal events. [3] Treatment of perioperative pain in setting of coronary artery bypass graft (CABG) surgery is contradictory. [4] It is contraindicated in patients who have experienced asthma, urticaria, or allergic-type reactions after taking aspirin or other NSAIDs [7].

20.8 CONCLUSIONS

In conclusion, nonnarcotic analgesics and antiinflammatory drugs are in wide use. They are available singly or in combination with many other drugs. Most of the drugs discussed here are safe when taken as directed. However, overdosing, due to easy availability of these drugs is common. Laboratory monitoring of these drugs is useful in therapeutic drug monitoring and overdose situations. Immunoassays are available for some but not all the drugs. Chromatographic methods remain reference methods and are the only methods for several NSAIDs. Also, chromatographic methods are the only methods to study the metabolism of these drugs.

ACKNOWLEDGMENT

The author thanks David Scott for his help in the preparation of the figures.

REFERENCES

1. Graham GG, Scott KF. 2005. Mechanism of action of paracetamol. *Am J Ther* 12:46–55.
2. Bridges RR, Kinniburgh DW, Keehn BJ, Jennison TA. 1983. An evaluation of common methods for acetaminophen quantitation for small hospitals. *J Toxicol Clin Toxicol* 20:1–17.
3. Hepler B, Weber J, Sutheimer C, Sunshine I. 1984. Homogeneous enzyme immunoassay of acetaminophen in serum. *Am J Clin Pathol* 81:602–10.
4. Lau GS, Critchley JA. 1994. The estimation of paracetamol and its major metabolites in both plasma and urine by a single high-performance liquid chromatography assay. *J Pharm Biomed Anal* 12:1563–72.
5. Whelpton R, Fernandes K, Wilkinson KA, Goldhill DR. 1993. Determination of paracetamol (acetaminophen) in blood and plasma using high performance liquid chromatography with dual electrode coulometric quantification in the redox mode. *Biomed Chromatogr* 7:90–93.
6. Damsten MC, Commandeur JN, Fidder A, Hulst AG, Touw D, Noort D, et al. 2007. Liquid chromatography/tandem mass spectrometry detection of covalent binding of acetaminophen to human serum albumin. *Drug Metab Dispos* 35:1408–17.
7. Broussard LA, McCudden CR, Garg U. 2007. Therapeutic drug monitoring of analgesics. In: Hammett-Stabler CA, Dasgupta A, eds. *Therapeutic Drug Monitoring Data*. Washington, DC: AACC Press, 193–208.
8. Trinder P. 1954. Rapid determination of salicylate in biological fluids. *Biochem J* 57:301–3.
9. Morris HC, Overton PD, Ramsay JR, Campbell RS, Hammond PM, Atkinson T, et al. 1990. Development and validation of an automated, enzyme-mediated colorimetric assay of salicylate in serum. *Clin Chem* 36:131–35.
10. Belanger PM, Lalande M, Dore F, Labrecque G. 1983. Rapid gas chromatographic determination of serum salicylates after silylation. *J Pharm Sci* 72:1092–93.
11. Levine B, Caplan YH. 1984. Liquid chromatographic determination of salicylate and methyl salicylate in blood and application to a postmortem case. *J Anal Toxicol* 8:239–41.
12. Brandon RA, Eadie MJ, Smith MT. 1985. A sensitive liquid chromatographic assay for plasma aspirin and salicylate concentrations after low doses of aspirin. *Ther Drug Monit* 7:216–21.
13. Chubb SA, Campbell RS, Price CP. 1986. Rapid method of measuring salicylate in serum by high-performance liquid chromatography. *J Chromatogr* 380:163–69.
14. Shen JJ, Wanwimolruk S, Roberts MS. 1991. Novel direct high-performance liquid chromatographic method for determination of salicylate glucuronide conjugates in human urine. *J Chromatogr* 565:309–20.
15. Seifert SA, Bronstein AC, McGuire T. 2000. Massive ibuprofen ingestion with survival. *J Toxicol Clin Toxicol* 38:55–57.
16. Hall AH, Smolinske SC, Stover B, Conrad FL, Rumack BH. 1992. Ibuprofen overdose in adults. *J Toxicol Clin Toxicol* 30:23–37.
17. Arranz I, Martin-Suarez A, Lanao JM, Mora F, Vazquez C, Escribano A, et al. 2003. Population pharmacokinetics of high dose ibuprofen in cystic fibrosis. *Arch Dis Child* 88:1128–30.
18. Sochor J, Klimes J, Sedlacek J, Zahradnicek M. 1995. Determination of ibuprofen in erythrocytes and plasma by high performance liquid chromatography. *J Pharm Biomed Anal* 13:899–903.
19. Lemko CH, Caille G, Foster RT. 1993. Stereospecific high-performance liquid chromatographic assay of ibuprofen: improved sensitivity and sample processing efficiency. *J Chromatogr* 619:330–35.
20. Castillo M, Smith PC. 1993. Direct determination of ibuprofen and ibuprofen acyl glucuronide in plasma by high-performance liquid chromatography using solid-phase extraction. *J Chromatogr* 614:109–16.
21. Canaparo R, Muntoni E, Zara GP, Della Pepa C, Berno E, Costa M, et al. 2000. Determination of Ibuprofen in human plasma by high-performance liquid chromatography: validation and application in pharmacokinetic study. *Biomed Chromatogr* 14:219–26.
22. Kepp DR, Sidelmann UG, Tjornelund J, Hansen SH. 1997. Simultaneous quantitative determination of the major phase I and II metabolites of ibuprofen in biological fluids by high-performance liquid chromatography on dynamically modified silica. *J Chromatogr B Biomed Sci Appl* 696:235–41.
23. Maurer HH, Kraemer T, Weber A. 1994. Toxicological detection of ibuprofen and its metabolites in urine using gas chromatography-mass spectrometry (GC-MS). *Pharmazie* 49:148–55.
24. Heikkinen L. 1984. Silica capillary gas chromatographic determination of ibuprofen in serum. *J Chromatogr* 307:206–9.
25. Lacy CF, Armstrong LL, Goldman MP, Lance LL, eds. 2003. *Drug Information Handbook*. Hudson, OH: Lexi-Comp, 735–37.

26. Al Za'abi MA, Dehghanzadeh GH, Norris RL, Charles BG. 2006. A rapid and sensitive microscale HPLC method for the determination of indomethacin in plasma of premature neonates with patent ductus arteriosus. *J Chromatogr B Analyt Technol Biomed Life Sci* 830:364–67.

27. Taylor PJ, Jones CE, Dodds HM, Hogan NS, Johnson AG. 1998. Plasma indomethacin assay using high-performance liquid chromatography-electrospray-tandem mass spectrometry: application to therapeutic drug monitoring and pharmacokinetic studies. *Ther Drug Monit* 20:691–96.

28. Vree TB, van den Biggelaar-Martea M, Verwey-van Wissen CP. 1993. Determination of indomethacin, its metabolites and their glucuronides in human plasma and urine by means of direct gradient high-performance liquid chromatographic analysis. Preliminary pharmacokinetics and effect of probenecid. *J Chromatogr* 616:271–82.

29. Nishioka R, Harimoto T, Umeda I, Yamamoto S, Oi N. 1990. Improved procedure for determination of indomethacin in plasma by capillary gas chromatography after solid-phase extraction. *J Chromatogr* 526:210–14.

30. Dawson M, Smith MD, McGee CM. 1990. Gas chromatography/negative ion chemical ionization/tandem mass spectrometric quantification of indomethacin in plasma and synovial fluid. *Biomed Environ Mass Spectrom* 19:453–58.

31. Helleberg I. 1976. Determination of indomethacin in serum and urine by electron-capture gas-liquid chromatography. *J Chromatogr* 117:167–73.

32. Sacerdote P, Carrabba M, Galante A, Pisati R, Manfredi B, Panerai AE. 1995. Plasma and synovial fluid interleukin-1, interleukin-6 and substance P concentrations in rheumatoid arthritis patients: effect of the nonsteroidal anti inflammatory drugs indomethacin, diclofenac and naproxen. *Inflamm Res* 44:486–90.

33. Vree TB, van den Biggelaar-Martea M, Verwey-van Wissen CP. 1992. Determination of naproxen and its metabolite O-desmethylnaproxen with their acyl glucuronides in human plasma and urine by means of direct gradient high-performance liquid chromatography. *J Chromatogr* 578:239–49.

34. Blagbrough IS, Daykin MM, Doherty M, Pattrick M, Shaw PN. 1992. High-performance liquid chromatographic determination of naproxen, ibuprofen and diclofenac in plasma and synovial fluid in man. *J Chromatogr* 578:251–57.

35. Andersen JV, Hansen SH. 1992. Simultaneous quantitative determination of naproxen, its metabolite 6-O-desmethylnaproxen and their five conjugates in plasma and urine samples by high-performance liquid chromatography on dynamically modified silica. *J Chromatogr* 577:325–33.

36. Tashtoush BM, Al-Taani BM. 2003. HPLC determination of naproxen in plasma. *Pharmazie* 58:614–15.

37. Rumack BH, Matthew H. 1975. Acetaminophen poisoning and toxicity. *Pediatrics* 55:871–76.

21 Therapeutic Drug Monitoring in Pain Management: Application of Chromatography and Mass Spectrometry

Christine L.H. Snozek and Loralie J. Langman
Mayo Clinic College of Medicine

CONTENTS

21.1   INTRODUCTION

The term "opioid" describes a wide range of compounds, encompassing the natural and semisynthetic opiates; essentially variations on a single structural theme as well as fully synthetic opioids with minimal structural homology to the natural alkaloids [1]. The defining characteristic of this class of drugs is their morphine-like antinociceptive activity stemming from interaction with opioid receptors, which play a major role in pain perception [2–5]. Other compounds that can be somewhat loosely referred to as "opioids" include receptor antagonists and mixed agonist/antagonists, as well as other opium-derived alkaloids such as papaverine that are not known to bind opioid receptors [6].

From the standpoint of pain management, opioid therapy is a mainstay of treating acute needs such as postsurgical analgesia, and of relieving moderate to severe chronic pain [7]. In the latter case, opioids are well accepted in the setting of cancer-related pain, but there is a great deal of controversy regarding the propriety and effectiveness of their use in nonmalignant chronic pain [7]. Most opioids have both substantial addictive capacity and potentially life-threatening side effects, thus the benefits of their use in nonend-stage patients must be carefully weighed against the chance of rather serious consequences [8]. In addition, the development of tolerance and the risk of prescription diversion complicate the process of monitoring long-term opioid therapy for compliance and efficacy even further.

A basic understanding of the physiology, pharmacology, and laboratory analysis of opioids is essential for management of patients receiving these medications. This chapter focuses on analysis by chromatography, but is also intended to provide sufficient background on opioids in vivo to assist in the interpretation of laboratory measurements in the setting of therapeutic drug management (TDM) of opioids.

21.2   OPIOID RECEPTORS

The hallmark of opioids is their ability to interact with the family of opioid receptors that are variably distributed throughout the body; opioid receptor agonists typically produce analgesia, while antagonists block this response [9,10]. The biochemistry of opioid receptor regulation and signaling is complex and has been reviewed in detail elsewhere [9–11], but a general overview is presented here.

The classical opioid receptors are divided into the mu, delta, and kappa (μ, δ, and κ, or MOR, DOR, and KOR, respectively) subfamilies [3–5], which exhibit considerable overlap in ligand specificity and downstream signaling [9,10]. A related protein, the ORL-1/nociceptin receptor, has also been described as an opioid receptor, though its characterization lags behind the other receptors [12]. Finally, the sigma receptor family can also interact with some opioids, but produce very different physiological responses including cardiac excitation and tachypnea; sigma receptors are now considered to be completely distinct from the classical opioid receptors [9].

Opioids can have preferential or selective binding to one or more of the different receptor classes. It is possible for a compound to stimulate one opioid receptor subtype while inhibiting another, as with mixed agonist/antagonist (MAA) compounds [9,10]. The effect of ligand binding varies between the receptor classes. Morphine-like analgesia is thought to be mediated primarily through stimulation of MOR, although compounds with preferential binding to DOR or KOR can also produce analgesia [9,10]. Other classical sequelae of opioid treatment are also attributable to MOR, including sedation and inhibition of respiratory function and gastrointestinal transit [8,10,13]. In contrast, neither DOR nor KOR is thought to affect respiration; DOR agonists do not produce sedation or reduce gastrointestinal motility [10].

In addition to analgesia, DOR shares some of the regulatory physiology attributed to MOR, such as regulation of growth hormone and dopamine [10,14,15]. Interestingly, DOR–MOR heterodimerization is thought to be involved in development of opioid tolerance, suggesting that DOR plays a role in regulation of MOR biochemistry [10,15,16]. KOR-mediated signaling tends to produce psychoactivity, thus, KOR-selective agonists (e.g., the hallucinogen salvinorin A) are less frequently used as analgesics. Interestingly, KOR and its endogenous ligand dynorphin are implicated in response to addiction to numerous drugs including opioids; KOR gene polymorphisms have also been linked to susceptibility to alcohol dependence, supporting a role for this receptor in addictive behavior [17–20].

Splice variants have been described for the opioid receptors; these alternate splice products appear to explain—at least in part—the functional characterization of receptor subtypes with differing ligand specificity and physiological response [10,21]. Some studies suggest that compounds with selectivity for a given receptor subtype may allow separation of the desired analgesic effect from adverse sequelae. However, the success of such attempts to tailor clinical response through targeting particular receptor subtypes has been limited and significant further investigation is needed before this means of avoiding adverse responses to opioid therapy will be feasible [22].

In addition to undesirable side effects, a major concern in long-term opioid therapy is the development of tolerance [9,10,23]. Tolerant individuals may require many-fold increases in dose to achieve the same level of analgesia, which can greatly complicate interpretation of TDM results and establishment of a therapeutic window. Interestingly, tolerance to a particular opioid is thought to be a consequence of altered regulation of the opioid receptor(s) to which that compound binds. Because of this reason, cross-tolerance can occur when multiple drugs interact with the same receptor [9,10,15,23]. In addition, several of the enzymes involved in opioid metabolism (see below) display substrate-dependent alterations in activity. Although substrate inhibition and induction represent different phenomena than tolerance, the clinical effect can be similar and may necessitate modification of the therapeutic regimen.

21.3 METABOLISM OF OPIOIDS

The metabolism of opioids is quite varied, but there are a number of biotransformations common to these drugs. Several of the most commonly used opiates can be formed in vivo by metabolism of other compounds, as is seen with codeine demethylation resulting in conversion to morphine [10,24]. This interconversion is a frequent source of confusion and must be considered when interpreting the results of opiate screens; specific details will be outlined below for key opioids with active metabolites.

Opioids, as with most xenobiotics, are metabolized by many different enzymes, including those of the cytochrome P450 (CYP) family [10,24–30]. One of the more important CYP enzymes, CYP2D6, is particularly notable for its role in variable clinical response to opioids, and will be discussed in more detail in a later section. CYP2D6 removes the 3-methyl group from codeine, dihydrocodeine, hydrocodone, and oxycodone, converting them into their respective active metabolites morphine, dihydromorphine, hydromorphone, and oxymorphone [10,24]. Tramadol is also

O-demethylated by CYP2D6 to form the M1 metabolite responsible for much of the opioid-like activity of this drug [10,24].

Many additional CYP enzymes are involved in opioid metabolism, including CYP3A and CYP2C isoforms, among others [24]. It is important to note that several of these enzymes are subject to substrate inhibition and/or induction, i.e., the apparent metabolic activity can decrease or increase, respectively, in response to substrate [31]. Although these alterations in metabolic rate are distinct from the development of tolerance, both phenomena can necessitate adjusting the dosage or choice of medication. In addition, substrate-dependent changes in metabolic activity can be affected by other drugs, herbal supplements, or endogenous compounds that are substrates of the same enzyme; for example, methadone levels may be lower than expected in a patient taking St. John's wort, a noted CYP3A4 inducer, but higher in patient ingesting a CYP3A4 inhibitor such as grapefruit juice [31].

CYPs are not the only metabolic enzymes associated with opioid biotransformation. Free hydroxyl groups, such as the 3- and 6-hydroxy moieties of morphine, are frequently glucuronidated by enzymes of the uridine diphosphate glucuronyl transferase (UGT) family [10,24]. Conjugation to glucuronide increases the solubility and excretion of the parent drug. This generally produces an inactive compound, though in some cases, such as morphine-6-glucuronide, the metabolite retains activity as an opioid receptor ligand [10,24]. UGT2B7 is the isoform primarily responsible for morphine glucuronidation in humans [32] while other UGT enzymes such as UGT1A1 and UGT1A8 can metabolize morphine in vitro but their relevance in vivo remains uncertain [33]. Most other opioids have not been studied as extensively with respect to the major UGT isoforms involved in their metabolism, though hydromorphone and oxymorphone both appear to be UGT2B7 and UGT1A3 substrates [34,35].

21.3.1 Pharmacogenetics Aspects

Polymorphic genes are found at several points in the in vivo handling of opioids, including receptors, transporters, metabolic enzymes and has been recently well-reviewed by Kadiev et al. [34]. Variant alleles have been described for MOR, DOR, and KOR, though reports differ as to their influence and importance in opioid therapy [36–43]. Similarly, polymorphisms of uncertain significance have been described for transporters such as P-glycoprotein and metabolic enzymes including UGT family members [44]. However, currently the only polymorphic genes with adequate evidence to support any degree of pharmacogenetic individualization of opioid therapy are the CYP enzymes [45–51].

Variant alleles of CYP3A, CYP2C, and CYP2D6 have been described, often with altered enzymatic activity [44]. Of these, CYP2D6 has been the most extensively characterized for its effects on opioid therapy. As outlined above, CYP2D6 plays a key role in the metabolism of several opioids, the best-studied of which is activation of the prodrug, codeine, via demethylation to morphine [24]. Over 60 alleles have been described for CYP2D6, with resultant enzymatic activity ranging from essentially zero, in the case of null alleles, to many times higher than normal, in the case of amplified alleles [52–56]. Thus, at the same codeine dose, patients with minimal CYP2D6 activity (poor metabolizers) would likely receive inadequate analgesia due to lack of conversion to morphine, while patients with very high CYP2D6 activity (ultra-rapid metabolizers) would be at risk for adverse responses to excessive morphine [10,57]. Without knowledge of the CYP2D6 genotype, these clinical presentations can be confusing; the possibility of pharmacogenetic effects is therefore important to consider when assessing appropriate dosing, patient compliance, and potential diversion or illicit use.

21.3.2 Therapeutic Drug Management (TDM) Considerations

One of the primary difficulties in treating pain with opioids is maintaining the fine balance between adequate control of pain and avoidance of negative outcomes, either toxicity or addiction [8]. TDM of opioids is quite different from management of many other types of drugs; for example for morphine there is no predictable relationship between morphine serum concentrations and analgesic response [58–60]. Although it is thought that a minimum analgesic drug level exists for most opioids [58–60], the minimum effective concentration varies from patient to patient. Interestingly, the relationship between serum drug levels and the incidence of adverse events is far from clear. Although higher concentrations are associated with greater risk [58–60], the definition of a "high" serum level varies greatly between individuals depending on factors such as age, prior therapy, medical condition, and psychological state [58–60].

The progressive development of tolerance and inter-individual variability make establishing an upper limit to the therapeutic range virtually impossible. Patients in pain management or addiction rehabilitation programs are typically monitored long-term to ascertain compliance, by assaying for the presence of the expected therapeutic agent and the absence of any other, nonprescribed opioids. However, as with any drug test, compliance assessment is not completely straightforward. The individual differences in metabolic rate, poor correlation between dose and urine drug levels and the detection window for the compound of interest all complicate the interpretation of compliance testing results. It is also important to recognize that many opiates are present in the same *in vivo* metabolic pathways and may therefore appear together when a precursor compound is administered [10,24,61].

Objectively assessing clinical response to opioids using TDM is, if anything, even more difficult than compliance testing. With many drugs, patient management is assisted by establishing a baseline drug level when the individual is known to be both compliant and clinically responsive. However, in long-term opioid treatment, baseline concentrations determined at the start of therapy become essentially meaningless over time as tolerance develops. Tolerance is a progressive phenomenon that can raise the drug level needed for clinical response well above the initial effective concentration; opioid-tolerant patients are often maintained on doses that would be lethal to opioid-naïve individuals [62]. Thus, even in fully compliant patients, establishing a true therapeutic range is simply not feasible. The situation is only made more difficult by the additional concerns of noncompliant patients, diversion of prescribed drugs, and interindividual variability in metabolism. Interpretation of TDM results requires consideration of all these factors, but frequently fails to provide definitive answers to the questions of compliance and efficacy.

The following sections provide basic information on select opioids, their physiological properties, and their measurement in the clinical laboratory.

21.4 NATURAL OPIUM ALKALOIDS

21.4.1 CODEINE

Due to its antitussive and analgesic properties, codeine is one of the most frequently prescribed opiates in the world. Codeine itself shows poor affinity for MOR, with only a fraction of the pain-relieving capacity of morphine, and is therefore generally considered a prodrug [63]. Analgesia is attributed to the small fraction (< 10%) of codeine converted to morphine by CYP2D6, though some studies suggest that the predominant (~80%) metabolite, codeine-6-glucuronide, may also be capable of mediating CNS effects independently of morphine [24]. Codeine is also converted to an inactive metabolite, norcodeine (10%), and to the active compounds hydrocodone (up to 10% with chronic administration) [24,64].

21.4.2 MORPHINE

The archetypical opiate, morphine is used as the basis of comparison for relative characterizations of the opioid class. Morphine interacts primarily with MOR to mediate its effects, but also shows some affinity for KOR [10]. The major metabolites of morphine are glucuronide conjugates formed primarily by UGT2B7 and UGT1A3: inactive morphine-3-glucuronide (M3G, ~60%), active morphine-6-glucuronide (M6G, ~10%), and a small amount of morphine-3,6-diglucuronide [32,65]. When morphine levels are high, a minor fraction can be converted to hydromorphone [66]. M6G has greater MOR agonist activity than morphine, and appears to be selective for the μ1 receptor subtype that is thought to contribute less to unwanted side effects [10,24,67,68]. However, the relative importance of morphine and M6G in analgesia and adverse responses remains controversial [65]; of note, morphine glucuronides do contribute to opioid toxicity in patients with renal insufficiency, as they are unable to excrete the water-soluble metabolites [69,70].

21.4.3 PAPAVERINE

Not thought to interact with opioid receptors, papaverine is used to treat vasospasm in settings such as cardiac surgery [10,63]. Its clinical use is typically short-term, so there has been little demand for its measurement in TDM; however, papaverine can be detected on some drug screens [71]. Because papaverine is relatively stable, it and other natural opium alkaloids have been proposed as markers of illicit use of opiates, notably heroin, though there are concerns that poppy seed consumption could produce false positives [72].

21.4.4 NOSCAPINE

Used clinically as an antitussive, noscapine also has and antitumor properties in vitro, but displays little if any analgesic potential [73]. Interestingly, noscapine may inhibit CYP2C9 and CYP3A4, reportedly affecting therapy with other substrates for these enzymes, notably warfarin [74,75]. Noscapine has also been suggested as marker for heroin use [76].

21.4.5 THEBAINE

Although it can be used as a synthetic base for other opioids, thebaine is not used therapeutically. However, its strychnine-like cytotoxicity has led to limited investigations as a possible antitumor agent [77]. Chromatography for thebaine is largely in the contexts of research, industry, or illicit drug analysis [78,79].

21.5 SEMISYNTHETIC OPIATES

21.5.1 DIHYDROCODEINE

Very similar in structure to codeine, dihydrocodeine has comparable antitussive and analgesic properties, and is frequently combined with other analgesics such as acetaminophen or aspirin [58,80]. In contrast to codeine, however, dihydrocodeine does not appear to rely heavily upon CYP2D6-mediated conversion to dihydromorphine for activity [24]. Because of its relatively short half-life, dihydrocodeine produces fewer negative withdrawal effects, leading to its increased use in opioid maintenance and detoxification programs as an alternative to methadone or buprenorphine, though it is not yet well-studied in this role [81].

21.5.2 HEROIN

A prodrug that is converted to morphine, heroin is also called diacetylmorphine or diamorphine. Heroin is no longer legally produced in the United States but still used elsewhere for fast-acting analgesia [82]. The two acetyl groups enhance CNS distribution [83], providing a rapid effect when first-pass metabolism is bypassed (e.g., intravenous administration). Heroin has an extremely short half-life that limits its detection in the laboratory; however, the presence of its unique metabolite 6-monoacetylmorphine (6-MAM) is definitive for heroin use. Aside from 6-MAM, its metabolic profile resembles that of morphine [84]. Heroin testing is typically performed for drug abuse screening rather than TDM; one interesting forensic application is the chromatographic analysis of minor impurities in seized heroin shipments to determine the site of origin [85].

21.5.3 HYDROCODONE

Like codeine, hydrocodone is metabolized by CYP2D6 to an active metabolite (hydromorphone), and therefore may be subject to pharmacogenetic variability in patients with abnormal CYP2D6 activity [44]. However, though studies are somewhat contradictory, hydrocodone may provide effective pain relief even in the absence of CYP2D6-mediated conversion to hydromorphone [86]. It remains unclear whether this is due primarily to the activity of hydrocodone itself, or of other, as yet unknown active metabolites. Hydrocodone is a metabolite of codeine, though the fraction of hydrocodone formed may depend on dose and length of treatment [64].

21.5.4 HYDROMORPHONE

Although it can be used as an analgesic in its own right with potency somewhat higher than hydrocodone [86], hydromorphone is also a primary metabolite of hydrocodone and a minor metabolite of morphine [66]. Like morphine, hydromorphone is metabolized in large part to an inactive 3-glucuronide by UGT2B7 and UGT1A3; hydromorphone lacks a free hydroxyl group at the 6-position, thus there is no metabolite analogous to M6G [35].

21.5.5 OXYCODONE

Poorly detected by most opiate screening assays, oxycodone is a potent analgesic with high oral bioavailability and a similar structure to hydrocodone [10,63]. Although its own strong analgesic activity precludes oxycodone from being considered a prodrug, it is also converted to a highly active metabolite, oxymorphone, through the activity of CYP2D6 [87]. This conversion appears to be less of a concern for CYP2D6 poor metabolizers, since oxycodone itself still provides analgesia, than for ultrarapid metabolizers who could be at increased risk for adverse effects [88].

21.5.6 OXYMORPHONE

Recently approved for oral administration, oxymorphone provides potent analgesia with minimal interaction with CYP enzymes, though it can be a substrate for CYP2C9 and CYP3A4 [89]. The majority of oxymorphone is metabolized by UGT2B7 to the 3-glucuronide; a minor metabolite, 6-hydroxyoxymorphone, is an active analgesic with a similar steady-state AUC to the parent compound. Oxymorphone is also a metabolite of oxycodone, formed via CYP2D6 [35].

21.6 SYNTHETIC OPIOIDS

21.6.1 FENTANYL

A lipophilic drug with numerous routes of administration, fentanyl is used in applications ranging from anesthesia to rapid management of breakthrough pain [90]. Fentanyl provides the structural backbone for a number of related, ultra-short-acting opioids used as anesthetics, including remifentanil and sufentanil. Transdermal fentanyl patches are used for longer-term administration and are gaining popularity amongst drug abusers, though nonstandard application of the patches (e.g., chewing or extraction) carries substantial risk for overdose [91]. Norfentanyl, the primary metabolite, is generated by CYP3A and is inactive [92]; the high potency of fentanyl and clinical insignificance of its metabolites make it a preferred analgesic for patients with major organ failure [90].

21.6.2 Dextromethorphan

Despite opioid-like antitussive properties, dextromethorphan and its active metabolites dextrorphan and 3-methoxymorphinan have minimal opioidergic analgesic effect, though they may have inhibitory effects at NMDA receptors [10]. Dextromethorphan also inhibits reuptake of serotonin and may lead to the serotonin syndrome in patients taking monoamine oxidase or serotonin reuptake inhibitors [93]. Formation of the metabolite dextrorphan is mediated by CYP2D6, thus dextromethorphan may be useful as a probe drug for CYP2D6 phenotyping [94]. In sufficient doses, dextromethorphan can produce euphoria and dissociative hallucination [93]; for this reason it is increasingly common as a recreational drug. The L-rotary isomer (levomethorphan) is an infrequently-used analgesic.

21.6.3 Levorphanol

Although it is structurally quite similar to morphine, levorphanol is considered a synthetic opioid because it lacks the furan (oxygen) bridge of the natural alkaloid [95,96]. The D-stereoisomer (dextrorphan) is a metabolite of dextromethorphan [10,63]. Levorphanol is a potent activator of all three opioid receptor types [96] and may inhibit uptake of norepinephrine and serotonin [95], but it is less commonly prescribed than many other analgesics [10].

21.6.4 Meperidine

Originally synthesized as an anticholinergic, meperidine has analgesic potency comparable to or somewhat lower than morphine [97]. One major metabolite, normeperidine, also has analgesic activity; normeperidine is thought to be responsible for the serotonergic toxicity of meperidine, particularly in patients receiving concomitant monoamine oxidase inhibitors [10,97]. Meperidine use has declined in recent years in favor of alternatives such as fentanyl.

21.6.5 Methadone

A relatively long-acting opiate, methadone is used both for analgesia and in treatment of opioid addiction [10]. It is thought to provide milder withdrawal, somewhat lower potential for abuse, and reduced exposure to the risks of illicit intravenous drug use [98]. Methadone has affinity for both MOR and DOR [99], the latter of which may explain its apparent utility in patients whose pain no longer responds to other opioids [100]. Methadone TDM is confounded by substantial inter- and intra-individual variability; both urine pH and seemingly self-inducible metabolism substantially influence the pharmacokinetics of this compound, as do commonly coadministered drugs such as benzodiazepines and antiretrovirals [10]. Although a large fraction of methadone is excreted unchanged, measurement of a metabolite such as 2-ethylidene-1,5-dimethyl-3,3-diphenylpyrrolidine (EDDP) in the setting of addiction treatment provides evidence for patient compliance rather than an exogenously spiked sample [101,102]. EDDP excretion is also less pH-dependent than is clearance of the parent drug [10,63,80]. Use of the methadone/EDDP ratio to assess compliance has been suggested but is complicated by the pharmacokinetic variability described above [101–103].

21.6.6 Propoxyphene

A relatively weak analgesic, propoxyphene is less potent than codeine but carries the risk of atypical adverse effects such as cardiac arrhythmia and seizure. The incidence of such negative responses is particularly high in the elderly, and has led to a decline in the number of prescriptions for this drug [104]. However, its nonmedical abuse remains common [105].

21.6.7 TRAMADOL

Unlike the majority of opioid agonists, tramadol has low abuse potential and is therefore it is not considered as a controlled substance in many countries [106]. It has low affinity for opioid receptors and mediates analgesia through opioid-independent regulation of neurotransmitter uptake; however, its main active metabolite (O-desmethyltramadol or M1) is a potent opioid receptor agonist [24]. These mechanisms are thought to work synergistically to provide greater total pain relief than the sum of each individual component. Metabolism to M1 occurs via CYP2D6, thus opioid-like effects are subject to genetic variability as with codeine [106]. However, because of its effects on neurotransmission, tramadol has the potential to cause serotonergic toxicity even in patients lacking CYP2D6 [24].

21.7 OPIOID ANTAGONISTS AND MIXED AGONIST/ANTAGONISTS (MAA)

These clinically useful compounds can produce very different physiological responses depending on the situation. For example, in opioid-naïve patients MAAs can provide MOR-mediated analgesia with less risk of an adverse reaction, while the same dose in an opioid-tolerant patient may precipitate immediate withdrawal. In medical usage, coadministration of low-dose antagonists or MAAs can alleviate minor opioid-induced side effects and appears useful in preventing opioid tolerance. In opioid addiction treatment, addition of a low-dose antagonist to maintenance therapy seems to minimize subjective "feel-good" effects without substantially worsening withdrawal symptoms.

21.7.1 BUTORPHANOL

Despite being only a partial agonist of MOR, butorphanol is a potent KOR agonist *in vitro*, though the question of which receptor predominates in humans remains incompletely answered [107]. Extensive first-pass metabolism leads to very poor oral bioavailability; the major metabolite is hydroxybutorphanol, with norbutorphanol and glucuronide conjugates also detectable [108].

21.7.2 BUPRENORPHINE

A semisynthetic derivative of thebaine, buprenorphine is a MOR partial agonist and KOR antagonist. Low doses provide analgesia through MOR activation, but unlike full agonists, there is a maximal threshold or "ceiling effect" to the pain relief [109]. Buprenorphine is available as sublingual tablets (with or without naloxone) for treatment of opioid dependence [105]. Buprenorphine is metabolized by CYP3A4 to the active compound, norbuprenorphine, both of which can be further conjugated to inactive glucuronides by UGT1A1 [86]. CYP3A4 and UGT1A1 are subject to environmental and genetic variability, though the effect of these factors on buprenorphine remain incompletely characterized [10].

21.7.3 NALBUPHINE

Thought to induce analgesia primarily through KOR [10], nalbuphine at low doses seems to increase pain in men, an effect that is reversed by the addition of naloxone [110]. Interestingly, low-dose nalbuphine in women retains analgesic potency, though it is enhanced with naloxone. This sexual dimorphism seems to be a general characteristic of KOR agonists, including butorphanol and pentazocine [110].

21.7.4 NALOXONE

The prototypical opioid antagonist, naloxone binds nonspecifically to all three receptor types, with the greatest effect at MOR and the least effect at DOR [10,111]. Its efficacy is much greater by intravenous administration as compared to oral or sublingual routes [105,112]. This characteristic is advantageous in deterring misuse of prescribed opioids: oral or sublingual opioid/naloxone formulations provide the desired benefit when taken properly, but when diverted for intravenous use cause opioid antagonism and may precipitate withdrawal [105,112].

21.7.5 NALTREXONE

Commonly used for treatment of alcoholism, naltrexone is a potent antagonist of all three opioid receptors [111]. Its combined formulation with opioid agonists is less common than are naloxone/ opioid combinations; however, the greater oral bioavailability of naltrexone suggests that it may be useful in applications where poor oral delivery limits the utility of naloxone [105].

21.7.6 PENTAZOCINE

A partial agonist of MOR, pentazocine is a full KOR agonist and appears to exert the majority of its effects through the latter receptor. Its previous popularity as a drug of abuse led to the inclusion of low-dose naloxone into current oral formulations, to deter illicit intravenous use with minimal effect on oral analgesia [105,112]. Structures and half-life of common opioids are summarized in Table 21.1.

TABLE 21.1
Structure and Half-Life of Common Opioids

	Structure	Half-Life
	Natural Opium Alkaloids	
Codeine		1.9–3.9 h
Morphine		1.3–6.7 h
	Semisynthetic Opiates	
Hydrocodone		3.4–8.8 h
Hydromorphone		1.5–3.8 h

(Continued)

TABLE 21.1 (Continued)

Oxycodone		4–6 h

Oxymorphone		

Fully Synthetic Opioids

Methadone		15–55 h

Propoxyphene		8–24 h

Tramadol		4.3–6.7 h

Fentanyl		3–12 h

Meperidine		2–5 h

Dextromethorphan		3.2–3.6 h (extensive metabolizer)

(Continued)

TABLE 21.1   (Continued)

	Structure	Half-Life
	Opioid Antagonists and Mixed Agonist/Antagonists	
Buprenorphine		2–4 h
Naloxone		30–80 m
Naltrexone		1–3 h (IV) 8–10 (oral)

Source: Baselt RC. *Disposition of Toxic Drugs and Chemicals in Man*, 7th Edition. Chemical Toxicology Institute, Foster City, CA, 2005.

21.8   ANALYTICAL CONSIDERATIONS

21.8.1   SCREENING VERSUS COMPOUND-SPECIFIC (CONFIRMATION) ASSAYS

Given the fact that opioids are both frequently-prescribed therapeutic agents and popular drugs of abuse, it is perhaps not surprising that immunoassays for this class of drugs are subject to the challenges of both areas of testing. Ideally, immunoassays designed for TDM should distinguish the analyte of interest from inactive metabolites or other similar drugs, while assays optimized to screen for abuse should provide equivalent detection of numerous compounds and their metabolites. Of course, these goals are difficult if not impossible to meet. Antibodies in opiate abuse screens commonly target morphine; there is wide variability in cross-reactivity to other congeners, thus some opiates with high abuse potential such as oxycodone are often poorly detected [113].

Given the relatively rapid turn-around time and ability to identify several opiates, immunoassays are the most commonly used screening tools. Immunoassays are also commercially available for several synthetic opioids such as dextromethorphan, and point of care devices are becoming more frequently used [114–116]. Other screening methodologies are available, including thin-layer chromatography, but these techniques are more labor intensive and may not provide adequate turn-around time for stat or emergency testing. It should be noted that commercial immunoassay development has largely been driven by abuse testing, thus many immunoassays either provide specific quantitation of compounds that do not require TDM (e.g., dextromethorphan), or provide only approximate quantitation for a group of compounds rather than distinguishing between specific opiates. Finally, the array of analytical interferences inherent to immunoassays can be a significant issue as well [113].

For compound-specific confirmation assays, gas chromatography (GC) with mass spectroscopic detection (GC-MS) has historically been considered the gold standard, and is still mandated for federal workplace testing in the United States. Typical GC-MS opiate assays simultaneously detect codeine, morphine, 6-hydro and 6-keto analogs, and sometimes 6-MAM. Interpretation of such panel assays must be performed with metabolic pathways in mind, as the presence of major (e.g., morphine from codeine) and minor (e.g., hydromorphone from morphine) metabolites that are also pharmaceutical agents can be a source of confusion.

Analysis of specific opioids can generally be performed using either GC or liquid chromatography (LC), depending on the inclination and experience of the developing laboratory. GC generally results in longer run times and is often incompatible with larger metabolites such as glucuronide conjugates. LC systems can be more expensive, require large quantities of organic solvents, and are not considered acceptable for federal testing. A wide variety of detectors are available for both GC and LC; mass spectroscopy (MS) or tandem MS are often preferred for the structural and mass-specific information provided. Analytical and technical considerations are discussed in detail below.

21.8.2 Sample Preparation and Extraction

The matrix and rationale for opioid testing influence the choice of methodology. Analysis of urine requires hydrolysis to recover glucuronide- or sulfate-conjugated metabolites of various opioids, notably codeine and morphine. Hydrolysis can be performed by acidification, e.g., concentrated hydrochloric acid at 115–120°C for 15 min [117–119], or by enzymatic treatment with β-glucuronidase alone [120–122] or in combination with arylsulfatase [123]. Acid hydrolysis is simpler, more rapid, and typically provides greater recovery than enzymatic methods, though a few studies have shown better recovery of some analytes with glucuronidase [124]. However, acidification destroys the metabolite 6-MAM, preventing conclusive determination of heroin use. Moreover, acid hydrolysis can also partially degrade morphine [125]. For this reason, drugs of abuse testing for opiates typically employ enzymatic hydrolysis regardless of the generally poorer analytical performance.

Serum analysis can be performed with or without a hydrolysis step; if a hydrolysis step is included, results reflect the sum of parent drug and metabolites, that is, "total" drug levels. For detection of illicit drug use, total concentrations are typically sufficient. However, omitting hydrolysis to preserve conjugated metabolites can be useful, for example when both the parent and metabolite are active compounds, as with morphine and M6G. As yet, few direct clinical applications exist for analyses of opioid metabolites (discussed below), but there has been much research interest in comparing differential responses, assessing likelihood of toxicity, and other areas of optimizing therapeutic use of opioids through metabolic studies.

Methods of analysis from serum or urine were initially developed using liquid–liquid extraction (LLE), though solid-phase extraction (SPE) is now often preferred. The latter is more expensive, but curtails the use of organic solvents and produces a cleaner extract [123] thus, reduces background, enhances mass spectral characteristics, improves identification of parent drugs and metabolites, and stabilizes day-to-day analytical performance [126]. A typical extraction begins with increasing the sample pH [118,120, 121,127] to suppress ionization of the amine moiety (typical pKa ~8–9); excessive alkalinity may cause ionization of the hydroxyphenyl group but the acceptable pH range is somewhat forgiving [126,128,129]. Glucuronide-conjugated metabolites, if present, remain ionized at high pH. Once the sample is alkaline, a variety of organic solvents for LLE [118,121,122,126,127,130–135] or columns for SPE [123,128,136–140] can be used to extract the compounds of interest. Most SPE cartridges consist of C18 or a similar hydrophobic organic matrix. However, a two-step SPE method was developed for morphine glucuronides [141], involving hydrophobic and charge-based isolation on carbon and ion-exchange resins, respectively; this extraction enhanced recovery of morphine metabolites from human plasma with fewer interferences compared to the C18 column alone.

After extraction, the organic phase can be purified by the acid-base method [118,126,127,133,142], or by organic phase partitioning [135], or it can simply be evaporated and then directly derivatized [121,132,143]. Some protocols do not derivatize prior to GC analysis [144,145], but this typically results in poor chromatographic properties. Derivatization converts polar hydroxyl groups into non-polar moieties, improving the chromatographic resolution and increasing the analytical sensitivity. Several agents are available for creating derivatives, including compounds that donate acetyl, propionyl, trimethylsilyl, or perfluoroester groups. Although the number of derivatizing agents described in the literature is relatively limited, there is great variability in the experimental conditions [118,119,121–123,126,127,132,134,136,142,143,146–152].

Acetyl-donating agents may provide incomplete derivatization, though acetyl derivatives have the advantage of being stable for up to 72 h when stored at room temperature in ethyl acetate [121,136]. Morphine and 6-MAM are both converted to diacetylmorphine (heroin), thus, acetyl derivatization does not permit distinction between morphine, 6-MAM, or heroin. In addition to diacetylmorphine, a small amount of 3-monoacetylmorphine (3-MAM) can be formed by acetylating agents; though clinically insignificant, 3-MAM shares the m/z 285 ion with deuterated (d_3) d_3-acetylcodeine, and can interfere with analysis of these compounds [143].

In contrast to acetylating agents, trimethylsilane (TMS) creates single derivatives for most opiates, although unfortunately TMS derivatives are sensitive to moisture [146]. There are also several analytical interferences associated with TMS: codeine and norcodeine derivatives coelute on GC, while 6-MAM produces an additional peak that coelutes with morphine and increases with room temperature storage [127]. Like TMS, pentafluoropropionic anhydride (PFP) derivatives are also moisture-sensitive; however, no breakdown products are detected after storage for 24 h [143]. The addition of pentafluoropropanol (PFPOH) improves the yield of PFP derivatives and allows morphine and 6-MAM to be clearly distinguished [136,138].

21.8.3   GAS CHROMATOGRAPHY–MASS SPECTROMETRY (GC/MS)

GC/MS is considered the reference method for determination of most natural and semisynthetic opiates, particularly in forensic settings, though other detectors are available and have been used for GC applications. MS detection provides structural information and allows use of deuterated (^{2}H-labeled) internal standards to overcome variability in recovery. In addition, nalorphine is also commonly used as an internal standard for opiate confirmation methods. Typically at least two ions are monitored for GC-MS identification of each compound, although three (one quantifying and two qualifying) ions are preferred.

Various GC-MS methods have been described for the identification and determination of opiates. Some investigators use chemical ionization [117,129,132,137], but electron impact mode is more common, generally at 70 eV. The GC is typically equipped with a 12- or 15-m fused-silica capillary column with a polar stationary phase of cross-linked dimethylsilicone, phenyl methyl silicone or 95% dimethyl-5% polysiloxane [120,121,123,131,136,146,153,154]. Most reports are focused on detection of illegal drug abuse, and therefore describe methods for the identification of morphine, codeine and 6-MAM, with additional characterization of a handful of semisynthetic opiates such as hydrocodone. However, Maurer and Pfleger described a screening procedure for the detection of 56 opioids, other analgesics, and metabolites [155]. GC-MS methods also exist for most opioids with forensic implications, as will be discussed below.

Due to the structural similarities between many opioids, particularly the natural and semisynthetic opiates, assays must be evaluated for interference from metabolites and congeners. The degree of overlap is such that the fragmentation patterns of various opioids can resemble one another greatly, as seen with the mass spectra of the TMS derivatives of hydromorphone, morphine, and norcodeine [156]. The chromatographic resolution of the compounds must be carefully optimized to provide reliable characterization, particularly since many structurally-related opiates are both commercially available and part of the same metabolic pathways.

21.8.4   Liquid Chromatography (LC)

Despite the long-standing role of GC in opiate analysis, LC methods are common and can be analytically advantageous. One notable example is the fact that LC provides the ability to analyze glucuronide-conjugated metabolites as well as parent compounds, thus adding information not available from a GC-derived total drug level. As with GC, there are a variety of detectors available for LC, though the use of MS detection is not as dominant with LC methods as it is with GC. In addition to MS or MS/MS techniques (tandem mass spectrometry), high-performance liquid chromatography (HPLC) methods for opioid analysis have been described using fluorescence (FD), ultraviolet-visible (UV), electrochemical (EC), and diode array detection (DAD), alone and in various combinations. HPLC-EC and HPLC-FD methods are comparable in sensitivity to GC–MS: reverse-phase HPLC with EC detection can detect opiates in the one labeled 5 ng/mL range. However, HPLC with non-MS detection lacks the specificity of GC–MS, thus sample preparation is critical to these methods. Both LLE and SPE methods are suitable for concentrating analytes and minimizing interferences.

MS detection provides greater specificity than most other detectors used for LC, but MS is relatively expensive and not universally available. There are also issues unique to LC-MS, including debates regarding the appropriate number of ions to assess and the definition of "acceptable" ion ratios. Unlike GC-MS, where clear guidelines exist, LC-MS and LC-MS/MS analyses suffer from the absence of formal recommendations from recognized experts regarding issues such as these. Early LC-MS studies frequently relied on only a single ion; however, monitoring two or more ions provides greater confidence in the identification, as the same concerns of overlapping fragmentation patterns discussed in the context of GC analysis also apply to LC methods. Tandem MS creates additional concerns, for example the observation that relying solely on product ions may lead to false identification [157]. Recommendations for acceptable compound characterization by LC-MS or LC-MS/MS are currently in development [158,159].

Apart from the issues of ions and ion ratios, there are a number of other considerations regarding sample preparation, chromatographic resolution and the value of including multiple analytes (e.g., metabolites) to support identification. One major concern regarding the application of MS to bioanalysis is the potential for matrix interference to affecting analyte signal variably in different samples. Electrospray ionization (ESI) is more susceptible to matrix effects than atmospheric pressure chemical ionization (APCI) to matrix effects, but ESI may be preferable for most opioids due to greater signal intensity [160]. Evaluation of matrix interference has been suggested as an important part of method validation for LC-MS/MS [161], although use of deuterated analogs as internal standards is thought to compensate for much of the influence of sample matrix.

Despite these concerns, LC-MS and LC-MS/MS can provide significant advantages over GC-based methods, beyond the ability to measure compounds like glucuronides that are unfavorable for GC analysis. With LC, preanalytical steps can often be simplified or eliminated, reducing both labor and solvent use. In addition, methods have been developed to determine polar metabolites without prior derivatization [162], while on-column extraction is possible with some LC systems. Dams et al. also demonstrated that preparation of urine samples by simple dilution is viable in LC-MS/MS [163]. These advantages explain the growing trend toward development of opioid assays using LC, particularly with MS/MS detection.

21.8.5   Analysis of Specific Opioids and Opioid Metabolites

Virtually all opioids have at least one published method for either GC or LC analysis; most have several reported protocols for each platform. In general, forensic applications have tended to utilize GC heavily, although this is not universally true, while TDM applications often incorporate LC for its added ability to measure conjugated metabolites. Morphine is essentially the archetype for opioids, thus it is fitting that the majority of analytical techniques limited to specific members of that drug class measure morphine and its metabolites. This section will discuss in detail several analytical methods for morphine measurement; other opioids will be discussed to a lesser extent.

A number of GC-MS methods have been developed to quantitate various combinations of morphine, other opiates, and their metabolites from extracts of human urine [164–166]. Long-standing use in forensic testing has made GC-MS the reference technique for determination of morphine and other frequently-abused opiates. However, HPLC is gaining in popularity for applications requiring faster turnaround or greater sensitivity than is typically feasible with GC. For example, a rapid and simple method described for analysis of morphine in plasma used Zeolite Y column extraction followed by reversed-phase HPLC-FD [167]; the assay provided reliable morphine quantitation up to five half-lives after last use. Similarly, an extremely sensitive (80 pg/mL) HPLC-ED method for detection of endogenous morphine in plasma has been described [168].

Although GC–MS is accepted as the reference technique for opiate analysis in biological fluids, there is still concern over the best methodology for direct determination of glucuronide metabolites. A recent review describes a number of HPLC methods for direct analysis of opiate glucuronides [169]. Ary and Rona reported a typical protocol for analysis of M3G and M6G: glucuronides were extracted using C18 column SPE with good recovery, then analyzed by reversed-phase (C8) HPLC-UV. The linear range spanned three orders of magnitude, with detection down to 10 ng/mL for both metabolites [170]. Most methods for morphine glucuronides are variations on a similar theme: a wide variety of techniques have been developed for several biological matrices, using different extraction methods, separation columns, and detectors. Bourquin et al. reported a reversed-phase HPLC-DAD method for analysis of plasma morphine metabolites including M3G and M6G, with quantitation to 25 ng/mL for each compound [171]. Wright et al. measured M3G and M6G in human cerebrospinal fluid and plasma using HPLC-ED after SPE preparation [172]. Other assays for plasma morphine glucuronides used HPLC-FD to take advantage of the compounds' native fluorescence without derivatization [173–176]. Reversed-phase ion-pair chromatography is also viable; morphine metabolites were measured in postmortem blood using this technique with both EC and UV detection [177].

The major advantage of these HPLC methods is that they make use of equipment that is less expensive and more readily available than LC-MS or LC-MS/MS platforms. However, three recent publications provided strong evidence that LC-MS is the method of choice for morphine glucuronide analysis [178–180]. Several analytical methods for morphine and its glucuronide metabolites exist for LC-MS or LC-MS/MS with different interfaces [178–191]. Tyrefors et al. reported detection of M3G and M6G using LC-ESI-MS in 1996; external standardization was applied, which according to the authors assured better accuracy and precision [178]. The first application of LC-APCI-MS for opiate analysis used C18 cartridges for SPE of urine samples, which were then analyzed for M3G and morphine in single-ion monitoring and full scan modes [191]. Most published assays for morphine glucuronides use reversed-phase HPLC; however, a normal-phase method using LC-APCI-MS was also reported [187]. Most recent work has centered on gaining sensitivity or improving performance factors such as cost and turnaround time. To these ends, sub-nanogram quantitation of morphine, M3G, and M6G was described using LC-ESI-MS/MS [192], while rapid and simple LC-MS methods have been developed using alternate sample preparation, such as protein precipitation, immunoaffinity extraction, or 96-well plate SPE [193–195].

The principles outlined above regarding measurement of morphine and its glucuronide metabolites are essentially applicable to most other compounds in this class of drugs. Closely related compounds (e.g., codeine, dihydrocodeine, oxycodone, and hydrocodone) can generally be detected using the same or very similar chromatographic conditions [63]. Some drugs are known to provide specific analytical challenges such as thermal decomposition at GC temperatures, as is seen with propoxyphene [196,197]. Methadone is also heat-sensitive, and can actually decompose to its physiological metabolite EDDP, making proper control of chromatographic parameters essential for valid results [101]. Certain opioids, such as meperidine, require formation of a derivative for reliable GC analysis [198,199]. Use of LC instrumentation can often bypass the need for derivatization or strict thermal control.

As knowledge of interindividual distinctions in drug response grows, TDM applications are becoming increasingly reliant upon measurement of both parent drug and metabolite(s), and therefore, trend toward measuring multiple compounds on LC-based platforms. Likewise, the cost savings and clinical utility of multianalyte assays have found favor in drug abuse testing as well, though GC methods remain a mainstay in that field. The oldest multicompound methods were largely designed for drug abuse analysis, and therefore measure several natural and semisynthetic opiates, including morphine, codeine, 6-MAM/heroin, and (separately or as total drug) morphine and codeine glucuronides by GC-MS [164–166], LC-MS [186,189–191], or LC-MS/MS [180,190]. Some protocols also include common antiabuse therapies such as methadone [200] or buprenorphine [201], or other nonopioid drugs of abuse including cocaine, amphetamines, and lysergic acid diethylamide (LSD) [162,202,203].

For TDM testing, recent reports have focused on quantitation of multiple opioids used therapeutically, e.g., in palliative care. Musshoff et al. report an LC-MS/MS method for analysis of 11 opioids and five metabolites, namely buprenorphine, codeine, fentanyl, hydromorphone, methadone, morphine, oxycodone, oxymorphone, piritramide, tilidine, and tramadol, with the metabolites bisnortilidine, morphine glucuronides, norfentanyl, and nortilidine [204]. The existence of subclasses of structurally related synthetic opioids is advantageous analytically: Thevis et al. developed a screening and confirmation method to identify fentanyl, alfentanil, remifentanil and sufentanil and their respective N-dealkylated or de-esterified metabolites by LC-MS/MS [205]. Metabolite profiling is another growing area in TDM testing, especially for compounds with known active metabolites such as tramadol [206].

21.9   CONCLUSIONS

In summary, the opioids are a structurally diverse class of drugs that are best-known for their analgesic effects, but which often possess additional physiological properties. Testing for these compounds is frequently used for both drug abuse and therapeutic applications, thus, understanding which analytes (parent and/or metabolite) are of greatest interest weighs heavily into determining the most appropriate methodology. Multidrug analyses have played and will continue to play an essential role in maximizing laboratory efficiency and clinical utility.

REFERENCES

1. Peat M. 2004. Workplace drug testing. In: Anthony M, Osselton MD, Brian W, eds. *Clarke's Analysis of Drugs and Poisons*, Vol. 3. London, UK: Pharmaceutical Press, 68–79.
2. Sora I, Takahashi N, Funada M, Ujike H, Revay RS, Donovan DM, et al. 1997. Opiate receptor knockout mice define mu receptor roles in endogenous nociceptive responses and morphine-induced analgesia. *Proceedings of the National Academy of Sciences of the United States of America* 94:1544–49.
3. Pert CB, Snyder SH. 1973. Opiate receptor: demonstration in nervous tissue. *Science* 79:1011–14.
4. Simon EJ, Hiller JM, Edelman I. 1973. Stereospecific binding of the potent narcotic analgesic (3H) Etorphine to rat-brain homogenate. *Proceedings of the National Academy of Sciences of the United States of America* 70:1947–49.
5. Terenius L. 1973. Stereospecific interaction between narcotic analgesics and a synaptic plasm a membrane fraction of rat cerebral cortex. *Acta Pharmacol Toxicol (Copenh)* 32:317–20.
6. Zollner C, Stein C. 2007. Opioids. *Handbook of Experimental Pharmacology* 177:31–63.
7. Harden RN. 2008. Chronic pain and opiates: a call for moderation. *Archives of Physical Medicine and Rehabilitation* 89:S72–76.
8. Gallagher RM, Rosenthal LJ. 2008. Chronic pain and opiates: balancing pain control and risks in long-term opioid treatment. *Archives of Physical Medicine and Rehabilitation* 89:S77–82.
9. Pasternak GW. 2004. Multiple opiate receptors: deja vu all over again. *Neuropharmacology* 47 Suppl 1:312–23.

10. Gutstein HB, Akil H. 2001. Opiod Analgesics. In: Hardman J, Limbird L, Gilman A, eds. *Goodman & Gilman's: The Pharmacological Basis of Therapeutics*, 10th ed. New York, NY: McGraw-Hill Professional, 569–619.

11. Waldhoer M, Bartlett SE, Whistler JL. 2004. Opioid receptors. *Annual Review of Biochemistry* 73:953–90.

12. Mollereau C, Parmentier M, Mailleux P, Butour JL, Moisand C, Chalon P, et al. 1994. ORL1, a novel member of the opioid receptor family. Cloning, functional expression and localization. *FEBS Letters* 341:33–38.

13. Noble M, Tregear SJ, Treadwell JR, Schoelles K. 2008. Long-term opioid therapy for chronic noncancer pain: a systematic review and meta-analysis of efficacy and safety. *Journal of Pain and Symptom Management* 35:214–28.

14. Mansour A, Meng F, Meador-Woodruff JH, Taylor LP, Civelli O, Akil H. 1992. Site-directed mutagenesis of the human dopamine D2 receptor. *European Journal of Pharmacology* 227:205–14.

15. Rozenfeld R, Abul-Husn NS, Gomez I, Devi LA. 2007. An emerging role for the delta opioid receptor in the regulation of mu opioid receptor function. *The Scientific World Journal* 7:64–73.

16. Rothman RB, Long JB, Bykov V, Jacobson AE, Rice KC, Holaday JW. 1988. beta-FNA binds irreversibly to the opiate receptor complex: in vivo and in vitro evidence. *The Journal of Pharmacology and Experimental Therapeutics* 247:405–16.

17. Maisonneuve IM, Kreek MJ. 1994. Acute tolerance to the dopamine response induced by a binge pattern of cocaine administration in male rats: an in vivo microdialysis study. *The Journal of Pharmacology and Experimental Therapeutics* 268:916–21.

18. Maisonneuve IM, Ho A, Kreek MJ. 1995. Chronic administration of a cocaine "binge" alters basal extracellular levels in male rats: an in vivo microdialysis study. *The Journal of Pharmacology and Experimental Therapeutics* 272:652–57.

19. Unterwald EM, Ho A, Rubenfeld JM, Kreek MJ. 1994. Time course of the development of behavioral sensitization and dopamine receptor up-regulation during binge cocaine administration. *The Journal of Pharmacology and Experimental Therapeutics* 270:1387–96.

20. Unterwald EM, Rubenfeld JM, Kreek MJ. 1994. Repeated cocaine administration upregulates kappa and mu, but not delta, opioid receptors. *Neuroreport* 5:1613–16.

21. Kilpatrick GJ, Dautzenberg FM, Martin GR, Eglen RM. 1999. 7TM receptors: the splicing on the cake. *Trends in Pharmacological Sciences* 20:294–301.

22. Pan YX. 2005. Diversity and complexity of the mu opioid receptor gene: alternative pre-mRNA splicing and promoters. *DNA and Cell Biology* 24:736–50.

23. DuPen A, Shen D, Ersek M. 2007. Mechanisms of opioid-induced tolerance and hyperalgesia. *Pain Management Nursing* 8:113–21.

24. Lotsch J. 2005. Opioid metabolites. *Journal of Pain and Symptom Management* 29:S10–24.

25. Wu D, Otton SV, Inaba T, Kalow W, Sellers EM. 1997. Interactions of amphetamine analogs with human liver CYP2D6. *Biochemistry and Pharmacology* 53:1605–12.

26. Shimada T, Yamazaki H, Mimura M, Inui Y, Guengerich FP. 1994. Interindividual variations in human liver cytochrome P-450 enzymes involved in the oxidation of drugs, carcinogens and toxic chemicals: studies with liver microsomes of 30 Japanese and 30 Caucasians. *The Journal of Pharamacology and Experimental Therapeutics* 270:414–23.

27. Zanger UM, Fischer J, Raimundo S, Stuven T, Evert BO, Schwab M, Eichelbaum M. 2001. Comprehensive analysis of the genetic factors determining expression and function of hepatic CYP2D6. *Pharmacogenetics* 11:573–85.

28. Smith DA, Abel SM, Hyland R, Jones BC. 1998. Human cytochrome P450s: selectivity and measurement in vivo. *Xenobiotica* 28:1095–128.

29. Evans WE, Relling MV. 1999. Pharmacogenomics: translating functional genomics into rational therapeutics. *Science* 286:487–91.

30. Eichelbaum M, Ingelman-Sundberg M, Evans WE. 2006. Pharmacogenomics and individualized drug therapy. *Annual Review of Medicine* 57:119–37.

31. Ferrari A, Coccia CP, Bertolini A, Sternieri E. 2004. Methadone--metabolism, pharmacokinetics and interactions. *Pharmacology Research* 50:551–59.

32. Coffman BL, Rios GR, King CD, Tephly TR. 1997. Human UGT2B7 catalyzes morphine glucuronidation. *Drug Metabolism and Disposition* 25:1–4.

33. Ohno S, Kawana K, Nakajin S. 2008. Contribution of UDP-glucuronosyltransferase 1A1 and 1A8 to morphine-6-glucuronidation and its kinetic properties. *Drug Metabolism and Disposition* 36:688–94.

34. Kadiev E, Patel V, Rad P, Thankachan L, Tram A, Weinlein M, et al. 2008. Role of pharmacogenetics in variable response to drugs: focus on opioids. *Expert Opinion on Drug Metabolism and Toxicology* 4:77–91.

35. Armstrong SC, Cozza KL. 2003. Pharmacokinetic drug interactions of morphine, codeine, and their derivatives: theory and clinical reality, Part I. *Psychosomatics* 44:167–71.

36. Bergen AW, Kokoszka J, Peterson R, Long JC, Virkkunen M, Linnoila M, Goldman D. 1997. Mu opioid receptor gene variants: lack of association with alcohol dependence. *Molecular Psychiatry* 2:490–94.

37. Bond C, LaForge KS, Tian M, Melia D, Zhang S, Borg L, et al. 1998. Single-nucleotide polymorphism in the human mu opioid receptor gene alters beta-endorphin binding and activity: possible implications for opiate addiction. *Proceedings of the National Academy of Sciences of the United States of America* 95:9608–13.

38. Berrettini WH, Hoehe MR, Ferraro TN, Demaria PA, Gottheil E. 1997. Human mu opioid receptor gene polymorphisms and vulnerability to substance abuse. *Addiction Biology* 2:303–8.

39. Hollt V. 2000. Allelic variation of delta and kappa opioid receptors and its implication for receptor function. *1999 Proceedings of the 61st Annual Scientific Meeting of the College on Problems of Drug Dependence*. National Institute of Drug Abuse, Bethesda, MD: Research Monograph Series (Harris LS ed). US Department of Health and Human Services, National Institutes of Health. NIH Publication No (ADM)00-4737, 50.

40. LaForge K, Kreek MJ, Uhl GR, Sora I, Yu L, Befort K, et al. 1999. Symposium XIII: allelic polymorphism of human opioid receptors: functional studies: genetic contributions to protection from, or vulnerability to, addictive diseases. *1999 Proceedings of the 61st Annual Scientific Meeting of the College on Problems of Drug Dependence*. National Institute of Drug Abuse, Bethesda, MD.: Research Monograph Series (Harris LS ed). US Department of Health and Human Services, National Institutes of Health. NIH Publication No (ADM)00-4737, 47–50,

41. Mayer P, Hollt V. 2001. Allelic and somatic variations in the endogenous opioid system of humans. *Pharmacology Therapy* 91:167–77.

42. Mayer P, Rochlitz H, Rauch E, Rommelspacher H, Hasse HE, Schmidt S, Hollt V. 1997. Association between a delta opioid receptor gene polymorphism and heroin dependence in man. *Neuroreport* 8:2547–50.

43. Gelernter J, Kranzler HR. 2000. Variant detection at the delta opioid receptor (OPRD1) locus and population genetics of a novel variant affecting protein sequence. *Human Genetics* 107:86–88.

44. Somogyi AA, Barratt DT, Coller JK. 2007. Pharmacogenetics of opioids. *Clinical Pharmacology Therapy* 81:429–44.

45. Stamer UM, Bayerer B, Stuber F. 2005. Genetics and variability in opioid response. *European Journal of Pain* 9:101–4.

46. Smith DA, Abel SM, Hyland R, Jones BC.1998. Human cytochrome P450s: selectivity and measurement in vivo. *Xenobiotica* 28:1095–128.

47. Linder MW, Prough RA, Valdes R, Jr. 1997. Pharmacogenetics: a laboratory tool for optimizing therapeutic efficiency. *Clinical Chemistry* 43:254–66.

48. Valdes R, Jr., Linder MW. 2004. Fine-tuning pharmacogenetics: paradigm for linking laboratory results to clinical action. *Clinical Chemistry* 50:1498–99.

49. Ingelman-Sundberg M, Oscarson M, McLellan RA. 1999. Polymorphic human cytochrome P450 enzymes: an opportunity for individualized drug treatment. *Trends in Pharmacological Sciences* 20:342–49.

50. Daly AK. 1995. Molecular basis of polymorphic drug metabolism. *Journal of Molecular Medicine (Berlin, Germany)* 73:539–53.

51. Daly AK, Fairbrother KS, Smart J. 1998. Recent advances in understanding the molecular basis of polymorphisms in genes encoding cytochrome P450 enzymes. *Toxicology Letters* 102–103:143–47.

52. http://www.cypalleles.ki.se/cyp2d6.htm. Accessed 8/13/2008.

53. Ingelman-Sundberg M. 2005. Genetic polymorphisms of cytochrome P450 2D6 (CYP2D6): clinical consequences, evolutionary aspects and functional diversity. *The Pharmacogenomics Journal* 5:6–13.

54. Kirchheiner J, Nickchen K, Bauer M, Wong ML, Licinio J, Roots I, Brockmoller J. 2004. Pharmacogenetics of antidepressants and antipsychotics: the contribution of allelic variations to the phenotype of drug response. *Molecular Psychiatry* 9:442–73.

55. Zanger UM, Raimundo S, Eichelbaum M. 2004. Cytochrome P450 2D6: overview and update on pharmacology, genetics, biochemistry. *Naunyn-Schmiedeberg's Archives of Pharmacology* 369:23–37.

56. Bernard S, Neville KA, Nguyen AT, Flockhart DA. 2006. Interethnic differences in genetic polymorphisms of CYP2D6 in the U.S. population: clinical implications. *The Oncologist* 11:126–35.

57. Eichelbaum M, Evert B. 1996. Influence of pharmacogenetics on drug disposition and response. *Clin Exp Pharmacol Physiol* 23:983–85.

58. *Physician's Desk Reference*, 61th ed. Montvale, NJ: Thomson PDR, 2007.

59. *MS CONTIN® (morphine sulfate controlled-release) Tablets Package Insert*. Stamford, CT: Purdue Pharma L.P., August 7, 2007.

60. *MSIR® Immediate-Release Oral Tablets CII (morphine sulfate) Package Insert*. Stamford, CT: Purdue Pharma L.P., October 29, 2004.

61. Sinatra R. 2006. Opioid analgesics in primary care: challenges and new advances in the management of noncancer pain. *The Journal of the American Board of Family Medicine* 19:165–77.

62. Kornbluth ID, Freedman MK, Holding MY, Overton EA, Saulino MF. 2008. Interventions in chronic pain management. 4. Monitoring progress and compliance in chronic pain management. *Archives of Physical Medicine and Rehabilitation* 89:S51–55.

63. Baselt RC. 2005. *Disposition of Toxic Drugs and Chemicals in Man*, 7th ed. Foster City, CA: Chemical Toxicology Institute.

64. Oyler JM, Cone EJ, Joseph RE, Jr., Huestis MA. 2000. Identification of hydrocodone in human urine following controlled codeine administration. *Journal of Analytical Toxicology* 24:530–35.

65. Wittwer E, Kern SE. 2006. Role of morphine's metabolites in analgesia: concepts and controversies. *The AAPS Journal* 8:E348–52.

66. Cone EJ, Heit HA, Caplan YH, Gourlay D. 2006. Evidence of morphine metabolism to hydromorphone in pain patients chronically treated with morphine. *Journal of Analytical Toxicology* 30:1–5.

67. Hanks GW, Hoskin PJ, Aherne GW, Turner P, Poulain P. 1987. Explanation for potency of repeated oral doses of morphine? *Lancet* 2:723–25.

68. Osborne R, Joel S, Trew D, Slevin M. 1990. Morphine and metabolite behavior after different routes of morphine administration: demonstration of the importance of the active metabolite morphine-6-glucuronide. *Clinical Pharmacology and Therapeutics* 47:12–19.

69. Osborne R, Joel S, Slevin M. 1996. Morphine intoxication in renal failure; the role of morphine-6-glucuronide. *British Medical Journal (Clinical Research Edition)* 293:1101.

70. Osborne RJ, Joel SP, Slevin ML. 1986. Morphine intoxication in renal failure: the role of morphine-6-glucuronide. *British Medical Journal (Clinical Research Edition)* 292:1548–49.

71. Langman LJ, Bjergum MW, Willis EA, Snozek CLH, Algeciras-Schimnich A, Santrach PJ. 2007. Quantitation of papaverine in blood salvaged for autotransfusion. *Therapeutic Drug Monitoring* 29:460–61.

72. Trafkowski J, Madea B, Musshoff F. 2006. The significance of putative urinary markers of illicit heroin use after consumption of poppy seed products. *Therapeutic Drug Monitoring* 28:552–58.

73. Jackson T, Chougule MB, Ichite N, Patlolla RR, Singh M. 2008. Antitumor activity of noscapine in human non-small cell lung cancer xenograft model. *Cancer Chemotheraphy and Pharmacology* 63:117–26.

74. Scordo MG, Melhus H, Stjernberg E, Edvardsson AM, Wadelius M. 2008. Warfarin-noscapine interaction: a series of four case reports. *The Annals of Pharmacotherapy* 42:448–50.

75. Ohlsson S, Holm L, Myrberg O, Sundstrom A, Yue QY. 2008. Noscapine may increase the effect of warfarin. *British Journal of Clinical Pharmacology* 65:277–78.

76. Klemenc S. 2000. Noscapine as an adulterant in illicit heroin samples. *Forensic Science International* 108:45–49.

77. Kawase M, Sakagami H, Furuya K, Kikuchi H, Nishikawa H, Motohashi N, et al. 2002. Cell death-inducing activity of opiates in human oral tumor cell lines. *Anticancer Research* 22:211–14.

78. Mohana M, Reddy K, Jayshanker G, Suresh V, Sarin RK, Sashidhar RB. 2005. Principal opium alkaloids as possible biochemical markers for the source identification of Indian opium. *Journal of Separation Science* 28:1558–65.

79. Zhang Z, Yan B, Liu K, Bo T, Liao Y, Liu H. 2008. Fragmentation pathways of heroin-related alkaloids revealed by ion trap and quadrupole time-of-flight tandem mass spectrometry. *Rapid Communications in Mass Spectrometry* 22:2851–62.

80. Kerrigan S, Goldberger BA. 2003. Opioids. In: Levine B, ed. *Principles of Forensic Toxicology*, 2nd ed. Washington DC: AACC Press, 187–205.

81. Banbery J, Wolff K, Raistrick D. 2000. Dihydrocodeine: a useful tool in the detoxification of methadone-maintained patients. *Journal of Substance Abuse Treatment* 19:301–5.

82. Giovannelli M, Bedforth N, 2008. Aitkenhead A. Survey of intrathecal opioid usage in the UK. *European Journal of Anaesthesiology* 25:118–22.

83. Rook EJ, van Ree JM, van den Brink W, Hillebrand MJ, Huitema AD, Hendriks VM, Beijnen JH. 2006. Pharmacokinetics and pharmacodynamics of high doses of pharmaceutically prepared heroin, by intravenous or by inhalation route in opioid-dependent patients. *Basic and Clinical Pharmacology and Toxicology* 98:86–96.

84. Rook EJ, Huitema AD, van den Brink W, van Ree JM, Beijnen JH. 2006. Population pharmacokinetics of heroin and its major metabolites. *Clinical Pharmacokinetics* 45:401–17.

85. Lurie IS, Toske SG. 2008. Applicability of ultra-performance liquid chromatography-tandem mass spectrometry for heroin profiling. *Journal of Chromatography* 1188:322–26.

86. Armstrong SC, Cozza KL. 2003. Pharmacokinetic drug interactions of morphine, codeine, and their derivatives: theory and clinical reality, Part II. *Psychosomatics* 44:515–20.

87. Riley J, Eisenberg E, Muller-Schwefe G, Drewes AM, Arendt-Nielsen L.2008. Oxycodone: a review of its use in the management of pain. *Current Medical Research and Opinion* 24:175–92.

88. de Leon J, Dinsmore L, Wedlund P. 2003. Adverse drug reactions to oxycodone and hydrocodone in CYP2D6 ultrarapid metabolizers. *Journal of Clinical Psychopharmacology* 23:420–21.

89. Chamberlin KW, Cottle M, Neville R, Tan J. 2007. Oral oxymorphone for pain management. *The Annals of Pharmacotherapy* 41:1144–52.

90. Pasero C. 2005. Fentanyl for acute pain management. *Journal of Perianesthesia Nursing* 20:279–84.

91. Thomas S, Winecker R, Pestaner JP. 2008. Unusual fentanyl patch administration. *American Journal of Forensic Medicine and Pathology* 29:162–63.

92. Tateishi T, Krivoruk Y, Ueng YF, Wood AJ, Guengerich FP, Wood M. 1996. Identification of human liver cytochrome P-450 3A4 as the enzyme responsible for fentanyl and sufentanil N-dealkylation. *Anesthesia and Analgesia* 82:167–72.

93. Olson KR. 2007. *Poisoning & Drug Overdose*, 5th ed. The McGraw-Hill Companies, 736.

94. Chou WH, Yan FX, Robbins-Weilert DK, Ryder TB, Liu WW, Perbost C, et al. 2003. Comparison of two CYP2D6 genotyping methods and assessment of genotype-phenotype relationships. *Clinical Chemistry* 49:542–51.

95. Prommer E. 2007. Levorphanol: the forgotten opioid. *Support Care Cancer* 15:259–64.

96. Prommer EE. 2007. Levorphanol revisited. *Journal of Palliative Medicine* 10:1228–30.

97. Latta KS, Ginsberg B, Barkin RL. 2002. Meperidine: a critical review. *American Journal of Therapeutics* 9:53–68.

98. Katzung BG (ed) 2006. *Basic & Clinical Pharmacology*, 10th ed. New York: The McGraw-Hill Medical, 489–526.

99. Mancini I, Lossignol DA, Body JJ. 2000. Opioid switch to oral methadone in cancer pain. *Current Opinion in Oncology* 12:308–13.

100. Crews JC, Sweeney NJ, Denson DD. 1993. Clinical efficacy of methadone in patients refractory to other mu-opioid receptor agonist analgesics for management of terminal cancer pain. Case presentations and discussion of incomplete cross-tolerance among opioid agonist analgesics. *Cancer* 72:2266–72.

101. Galloway FR, Bellet NF. 1999. Methadone conversion to EDDP during GC-MS analysis of urine samples. *Journal of Analytical Toxicology* 23:615–19.

102. George S, Gill L, Braithwaite RA. 2007. Simple high-performance liquid chromatographic method to monitor vigabatrin, and preliminary review of concentrations determined in epileptic patients. *Annals of Clinical Biochemistry* 37 (Pt 3):338–42.

103. George S, Braithwaite RA. 1999. A pilot study to determine the usefulness of the urinary excretion of methadone and its primary metabolite (EDDP) as potential markers of compliance in methadone detoxification programs. *Journal of Analytical Toxicology* 23:81–85.

104. Barkin RL, Barkin SJ, Barkin DS. 2006. Propoxyphene (dextropropoxyphene): a critical review of a weak opioid analgesic that should remain in antiquity. *American Journal of Therapeutics* 13:534–42.

105. Fudala PJ, Johnson RE. 2006. Development of opioid formulations with limited diversion and abuse potential. *Drug and Alcohol Dependence* 83 Suppl 1:S40–47.

106. Raffa RB 2008. Basic pharmacology relevant to drug abuse assessment: tramadol as example. *Journal of Clinical Pharmacy and Therapeutics* 33:101–8.

107. Walsh SL, Chausmer AE, Strain EC, Bigelow GE. 2008. Evaluation of the mu and kappa opioid actions of butorphanol in humans through differential naltrexone blockade. *Psychopharmacology (Berlin)* 196:143–55.

108. Vachharajani NN, Shyu WC, Greene DS, Barbhaiya RH. 1997. The pharmacokinetics of butorphanol and its metabolites at steady state following nasal administration in humans. *Biopharmaceutics & Drug Disposition* 18:191–202.

109. Walsh SL, Preston KL, Stitzer ML, Cone EJ, Bigelow GE. 1994. Clinical pharmacology of buprenorphine: ceiling effects at high doses. *Clinical Pharmacology and Therapeutics* 55:569–80.
110. Gear RW, Gordon NC, Miaskowski C, Paul SM, Heller PH, Levine JD. 2003. Sexual dimorphism in very low dose nalbuphine postoperative analgesia. *Neuroscience Letters* 339:1–4.
111. Trescot AM, Datta S, Lee M, Hansen H. 2008. Opioid pharmacology. *Pain Physician* 11:S133–53.
112. Fudala PJ, Bridge TP, Herbert S, Williford WO, Chiang CN, Jones K, et al. 2003. Office-based treatment of opiate addiction with a sublingual-tablet formulation of buprenorphine and naloxone. *The New England Journal of Medicine* 349:949–58.
113. Reisfield GM, Salazar E, Bertholf RL. 2007.Rational use and interpretation of urine drug testing in chronic opioid therapy. *Annals of Clinical and Laboratory Science* 37:301–14.
114. Crouch DJ, Frank JF, Farrell LJ, Karsch HM, Klaunig JE. A 1998. multiple-site laboratory evaluation of three on-site urinalysis drug-testing devices. *Journal of Analytical Toxicology* 22:493–502.
115. Moeller KE, Lee KC, Kissack JC. 2008. Urine drug screening: practical guide for clinicians. *Mayo Clinic Proceedings* 83:66–76.
116. Wu AH, Wong SS, Johnson KG, Callies J, Shu DX, Dunn WE, Wong SH. 1993. Evaluation of the triage system for emergency drugs-of-abuse testing in urine. *Journal of Analytical Toxicology* 17:241–45.
117. Cone EJ, Darwin WD, Buchwald WF. 1983. Assay for codeine, morphine and ten potential urinary metabolites by gas chromatography-mass fragmentography. *Journal of Chromatography* 275:307–18.
118. Paul BD, Mell LD, Jr., Mitchell JM, Irving J, Novak AJ. 1985. Simultaneous identification and quantitation of codeine and morphine in urine by capillary gas chromatography and mass spectroscopy. *Journal of Analytical Toxicology* 9:222–26.
119. Struempler RE. 1987. Excretion of codeine and morphine following ingestion of poppy seeds. *Journal of Analytical Toxicology* 11:97–99.
120. Lora-Tamayo C, Tena T, Tena G. 1987. Concentrations of free and conjugated morphine in blood in twenty cases of heroin-related deaths. *Journal of Chromatography* 422:267–73.
121. Bowie LJ, Kirkpatrick PB. 1989. Simultaneous determination of monoacetylmorphine, morphine, codeine, and other opiates by GC/MS. *Journal of Analytical Toxicology* 13:326–29.
122. Combie J, Blake JW, Nugent TE, Tobin T. 1982. Morphine glucuronide hydrolysis: superiority of beta-glucuronidase from Patella vulgata. *Clinical Chemistry* 28:83–86.
123. Bermejo AM, Ramos I, Fernandez P, Lopez-Rivadulla M, Cruz A, Chiarotti M, et al. 1992. Morphine determination by gas chromatography/mass spectroscopy in human vitreous humor and comparison with radioimmunoassay. *Journal of Analytical Toxicology* 16:372–74.
124. Delbeke FT, Debackere M. 1993. Influence of hydrolysis procedures on the urinary concentrations of codeine and morphine in relation to doping analysis. *Journal of Pharmaceutical and Biomedical Analysis* 11:339–43.
125. Fish F, Hayes TS. 1974. Hydrolysis of morphine glucuronide. *Journal of Forensic Science* 19:676–83.
126. Paul BD, Mitchell JM, Mell LD, Jr., Irving J. 1989. Gas chromatography/electron impact mass fragmentometric determination of urinary 6-acetylmorphine, a metabolite of heroin. *Journal of Analytical Toxicology* 13:2–7.
127. Christophersen AS, Biseth A, Skuterud B, Gadeholt G. 1987. Identification of opiates in urine by capillary column gas chromatography of two different derivatives. *Journal of Chromatography* 422:117–24.
128. Huang W, Andollo W, Hearn WL. 1992. A solid phase extraction technique for the isolation and identification of opiates in urine. *Journal of Analytical Toxicology* 16:307–10.
129. Pawula M, Barrett DA, Shaw PN. 1993. An improved extraction method for the HPLC determination of morphine and its metabolites in plasma. *Journal of Pharmaceutical and Biomedical Analysis* 11:401–6.
130. Dutt MC, Lo DS, Ng DL, Woo SO. 1983. Gas chromatographic study of the urinary codeine-to-morphine ratios in controlled codeine consumption and in mass screening for opiate drugs. *Journal of Chromatography* 267:117–24.
131. elSohly HN, Stanford DF, Jones AB, elSohly MA, Snyder H, Pedersen C. 1988. Gas chromatographic/mass spectrometric analysis of morphine and codeine in human urine of poppy seed eaters. *Journal of Forensic Science* 33:347–56.
132. Clarke PA, Foltz RL. 1974. Quantitative analysis of morphine in urine by gas chromatography-chemical ionization-mass spectrometry, with (N-C2H3)morphine as an internal standard. *Clinical Chemistry* 20:465–69.
133. Jones AW, Blom Y, Bondesson U, Anggard E. 1984. Determination of morphine in biological samples by gas chromatography-mass spectrometry. Evidence for persistent tissue binding in rats twenty-two days post-withdrawal.*Journal of Chromatography* 309:73–80.

134. Wu Chen NB, Schaffer MI, Lin RL, Stein RJ. 1982. Simultaneous quantitation of morphine and codeine in biological samples by electron impact mass fragmentography. *Journal of Analytical Toxicology* 6:231–34.

135. Lee HM, Lee CW. 1991. Determination of morphine and codeine in blood and bile by gas chromatography with a derivatization procedure. *Journal of Analytical Toxicology* 15:182–87.

136. Fehn J, Megges G. 1985. Detection of O6-monoacetylmorphine in urine samples by GC/MS as evidence for heroin use. *Journal of Analytical Toxicology* 9:134–38.

137. Drost RH, van Ooijen RD, Ionescu T, Maes RA. 1984. Determination of morphine in serum and cerebrospinal fluid by gas chromatography and selected ion monitoring after reversed-phase column extraction. *Journal of Chromatography* 310:193–98.

138. Schuberth J, Schuberth J. 1989. Gas chromatographic-mass spectrometric determination of morphine, codeine and 6-monoacetylmorphine in blood extracted by solid phase. *Journal of Chromatography* 490:444–49.

139. Gjerde H, Fongen U, Gundersen H, Christophersen AS. 1991. Evaluation of a method for simultaneous quantification of codeine, ethylmorphine and morphine in blood. *Forensic Science International* 51:105–10.

140. Wasels R, Belleville F, Paysant P, Nabet P, Krakowski I. 1989. Determination of morphine in plasma by gas chromatography using a macrobore column and thermoionic detection after Extrelut column extraction: application to follow-up morphine treatment in cancer patients. *Journal of Chromatography* 489:411–18.

141. Meng QC, Cepeda MS, Kramer T, Zou H, Matoka DJ, Farrar J. 2000. High-performance liquid chromatographic determination of morphine and its 3- and 6-glucuronide metabolites by two-step solid-phase extraction. *Journal of Chromatography B: Biomedical Sciences and Applications* 742:115–23.

142. Delbeke FT, Debackere M. 1991. Urinary concentrations of codeine and morphine after the administration of different codeine preparations in relation to doping analysis. *Journal of Pharmaceutical and Biomedical Analysis* 9:959–64.

143. Grinstead GF. 1991. A closer look at acetyl and pentafluoropropionyl derivatives for quantitative analysis of morphine and codeine by gas chromatography/mass spectrometry. *Journal of Analytical Toxicology* 15:293–8.

144. Caldwell R, Challenger H. 1989. A capillary column gas-chromatographic method for the identification of drugs of abuse in urine samples. *Annals of Clinical Biochemistry* 26 (Pt 5):430–43.

145. Masumoto K, Tashiro Y, Matsumoto K, Yoshida A, Hirayama M, Hayashi S. 1986. Simultaneous determination of codeine and chlorpheniramine in human plasma by capillary column gas chromatography. *Journal of Chromatography* 381:323–29.

146. Chen BH, Taylor EH, Pappas AA. 1990. Comparison of derivatives for determination of codeine and morphine by gas chromatography/mass spectrometry. *Journal of Analytical Toxicology* 14:12–17.

147. Mule SJ, Casella GA. 1988. Rendering the "poppy-seed defense" defenseless: identification of 6-monoacetylmorphine in urine by gas chromatography/mass spectroscopy. *Clinical Chemistry* 34:1427–30.

148. Hayes LW, Krasselt WG, Mueggler PA. 1987. Concentrations of morphine and codeine in serum and urine after ingestion of poppy seeds. *Clinical Chemistry* 33:806–8.

149. Saady JJ, Narasimhachari N, Blanke RV. 1982. Rapid, simultaneous quantification of morphine, codeine, and hydromorphone by GC/MS. *Journal of Analytical Toxicology* 6:235–7.

150. Phillips WH, Jr., Ota K, Wade NA. 1989. Tandem mass spectrometry (MS/MS) utilizing electron impact ionization and multiple reaction monitoring for the rapid, sensitive, and specific identification and quantitation of morphine in whole blood. *Journal of Analytical Toxicology* 13:268–73.

151. Mule SJ, Casella GA. 1988. Confirmation of marijuana, cocaine, morphine, codeine, amphetamine, methamphetamine, phencyclidine by GC/MS in urine following immunoassay screening. *Journal of Analytical Toxicology* 12:102–7.

152. Lewis KW. 1983. GLC of morphine and co-extractants in the rapid analysis of post mortem blood. *Journal of Chromatographic Science* 21:521–23.

153. Goldberger BA, Caplan YH, Maguire T, Cone EJ. 1991. Testing human hair for drugs of abuse. III. Identification of heroin and 6-acetylmorphine as indicators of heroin use. *Journal of Analytical Toxicology* 15:226–31.

154. Inturrisi CE, Max MB, Foley KM, Schultz M, Shin SU, Houde RW. 1984. The pharmacokinetics of heroin in patients with chronic pain. *The New England Journal of Medicine* 310:1213–17.

155. Maurer H, Pfleger K. 1984. Screening procedure for the detection of opioids, other potent analgesics and their metabolites in urine using a computerized gas chromatographic-mass spectrometric technique. *Fresenius' Journal of Analytical Chemistry* 317:42–52.

156. Goldberger BA, Cone EJ. 1994. Confirmatory tests for drugs in the workplace by gas chromatography-mass spectrometry. *Journal of Chromatography* 674:73–86.

157. Nordgren HK, Holmgren P, Liljeberg P, Eriksson N, Beck O. 2005. Application of direct urine LC-MS-MS analysis for screening of novel substances in drug abusers. *Journal of Analytical Toxicology* 29:234–39.

158. Maralikova B, Weinmann W. 2004. Confirmatory analysis for drugs of abuse in plasma and urine by high-performance liquid chromatography-tandem mass spectrometry with respect to criteria for compound identification. *Journal of Chromatography B: Analytical Technologies in the Biomedical Life Sciences* 811:21–30.

159. Rivier L. 2003. Criteria for the identification of compounds by liquid chromatography–mass spectrometry and liquid chromatography–multiple mass spectrometry in forensic toxicology and doping analysis *Analytica Chimica Acta* 492:69–82.

160. Edinboro LE, Backer RC, Poklis A. 2005. Direct analysis of opiates in urine by liquid chromatography-tandem mass spectrometry. *Journal of Analytical Toxicology* 29:704–10.

161. Matuszewski BK, Constanzer ML, Chavez-Eng CM. 2003. Strategies for the assessment of matrix effect in quantitative bioanalytical methods based on HPLC-MS/MS. *Analytical Chemistry* 75:3019–30.

162. Bogusz MJ, Maier RD, Kruger KD, Kohls U. 1998. Determination of common drugs of abuse in body fluids using one isolation procedure and liquid chromatography--atmospheric-pressure chemical-ionization mass spectrometry. *Journal of Analytical Toxicology* 22:549–58.

163. Dams R, Huestis MA, Lambert WE, Murphy CM. 2003. Matrix effect in bio-analysis of illicit drugs with LC-MS/MS: influence of ionization type, sample preparation, and biofluid. *Journal of the American Society for Mass Spectrometry* 14:1290–94.

164. Cone EJ, Darwin WD, Wang WL. 1993. The occurrence of cocaine, heroin and metabolites in hair of drug abusers. *Forensic Science International* 63:55–68.

165. Fuller DC, Anderson WH. 1992. A simplified procedure for the determination of free codeine, free morphine, and 6-acetylmorphine in urine. *Journal of Analytical Toxicology* 16:315–8.

166. Montagna M, Stramesi C, Vignali C, Groppi A, Polettini A. 2000. Simultaneous hair testing for opiates, cocaine, and metabolites by GC-MS: a survey of applicants for driving licenses with a history of drug use. *Forensic Science International* 107:157–67.

167. Ghazi-Khansari M, Zendehdel R, Pirali-Hamedani M, Amini M. 2006. Determination of morphine in the plasma of addicts in using Zeolite Y extraction following high-performance liquid chromatography. *Clin Chimica Acta* 364:235–38.

168. Liu Y, Bilfinger TV, Stefano GB. 1997. A rapid and sensitive quantitation method of endogenous morphine in human plasma. *Life Science* 60:237–43.

169. Kaushik R, Levine B, LaCourse WR. 2006. A brief review: HPLC methods to directly detect drug glucuronides in biological matrices (Part I). *Analytica Chimica Acta* 556:255–66.

170. Ary K, Rona K. 2001. LC determination of morphine and morphine glucuronides in human plasma by coulometric and UV detection. *Journal of Pharmaceutical and Biomedical Analysis* 26:179–87.

171. Bourquin D, Lehmann T, Hammig R, Buhrer M, Brenneisen R. 1997. High-performance liquid chromatographic monitoring of intravenously administered diacetylmorphine and morphine and their metabolites in human plasma. *Journal of Chromatography B: Biomedical Sciences and Applications* 694:233–8.

172. Wright AW, Watt JA, Kennedy M, Cramond T, Smith MT. 1994. Quantitation of morphine, morphine-3-glucuronide, and morphine-6-glucuronide in plasma and cerebrospinal fluid using solid-phase extraction and high-performance liquid chromatography with electrochemical detection. *Therapeutic Drug Monitoring* 16:200–8.

173. Glare PA, Walsh TD, Pippenger CE. 1991. A simple, rapid method for the simultaneous determination of morphine and its principal metabolites in plasma using high-performance liquid chromatography and fluorometric detection. *Therapeutic Drug Monitoring* 13:226–32.

174. Hartley R, Green M, Quinn M, Levene MI. 1993. Analysis of morphine and its 3- and 6-glucuronides by high performance liquid chromatography with fluorimetric detection following solid phase extraction from neonatal plasma. *Biomedical Chromatography* 7:34–37.

175. Huwyler J, Rufer S, Kusters E, Drewe J. 1995. Rapid and highly automated determination of morphine and morphine glucuronides in plasma by on-line solid-phase extraction and column liquid chromatography. *Journal of Chromatography B: Biomed Appl* 674:57–63.

176. Aderjan R, Hofmann S, Schmitt G, Skopp G. 1995. Morphine and morphine glucuronides in serum of heroin consumers and in heroin-related deaths determined by HPLC with native fluorescence detection. *Journal of Analytical Toxicology* 19:163–8.

177. Gerostamoulos J, Drummer OH. 1996. Solid phase extraction of morphine and its metabolites from post-mortem blood. *Forensic Science International* 77:53–63.

178. Tyrefors N, Hyllbrant B, Ekman L, Johansson M, Langstrom B. 1996. Determination of morphine, morphine-3-glucuronide and morphine-6-glucuronide in human serum by solid-phase extraction and liquid chromatography-mass spectrometry with electrospray ionisation. *Journal of Chromatography* 729:279–85.

179. Schanzle G, Li S, Mikus G, Hofmann U. 1999. Rapid, highly sensitive method for the determination of morphine and its metabolites in body fluids by liquid chromatography-mass spectrometry. *Journal of Chromatography B: Biomedical Sciences and Applications* 721:55–65.

180. Zuccaro P, Ricciarello R, Pichini S, Pacifici R, Altieri I, Pellegrini M, D'Ascenzo G. 1997. Simultaneous determination of heroin 6-monoacetylmorphine, morphine, and its glucuronides by liquid chromatography--atmospheric pressure ionspray-mass spectrometry. *Journal of Analytical Toxicology* 21:268–77.

181. Pacifici R, Pichini S, Altieri I, Caronna A, Passa AR, Zuccaro P. 1995. High-performance liquid chromatographic-electrospray mass spectrometric determination of morphine and its 3- and 6-glucuronides: application to pharmacokinetic studies. *Journal of Chromatography B: Biomedical Applications* 664:329–34.

182. Blanchet M, Bru G, Guerret M, Bromet-Petit M, Bromet N. 1999. Routine determination of morphine, morphine 3-beta-D-glucuronide and morphine 6-beta-D-glucuronide in human serum by liquid chromatography coupled to electrospray mass spectrometry. *Journal of Chromatography* 854:93–108.

183. Katagi M, Nishikawa M, Tatsuno M, Miki A, Tsuchihashi H. 2001. Column-switching high-performance liquid chromatography-electrospray ionization mass spectrometry for identification of heroin metabolites in human urine. *Journal of Chromatography B: Biomedical Sciences and Applications* 751:177–85.

184. Mortier KA, Maudens KE, Lambert WE, Clauwaert KM, Van Bocxlaer JF, Deforce DL, et al. 2002. Simultaneous, quantitative determination of opiates, amphetamines, cocaine and benzoylecgonine in oral fluid by liquid chromatography quadrupole-time-of-flight mass spectrometry. *Journal of Chromatography B: Analytical Technologies in the Biomedical and Life Sciences* 779:321–30.

185. Zheng M, McErlane KM, Ong MC. 1998. High-performance liquid chromatography-mass spectrometry-mass spectrometry analysis of morphine and morphine metabolites and its application to a pharmacokinetic study in male Sprague-Dawley rats. *Journal of Pharmaceutical and Biomedical Analysis* 16:971–80.

186. Bogusz MJ. 2000. Liquid chromatography-mass spectrometry as a routine method in forensic sciences: a proof of maturity. *Journal of Chromatography B: Biomedical Sciences and Applications* 748:3–19.

187. Naidong W, Lee JW, Jiang X, Wehling M, Hulse JD, Lin PP. 1999. Simultaneous assay of morphine, morphine-3-glucuronide and morphine-6-glucuronide in human plasma using normal-phase liquid chromatography-tandem mass spectrometry with a silica column and an aqueous organic mobile phase. *Journal of Chromatography B: Biomedical Sciences and Applications* 735:255–69.

188. Shou WZ, Pelzer M, Addison T, Jiang X, Naidong W. 2002. An automatic 96-well solid phase extraction and liquid chromatography-tandem mass spectrometry method for the analysis of morphine, morphine-3-glucuronide and morphine-6-glucuronide in human plasma. *Journal of Pharmaceutical and Biomedical Analysis* 27:143–52.

189. Bogusz MJ, Maier RD, Driessen S. 1997. Morphine, morphine-3-glucuronide, morphine-6-glucuronide, and 6-monoacetylmorphine determined by means of atmospheric pressure chemical ionization-mass spectrometry-liquid chromatography in body fluids of heroin victims. *Journal of Analytical Toxicology* 21:346–55.

190. Bogusz MJ, Maier RD, Erkens M, Driessen S. 1997. Determination of morphine and its 3- and 6-glucuronides, codeine, codeine-glucuronide and 6-monoacetylmorphine in body fluids by liquid chromatography atmospheric pressure chemical ionization mass spectrometry. *Journal of Chromatography B: Biomedical Sciences and Applications* 703:115–27.

191. Tatsuno M, Nishikawa M, Katagi M, Tsuchihashi H. 1996. Simultaneous determination of illicit drugs in human urine by liquid chromatography-mass spectrometry. *Journal of Analytical Toxicology* 20:281–6.

192. Slawson MH, Crouch DJ, Andrenyak DM, Rollins DE, Lu JK, Bailey PL. 1999. Determination of morphine, morphine-3-glucuronide, and morphine-6-glucuronide in plasma after intravenous and intrathecal morphine administration using HPLC with electrospray ionization and tandem mass spectrometry. *Journal of Analytical Toxicology* 23:468–73.

193. Projean D, Minh Tu T, Ducharme J. 2003. Rapid and simple method to determine morphine and its metabolites in rat plasma by liquid chromatography-mass spectrometry. *Journal of Chromatography B: Analytical Technologies in the Biomedical and Life Sciences* 787:243–53.

194. Beike J, Kohler H, Brinkmann B, Blaschke G. 1999. Immunoaffinity extraction of morphine, morphine-3-glucuronide and morphine-6-glucuronide from blood of heroin victims for simultaneous high-performance liquid chromatographic determination. *Journal of Chromatography B: Biomedical Sciences and Applications* 726:111–19.
195. Whittington D, Kharasch ED. 2003. Determination of morphine and morphine glucuronides in human plasma by 96-well plate solid-phase extraction and liquid chromatography-electrospray ionization mass spectrometry. *Journal of Chromatography B: Analytical Technologies in the Biomedical and Life Sciences* 796:95–103.
196. Sparacino CM, Pellizzari ED, Cook CE, Wall MW. 1973. A re-examination of the gas chromatographic determination of d-propoxyphene. *Journal of Chromatography* 77:413–18.
197. Millard BJ, Sheinin EB, Benson WR. 1980. Thermal decomposition of propoxyphene during GLC analysis. *Journal of Pharmaceutical Sciences* 69:1177–79.
198. Todd EL, Stafford DT, Bucovaz ET, Morrison JC. 1989. Pharmacokinetics of meperidine in pregnancy. International Journal of Gynaecology and Obstetrics: The Official Organ of the International Federation of Gynaecology and Obstetrics 29:143–46.
199. Verbeeck RK, James RC, Taber DF, Sweetman BJ, Wilkinson GR. 1980. The determination of meperidine, noremeperidine and deuterated analogs in blood and plasma by gas chromatography mass spectrometry selected ion monitoring. *Biomedical Mass Spectrometry* 7:58–60.
200. Rook EJ, Hillebrand MJ, Rosing H, van Ree JM, Beijnen JH. 2005. The quantitative analysis of heroin, methadone and their metabolites and the simultaneous detection of cocaine, acetylcodeine and their metabolites in human plasma by high-performance liquid chromatography coupled with tandem mass spectrometry. *Journal of Chromatography B: Analytical Technologies in the Biomedical and Life Sciences* 824:213–21.
201. Al-Asmari AI, Anderson RA. 2007. Method for quantification of opioids and their metabolites in autopsy blood by liquid chromatography-tandem mass spectrometry. *Journal of Analytical Toxicology* 31:394–408.
202. Weinmann W, Svoboda M. 1998. Fast screening for drugs of abuse by solid-phase extraction combined with flow-injection ionspray-tandem mass spectrometry. *Journal of Analytical Toxicology* 22:319–28.
203. Concheiro M, de Castro A, Quintela O, Lopez-Rivadulla M, Cruz A. 2006. Determination of drugs of abuse and their metabolites in human plasma by liquid chromatography-mass spectrometry. An application to 156 road fatalities. *Journal of Chromatography B: Analytical Technologies in the Biomedical Life Sciences* 832:81–89.
204. Musshoff F, Trafkowski J, Kuepper U, Madea B. 2006. An automated and fully validated LC-MS/MS procedure for the simultaneous determination of 11 opioids used in palliative care, with 5 of their metabolites. *Journal of Mass Spectrometry* 41:633–40.
205. Thevis M, Geyer H, Bahr D, Schanzer W. 2005. Identification of fentanyl, alfentanil, sufentanil, remifentanil and their major metabolites in human urine by liquid chromatography/tandem mass spectrometry for doping control purposes. *European Journal of Mass Spectrometry (Chichester, England)* 11:419–27.
206. Hakala KS, Kostiainen R, Ketola RA. 2006. Feasibility of different mass spectrometric techniques and programs for automated metabolite profiling of tramadol in human urine. *Rapid Communications in Mass Spectrometry* 20:2081–90.

22 Investigation of Drug–Herb Interactions: Application of various Chromatographic Techniques for Analysis of Active Components of Herbal Supplements

Amitava Dasgupta
University of Texas Medical School

CONTENTS

22.1   INTRODUCTION

Herbal remedies are widely used by the general population in the United States, Europe, and other parts of the world. In the United States, the sale of herbal medicine increased from $200 million in 1988 to over $3.3 billion in 1997 [1]. The majority of the population using herbal medicines in the United States has a college degree and belongs to the 25–49 age group. In one study, 65% of people thought that herbal remedies were safe and effective [1]. Race and ethnic origin also play major roles in the demographic of usage of complementary and alternative medicine. In another recent study involving 13,436 subjects, the authors found that prevalence of using herbal or natural supplements was lowest among African Americans (9.5%), intermediate in Hispanics (12%) and highest among Whites (19%). More women use complementary and alternative medicines compared to men and the use were also higher for subjects between 45 and 64 years of age regardless of race and ethnicity. The use of these products also increased with increasing years of education [2]. Gulla et al. performed a survey of 369 patient-escort pairs and found that ginseng was most commonly used (20%) followed by echinacea (19%), *ginkgo biloba* (15%) and ST John's wort (14%) [3]. Although there is a general perception often portrayed in marketing and the media that anything natural is safe, this concept is wrong. Herbal remedies can be toxic and inappropriate use or overuse may even cause fatality. Deaths have been reported from use of dietary supplements containing ephedra alkaloids and kava-kava [4,5]. The United States Food and Drug administration (FDA) regulates drugs and requires that they be both safe and effective. Most herbal products are classified as dietary supplements and are marketed pursuant to the Dietary Supplement Health and Education Act of 1994. In other countries local laws regulate sale of herbal supplements although in many countries worldwide there are minimal regulations for marketing of herbal supplements.

22.2   DRUG–HERB INTERACTIONS

Mechanism of drug–herb interactions can be classified under two main categories:

1. Herbal product may increase the clearance of a Western drug leading to unexpected lower concentration of a therapeutic drug. St John's wort, a herbal antidepressant increased clearance of many Western drugs.
2. An herbal remedy may have a synergistic effect of increasing pharmacological activity of a Western drug or may decrease therapeutic efficacy of a drug.

Herbal supplements which have clinically significant drug interactions with Western drugs include St John's wort, *ginkgo biloba*, dong qui, fenugreek, garlic, ginseng, and kava.

22.3   ST JOHN'S WORT

Herbal remedies are often taken in conjunction with therapeutic drugs. St John's wort is a popular herbal antidepressant which is used worldwide by the general population. Patients diagnosed with cancer or HIV often prefer various herbal antidepressants such as St John's wort and energy pills. Cho et al. recently reported that in their study population of patients visiting outpatient HIV clinics, 74% use herbal supplements or visit herbalists and St John's wort was used among these patients [6]. Most commercially available St John's wort preparations in the United States are dried alcoholic extract of the *Hypericum perforatum* plant. St John's wort is licensed in Europe for treatment of depression and anxiety and is sold over the counter in the United Kingdom [7]. The antidepressant activity of St John's wort is mostly attributed to the active component hyperforin although other components such as hypericin and pseudohypericin may also play important roles. Hyperforin probably acts through the inhibition of neuronal reuptake of serotonin, dopamine and noradrenaline. In addition, hyperforin may also inhibit the reuptake of gamma-aminobutyric acid (GABA) and L-glutamate [8]. The chemical structure of hypericin and hyperforin are given in Figure 22.1.

Although the adverse effects of St John's wort appear to be limited, fair skinned persons should be cautious about exposure to bright sun light because the active components of St John's wort have photosensitivity. Photosensitivity may also be present as neuropathy, possibly due to demyelination of cutaneous axons by photo-activated hypericins. After taking St John's wort for four weeks, a 35-year-old woman complained about stinging pain on sun exposed areas. The neuropathy resolved two months after she discontinued the product [9]. There are few case reports describing episodes of hypomania (irritability, agitation, anger, insomnia, and difficulty in concentrating) after using St John's wort. O'Breasail and Argouarch reported two cases of hypomania occurring six weeks and after three months usage of St John's wort [10]. Other adverse effects reported with St John's wort include gastrointestinal irritations, headache, allergic reactions, tiredness and restlessness. Demiroglu et al. described a case where hematological toxicity and bone marrow necrosis due to use of St John's wort (100 mg/day) for three weeks caused death in a patient [11].

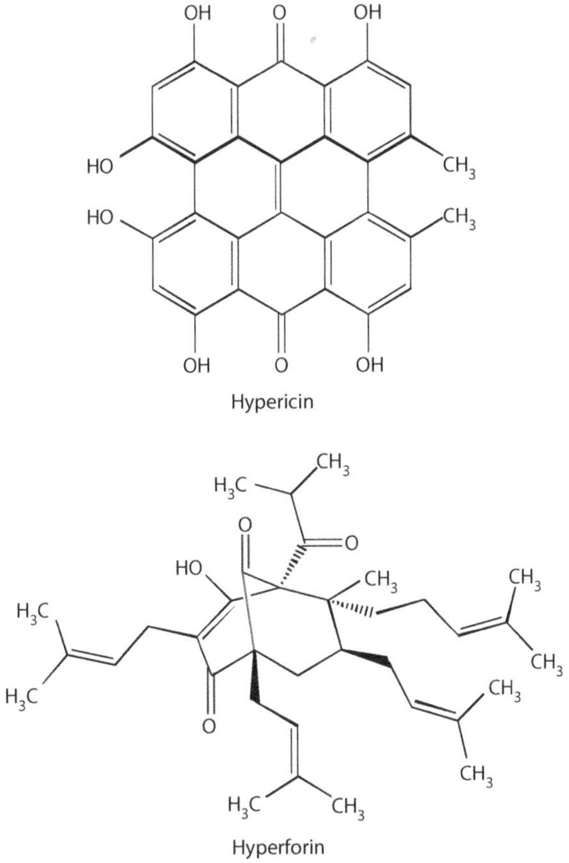

FIGURE 22.1   Chemical structures of hypericin and hyperforin.

22.4 MECHANISM OF INTERACTION OF ST JOHN'S WORT WITH WESTERN DRUGS

The primary mechanism of interaction of St John's wort with Western drugs involves induction of hepatic metabolism of drugs by cytochrome P450 (CYP) mixed function oxidase. In addition, component of St John's wort also modulate activity of drug efflux pumps including P-glycoprotein and multiple resistance proteins (MRS). There are many isoform of CYP but the CYP3A4 is the most abundant isoenzyme which is responsible for metabolism of more than 73 drugs and numerous endogenous compounds [12]. The active components of St John's wort particularly hyperforin induce CYP3A4 and CYP2B6 probably through activation of a nuclear steroid/pregnane and xenobiotic receptor [13–15]. Another component of St John's Wort, hypericin, also induces P-glycoprotein drug transporter and may reduce efficacy of drugs where hepatic metabolism may not be the major pathway of clearance. [16]. However, not all drugs interact with St John's wort [17].

22.5 LOWER LEVELS OF THERAPEUTIC DRUGS DUE TO CONCURRENT USE OF ST JOHN'S WORT

Unrecognized use of St John's wort is frequent among patients and may have important influences on the effectiveness and safety of drug therapy during hospital stay [18]. Published reports indicate that St John's wort significantly reduces steady state plasma concentrations of many drugs including amitriptyline, cyclosporine, digoxin, fexofenadine, indinavir, methadone, midazolam, nevirapine, oral contraceptives, phenprocoumon, tacrolimus, theophylline saquinavir, simvastatin, and warfarin [19,20]. In addition, pharmacodynamic interactions of St John's wort with selective serotonin reuptake inhibitors (SSRIs) has also been documented [21]. Drugs that undergo clinically significant interactions with St John's wort are listed in Table 22.1. Some drugs such as carbamazepine and mycophenolic acid have no reported interaction with St John's wort.

Interactions of St John's wort with various drugs also depend on concentrations of active components. Herbal remedies are not prepared following rigorous pharmaceutical standards. Wide variations in the active component of St John's wort in various commercial preparations have been reported. Draves and Walker reported that in commercial tablets of St John's wort, the percentage of active components varied from 31.3% to 80.2% of the claim of active ingredients based on labeling of the bottle [22]. Studies have demonstrated that cytochrome P450 enzyme induction by St John's wort depends on the hyperforin content and products that do not contain substantial amount of

TABLE 22.1
Important Drug–Herb Interaction Involving St John's Wort

Class of Drug	Name of the Drug	Reference
Immunosuppressants	Cyclosporine, tacrolimus	30,31,32
Protease inhibitors	Atazanavir, lopinavir, indinavir	35,36,37,38
Cardioactive	Digoxin, verapamil	40,41,42,57
Benzodiazepines	Alprazolam, midazolam	45
Anticancer	Irinotecan, imatinib	48,50
Tricyclic antidepressant	Amitriptyline	43
SSRI	Fluoxetine, sertraline, paroxetine	44
Cholesterol lowering drug	Simvastatin	55
Synthetic opioid	Methadone	47
Oral contraceptives	Norethindrone, ethinyl estradiol	54
Proton pump inhibitor	Omeprazole	56
Antidiabetic	Gliclazide	58

hyperforin (<1%) may not show clinically significant interactions with drugs [23]. Arold et al. demonstrated that low hyperforin containing St John's wort had no significant interaction with alprazolam, caffeine, tolbutamide and digoxin [24]. Moreover hyperforin is photosensitive and unstable in aqueous solution while degradation is dependent on the pH of the solution [25]. Important interactions of various Western drugs with St John's wort are given in Table 22.1.

However, St John's wort does not interact with carbamazepine probably due to already established auto-induction of liver cytochromes responsible for metabolism of carbamazepine [26]. Bell et al. observed no interaction between prednisone and St John's wort in healthy male subjects [27]. We recently reported that St John's wort does not alter metabolism of procainamide in mouse model probably because components of St John's wort do not induce N-acetyltransferase [28].

22.5.1 INTERACTIONS OF IMMUNOSUPPRESSANTS WITH ST JOHN'S WORT

Interaction of St John's wort with immunosuppressants such as cyclosporine and tacrolimus is of clinical significance because subtherapeutic level of such immunosuppressants due to concurrent administration of St John's wort may cause organ rejection. Barone et al. reported two cases where renal transplant recipients started self-medication with St John's wort. Both patients experienced subtherapeutic concentrations of cyclosporine and one patient developed acute graft rejection due to low cyclosporine concentration. Fortunately, upon termination of use of St John's wort, both patients' cyclosporine concentrations returned to therapeutic levels [29]. Alschner and Klotz reported a case study where a 57-year-old kidney transplant patient taking cyclosporine [125–150 mg/day] and prednisolone (5 mg/day) for a long time showed cyclosporine trough level [100–130 ng/ml) over the past two years. This patient suddenly demonstrated a drop in cyclosporine blood level to 70 ng/ml despite the daily cyclosporine dose being increased to 250 mg per day. The patient admitted taking a herbal tea mixture for depression which contained St John's wort. Five days after discontinuing the herbal tea his cyclosporine level was increased from 70 ng/ml to 170 ng/ml (250 mg of cyclosporine per day). Then the dose was reduced to 175 mg per day to readjust his cyclosporine whole blood concentration and his trough cyclosporine level again returned to 130 ng/ml [30]. Mai et al. reported that hyperforin content of St. John's wort determines the magnitude of interaction between St John's wort and cyclosporine. Patients who received low hyperforin containing St John's wort showed minimal changes in pharmacokinetic parameters and needed no dose adjustment. In contrast, the patients who received high amounts of hyperforin containing St John's wort needed dose increases within three days in order to maintain trough therapeutic concentration of cyclosporine [31].

Significant reduction in area under the curve (AUC) for tacrolimus was also observed in 10 stable renal transplant patients receiving St John's wort. The maximum concentration of tacrolimus was also reduced from a mean value of 29.0 ng/ml to 22.4 ng/ml following coadministration of St John's wort [32]. Bolley et al. reported a case where a 65-year-old patient who received a renal transplant in November 1998 had a trough whole blood level tacrolimus concentration between 6 ng/ml and 10 ng/ml. The patient started self-medication with St John's wort in July 2000 (600 mg per day) because of depression and in August 2000 showed an unexpected low tacrolimus concentration of 1.6 ng/ml. The serum creatinine was also decreased to 0.8 mg/dL from an initial value of between 1.6 and 1.7 mg/dL. When the patient stopped taking St John's wort, tacrolimus level returned to the previous range of 6–10 ng/ml. After one month, the creatinine value was also gradually increased to 1.3 ng/ml. Because the patient showed no rejection episode the new tacrolimus target level was set to 4–6 ng/ml [33]. Mai et al. studied interaction of St John's wort with tacrolimus and mycophenolic acid using 10 stable renal transplant patients. Coadministration of St John's wort significantly reduced the AUC as well as both peak and trough blood concentrations of tacrolimus. In order to achieve sufficient immunosuppression, tacrolimus doses were increased in all patients (median 4.5 mg per day to 8.0 mg/day). The tacrolimus trough levels after corrected for dose, decreased from a median value of 10.8 ng/ml (pre St John's wort) to 3.8 ng/ml two weeks after initiation of use of

St John's wort. Two weeks after discontinuation of St John's wort treatment, trough concentrations were increased again to 7.6 ng/ml and patients were adjusted to their previous doses approximately four weeks after the end of the study. Interestingly pharmacokinetic parameters of mycophenolic acid, another immunosuppressant were not affected by coadministration of St John's wort [34].

22.5.2 INTERACTIONS OF ANTIRETROVIRAL AGENTS WITH ST JOHN'S WORT

A patient positive for HIV and taking antiviral agents should not consume St John's wort, echinacea, garlic, ginkgo, and milk thistle because of significant interactions between these herbal remedies and antiretroviral drugs that may cause treatment failure. Clinically significant interactions of antiretroviral agents with St John's wort have been documented. Therefore, patients with AIDS taking amprenavir, atazanavir, zidovudine, efavirenz, indinavir, lopinavir, nelfinavir, nevirapine, ritonavir, and saquinavir must avoid concomitant use of St John's wort [35]. St John's wort was shown to reduce the AUC of the HIV-1 protease inhibitor indinavir by a mean of 57% and decreased the extrapolated trough by 81%. The subjects received 300 mg of St John's wort three times a day for 14 days. The mean peak concentration (Cmax) decreased from 12.3 µg/ml to 8.9 µg/ml in healthy volunteers taking both indinavir and St John's wort. A more significant effect was observed in C8 concentrations (indinavir concentration 8 h after dose) where the mean value was reduced from 0.494 µg/ml to 0.048 µg/ml in the group taking both St John's wort and indinavir. Reduction in indinavir concentrations of these magnitudes are clinically significant and could lead to treatment failure [36]. Reduced concentration of nevirapine due to administration of St John's wort has also been reported [37]. Busti et al. reported that atazanavir therapy can also be affected due to simultaneous use of St John's wort [38]. Coadministration of lopinavir/ritonavir with St John's wort is also not recommended because of substantial reduction in lopinavir plasma concentrations [39].

22.5.3 DIGOXIN AND ST JOHN'S WORT

Interaction between St John's Wort and digoxin is of clinical significance. Johne et al. reported that 10 days usage of St John's wort resulted in a 33% decrease of peak and 26% decrease in trough serum digoxin concentrations. The mean peak digoxin concentration was 1.9 ng/ml in the placebo group and 1.4 ng/ml in the group taking St John's wort. The AUC between zero and 24 h was 25% lower in the group consuming St John's wort compared to the placebo group [40]. Digoxin is a substrate for P-glycoprotein, which is induced by St John's wort. Durr D et al. also confirmed the lower digoxin concentrations in healthy volunteers who concurrently took St John's Wort [41]. The dosage of St John's wort as well as preparation also affect pharmacokinetics of digoxin. Muller et al. reported that low daily dose of hyperforin containing St John's wort does not affect the pharmacokinetics of digoxin. In contrast, comedication with high dose hyperforin rich extract resulted in a 24.8 % decrease in AUC from time zero to 24 h. A reduction of 37% was also observed in digoxin maximal plasma concentrations [42]. Therefore, patients taking digoxin should not self-medicate themselves with any preparation of St John's wort.

22.5.4 ANTIDEPRESSANTS AND ST JOHN'S WORT

When 12 depressed patients taking amitriptyline also took St John's wort for two weeks, a 22% reduction in AUC (between 0 and 12 h) of amitriptyline was observed due to concurrent therapy with St John's wort. For nortriptyline, the AUC was reduced by 41%. The mean peak concentration of amitriptyline was reduced from 69.8 ng/ml to 54.1 ng/ml in patients also receiving St John's wort and significant reductions were also observed in peak nortriptyline concentrations among subjects taking St John's wort [43]. The demethylation of amitriptyline to nortriptyline is catalyzed by CYP3A4 and CYP2C19 while further metabolism of nortriptyline through hydroxylation at position 10 is mediated by CYP3A4 and CYP2D6.

There is also an increased risk of interactions between St John's wort and selective serotonin reuptake inhibitor (SSRI) agents such as fluoxetine, sertraline, and paroxetine. Such pharmacodynamic interactions may lead to "serotonin syndrome" which may also lead to seizure and come [44].

22.5.5 Interactions of Benzodiazepines and Fexofenadine with St John's Wort

Benzodiazepines such as alprazolam and midazolam are metabolized by CYP3A4. Although short term ingestion of St John's wort (900 mg/day for one to three days) does not alter the pharmacokinetics of alprazolam and midazolam in healthy volunteers, long term ingestion (900 mg per day for two weeks) significantly increased oral clearance of midazolam and decreased oral bioavailability by 39.3% [45]. Fexofenadine is a nonsedating antihistamine. A single dose of St John's wort (900 mg) significantly increased the maximum plasma concentration of fexofenadine by 45% and significantly decreased the oral clearance by 20% without any significant change in half-life or renal clearance. However, long term use of St John's wort (two weeks) caused a significant decrease of 35% in maximum plasma concentration and a significant increase (47%) in oral clearance. This is probably due to inhibition of intestinal P-glycoprotein when a single dose of St John's wort was given but a long time use reversed the changes in fexofenadine disposition [46].

22.5.6 Methadone and St John's Wort

Reduced plasma level of methadone was also observed in the presence of St John's wort. Long term treatment with St John's wort (900 mg/day) for a median period of 31 days (range 14–47 days) decreased the trough concentrations of methadone by an average of 47% in four patients. Two patients experienced withdrawal symptoms due to reduced plasma levels of methadone [47].

22.5.7 Anticancer Agents and St John's Wort

Clearance of imatinib mesylate, an anticancer drug is also increased due to administration of St John's wort resulting in reduced clinical efficacy of the drug. Imatinib is used in the treatment of Philadelphia chromosome positive chronic myeloid leukemia and gastrointestinal stromal tumors. In one study involving 10 healthy volunteers, two weeks treatment with St John's wort significantly reduced maximum plasma concentration by 29%, AUC by 32%. The half-life of the drug was reduced by 21% [48]. St John's wort also showed significant interaction with another anticancer drug irinotecan. In one study involving five patients ingestion of St John's wort (900 mg per day) for 18 days resulted in an average 42% reduction in concentration of SN-38, the active metabolite of irinotecan. This reduction also caused decreased myelosuppression [49]. Hu et al. reported that aqueous and ethanolic extract of St John's wort markedly alter glucuronidation of irinotecan metabolite SN-38 as well as intracellular accumulation of irinotecan and SN-38. This pharmacokinetic interaction may be related to the marked protective effect of St John's wort on irinotecan induced blood and gastrointestinal toxicity [50].

22.5.8 Oral Contraceptives and St John's Wort

Oral contraceptives are divided into two types; progestogen only and combined estrogen and progestogen. Most oral contraceptives are substrates for CYP3A4 [51]. 17-Ethynylestradiol is a major component of the oral contraceptive pill and is also used in hormonal replacement therapy in postmenopausal women. It is metabolized through hydroxylation in position 2 by CYP3A4 [52]. St John's wort has significant interaction with oral contraceptives [53]. Murphy et al. studied interaction between St John's wort and oral contraceptives by investigating pharmacokinetics of norethindrone and ethinyl estradiol using 16 healthy women. Treatment with St John's wort (300 mg three times a day for 28 days) resulted in a 13–15% reduction in dose exposure from oral contraceptives. Breakthrough bleeding increased in treatment cycle as did evidence of follicle growth and probable ovulation. Authors concluded that St John's wort increased metabolism of norethindrone and ethinyl estradiol and thus interfered with contraceptive effectiveness [54].

22.5.9 MISCELLANEOUS OTHER DRUG INTERACTIONS WITH ST JOHN'S WORT

Sugimoto et al. reported interactions of St John's wort with cholesterol lowering drugs simvastatin and pravastatin. In a double blind cross over study using 16 healthy male volunteers, the authors demonstrated that use of St John's wort (900 mg per day) for 14 days decreased peak serum concentration of simvastatin hydroxyl acid, the active metabolite of simvastatin from an average of 2.3 ng/ml in the placebo group to 1.1 ng/ml in the group taking St John's wort. The AUC was also reduced in the group of volunteers taking St John's wort compared to the placebo group. Simvastatin is extensively metabolized by CYP3A4 in the intestinal wall and liver and St John's wort induces this enzyme. On the other hand St John's wort did not influence plasma pravastatin concentration [55]. St John's wort also induces both CYP3A4 catalyzed sulfoxidation and 2C19 dependent hydroxylation of omeprazole. In a study involving 12 healthy adult men, a group of volunteers received St John's wort (900 mg per day) for 14 days. Then both control groups and volunteers taking St John's wort consumed a single dose of omeprazole (20 mg) orally. Significant decreases in peak plasma concentrations of omeprazole were observed in volunteers taking St John's wort indicating significant interactions between St John's wort and omeprazole [56]. Tannergren et al. reported that repeated administration of St John's wort significantly decreases bioavailability of R- and S-verapamil. This effect is caused by induction of first pass metabolism by CYP3A4 most likely in the gut [57]. Recently, Xu et al. reported that treatment with St John's wort significantly increases the apparent clearance of gliclazide, a drug which is used in treating patients with Type II diabetes mellitus [58].

Interestingly, St John's wort does not interact with carbamazepine. Burstein et al. reported that intake of St John's wort (900 mg per day) for two weeks did not alter pharmacokinetics of the antiepileptic drug carbamazepine [59]. Carbamazepine is metabolized by CYP3A4 but the lack of interaction may be due to the inducing property of carbamazepine itself on cytochrome P450 enzymes and therefore further induction by St John's wort may not occur.

A patient taking paroxetine (Paxil, 40 mg) for eight months stopped taking paroxetine and started taking St John's wort (600 mg per day). She experienced no adverse effect from switching medication. However, one night when she felt tired she took 20 mg of paroxetine. She felt lethargic and ended up in a hospital. The authors conclude that St John's wort is a monoamine oxidase inhibitor and interacted with paroxetine, a SSRI [60].

22.6 MEASUREMENT OF ACTIVE COMPONENTS OF ST JOHN'S WORT IN COMMERCIAL EXTRACTS

There is no commercially available immunoassay for analysis of components of St John's wort. Therefore high performance liquid chromatography (HPLC) combined with ultraviolet (UV) detection or electrochemical detection is used for determination of active components of St John's wort in commercially available extracts. Li and Fitzloff described a rapid reverse phase HPLC method for determination of the major constituents of St John's wort: rutin, hyperoside, isoquercitrin, quercitrin, quercetin, pseudohypericin, hypericin, and hyperforin. The authors extracted active components of St John's wort from the specimens using methanol by two sonication steps (30 min each) at low temperature. Extraction efficiency for the major active ingredients of St John's wort was around 99%. HPLC analysis was carried out using a reverse phase C-18 column and a mobile phase gradient of water-acetonitrile-methanol-trifluoroacetic acid. The run time was 60 min and the analytes were measured with photodiode array detector [61]. Ruckert et al. described a HPLC method with electrochemical detection for the determination of hyperforin in St John's wort preparations. The authors used an isocratic mobile phase consisting of 10% ammonium acetate buffer (0.5 M, pH: 3.7) methanol-acetonitrile (10:40:50 by volume) and a flow rate of 0.8 ml/min. Hyperforin was detected ampherometrically with a glassy carbon electrode at a potential of +1.1 V versus silver/silver chloride/3M potassium chloride reference electrode. The limit of detection was 0.05 ng of hyperforin on column [62]. Mauri and Pietta used HPLC coupled simultaneously with a diode array detector and electrospray mass spectrometry for the analysis of hypericum extract. Hypericin, pseudohypericin, hyperforin, and adhyperforin were separated and identified based on their UV and mass spectra [63].

Although HPLC, as well as HPLC combined with mass spectrometry, is the most common method for analysis of active components of St John's wort, Seger et al. used both HPLC combined with mass spectrometry and gas chromatography combined with mass spectrometry for the analysis of supercritical fluid extract of St John's wort. Supercritical fluid extraction of plant material with carbon dioxide yields extracts enriched with lipophilic components. Besides the dominating phloroglucinols hyperforin (36.5±1.1%) and adhyperforin (4.6%±0.1%), the extracts mainly contained alkanes (predominately nonacosane) fatty acids and wax esters. The nonpolar components tended to accumulate in a waxy phase resting at the top of the hyperforin enriched phase. Highly polar compounds (napthodianthrones) were not found. For the gas chromatography/mass spectrometric analysis, the authors used electron impact mass spectrometric analysis (scan range: 40–640 amu). Ten oxygenated hyperforin derivatives were identified [64].

22.7 MEASURING HYPERICIN AND HYPERFORIN IN SERUM OR PLASMA

Hyperforin concentration in human plasma can be measured using HPLC combined with UV detection at 287 nm. In one report, a Luna C-18 column (150 × 4.6 mm, 3 μm particle size, Phenomenex) was used and the mobile phase was prepared by adding a methanol-acetonitrile organic phase (3:2 by volume) to water so that the final composition of organic phase was 92% and to aqueous phase was 8%. Finally 2 ml formic acid and 2 ml triethylamine were added to 1000 ml of mobile phase and the pH of the final mobile phase was 3.2. Hyperforin-containing or spiked plasma was mixed with acetonitrile and finally hyperforin was extracted using a solid phase extraction column. Benzo[k] fluoranthene was used as the internal standard. The limit of detection was 4 ng/ml and limit of quantitation was 10 ng/ml [65]. Bauer et al. also described HPLC combined with UV detection for determination of hyperforin and HPLC combined with fluorimetric detection for analysis of hypericin and pseudohypericin in human plasma. The authors used liquid-liquid extraction. The limit of quantitation for hyperforin was 10 ng/ml, while the limit of quantitation was 0.25 ng/ml for both hypericin and pseudohypericin [66]. Gioti et al. also used HPLC combined with UV and fluorescence detection for determination of hypericin, pseudohypericin and hyperforin in human urine and plasma using single drop liquid phase micro-extraction. The limit of quantitation was 3.0 ng/ml for pseudohypericin in human urine while the corresponding limits were 6 ng/ml and 12 ng/ml, respectively for hypericin and hyperforin. The limits were 5, 12 and 20 ng/ml, respectively in human plasma for pseudohypericin, hypericin and hyperforin [67].

HPLC combined with mass spectrometry can also be utilized for analysis of active components of St John's wort in human plasma. Pirker et al. used liquid–liquid extraction and HPLC combined with tandem mass spectrometry for simultaneous determination of hypericin and hyperforin in both human plasma and serum. For sample preparation, the authors mixed 1 ml plasma with 0.4 ml of dimethyl sulfoxide (DMSO) and 0.15 ml of acetonitrile, followed by mixing for 30 sec and extraction into 1 ml of ethyl acetate-hexane (70:30 by vol). After removing ethyl acetate-hexane layer, residue was extracted again and both organic phases were combined and concentrated under nitrogen for further analysis. Recovery of hyperforin was much higher (89.9–100.1%) than hypericin (32.2–35.6 %). The assay was linear for hypericin concentrations between 8.4 ng/ml and 28.7 ng/ml and for hyperforin the linearity was from 21.6 ng/ml to 242.6 ng/ml [68]. Riedel et al. described a

TABLE 22.2
Chromatographic Techniques to Determine Concentrations of Active Ingredients of St John's Wort in Human Serum or Plasma

Name of the Ingredient	Comments	Reference
Hyperforin	HPLC with UV detection.	65
Hyperforin	HPLC combined with UV detection	66
Hypericin	HPLC combined with fluorometric detection	66
Hypericin, pseudohypericin, and hyperforin	HPLC combined with UV and fluorescence detection	67
Hypericin and hyperforin	HPLC combined with mass spectrometry	68
Hypericin and hyperforin	HPLC combined with tandem mass spectrometry	69

HPLC method combined with tandem mass spectrometry for the determination of hypericin and hyperforin concentrations in human plasma. The authors used liquid-liquid extraction with ethyl acetate and hexane, and used a reverse phase (RP-18) column for their analysis. The limit of quantitation was 0.05 ng/ml for hypericin and 0.035 ng/ml for hyperforin. The hypericin method was linear between 0.05 ng/ml and 10 ng/ml. The linearity of the hyperforin assay was from 0.035 ng/ml to 100 ng/ml [69]. A summary of these methods are given in Table 22.2.

Measuring concentration of hypericin and hyperforin in human plasma or serum may be beneficial to evaluate a suspected interaction of a Western drug with St John's wort in patients receiving that particular drug and self-medicated with St John's wort.

22.8   INTERACTION OF VARIOUS DRUGS WITH KAVA

Kava is a herbal remedy with has both sedative and calming effect. Kava is prepared from a South Pacific plant (*Piper mesthysticum*). Kava drink is prepared by mixing fresh or dried root with cold water or coconut milk. Kava is available from a variety of manufacturers. The neurological effects of kava are probably related to a group of substituted dihydropyrones called kava lactones.

Heavy consumption of kava has been associated with hepatotoxicity as revealed by increases in liver enzymes such as γ-glutamyltransferase (GGT), alanine aminotransferase (ALT) and aspartate aminotransferase (AST). Escher et al. described a case where a 50-year-old man who took three to four kava capsules daily for two months demonstrated a 60–70-fold increases in AST and ALT. All tests for viral hepatitis were negative as well as tests for cytomegalovirus (CMV) and human immunodeficiency virus (HIV). The patient eventually received a liver transplant [70]. In January 2003, kava extracts were banned in the European Union, and Canada. In the United States the FDA strongly cautioned the general public against using kava. There are at least 11 cases of serious hepatic failure and four deaths directly linked to kava extract consumption and there are also 23 reports indirectly linking kava with hepatotoxicity [71]. However, for centuries the South Pacific islanders have consumed aqueous extracts of kava in ceremonies but no serious toxicity from consumption of such beverages have been documented. Cote et al. observed that there was a significant difference between kava lactones present in aqueous extract versus kava lactones present in commercial organic extract. Moreover, inhibitions of liver enzymes CYP3A4, CYP1A2 and CYP2C19 were more pronounced in commercial extracts compared to traditional aqueous extracts. The authors concluded that variation of health effects reported for kava extracts may be related to different protocols of preparation [72].

Because several kava lactones are potent inhibitor of various enzymes of cytochrome P450 system (CYP1A2, CYP2C19, CYP2C9, CYP2D6, CYP3A4, and CYP4A9/11), there is a potential of drug interaction with kava especially for drugs that are metabolized by cytochrome P450 system [73]. One study involving six healthy human volunteers who consumed traditional aqueous extract of kava indicated that caffeine metabolic ratio increased from 0.3 with consumption of kava to 0.6 at 30 days after the subjects stopped using kava. The later value corresponds to metabolic ratios in healthy subjects. The authors concluded that kava drinking inhibits CYP1A2 [74].

Kava has known sedative effect and it is speculated that kava may interact with central nervous system (CNS) depressants such as benzodiazepines, alcohol and barbiturates. There is a case report describing interaction of kava with alprazolam. A 54-year-old patient taking alprazolam, cimetidine and terazosin started self-medication with kava for three days and was hospitalized. The authors suggested that both kava lactones and alprazolam have additive effect because both act on the same GABA receptors. Moreover kava lactones are potent inhibitor of CYP3A4 which metabolizes alprazolam [75].

22.9 ANALYSIS OF ACTIVE COMPONENTS OF KAVA

Gaub et al. used HPLC combined with coordination ion spray mass spectrometry, where charged complexes are formed through addition of central complexing ions such as sodium, silver, and cobalt, for analysis of kava extracts [76]. Hu et al. analyzed six kava lactones; methysticin, dihydomethysticin, kavain, dihydrokavain, yangonin, and desmethoxyyangonin in various kava preparations using liquid chromatography. The authors used 5,7-dihydroxyflavone as the internal standard, a Luna-C18-2 column heated at 60°C and an isocratic mobile phase consisting of 2-propanol, acetonitrile, water and acetic acid (16:16:68:0.1 by vol) in order to achieve a complete separation of kava lactones in 30 min [77]. Duffield et al. used gas chromatography combined with chemical ionization mass spectrometry for identification of human urinary metabolites of kava lactones following ingestion of kava prepared by the traditional method of aqueous extraction from the plant *Piper methysticum*. All seven major and several minor kava lactones were identified in human urine. Metabolic transformations include reduction of 3,4-double bond and/or demethylation. Ring opening products of kava lactones were also detected in human urine [78].

22.10 DRUG–HERB INTERACTIONS INVOLVING *GINKGO BILOBA*

Ginkgo biloba is prepared from dried leaves of the ginkgo tree by organic extraction (acetone/ water). After the solvent is removed, the extract is dried and standardized. Most commercial dosage forms contain 40 mg of this extract. *Ginkgo biloba* is sold in the United States as a dietary supplement in order to sharpen mental focus and to improve diabetes related circulatory disorder. The German Commission E approved the use of ginkgo for memory deficit, disturbances in concentration, depression, dizziness, vertigo and headache. Ginkgo leaf contains kaempterol-3-rhamnoglucoside, ginkgetin, isoginketin and bilobetin. Several glycosides have also been isolated (ginkgolide A and B) from *ginkgo biloba*. Several chemicals found in ginkgo extracts, especially ginkgolide B are potent antagonist of platelet activity factor and also have antioxidant effect.

Ginkgo biloba induces CYP2C19 activity. Yin et al. investigated interaction of *ginkgo biloba* with omeprazole using 18 healthy subjects. All subjects received a single dose of omeprazole (40 mg) at baseline following 12 days treatment with *ginkgo biloba* (140 mg, twice daily). The authors observed that plasma concentrations of omeprazole and omeprazole sulfone were significantly reduced and concentration of 5-hydroxyomeprazole was significantly increased following treatment with *ginkgo biloba*. This interaction was related to increased omeprazole hydroxylation in a CYP2C19 genotype-dependent manner [79]. However, *Ginkgo biloba* has no significant interaction with digoxin [80].

Yang et al. studied bioavailability of cyclosporine in the presence of ginkgo and onion in rats. Cyclosporine was administered both orally and intravenously with or without ginkgo or onion in crossover design. Oral administration of ginkgo and onion significantly reduced Cmax by 62 and 60% and also reduced the AUC by 51 and 68%, respectively. The observed average maximum serum concentration of cyclosporine in the control group was 169.4 ng/ml and in the group receiving ginkgo was 65.2 ng/ml. In contrast, no effect was seen on pharmacokinetics of cyclosporine in the presence of ginkgo and onion when cyclosporine was given intravenously [81].

One case report indicated fatal seizures in a 55-year-old male possibly due to interaction of *ginkgo biloba* with antiepileptic drugs. The patient suffered a fatal breakthrough seizure with no evidence of noncompliance with anticonvulsant medications. The post mortem femoral blood concentrations of phenytoin (2.5 µg/ml) and valproic acid (<26 µg/ml) were subtherapeutic. In contrast, his phenytoin serum concentrations were within therapeutic in the last six months (range: 9.6–21.2 µg/ml) while the last phenytoin value prior to his death was 13.9 µg/ml. The patient was taking a variety of herbal supplements but mainly *ginkgo biloba*. Phenytoin is primarily metabolized by CYP2C9 and secondarily by CYP2C19 while valproic acid metabolism is also modulated by CYP2C9 and CYP2C19. *Ginkgo biloba* induces CYP2C19 activity and may be responsible for subtherapeutic levels of anticonvulsant medications due to increased metabolism in this patient [82]. Granger reported cases of two patients who were stable with valproic acid but developed seizure within two weeks of using ginkgo products. After discontinuation of ginkgo, both patients were again seizure free without any increases in dose of valproic acid [83]. Using a rat model, Kubota et al. demonstrated that *ginkgo biloba* extract when orally administered to rats for two weeks reduced the hypotensive effect of nicardipine. This may be due to increased hepatic metabolism of nicardipine [84]. Sugiyama et al. reported that intake of ginkgo attenuated hypoglycemic action of tolbutamide in aged rats [85]. Robertson et al. reported that *ginkgo biloba* modulated CYP3A4 activity and decreases serum concentration of midazolam. However, there is no change in the exposure of lopinavir when lopinavir is used in combination with ritonavir because of potential inhibition of CYP3A4 activity by ritonavir. Authors further speculated that *ginkgo biloba* may affect clearance of lopinavir if used not in combination with ritonavir. The pharmacokinetics of fexofenadine was not affected due to administration of *ginkgo biloba* in healthy subjects [86].

There are reports describing bleeding associated with the use of *ginkgo biloba*. Bent et al. based on a case report and review of literature data found 15 published case reports describing a temporal association between using *ginkgo biloba* and bleeding event. Most cases reported involved serious medical conditions. Only six reports clearly demonstrated that after discontinuation of ginkgo bleeding did not occur. The authors concluded that patients using ginkgo particularly those with known bleeding risk should be counseled about increased bleeding risk associated with the use of *ginkgo biloba* [87]. Gardner et al. studied the effect of *ginkgo biloba* and aspirin on platelet aggregation and platelet function analysis among older adults at risk of cardiovascular disease and concluded that in these older adults a relatively high dose of *ginkgo biloba* combined with 325 mg of daily aspirin did not have a clinically or statistically detectable impact on indices of coagulation examination over four weeks compared with the effect of only aspirin. In addition, the authors did not observe any adverse bleeding event in any patient [88].

22.11 ANALYSIS OF COMPONENTS OF *GINKGO BILOBA* FROM COMMERCIAL EXTRACTS AND HUMAN SERUM BY HIGH PERFORMANCE LIQUID CHROMATOGRAPHY (HPLC)

Ginkgolic acids from *ginkgo biloba* extract can be analyzed by HPLC after liquid-liquid extraction of aqueous commercially available extract using ethyl acetate or aliphatic hydrocarbons such as hexane. Analysis can be carried out using HPLC combined with UV detection with a photo diode array (200–550 nm) or combining HPLC with mass spectrometry [89]. Tang et al. used reverse phase HPLC (C-18 column) and a mobile phase composed of methanol and water (33:67 by vol) for analysis of ginkgolides and bilobalide from *ginkgo biloba* extract. Samples were extracted with ethyl acetate and purified by passage through an aluminum oxide column. The authors used evaporative light scattering technology for detection of the compounds eluting from the column [90]. On-line dialysis is an alternative to the conventional extraction technique for isolating compounds of interest from a complex matrix. Chiu et al. have developed a method for measuring ginkgolide

A and B, and bilobalide from *ginkgo biloba* extract using a self assembled microdialysis device coupled to an HPLC instrument. The dialysis efficiencies for ginkgolide A and B and bilobalide were between 97.8 and 100.7%. The authors used a Zorbax SB-C18 column (150 × 4.6 mm, particle size 5 μm) and the detection wavelength was set at 219 nm. The composition of the mobile phase was methanol, acetonitrile and 0.01 M phosphate buffer (30:5:65 by volume) [91]. HPLC combined with photodiode array detection can be used for quantitative determination of five selected flavonol compounds which are used as marker for quality control of *ginkgo biloba* extracts. These compounds include rutin, quercitrin, quercetin, kaempferol, and isorhamnetin. Separation of these compounds can be achieved using a Phenomenex Luna C-18 [2] column (250 × 2.0 mm, particle size: 5 μm). For optimal separation, the temperature of the column was maintained at 45°C by the authors and the composition of the mobile phase was acetonitrile: formic acid (0.3%) with a one step linear gradient and a flow rate of 0.4 ml/min. The limits of detections were 2.76, 0.77, 1.11, 1.55, and 1.03 μg/ml for rutin, quercitrin, quercetin, kaempferol and isorhamnetin, respectively [92]. Dubber et al. combined HPLC with tandem mass spectrometry (LC-MS-MS) for accurate determination of two flavonolglycosides along with quercetin, kaempferol and isorhamnetin in several *ginkgo biloba* commercial preparations. A one step gradient of acetonitrile-formic acid (0.3%) at a flow rate of 0.5 ml/min was used and the column temperature was maintained at 45°C. Baseline separations of these compounds were achieved within 20 min [93]. Ding et al. used a reverse phase HPLC combined with electrospray ionization mass spectrometry for simultaneous determination of 10 active major components of *ginkgo biloba* extract (bilobalide, ginkgolides A, B, and C, quercetin, kaempferol, isorhamnetin, rutin hydrate, quercetin-3-beta-D-glucoside, and quercitrin hydrate). The authors achieved baseline separation of these ten components in 50 min using a C-18 column. Quantitation was achieved using negative electrospray ionization in selected ion monitoring mode [94]. Later the same authors developed a fingerprint profile method using capillary HPLC combined with tandem mass spectrometry to identify more than 70 compounds from *ginkgo biloba* extract [95].

Wang et al. studied disposition of quercetin and kaempferol in ten adult volunteers following oral administration of *ginkgo biloba* extract. Quercetin and kaempferol were determined in human urine using reverse phase HPLC. Quercetin and kaempferol were excreted from urine mainly as glucuronides [96]. An HPLC protocol using the ion-pairing technique has been reported for rapid analysis of 4-O-methylpyridoxine in human serum. This compound is present in ginkgo seeds, and when consumed in larger quantities can cause vomiting and convulsions. The authors used fluorescence detection (excitation wavelength 290 nm, emission wavelength 400 nm) and observed a detection limit of 5 pg. The analysis time was 30 min [97]. This method can be applied to the detection of 4-O-methylpyridoxine in human serum. Ding et al. developed a capillary HPLC combined with mass spectrometry for determination of active components of *ginkgo biloba* in human urine after ingestion of ginkgo extract. The authors used C-18 column and precolumn with column switching method for separation of active components of *ginkgo biloba*. A limit of detection between 1 ng/ml and 18 ng/ml as well as high selectivity for components of *ginkgo biloba* in human urine was achieved by using a selected ion monitoring scan in negative ion mode [98].

22.12   DRUG–HERB INTERACTIONS INVOLVING VARIOUS GINSENGS

There are different types of ginseng such as Asian ginseng, American ginseng, Siberian ginseng and Indian ginseng also known as Ashwagandha, an Ayurvedic medicine. Asian ginseng is the most popular ginseng used in the United States. Asian ginseng is also widely used as an herbal product in China, other Asian countries and various other parts of the world. For thousands of years the common people in China have used ginseng as a tonic. The Chinese ginseng that grows in Manchuria is *Panax ginseng*. However, the ginseng that grows in North America is *Panax quinquefolius*. The common preparation of ginseng is ginseng root. Ginseng is promoted as a tonic and also as a reliever of stress. Ginseng may also be effective in the treatment of mild hyperglycemia. In Germany, it is indicated to combat lack of energy. Ginseng contains saponins known as ginsenosides. Panax ginseng is well tolerated and its adverse effects are mild and reversible. Associated adverse effects include nausea, diarrhea, euphoria, headaches, hypertension, and vaginal bleeding [99].

Lee et al. studied interaction between Panax ginseng and alcohol in 14 healthy male volunteers utilizing each subject as their own control. At 40 min after the last drink, the blood alcohol in the test group receiving ginseng extract (3 g/65 kg body weight) along with alcohol (72 g/65 kg body weight) was about 35% lower than the control value [100]. A study using mice indicated that decreased plasma concentrations of alcohol in the presence of ginseng may be due to a delay in gastric emptying [101]. Interaction between ginseng and phenelzine, a monoamine oxidase inhibitor has been reported. The interaction may be related to the psychoactive effect of ginseng [102]. Panax ginseng may interact with caffeine to cause hypertension. Ginseng may also decrease efficacy of warfarin [103].

22.13 ANALYSIS OF ACTIVE COMPONENTS OF GINSENG BY HIGH PERFORMANCE LIQUID CHROMATOGRAPHY (HPLC)

Analysis of active components of ginseng using HPLC combined with UV detection or mass spectrometry has been extensively studied. Harkey et al. analyzed 25 commercial ginseng products available in the United States for the presence of marker compound using HPLC and tandem mass spectrometry. The authors concluded that although all products were labeled correctly and marker compounds were found in all preparations, there was wide variation in concentrations of marker products, suggesting poor quality control and standardization in manufacturing such products [104]. Bonfill et al. described a reverse-phase HPLC assay for simultaneous quantitative determination of seven ginsenosides, Rb (1), Rb (2), Rc, Rg(1), Re, and Rf in ginseng products. Chromatographic separation can be achieved in less than 20 min using a diol column and UV detection at 203 nm [105]. Another method employed HPLC combined with negative ion electrospray mass spectrometry for determination of three ginsenosides (Rb 1, Rc, and Re) in six different samples of ginseng including a liquid extract, capsules, tea bags, and one instant tea. The authors found at least one ginsenoside in four of the six products studied [106]. Zhu et al. reported a comparative study on the triterpene saponins of 47 samples of ginseng using HPLC. The authors selected 11 ginsenosides as markers and found ten-fold variations in ginsenoside concentrations between different products [107]. Chen et al. studied metabolism of ginsenoside Rb (1) in rat using HPLC combined with mass spectrometry. Ten metabolites of Rb (1) were detected [108].

22.14 INTERACTION OF GARLIC (ALLIUM SATIVUM) WITH VARIOUS DRUGS

Garlic is believed to lower serum cholesterol and blood pressure. Garlic is rich in the sulfur containing compounds allicin and alliin. Piscitelli et al. studied the effect of garlic on pharmacokinetics of saquinavir, a protease inhibitor using ten health volunteers. In the presence of garlic, the mean saquinavir AUC during 8-h dosing intervals decreased by 51% and trough serum concentration 8 h after dosing reduced by 54%. After a 10-day washout period, the AUC and trough serum concentrations returned to 60–70% of the baseline values. The altered pharmacokinetics of saquinavir was considered to be related to decreased bioavailability of saquinavir [109]. Although garlic may enhance pharmacological effects of anticoagulants (warfarin, fluindione) [110], another report observed no significant pharmacokinetic or pharmacodynamic effect of garlic on warfarin although cranberry altered pharmacodynamics of warfarin with potential to increase the effect of warfarin [111].

Hypersensitivity to garlic has been reported. Topically-applied garlic can cause garlic burn as well as an allergic dermatitis. Use of garlic should be stopped seven to ten days before surgery because garlic can prolong bleeding time. Postoperative bleeding has been reported with garlic alone [112].

22.15   MEASUREMENT OF ACTIVE COMPONENTS OF GARLIC BY HIGH PERFORMANCE LIQUID CHROMATOGRAPHY (HPLC)

Arnault et al. described an ion-pair chromatographic method for simultaneous analysis of allin, deoxyallin, allicin and dipeptide precursors in garlic products. The authors developed a rapid HPLC protocol using a mobile phase containing heptanesulfonate as an ion-pairing reagent and photo-diode array UV and electrospray ionization ion trap mass spectrometry for detection [113]. Rosen et al. determined allicin, S-allylcysteine and volatile metabolites of garlic in breath, plasma, and stimulated gastric fluid using head space sampling and gas chromatography-mass spectrometry for analysis of volatiles from breath, and HPLC combined with mass spectrometry for determination of S-allylcysteine in plasma. For determination of concentrations of volatiles in breath, a short path thermal desorption device was used to volatilize the analytes. The absorption trap was spiked with d_8-toluene and d_8-naphthalene as internal standards. The desorption time was 3 min and the desorption temperature was 150°C. The gas chromatography column used was DB-1 methyl silicone capillary column (0.25 μm film thickness, 60 m × 0.32 mm id), and the mass spectrometer was operated in electron ionization mode (70 eV). The mass scanning range was 35–450 amu. The HPLC system for analysis of allicin used a Supelco 25 cm × 4.6 mm id C-18 column with a photodiode array (195 nm detection) and a isocratic mobile phase composition of acetonitrile/water (30:70 by vol). The major volatile component found in the breath was allyl methyl sulfide. After consumption of raw garlic, limonene and p-cymene were also detected in breath [114].

22.16   CLINICALLY SIGNIFICANT INTERACTION OF WARFARIN WITH HERBAL SUPPLEMENTS

Warfarin acts by antagonizing the cofactor function of vitamin K. Variability in the anticoagulant response to warfarin is an ongoing clinical dilemma. Although clinical efficacy of warfarin varies with intake of vitamin K and genetic polymorphisms that modulate expression of CYP2C9, the isoform responsible for clearance of S-warfarin, several herbal supplements also have significant effects on metabolism of warfarin. One report indicates that St John's wort increases clearance of both R and S-warfarin [115].

The anticoagulant effect of warfarin increases if combined with coumarin containing herbal remedies such as fenugreek and dong quai or with antiplatelet herbs such as danshen, garlic and *ginkgo biloba*. Conversely, a vitamin K containing supplement such as green tea may antagonize the anticoagulant effect of warfarin. The international normalization ratio (INR) was increased in a patient treated with warfarin for atrial fibrillation when he started taking coumarin containing herbal products boldo and fenugreek. After discontinuation of herbal supplements, his INR returned to normal after one week [116,117]. Increased anticoagulation due to interaction between warfarin and danshen has been reported [118]. There is a case report of a 87-year-old African American man receiving warfarin therapy who was admitted to hospital with an INR of 6.88. The INR was increased to 7.29 during hospital stay although his previous INR values ranged from 1.9 to 2.4 (therapeutic range: 2–3). The patient admitted taking a herbal supplement called royal jelly a week prior to his hospital admission and the elevated INR in this patient was probably related to the use of royal jelly [119]. Consumption of coenzyme Q10 and ginger also appear to increase the risk of bleeding with warfarin therapy [120]. Recently Cheng reported that both green tea and green leafy vegetables (turnip green, broccoli, lettuce, cabbage, spinach, green beans, and potatoes) inhibit the action of warfarin because these green vegetables especially turnip green and broccoli are rich in vitamin K [121].

22.17   CONCLUSIONS

Although many alternative remedies may have clinically significant interactions with Western drugs, at present interaction of herbal antidepressant St John's wort with various Western drugs has been well documented in the literature. The magnitude of interaction depends on the hyperforin content of the herbal extract. Transplant recipients and patients in warfarin should refrain from taking any herbal remedies due to potential of life threatening interactions of immunosuppressants and warfarin with various herbal supplements. Moreover, *ginkgo biloba*, garlic and other related herbal supplements may increase the risk of bleeding and patients with bleeding disorder should avoid taking herbal supplements. Currently, there is no commercially available immunoassay for measuring concentrations of active ingredients of various herbal supplements and only chromatographic techniques are used for investigating concentrations of these components in herbal extract or biological matrix after ingestion of a suspected herbal supplement.

REFERENCES

1. Mahady GB. 2001. Global harmonization of herbal health claims. *J Nutr* 131: 1120 S11–23S.
2. Kelly JP, Kaufman DW, Kelley K, Rosenberg L, Mitchell AA. 2006. Use of herbal/natural supplements according to racial/ethnic group. *J Altern Complement Med* 12: 555–561.
3. Gulla J, Singer AJ, Gaspari R. 2001. Herbal use in ed patients. *Acad Emerg Med* 8: 450.
4. Haller CA and Benowitz NL. 2000. Adverse cardiovascular and central nervous system events associated with dietary supplements containing ephedra alkaloids. *N Eng J Med* 343: 1833–1838.
5. Gow PJ, Connelly NJ, Hill RL, Crowley P, Angus PW. 2003. Fatal fulminant hepatic failure induced by a natural therapy containing kava. *Med J Aust* 178: 442–442.
6. Cho M, Ye X, Dobs A, and Cofrancesco J. 2006. Prevalence of complementary and alternative medicine use among HIV patients for perceived lipodystrophy. *J Altern Complement Med* 12: 475–482.
7. Schwarz JT and Cupp MJ. 2000. *St John's Wort in Toxicology and Clinical Pharmacology of Herbal Products*. Cupp MJ Ed. Totowa, New Jersey: Humana Press, 67–78.
8. Wille SM, Cooreman SG, Neels HM and Lambert WE. 2008. Relevant issues in the monitoring and the toxicology of antidepressants. *Crit Rev Clin Lab Sci* 45: 25–89.
9. Bove GM. 1998. Acute neuropathy after exposure to sun in a patient treated with St. John's Wort. *Lancet* 352: 1121–1122.
10. O'Breasail AM and Argouarch A. 1998. Hypomania and St. John's wort. *Can J Psychiatry* 43: 746–747.
11. Demiroglu YZ, Yeter TT, Boga C, Ozdogu H, et al. 2005. Bone marrow necrosis: a rare complication of herbal treatment with Hypericum perforatum (St. John's wort). *Acta Medica (Hradec Kralove)* 48: 91–94.
12. Landrum-Michalets E. 1998. Update: clinically significant cytochrome P450 drug interactions. *Pharmacotherapy* 18: 84–112.
13. Krusekopf S, Roots I. 2005. St. John's wort and its constituent hyperforin concordantly regulate expression of genes encoding enzymes involved in basic cellular pathways. *Pharmacogenet Genom* 15: 817–829.
14. Hu Z, Yang X, Ho PC, Chan SY, et al. 2005. Herb-drug interactions: a literature review. *Drugs* 65: 1239–1282.
15. Wentworth JM, Agostini M, Love J, Schwabe JW, Chatterjee VK. 2000. St John's wort, a herbal antidepressant. Activates the steroid X receptor. *J Endocrinol* 166: R11–16.
16. Raffa R. 1998. Screen of receptor and uptake site activity of hypericin components of St John's Wort reveal σ receptor binding. *Life Sci* 62: PL265–270.
17. Madabushi R, Frank B, Drewelow B, Derendorf H, Butterweck V. 2006. Hyperforin in St. John's wort drug interactions. *Eur J Clin Pharmacol* 62: 225–233.
18. Martin-Facklam M, Rieger K, Riedel KD, Burhenne J, et al. 2004. Undeclared exposure of St. John's wort in hospitalized patients. *Br J Clin Pharmacol* 58: 437–441.
19. Zhou S, Chan E, Pan SQ, Huang M, Lee EJ. 2004. Pharmacokinetic interactions of drugs with St. John's wort. *J Psychopharmacol* 18: 262–276.
20. Dasgupta A. 2008. Herbal supplements and therapeutic drug monitoring: focus on digoxin immunoassays and interaction with St. John's wort. *Ther Drug Monit* 30: 212–217.
21. Zhou SF, Lai X. 2008. An update on clinical drug interactions with herbal antidepressant St. John's wort. Curr Drug Metab 9: 394–409.
22. Draves AH, Walker SE. 2003. Analysis of hypericin and pseudohypericin content of commercially available St. John's wort preparation. *Can J Clin Pharmacol* 10: 114–118.

23. Madabushi R, Frank B, Drewlow B, Derendirf H et al. 2006. Hyperforin in St. John's wort drug interactions. *Eur J Clin Pharmacol* 62: 225–233.
24. Arold G, Donath F, Maurer A, Diefenbach K et al. 2005. No relevant interaction with alprazolam, caffeine, tolbutamide and digoxin by treatment with a low hyperforin St. John's wort extract. *Planta Med* 71: 331–337.
25. Ang CY, Hu L, Heinze TM, Cui Y et al. 2004. Instability of St. John's wort (*Hypericum perforatum* L) and degradation of hyperforin in aqueous solutions and functional beverage. *J Agric Food Chem* 52: 6156–6164.
26. Burstein AH, Hortan RL, Dunn T, Alfaro RM et al. 2000. Lack of effect of St. John's wort on carbamazepine pharmacokinetics in healthy volunteers. *Clin Pharmacol Ther* 68: 605–612.
27. Bell EC, Ravis WR, Chan HM, Lin YJ. 2007. Lack of pharmacokinetic interaction between St. John's wort and prednisone. *Ann Pharmacother* 41: 1819–1924.
28. Dasgupta A, Hovanetz M, Olsen M, Wells A, Actor JK. 2007. Drug-herb interaction: effect of St. John's wort on bioavailability and metabolism of procainamide in mice. *Arch Pathol Lab Med* 131: 1094–1098.
29. Barone GW, Gurley BJ, Ketel BL, Abul-Ezz SR. 2001. Herbal supplements; a potential for drug interactions in transplant recipients. *Transplantation* 71: 239–241.
30. Alscher DM, klotz U. 2003. Drug interaction of herbal tea containing St. John's wort with cyclosporine [Letter]. *Transpl Int* 16: 543–544.
31. Mai I, Bauer S, Perloff ES, Johne A, et al. 2004. Hyperforin content determines the magnitude of the St. John's wort-cyclosporine drug interaction. *Clin Pharmacol* 76: 330–340.
32. Hebert MF, Park JM, Chen YL, Akhtar S, Larson AM. 2004. Effects of St John's wort (Hypericum perforatum) on tacrolimus pharmacokinetics in healthy volunteers. *Clin Pharmacol* 44: 89–94.
33. Bolley R, Zulke C, Kammerl M, Fischereder M, Kramer BK. 2002. Tacrolimus induced nephrotoxicity unmasked by induction of CYP3A4 system with St. John's wort [Letter]. *Transplantation* 73: 1009.
34. Mai I, Stormer E Bauer S, Kruger H et al. 2003. Impact of St. John's wort treatment on the pharmacokinetics of tacrolimus and mycophenolic acid in renal transplant patients. *Nephrol Dial Transplant* 18: 819–822.
35. van den Bout-van den Beukel CJ, Koopmans PP, van der Ven AJ, De Smet PA, Burtger DM. 2006. Possible drug metabolism interactions of medicinal herbs with antiretroviral agents. *Drug Metab Rev* 38: 477–514.
36. Piscitelli SC, Burstein AH, Chaitt D, Alfaro RM, Fallon J. 2000. Indinavir concentrations and St. John's Wort. *Lancet* 355: 547–548.
37. de Maat MM, Hoetelmans RM, Math t RA. Van Gorp EC et al. 2001. Drug interaction between St. John's wort and nevirapine. *AIDS* 15: 420–421.
38. Busti AJ, Hall RJ, Margolis DM. 2004. Atazanavir for the treatment of human immunodeficiency virus infection. *Pharmacotherapy* 24: 1732–1747.
39. Cvetkovic RS, Goa KL. 2003. Lopinavir/ritonavir: a review of its use in the management of HIV infection. *Drugs* 63: 769–802.
40. Johne A, Brockmoller J, Bauer S, Maurer A, et al. 1999. Pharmacokinetic interaction of digoxin with an herbal extract from St John's Wort (Hypericum perforatum). *Clin Pharmacol Ther* 66: 338–345.
41. Durr D, Stieger B, Kullak-Ublick GA, Rentsck KM et al. 2000. St John's Wort induces intestinal P-glycoprotein/MDR1 and intestinal and hepatic CYP3A4. *Clin Pharmacol Ther* 68: 598–604.
42. Muller SC, Uehleke B, Woehling H, Petzsch M et al. 2004. Effect of St. John's wort dose and preparation on the pharmacokinetics of digoxin. *Clin Pharmacol Ther* 75: 546–557.
43. Johne A, Schmider J, Brockmoller J, Stadelman AM, et al. 2002. Decreased plasma levels of amitriptyline and its metabolites on comedication with an extract from St. John's wort (*Hypericum perforatum*). *J Clin Psychopharmacol* 22: 46–54.
44. Singh YN. 2005. Potential for interaction of kava and St. John's wort with drugs. *J Ethnopharmacol* 100: 108–113.
45. Wang Z, Gorski JC, 2001. Hamman MA, Huang SM, et al. The effects of St. John's wort (Hypericum perforatum) on human cytochrome P450 activity. *Clin Pharmacol Ther* 70: 317–326.
46. Wang Z, Hamman MA, Huang SM, Lesko LJ, Hall SD. 2002. Effect of St. John's wort on the pharmacokinetics of fexofenadine. *Clin Pharmacol* 71: 411–420.
47. Eich-Hochli D, Oppliger R, Golay KP, Baumann P, Eap CB. 2003. Methadone maintenance treatment and St. John's wort-a case study. *Pharmacopsychiatry* 36: 35–37.
48. Smith P. 2004. The influence of St. John's wort on the pharmacokinetics and protein binding of imatinib mesylate. *Pharmacotherapy* 24: 1508–1514.

49. Mathijssen RH, Verweij J, de Bruijn P, Loos WJ, Sparreboom A. 2002. Effects of St. John's wort on irinotecan metabolism. *J Natl Cancer Inst* 94: 1247–1249.
50. Hu ZP, Yang XX, Chen X, cao J et al. 2007. A mechanistic study on altered pharmacokinetics of irinotecan by St. John's wort. *Curr Drug Metab* 8: 157–171.
51. Thummel KE, Wilkinson GR. 1998. In vitro and in vivo drug interactions involving human CYP3A. *Annu Rev Pharmacol Toxicol* 38: 389–430.
52. Guengerich FP. 1998 Oxidation of 17-ethynylestradiaol by human liver cytochrome P 450. *Mol Pharmacol* 33: 500–508.
53. Hill SD, Wang Z, Huang SM, Hamman MA et al. 2003. The interaction between St. John's wort and oral contraceptives. *Clin Pharmacol* 74: 525–535.
54. Murphy PA, Kern SE, Stanczyk FZ, Westhoff CL. 2005. Interaction of St. John's wort with oral contraceptives: effects on the pharmacokinetics of norethindrone and ethinyl estradiol, ovarian activity and breakthrough bleeding. *Contraception* 71: 4102–408.
55. Sugimoto K, Ohmori M, Tsuruoka S, Nishiki K et al. 2001. Different effect of St. John's wort on the pharmacokinetics of simvastatin and pravastatin. *Clin Pharmacol Ther* 70:518–524.
56. Wang LS, Zhou G, Zhu B, Wu J et al. 2004. St. John's wort induces both cytochrome P450 3A4 catalyzed sulfoxidation and 2 C19 dependent hydroxylation of omeprazole. *Clin Pharmacol Ther* 75: 191–197.
57. Tannergren C, Engman H, Knutson L, Hedeland M et al. 2004. St John's wort decreases the bioavailability of R and S-verapamil through induction of the first pass metabolism. *Clin Pharmacol Ther* 5: 298–309.
58. Xu H, Williams KM, Liauw WS, Murray M et al. 2008. Effects of St. John's wort and CYP2C9 genotype on the pharmacokinetics and pharmacodynamics of gliclazide. *Br J Pharmacol* 153: 1579–1586.
59. Burstein AH, Horton RL, Dunn T, Alfaro RM, et al. 2000. Lack of effect of St. John's wort on carbamazepine pharmacokinetics in healthy volunteers. *Clin Pharmacol Ther* 68: 605–612.
60. Gordon JB. 1998. SSRIs and St. John's wort: possible toxicity? [Letter] *Am Fam Physician* 57: 950–953.
61. Li W, Fitzloff JF. 2001. High performance liquid chromatographic analysis of St. John's wort with photodiode array detection. *J Chromatogr B Biomed Sci Appl* 765: 99–105.
62. Ruckert U, Eggenreich K, Wintersteiger R, Wurglics M, Likussar W, Michelitsch A. 2004. Development of a high performance liquid chromatographic method with electrochemical detection for the determination of hyperforin. *J Chromatogr A* 1041: 181–185.
63. Mauri P, Pietta P. 2000. High performance liquid chromatography/electrospray mass spectrometry of Hypericum perforatum extract. *Rapid Commun Mass Spectrom* 14: 95–99.
64. Seger C, Rompp H, Sturm S, Haslinger E, Schmidt PC, Hadacek F. 2004. Characterization of supercritical fluid extracts of St. John's wort (Hypericum perforatum L) by HPLC-MS and GC-MS. *Eur J Pharm Sci* 21: 453–463.
65. Cui Y, Gurley B, Ang CYW, Leakey J. 2002. Determination of hyperforin in human plasma using solid-phase extraction and high performance liquid chromatography with ultraviolet detection. *J Chromatogr B* 780: 129–135.
66. Bauer S, Stormer E, Graubaum HJ, Roots I. 2001. Determination of hyperforin, hypericin and pseudohypericin in human plasma using high-performance liquid chromatography analysis with fluorescence and ultraviolet detection. *J Chromatogr B Biomed Sci Appl* 765: 29–35.
67. Gioti EM, Skalkos DC, Fiamegos YC and Stalikas CD. 2005. Single drop liquid-phase microextraction for the determination of hypericin, pseudohypericin and hyperforin in biological fluids by high performance liquid chromatography. *J Chromatogr A* 1093: 1–10.
68. Pirker R, Huck CW, Bonn GK. 2002. Simultaneous determination of hypericin and hyperforin in human plasma and serum using liquid-liquid extraction, high performance liquid chromatography-tandem mass spectrometry. *J Chromatogr B Analyt Technol Biomed Life Sci* 777: 147–153.
69. Riedel KD, Rieger K, Martin-Facklam M, Mikus G, Haefeli WE, Burhenne J. 2004. Simultaneous determination of hypericin and hyperforin in human plasma with liquid chromatography-tandem mass spectrometry. *J Chromatogr B Analyt Technol Biomed Life Sci* 813: 27–33.
70. Escher M, Desmeules J. 2001.Hepatitis associated with kava, a herbal remedy. *Br Med J* 322: 139.
71. Clouatre DL. 2004. Kava Kava: examining new reports of toxicity. *Toxicol Lett* 150: 85–96.
72. Cote CS, Kor C, Cohen J and Auclair K. 2004. Composition and biological activity of traditional and commercial kava extracts. *Biochem Biophys Res Commun* 322: 147–152.
73. Anke J, Ramzan I. 2004. Pharmacokinetic and pharmacodynamic drug interactions with Kava (*Piper methysticum* Forst.f). *J Ethnopharmacol* 93: 153–160.

74. Russmann S, Lauterburg BH, Barguil Y, Choblet E et al. 2005. Traditional aqueous kava extracts inhibit P450 1A2 in humans: Protective effect against environmental carcinogens? [Letter]. *Clin Pharmacol Ther* 77: 453–454.

75. Almeida JC, Grimsley EW. 1996. Coma from the health food store: Interaction between Kava and alprazolam. *Ann Intern Med* 125: 940–941.

76. Gaub M, von Brocke A, Ross G, Kovar KA. 2004. High-performance liquid chromatography-coordination ion spray mass spectrometry (HPLC-CIS/MS): a new tool for the analysis of non polar compound classes in plant extract using the example of *Piper methysticum* Forst. *Phytochem Anal* 15: 300–305.

77. Hu L, Jhoo JW, Ang CY, Dinovi M et al. 2005. Determination of six kavalactones in dietary supplements and selected functional foods containing *Piper methysticum* by isocratic liquid chromatography with internal standard. *J AOAC Int* 88: 16–25.

78. Duffield AM, Jamieson DD, Lidgard RO, Duffield PH, Bourne DJ. 1989. Identification of some urinary metabolites of the intoxicating beverage kava. *J Chromatogr* 475: 273–281.

79. Yin OQ, Tomlinson B, Waye MM, Chow AH, Chow MS. 2004. Pharmacogenetics and herb-drug interactions: experience with ginkgo. *Pharmacogenetics* 14: 841–850.

80. Mauro VF, Mauro LS, Kleshinski JF, Khuder SA et al. 2003. Impact of ginkgo biloba on the pharmacokinetics of digoxin. *Am J Ther* 10: 247–252.

81. Yang CY, Chao PD, Hou YC, Tsai SY et al. 2006. Marked decrease of cyclosporine bioavailability caused by coadministration of ginkgo and onion. *Food Chem Toxicol* 44: 1672–1578.

82. Kupiec T, Raj V. 2005. Fetal seizures due to potential herb-drug interactions with ginkgo biloba. *J Anal Toxicol* 29: 755–758.

83. Granger AS. 2001. Ginkgo biloba precipitating epileptic seizures. *Age Ageing* 30: 523–525.

84. Kubota Y, Kobayashi K, Tanaka N, Nakamura K et al. 2003. Interaction of ginkgo biloba extract (GBE) with hypotensive agent nicardipine in rats. *In Vivo* 17: 409–412.

85. Sugiyama T, Kubota Y, Shinozuka K, Yamada S et al. 2004. Ginkgo biloba extract modifies hypoglycemic action of tolbutamide via hepatic cytochrome P450 mediated mechanism in aged rats. *Life Sci* 75: 1113–1132.

86. Robertson SM, Davey RT, Voell J, Formentini E. 2008. Effect of ginkgo biloba extract on lopinavir, midazolam and fexofenadine pharmacokinetics in healthy subjects. *Curr Med Res Opin* 24: 591–599.

87. Bent S, Goldberg H, Padula A and Avins AL. 2005. Spontaneous bleeding associated with ginkgo biloba: a case report and systemic review of the literature. *J Gen Intern Med* 20: 657–661.

88. Gardner CD, Zehnder JL, Rigby AJ, Nicholus JR et al. 2007. Effect of ginkgo biloba (EGb 761) and aspirin on platelet aggregation and platelet function analysis among older adults at risk of cardiovascular disease: a randomized clinical trial. *Blood Coagul Fibrinolysis* 18: 787–793.

89. Fuzzati N, Pace R, Villa F. 2003. A simple HPLC-UV method for the assay of ginkgolic acid in ginkgo biloba extract. *Fitoterapia* 74: 247–256.

90. Tang C, Wei X, Yin C. 2003. Analysis of ginkgolides and bilobalide in Ginkgo biloba L extract injections by high performance liquid chromatography with evaporative light scattering detection. *J Pharm Biomed Anal* 33: 811–817.

91. Chiu HL, Lin HY, Yang TCC. 2004. Determination of ginkgolide A, B and bilobalide in biloba L extracts by microdialysis-HPLC. *Anal Bioanal Chem* 379: 445–448.

92. Dubber MJ, Kanfer I. 2004. High-performance liquid chromatographic determination of selected flavonols in *Ginkgo biloba* solid oral dosage forms. *J Pharm Pharm Sci* 7: 303–309.

93. Dubber MJ, Sewram V, Mshicileli N, Shephard GS, Kanfer I. 2005. The simultaneous determination of selected flavonol glycosides and aglycones in ginkgo biloba oral dosage forms by high performance liquid chromatography-electrospray ionization mass spectrometry. *J Pharm Biomed Anal* 37: 723–731.

94. Ding S, Dudley E, Plummer S, Tang J et al. 2006. Quantitative determination of major active components of ginkgo biloba dietary supplement by liquid chromatography/mass spectrometry. *Rapid Commun Mass Spectrom* 20: 2753–2760.

95. Ding S, Dudley E, Plummer S, Tang J et al. 2008. Fingerprint profile of ginkgo biloba nutritional supplements by LC/ESI-MS/MS. *Phytochemistry* 69: 1555–1564.

96. Wang FM. Yao TW, Zeng S. 2003. Disposition of quercetin and kaempferol in human following an oral administration of ginkgo biloba extract tablets. *Eur J Drug Metab Phramacokinetic* 28: 173–177.

97. Hori Y, Fujisawa M. Shimada K, Oda A. 2004. Rapid analysis of 4-O-methylpyridoxine in serum of patients with ginkgo biloba seed poisoning by ion-pair high performance liquid chromatography. *Bio Pharm Bull* 27: 486–491.

98. Ding S, Dudley E, Chen L, Plummer S et al. 2006. Determination of active components of ginkgo biloba in human urine by capillary high-performance liquid chromatography/mass spectrometry with on-line column switching purification. *Rapid Commun Mass Spectrom* 20: 3619–3624.

99. Coon Jt and Ernst E. 2002. Panax ginseng, a systematic review of adverse effects and drug interactions. *Drug Saf* 25: 323–344.

100. Lee FC, Ko JH, Park JK, Lee JS. 1987. Effects of Panax ginseng on blood alcohol clearance in man. *Clin Exp Pharmacol Physiol* 14: 543–546.

101. Koo MW. 1999. Effects of ginseng on ethanol induced sedation in mice. *Life Sci* 64: 153–160.

102. Jones BD, Runikis AM. 1987. Interaction of ginseng with phenelzine. *J Clin Psychopharmacol* 3: 201–202.

103. Kiefer D and Pantuso T. 2003. Panax ginseng. *Am Fam Physician* 68: 1539–1542.

104. Harkey MR, Henderson GL, Gershwin ME, Stern ME, Stern JS, Hackman RM. 2001. Variability in commercial ginseng products: an analysis of 25 preparations. *Am J Clin Nutr* 73: 1101–1106.

105. Bonfill M, Casals I, Palazon J, Mallol A, Morales C. 2002. Improved high performance liquid chromatographic determination of ginsenosides in Panax ginseng based pharmaceuticals using a diol column. *Biomed Chromatogr* 16: 68–72.

106. Luchtefeld R, Kostoryz E, Smith RE. 2004. Determination of ginsenosides Rb1,Rc, and Re in different dosage forms of ginseng by negative ion electrospray liquid chromatography-mass spectrometry. *J Agri Food Chem* 52: 1953–1956.

107. Zhu S, Zou K, Fushimi H, Cai S, Komatsu K. 2004. Comparative study on triterpene saponins of ginseng drugs. *Planta Med* 70:666–677.

108. Chen G, Yang M, Song Y, Lu Z et al. 2008. Comparative analysis of microbial and rat metabolism of ginsenoside Rb(1) by high performance liquid chromatography coupled with tandem mass spectrometry. *Biomed Chromatogr* 22: 779–785.

109. Piscitelli SC, Brustein AH, Welden N, Gallicano KD, Falloon J. 2002. The effect of garlic supplements on the pharmacokinetics of saquinavir. *Clin Infect Dis* 34: 234–238.

110. Borrelli F, Capasso R and Izzoo AA. 2007. garlic (Allium sativum L.): adverse effects and drug interactions in humans. *Mol Nutr Food Res* 51: 1386–1397.

111. Mohammed Abdul MI, Jiang X, Williams KM, Day RO et al. 2008. Pharmacological interaction of warfarin with cranberry but not with garlic in healthy subjects. *Br J Pharmacol* 154: 1691–1700.

112. Petry JJ. 1995. Garlic and postoperative bleeding [Letter]. *Plast Reconstr Surg* 96: 483–484.

113. Arnault I, Christides JP, Mandon N, Haffner T, Kahane R, Auger J. 2003. High-performance ion pair chromatography method for simultaneous analysis of allin, deoxyallin, allicin and dipeptide precursors in garlic products using multiple mass spectrometry and UV detection. *J Chromatogr A* 991: 69–75.

114. Rosen RT, Hiserodt RD, Fukuda EK, Ruiz RJ et al. 2001. Determination of allicin, S-allylcysteine and volatile metabolites of garlic in breath, plasma or simulated gastric fluid. *J Nutr* 131: 968S–971S.

115. Heck AM, DeWitt BA, Lukes AL. 2000. Potential interactions between alternative therapies and warfarin. *Am J Health-Syst Pharm* 57: 1221–1227.

116. Lambert JP, Cormier A. 2002. Potential interaction between warfarin and boldo-fenugreek. *Pharmacotherapy* 21: 509–512.

117. Tam LS, Chan Tym Leung WK, Critchley JA.1995. Warfarin interaction with Chinese traditional medicines: danshen and methyl salicylate medicated oil. *Aust NZ J Med* 25: 238.

118. Yu CM, Chan JC, Sanderson JE.1997. Chinese herbs and warfarin potentiation by danshen. *J Intern Med* 25: 337–339.

119. Lee NJ and Fermo JD. 2006. Warfarin and royal jelly interaction. *Pharmacotherapy* 26: 583–586.

120. Shalansky S, Lynd L, Richardson K, Ingaszewski A et al. 2007. Risk of warfarin related bleeding events and supra therapeutic international normalized ratios associated with complementary and alternative medicines: a longitudinal study. *Pharmacotherapy* 27: 1237–1247.

121. Cheng TO. 2008. Not only green tea but also green leafy vegetables inhibit warfarin [Letter]. *Int J Cardiol* 125: 101.

Index